Fourth Edition

OUR GLOBAL ENVIRONMENT
A Health Perspective

Anne Nadakavukaren
Illinois State University

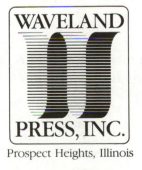

WAVELAND
PRESS, INC.
Prospect Heights, Illinois

D0166070

For information about this book, write or call:
Waveland Press, Inc.
P.O. Box 400
Prospect Heights, Illinois 60070
(847) 634-0081

Copyright © 1995, 1990, 1986, 1984 by Anne Nadakavukaren

ISBN 0-88133-831-1

Printed in the United States of America

7   6   5   4

Contents

PART III ENVIRONMENTAL DEGRADATION
How We Foul Our Own Nest   417

viii   Contents

Preface

Our Global Environment: A Health Perspective is intended as a text for introductory level courses in environmental health or human ecology, presenting a broad survey of the major environmental issues facing society at the end of the 20th century. The book combines an overall ecological concern with specific elements related to personal and community health, emphasizing the interrelatedness of the two and conveying to students an awareness of how current environmental issues directly affect their own lives.

Commencing with a rudimentary discussion of general ecological principles, the text focuses primarily on our present population-resources-pollution crisis and explains why human health and welfare depend on a successful resolution of these challenges. Intended for a one-semester course, the text consists of 16 chapters and is divided into three main sections, each with its own introduction. Discussion within each chapter covers general aspects of the subject in question, while specific illustrative examples are treated in box inserts. In order to give students a perspective on the kinds of actions being taken to deal with identified problems, a brief description of federal statutes dealing with particular environmental issues is included wherever appropriate. Appendices at the end of the book describe the various federal agencies dealing with environmental and health issues and list names and addresses of major nongovernmental environmental organizations for the benefit of those students who wish to obtain further information or to become actively affiliated with such groups. The ability of citizens to influence public policy is stressed throughout the book, a basic purpose of the text being to provide students with sufficient information and insight into environmental problems to enable them to understand and participate in the public decision-making processes which will profoundly influence health and environmental quality in the decades ahead.

I would like to express my sincere gratitude to those who helped me make this book possible: to Heinz Russelmann, former Director of the Environmental Health Program at Illinois State University, whose encouragement, suggestions, and painstaking review of the manuscript were of invaluable assistance; to my colleagues Steve Arnold and Tom Bierma whose critical review of the sections on noise and radon was extremely helpful; to Becky Anderson whose classroom experience using the text enabled her to give valuable suggestions on content and scope of this revision, especially on issues pertaining to ecology and biodiversity; to Patrick Waller, at Massachusetts Institute of Technology, and Herman Brockman, Professor of Genetics at Illinois State University, for their insightful comments on the section dealing with cancer; to former colleague Phil Kneller, now at Western Carolina University, and to Tom Anderson of the McLean County Health Department for their suggestions and review of material on foodborne disease; to Linn Haramis at the Illinois Department of Public Health for his review of the passage on Lyme Disease; to Art Carlson at Illinois Department of Nuclear Safety for reviewing coverage of medical X-rays; to Laurie Prossnitz, Waveland Press, whose friendly cooperation and painstaking editorial efforts have been sincerely appreciated; to Neil Rowe, publisher of Waveland Press, for his cooperation and help; and especially to my husband and daughters for their loving support and understanding during the course of this project.

Anne Nadakavukaren

PART I

People, Progress, and Nature
Is Conflict Inevitable?

Only within the moment of time represented by the present century has one species—man—acquired significant power to alter the nature of his world.

—Rachel Carson

Human beings, as a species, are unquestionably the dominant form of life on earth today. Inhabiting every continent, roaming the seas, exploring space, creating glittering cities and festering slums, taming rivers, bringing water to the desert, harnessing the atom, tinkering with the gene—people often deceive themselves into believing they are all-powerful, creatures apart from the rest of nature. Yet a half-million years of cultural evolution cannot alter the fact that humans, like all other living organisms, are inextricably bound up in the web of interdependency and interrelationships that characterize life on this planet. Human health, well-being, and indeed survival are ultimately dependent on the health and integrity of the whole environment in which we live. Today the natural world that we share with all other forms of life on this planet is under unprecedented attack, not by outside forces of evil, as in a science fiction movie, but rather by a wide range of human activities and the sheer pressure of human numbers. Sometimes unwittingly, sometimes with full awareness of the consequences of our actions, we are rapidly altering the basic foundations of the environment that sustains us.

Will the abuses we are currently heaping upon the environment ultimately lead to the collapse of the entire system? This question has been a hot topic of debate for at least the past two decades as levels of pollution, depletion of resources, destruction of land, and the population spiral continue to mount. On June 3, 1992, representatives of 178 nations converged on Rio de Janeiro, Brazil, for an extraordinary 12-day gathering to wrestle with these issues. Political leaders, journalists, and citizen activists from around the world joined forces to demonstrate their hopes and concerns for the future health and habitability of our planet. More than one hundred heads of state, the largest number of world leaders ever assembled for a single purpose, attempted to forge an international accord to deal with environmental problems so pervasive that they can no longer be solved solely by national efforts.

Widely referred to as the "Earth Summit," the Rio conference, officially designated as the United Nations Conference on Environment and Development (UNCED), marked the second time the world organization had sponsored a major international gathering to focus on environmental concerns. The first such meeting had been held 20 years earlier in Stockholm, Sweden. Coming at a time when the environmental movement was in its infancy, this event stimulated the formation of thousands of grass-roots ecological groups around the world and prompted over one hundred nations to establish official environmental agencies to confront national problems of pollution and resource depletion. During the years following the Stockholm conference, global environmental awareness gradually increased, but Cold War tensions and East-West ideological divisions relegated international cooperation on ecological issues to the sidelines.

With the collapse of the Soviet empire in the late 1980s, it has become increasingly obvious that the major division in the world today is not one separating Communists from capitalists, but is rather a North-South split in which the affluent consumer societies of Europe, North America, and Japan view with apprehension the rapidly growing, resource-hungry populations of the Third World who demand their share of the "good life" enjoyed by their neighbors in the industrialized world. It also has become obvious that if the developing nations of Asia, Africa, and Latin America attempt to copy the model of development followed by Western nations, the resulting pollution and depletion of resources would lead to ecological destruction of enormous proportions, affecting the entire planet. Thus the main goal at the Earth Summit was to try to convince the world's governments to abandon development policies that lead ultimately to eco-catastrophe and to adopt instead programs of "sustainable development"— those which balance valid economic considerations with environmental realities, satisfying reasonable human needs without jeopardizing the well-being of future generations. The urgency of the environmental challenge facing the world's people was aptly described by U.N. Secretary-General Boutros Boutros-Ghali who opened the Earth Summit with an appeal to delegates to redirect their military spending to programs of environmental protection, suggesting that the Rio conference might well be remembered by future generations as the time when humans recognized that "nature no longer exists in the classic sense of the term" but "lies within the hands of man."

The major issues tackled by Earth Summit delegates were global in scope: loss of biodiversity, tropical deforestation, climate change, eradication of poverty. More local concerns dealing with air and water pollution, the toxic wastes trade, rights of indigenous peoples, and a broad host of other concerns were hotly debated, not only by official dignitaries but also by the thousands of citizens from around the world who flocked to Rio as representatives of nongovernmental organizations. Disappointingly, there were several major policy issues on which participants failed to reach agreement—or refused even to address. Conspicuously absent from the main agenda was serious discussion of how to reverse the population explosion that many observers are convinced is the underlying cause of much, if not most, of the pressure leading to rampant environmental degradation. The combined opposition of the Vatican and the conservative Islamic nations to any meaningful deliberation of family-planning strategies was but one of many examples of politics obstructing effective action. North-South wrangling over who should provide the enormous sums (estimated at $125 billion annually) required to clean up pollution and alleviate poverty in the Third World frequently imparted a rich nations versus poor nations aspect to UNCED sessions. Perhaps most disappointing to those who had envisioned the Rio conference as a major turning point in the "race to save the planet" was the obstructionist position taken by the U.S. delegation which, under orders from President Bush, refused to sign an international convention to protect endangered species and fatally weakened the agreement on global warming by insisting that specific targets and timetables for reducing carbon dioxide emissions be deleted from the final document. Most significantly, American refusal to provide a major increase in funding for Third World development and pollution abatement programs guaranteed that many of the lofty goals adopted at the conference would never be realized. While preaching the virtues of sustainable development to Southern Hemisphere governments, the United States and other nations of the North made it clear that they are unwilling to accept economic limits at home to promote global environmental stability. Reflecting his government's position, an American delegate bluntly pointed out that "the United States standard of living is not up for negotiation."

As the 12-day conference ended and the participants headed homeward, some disillusioned observers denounced Rio's results as ineffectual, "business as usual," or "a failure to set a new direction for life on earth." The gathering dramatized a vivid rise in North-South antagonism over money and clarified the difficulties of setting aside national differences even when the stakes involved are as fundamental as planetary survival. Nevertheless, most delegates departed with the conviction that Rio had marked the beginning of something very important—a new era of awareness that human development and well-being is inextricably bound to protection of the earth's environment. As Prime Minister Felipe Gonzales of Spain remarked, "Five hundred years ago men set out to discover the size of the earth. At this meeting we discovered its limits."

In the months since the Earth Summit, numerous crises, both domestic and international, have displaced the concerns raised at Rio from the forefront of world attention. Such issues are not forgotten, however. Beyond the glare of media spotlights, the United Nations Commission on Sustainable Development—a body created at Rio to integrate the environment and development activities of the U.N. with those of other agencies and to monitor followup on Earth Summit treaty commitments—meets regularly and prods governments to fulfill pledges made. In November of 1992 American voters elected a new President and Vice-President whose stated positions were much more "environmentally friendly" than the Administration they replaced. Among environmentalists hope soared that a new era of government commitment to the principles expressed at Rio would soon become reality and that the United States would regain its former role as the world leader in environmental protection.

However, the strongest reason for optimism about humanity's chances of reversing the current downward spiral of environmental degradation is the worldwide proliferation of small grassroots organizations made up of committed citizens, working independently on their own local problems but united in their determination to save our natural heritage for future generations. Inspired and energized by the spectacle at Rio, they have recognized that we don't have to sit back as passive spectators to the despoliation of our environment and the impoverishment of our society. They realize that much can be done to limit the impact of advanced technology on the natural world and to incorporate environmental considerations into national policy-making. These activists, ordinary people from all walks of life, have an important message for the rest of us: to a great extent the technical know-how to prevent further deterioration exists—what is needed most is a societal commitment to get the job done. The most important decisions being made in the environmental health arena today are political decisions, balancing ecological concerns with economic and social considerations. Individuals wishing to become involved in protecting and enhancing environmental quality will find their efforts most effective when directed toward influencing environmental policy-making bodies at every level of government. To be a successful eco-advocate, however, requires a thorough understanding of the nature of our environmental crisis, how the present situation developed, what the human impact of these threats may be, and what actions have already been taken in an attempt to restore and maintain a quality environment. These are the issues this book will attempt to address in the belief that a well-informed, politically active citizenry is an essential ingredient for attaining the worthy goals so eloquently articulated at the Earth Summit■

CHAPTER 1

Introduction to Ecological Principles

> *The most important fact about Spaceship Earth: an instruction book didn't come with it.*
>
> —Buckminster Fuller

When astronauts Neil Armstrong and "Buzz" Aldrin became the first humans to land on the moon and gazed back at their home planet more than 200,000 miles away, they were filled with a sense of wonder at the beauty and uniqueness of Earth. Of all the heavenly bodies of which we are aware, our planet is neither the largest nor the smallest, the hottest nor the coldest, yet it *is* extraordinary in one vital respect—in all the universe Earth is the only planet known to support life. Within that narrow film of air and water which envelops the surface of the globe, extending vertically from the deepest ocean trenches more than 36,000 feet below sea level to about 30,000 or more feet above sea level, exists what ecologists call the **biosphere**—that portion of the Earth where life occurs.

For all practical purposes, the physical extent of the biosphere is even more limited than just described. Even though the deep ocean trenches do possess a number of bizarre aquatic species and certain fungal spores and pollen grains may be found floating in the upper reaches of the atmosphere, by far the greatest number of living things are found in the region extending from the permanent snow line of tropical and subtropical mountain ranges (about 20,000 feet above sea level) to the limit of light penetration in the clearest oceans (about 600 feet deep). Here a vast assemblage of plant, animal, and microbial life can be found—perhaps as many as 10 million different species living today. These species interact both with each other and with their physical environment; over very long periods of time they become modified in response to environmental pressures and, in turn, they themselves modify their physical surroundings.

The first living organisms on earth (probably forms similar to bacteria) are now thought to have arisen more than 3.5 billion years ago on a planet whose environment was considerably different from that of the present-day world. The life activities of those early organisms, feeding upon and reacting with the chemical compounds in the waters where they first arose, were responsible for the creation of the modern atmosphere, which made possible the emergence of higher forms of life. The first primitive organisms evolved in a world devoid of atmospheric oxygen but rich in carbon dioxide. This carbon dioxide in turn provided a carbon source for the evolutionarily more advanced photosynthetic organisms which could produce their own food by utilizing the sun's energy to convert carbon dioxide and water into carbohydrates, releasing oxygen as a waste product. It was through the action of such photosynthetic organisms that the earth's atmosphere gradually became an oxygen-rich one, permitting the development of the types of life with which we are familiar today. In this way, the life activities of one group of organisms profoundly altered the environment and created conditions which facilitated the emergence of other forms of life. The ability of living things to modify their surroundings and the tendency of other organisms to respond positively or negatively to such changes has been a constant feature of evolutionary progression throughout the ages and remains so today.

Ecosystems

The concept of nature as divided into basic functional units called **ecosystems** reflects scientists' recognition of the complex manner in which living organisms interact with each other and with the nonliving (or abiotic) components of their environment to process energy and cycle nutrients. The concept is admittedly imprecise, since few ecosystems have definitive spatial boundaries or exist in splendid isolation. Adjacent ecosystems commonly influence each other, as when a pond ecosystem is altered by materials washing into it from surrounding terrestrial ecosystems, and certain components (e.g. water birds, insects) may be moving in and out on a regular basis (Smith, 1986). Similarly, the concept of ecosystems is a broad one, its main usefulness being to emphasize the interdependence of the biotic and abiotic components of an area. An ecosystem has no defining size limitations: an abandoned tire casing containing trapped rainwater, microorganisms, and swarms of mosquito larvae can be regarded as an ecosystem; so can a family-room aquarium, a city park, a cornfield, a tidepool, a cow pasture, or, indeed, the entire Planet Earth. Any of these widely diverse situations can be considered an ecosystem so long as living and nonliving elements are present and interacting to process energy and cycle materials (Stiling, 1992).

Biotic Community

The most familiar classification system used for grouping plants and animals is one based upon presumed evolutionary relationships—lions, tigers, and leopards being grouped in the cat family; wheat, corn, and rice in the grass family, and so forth. However, ecologists tend to arrange species on the basis of their functional association with each other. A natural grouping of different kinds of plants and animals within any given habitat is termed by ecologists a **biotic community**.

"Biotic community," like "ecosystem," is a broad term which can be used to describe natural groupings of widely differing sizes, from the various microscopic diatoms and zooplankton swimming in a drop of pond water to the hundreds of species of trees, wild flowers, ferns, insects, birds, mammals, and so forth, found in an Appalachian forest. Biotic communities have characteristic trophic structures and energy flow patterns and also have a certain taxonomic unity, in the sense that certain species tend to exist together.

Individuals of the same species living together within a given area are collectively referred to as a **population**. Such populations constitute groups more or less isolated from other populations of the same species. A population within the biotic community of a region is not a static entity but is continually changing in size and reshuffling its hereditary characteristics in response to environmental changes and to fluctuations in the populations of other members of the community.

The community concept is one of the most important ecological principles because 1) it emphasizes the fact that different organisms are not arbitrarily scattered around the earth with no particular reason as to why they live where they do, but rather that they dwell together in an orderly manner; and 2) by illuminating the importance of the community as a whole to any of its individual parts, the community concept can be used by humans to manage a particular organism, in the sense of increasing or decreasing its numbers. Emphasizing biotic communities as a whole, rather than focusing on their constituent species, is helpful also in demonstrating why removing one species from a community (or, conversely, introducing a nonnative species into a community) can often have unintended—and sometimes disastrous—consequences.

European settlement of the sparsely populated North American continent launched a gigantic experiment in human interference with natural ecosystems. One dramatic example of how a stable biotic community can unravel simply by elimination of one of its members is the sad tale of beaver exploitation. In the late 17th century French traders began trapping these once-abundant mammals, shipping enormous numbers of valuable pelts back to Europe to accommodate the insatiable demands of the hat-making industry. So extensively and heavily were they hunted that within 150 years beavers faced extinction from the Great Lakes region all the way to Oregon and California. Only as their numbers plummeted did the beavers' role within their biotic community become apparent. With the demise of their architects, beaver dams were no longer maintained and eventually washed away. As a result, rates of stream flow sharply accelerated, destroying the spawning beds of fish species which relied on the quiet waters behind the dams for breeding. Marshy areas created by the dams were either drained or flooded, depending on location, and waterfowl populations declined as nesting sites were lost. Flooding increased in frequency and intensity, streamside erosion worsened, and siltation of river channels accelerated. Disappearance of the beaver, perceived by the trappers as a creature that was "going to waste" in the wilderness, thus led to surprisingly far-reaching effects (Ashworth, 1986).

Introducing a nonnative species (i.e. an exotic) into an established biotic community can be every bit as destabilizing as removing a component species. Time and again, accidentally or deliberately, humans have released plants or animals into a new environment only to see them quickly attain major pest status, usually due to the absence of natural predators which could keep their numbers under control. The zebra mussel (see Box 1-1) is but the most recent in a host of unwanted aliens to invade our shores—gypsy moths, European starlings, carp, kudzu, water hyacinths, sea lampreys—to mention but a few of the most notorious. In our attempts to "control nature" we must never forget that the intricate interdependencies which have evolved over the millennia among the biotic

BOX 1-1

Striped Invaders

In the spring of 1988, two Canadian biology students conducting investigations in Lake St. Clair (east of Detroit midway between Lake Huron and Lake Erie) came across a distinctively marked tiny mollusk that had never been seen in the lake before. The new find was subsequently identified as a European species called the zebra mussel (*Dreissena polymorpha*), so named because its coloration features dark brown stripes against a light tan background. Though the students had no way of knowing it at the time, they had just discovered the vanguard of an invading horde which, within a few years, would spread rapidly throughout the Great Lakes, eastward into the St. Lawrence Seaway and New York's Finger Lakes, southwestward into the Illinois River and thence to the Mississippi and its tributaries as far west as the Rocky Mountains. Indeed,

the only known factor possibly limiting the geographic expansion of these creatures is water temperature; zebra mussels thrive in cool, fresh water ranging from 68° to 77° F and die off quickly when water temperatures exceed 104°F. Observers now glumly acknowledge the virtual inevitability of the zebra mussels' dispersal through most of the inland waterways in the United States. And where the zebra mussel goes, mega-problems follow in its wake.

The diminutive bivalve doesn't look like a villain. An average adult is only 1–1½ inches in length and weighs about an ounce. One such creature would pose no concern, but zebra mussels like company—lots of company—and tend to cluster in colonies where population densities may be as high as 70,000/yd^3. Because they prefer to attach themselves to a solid substrate

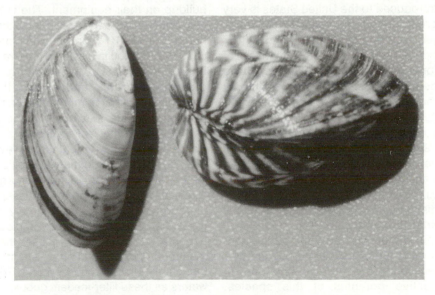

The average zebra mussel is 1–1½ inches in length and weighs an ounce. [J. Ellen Marsden, Illinois Natural History Survey]

rather than burrowing in sand or mud, zebra mussels may settle in enormous numbers on boat hulls, docks, fishing gear, rocky shorelines, and, perhaps most objectionably, on the water supply pipes serving industries, power plants, and public water filtration plants. In the latter case, the proliferation of mussels inside the pipes narrows their diameter to such an extent that water intake capacity can be reduced by as much as 50%.

Native to the Caspian Sea in central Asia, zebra mussels began spreading westward to freshwater ports all over Europe in the late 1700s, traveling along inland waterways as inconspicuous hitchhikers on the hulls of sailing vessels. For many decades the salty expanse of the Atlantic prevented these fresh- and brackish-water mollusks from making the transoceanic journey to North America, but the potential threat caused considerable anxiety among American zoologists aware of the problems they were causing in western Europe. As early as 1921, one worried observer remarked that ''the possibility of the zebra mussel being introduced to the United States is very great. There is entirely too much reckless dumping of aquaria into our ponds and streams. A number of foreign freshwater shells, etc., have been introduced in this way. Why not the mussel?'' (Nalepa and Schloesser, 1993). He was right. The specimen discovered by the Canadian students in 1988 is thought to have arrived two years earlier as a free-floating larva transported in the ballast water of a European ship which subsequently discharged this water from its bilges prior to docking.

The mussels' rapid spread throughout the Great Lakes and beyond was facilitated by the enormous reproductive potential of this species. Reaching sexual maturity at about two years of age, a female zebra mussel produces 30,000–40,000 eggs at one spawning. Eggs hatch soon after fertilization into microscopic larvae which are easily transported by water currents throughout a lake or river. They also can be spread from one waterway to another when they make their way, unnoticed, into bait buckets, engine cooling systems, boat bilges— or possibly by riding along in the water droplets trapped on the plumage of aquatic birds. After about three weeks, these larvae begin to develop shells, the weight of which causes them to sink and settle onto a solid substrate where they attach themselves by means of strong adhesive fibers. During their first year of life, young adult mussels can detach and move to another substrate; older individuals are immobile, but they may be carried from one waterway to another by unwary navigators on boat hulls and trailers.

Damage caused by zebra mussels is not limited to the multimillion dollar impact they are having on the factories, power plants, and water treatment facilities that are currently spending enormous sums to combat mussel buildup on their equipment. The U.S. Fish and Wildlife Service estimates that during the 1990s, zebra mussels may cause $2.7 billion in losses to the Great Lakes fisheries by consuming a disproportionate share of the phytoplankton that comprise the basic link in the aquatic food chain. As early as 1989, both the United States and Canada were reporting that walleye pike, an important commercial species, were declining both in number and size—an indication of the mussels' interference with the food supply of these fish. (Ironically, the voracious appetite of the zebra mussel has resulted in noticeable improvement in the clarity of once-murky Lake Erie waters as these filter-feeders gobble up the previously over-abundant algal cells. Zebra mussels have at least *some* redeeming social value!) Even from an aesthetic perspective zebra mussels can be a nuisance when they wash up along the shore in enormous numbers, their decaying shells creating an unpleasant stench and presenting a risk of painful cuts to barefoot strollers along the beach.

Currently extensive research efforts are underway in hopes of finding an effective weapon to repel the mussels' onslaught. Chlorination is lethal against zebra mussels and constitutes the most common method of control, but safety considerations and environmental side effects render chlorination a problematic solution. Several molluskicides and toxic metallic ions have been employed as control agents, but these are expensive, can be difficult to apply, and are toxic to other aquatic organisms as well. Physical controls such as scraping mussels off surfaces to which they are attached, creating anaerobic conditions to suffocate the mussels, or heating the water to temperatures above 104 °F can be effective in some situations and entail no risk of toxic discharges. Natural enemies, successfully employed against other alien invaders, don't appear to offer grounds for optimism. In Europe both water birds and crayfish have been utilized in control efforts with only limited success.

Researchers are hopeful that, in time, newer, environmentally sound treatment methods will be developed, permitting the explosive growth of zebra mussel populations to be brought under control. *Eradication* of these hardy newcomers is unlikely, however. Zebra mussels have established themselves as an enduring part of the Great Lakes ecosystem and provide a dramatic—and costly—example of how human interference with biotic communities can have unintentional and far-reaching implications (Turner, 1990).

References

Nalepa, Thomas F., and Donald W. Schloesser, eds. 1993. *Zebra Mussels: Biology, Impacts, and Control*. Lewis Publishers.

Turner, Suzanne K. 1990. *Zebra Mussels: The Great Lakes' Latest Menace*. The New York State Majority Task Force on Zebra Mussels.

communities of the earth cannot be altered without provoking a corresponding change somewhere else in the ecosystem.

Ecological Dominants

Although all members of a biotic community have a role to play in the life of that community, it is obvious that certain plants or animals exert more of an influence on the ecosystem as a whole than do others. As George Orwell might have put it, "All animals are equal, but some animals are more equal than others." Those organisms which exert a major modifying influence on the community are known as **ecological dominants**. Such dominants generally comprise those species that control the flow of energy through the community; if they were to be removed from the community, much greater changes in the ecosystem would result than if a nondominant species were to be removed. For example, when farmers chop down the dominant hardwood trees in an eastern forest to clear the land for cultivation, the changes produced by this removal (i.e. loss of animal species which depend on the trees for food and shelter, loss of shade-loving plants which proliferate under the canopy, change in soil microbiota, raising of soil temperature, increase in soil erosion, and so forth) are much more pronounced than would be the changes brought about when the farmers' children wander into the forest and pick all of the trilliums and lady slippers they find growing there. In either case, the stability of the ecosystem is upset, but the loss of several species of spring wildflowers, while unfortunate, has much less effect on the forest community as a whole than does the loss of the dominant oaks, maples, and beeches.

In most terrestrial biotic communities certain plants comprise the dominant species because not only do they provide food and shelter for other organisms but also because they directly affect and modify their physical environment. That is, they contribute to a build-up of topsoil, moderate fluctuations of temperature, improve moisture retention, affect the pH of the soil, and so on. As a general rule, the number of dominant species within a community becomes progressively fewer as one moves toward the poles and greater the closer the community is to the tropics. While a northern coniferous forest may consist of only spruces or firs, a jungle in Sumatra may have a dozen or more tree species that could be considered dominants. In addition to the effects of latitude on number of

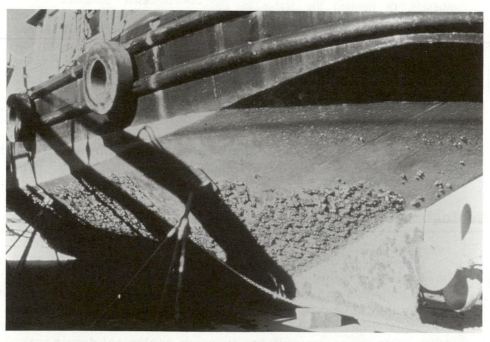

Zebra mussels attach themselves in enormous numbers to a solid surface, such as this boat hull. [Great Lakes Sea Grant Network, Exotic Species Graphics Library]

dominants in a community, one can also generalize that dominant species are fewer in regions where climatic conditions are extreme, i.e. tundra and deserts (Odum, 1959).

Biomes

The species composition of any particular biotic community is profoundly affected by the physical characteristics of the environment, particularly temperature and rainfall. The kinds of plants and animals one would see while touring Yellowstone National Park would differ significantly from those found on a trek through the Amazon. Ecologists have divided the terrestrial communities of the world into general groupings called **biomes**, areas which can be recognized by the distinctive life forms of their dominant species. In most cases, the key characteristic of a biome is its dominant type of vegetation. We might define a biome as a complex of communities characteristic of a regional climatic zone. Each biome has its own pattern of rainfall, its own seasons, its own maximum and minimum temperatures, and its own changes of day length, all of which combine to support a certain kind of vegetation. Since climatic zones change in a relatively uniform pattern as one moves from the poles toward the equator, the earth's biomes form more or less continuous latitudinal bands around the globe. Starting at the polar regions, let's take a brief look at the major biomes of the earth (Note: ecologists list numerous subdivisions of the biomes described here, but for our purposes these general groupings will suffice).

Tundra

The northernmost of the world's land masses, tundra is characterized by permanently frozen subsoil called **permafrost**. In this biome rainfall is quite low, about 8 inches annually, but because the permafrost doesn't allow moisture to penetrate beyond the upper few inches of soil, the tundra in summer is dotted with numerous lakes and bogs—and probably the world's most voracious mosquitoes! The tundra is windy, with only a few stunted trees. The dominant vegetation here consists of moss, lichens, grass, and some small perennials. Animal life is limited in the number of species but very abundant in the number of individuals. These include caribou or reindeer, birds, insects, polar bears, lemmings, foxes, rabbits, and fish. Reptiles and amphibians are absent. The tundra is basically a very fragile environment. Because of the slow rates at which tundra plants grow and decompose (due to the low temperatures and the characteristics of permafrost), the thick, spongy matting of lichens, grasses, and sedges that typify tundra is especially slow to recover from disturbance. Tracks of vehicles or animals can remain visible for decades. Great care must be taken in building on tundra because heat from structures will melt the permafrost and cause uneven settling, which often badly distorts the buildings. Until recently the tundra was relatively unexploited, but with the construction of the Alaska oil pipeline and similar kinds of mineral development in Canada and Siberia, that situation has changed.

Taiga

A Russian word for "swamp forest," the taiga is sometimes called the **northern coniferous forest**. This biome covers much of Canada, Scandinavia, and Russia. As the name implies, the dominant vegetation here consists of conifer trees that have needlelike leaves which stay on the trees for three to five years. These include spruces, firs, hemlocks, and pines. Some deciduous trees such as aspens, alders, and larches are also prominent. In general, the trees are much less diverse in number of species than those in the deciduous forests farther south and the soils have a different kind of humus and are more acid. Precipitation in the taiga is only moderate, but because drainage is poor lakes, ponds, and bogs are common here. Animals of the taiga include bears, moose, lynxes, weasels, wolverines, and a variety of birds. Because of the huge stands of just one or two species of conifers, the taiga provides an opportunity for periodic outbreaks of pests like the spruce budworm which can defoliate huge areas of forest. Perhaps because of the lack of diversity of species, taiga populations tend to undergo "boom or bust" cycles fairly regularly.

Temperate Deciduous Forest

This biome occurs in a belt south of the taiga where climate is milder and where rainfall is abundant relative to the amount of evaporation. This is the biome familiar to most of us because it is the one in which Western, as well as Chinese and Japanese, civilization developed. Soil types and elevations vary widely within this biome. Maples, beech, oaks, and hickories are common trees; many species of ferns and flowering herbaceous plants are found also. The deciduous forest has a great variety of mammals, birds, and insects, as well as a modest number of reptiles and amphibians. Because of the annual leaf drop, deciduous forests generate soils rich in nutrients, which in turn support a multitude of soil microbes. When such forests are cleared, the richness of the soils can be maintained if great care is taken to see that their supplies of nutrients and decaying organic matter are preserved (in a sense, raising crops or grazing animals is akin to mining the soil, since the nutrients leave along with the crops, meat, wool, or whatever is removed). All too often, however, short-term careless exploiters have allowed soils to deteriorate or have ignored opportunities to improve them. Unfortunately, economic considerations often lead individuals who are exploiting an ecosystem to use short-term strategies that are disastrous for humanity in the long run.

Grasslands

In regions where annual rainfall is not sufficient to sustain the growth of trees and evaporation rates are high, we find the grasslands of the world.

Figure 1-1

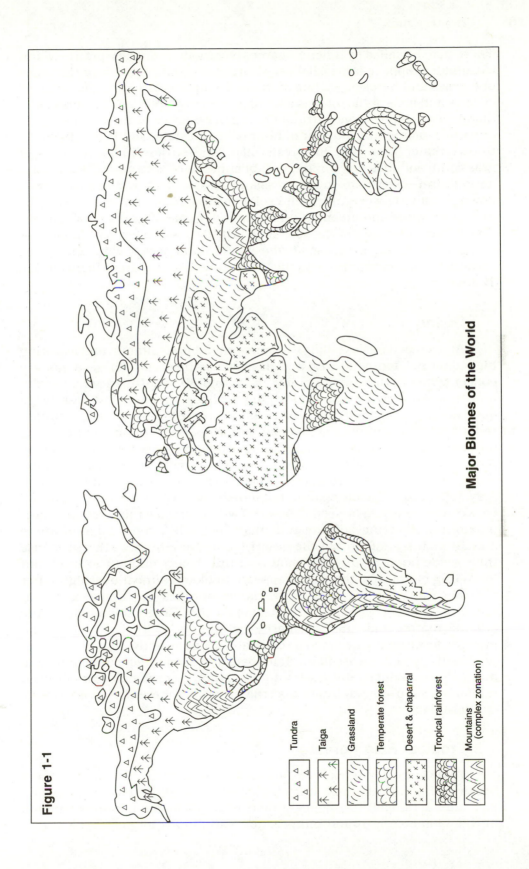

Tundra

Taiga

Grassland

Temperate forest

Desert & chaparral

Tropical rainforest

Mountains
(complex zonation)

Major Biomes of the World

These may be called by different names in various countries: prairie, veldt, savannah, steppe, pampas, llanos. All are characterized by the dominance of grasses and herds of grazing animals. Carnivores also abound, such as coyotes and lions, as do rodents and many species of reptiles. The grassland biome has a higher concentration of organic matter in its soil than does any other biome, the amount of humus in grassland soil being about 12 times greater than that in forest soils. The extraordinary richness of grassland soil has led to the establishment of extremely successful agricultural ecosystems in the grassland areas. These systems can break down rapidly, however, if careful soil conservation is not practiced. The interlaced roots and creeping underground stems of grasses form a turf that prevents erosion of the soil. When the turf is broken with a plow or overgrazed, the soil is exposed to the erosive influences of wind and water, resulting in such calamities as the "Dust Bowl" of the Great Plains in the 1930s.

Desert

Areas receiving less than 10 inches annual precipitation and featuring high daytime temperatures are classified as deserts. These areas are concentrated in the vicinity of 30° north and 30° south latitude. Lack of moisture is the essential factor shaping the desert biome. Most deserts are quite hot in the daytime and, because of the sparse vegetation and resultant rapid reradiation of heat, quite cold at night. Desert plants and animals are characterized by species that can withstand prolonged drought. Among plants such adaptations include waxy cuticle on stems or leaves, reduction in leaf size, and spiny growths to repel moisture-seeking animals. Plants may appear to be widely spaced, but if their roots were visible, the ground between them would be seen to be laced with a shallow root system to take maximum advantage of any rain that does fall. Proportionately more annual plants are found in the desert biome than in any other; because their seeds often require abrasion or a rain heavy enough to leach out inhibiting chemicals, the desert appears to bloom almost overnight after a heavy rain. For the most part, desert animals are active at night, remaining under cover during the heat of the day. Desert soils contain little organic matter and must ordinarily be supplied with both water and nitrogen fertilizer if they are to be cultivated. Human activities have already produced a great increase in the amount of desert and wasteland, removing many once-productive acres from cultivation. Occasional years of good rainfall cause people to forget that the desert is inherently a very fragile environment.

Tropical Rain Forest

This biome is found in Central and South America, central Africa, and South and Southeast Asia. It is characterized by high temperatures and high annual rainfall; 100 inches or more of annual precipitation is common in this biome. Year-round temperature variation is slight. Tropical rain forests are characterized by a great diversity of plant and animal species and by four distinct layers of plant growth—the top canopy of trees reaching 200 feet or more; a lower canopy of densely intertwined treetops at about 100 feet; a sparse understory, and only a very few plants growing at ground level. A wide variety of epiphytic plants can be found. Both plant and animal species exist in greater diversity in the tropical rain forest than anywhere else in the world, though numbers of individuals of a particular species are usually limited. To most people, the luxuriant growth of a tropical jungle implies a rich soil, and one hears many glowing promises of the agricultural riches to be reaped by turning the Amazon or Congo River basins into farmland. The truth of the situation is far different, however. Tropical forest soils in general are exceedingly thin and nutrient-poor. They cannot maintain large reserves of minerals needed for plant growth, primarily because heavy rainfall and a high rate of water flow through the ground to the water table leach them from the soil. The leaching process leaves large residues of insoluble iron and aluminum oxides in the upper levels of tropical forest soils, a process termed "laterization." With the exception of certain fertile river valleys, primitive slash-and-burn agriculture is the only type suitable to most areas of the tropical rain forest. Unfortunately, this fragile ecosystem is being destroyed more rapidly than any other biome under the pressure of expanding human populations and in some cases, such as in Brazil, as a direct consequence of governmental actions.

Note: In areas where there are substantial variations in altitude, the biomes differ at different elevations. This is primarily because the temperature of the air decreases about 6 °C for every 1000 meter increase in altitude and because, especially in desert areas, rainfall increases with altitude.

This brief survey of biome characteristics should make it obvious that various regions differ in their ability to return to an ecologically stable condition once they have been disrupted by human activities. Thus it should not be surprising that certain practices are far more devastating to the local ecology in some areas than they are in others. For example, strip mining in the flat or gently-rolling lands of Illinois, Indiana, and Ohio is certainly disruptive to the environment, yet with proper soil reclamation practices the land can be restored to productive uses once mining has ceased. In the arid regions of the High Plains and Southwest, however, exploitation of fossil fuel reserves by strip mining presents a real threat that the acres thus despoiled could never recover and would remain permanent wastelands.

Ecological Niches

Within any biotic community each species is defined by its own unique position, or **niche**, different from that of any other member of the community and determined largely by its size and food habits. Through the processes of evolution and natural selection, plants and animals have become increasingly better adapted to the specific environments in which they live. In order to reduce competition among species for food and living space, organisms have become more specialized in terms of the foods they utilize, period of the day or night during which they are active, and/or the types of microhabitats they exploit. Thus, in an ecological context, the term niche denotes not simply the physical space that a species occupies but, more importantly, what that species *does* (Pianka, 1988). The **Principle of Competitive Exclusion**, basic to ecological theory, holds that when two species are competing for the same limited resources, only one will survive. Only when the environmental resources in a given community are partitioned among the co-inhabiting species by means of niche diversification is direct competition minimized, thus permitting coexistence of species.

The benefits of niche diversification can be well illustrated by several species of lice which peacefully coexist on a human host by restricting their activities to different anatomical regions. The body louse, notorious in history as the vector of typhus fever, feeds on parts of the body below the neck; the closely related head louse confines its activities to the head and neck. The fact that the two are quite similar in appearance and occasionally interbreed indicates their close relationship, but niche diversification is quite apparent in their different behavioral patterns. Head lice cement their eggs ("nits") to hairs of the scalp, while body lice usually glue theirs to fibers of clothing; in fact, body lice spend most of their time on clothing, coming into contact with the human body only when taking a blood meal. A third type, the crab louse, is morphologically specialized for life among the widely spaced, coarse hairs of the pubic areas. Unlike body and head lice which constantly move about, crab lice tend to settle in one spot and feed off and on for many hours at a time. Through behavioral and territorial specialization, these species avoid competition and thrive in their own unique ecological niche.

In other situations species may utilize the same physical space but minimize competition by restricting their feeding activities to different times of the day. Within any given area one can find some species which are diurnal (active during the day), such as most birds, grazing animals, primates, and so on; other species which are nocturnal (active at night), including most snakes, many predators such as lions, foxes, owls, and so on; and still others such as deer and rabbits which prefer the in-between hours of dawn and dusk. Structural modifications among species allow animals inhabiting the same general area to utilize different foods. The finches of the Galapagos Islands, immortalized by Charles Darwin, were very similar in appearance and obviously evolved from the same parental stock, but modifications in their beak structure permitted each species to utilize a different type of food—insects, small seeds, medium-sized seeds, or large seeds, depending on the size and shape of beak—and thus to coexist within the same geographic area.

Examples of niche diversification illustrate the fact that throughout evolutionary history ecosystems have become exceedingly complex through increasingly effective adaptation of organisms within any natural community. Such a complex ecosystem is generally quite stable unless something happens to change that environment to which the organisms have become so well adapted. The processes of natural selection and adaptation are too slow to permit the vast majority of organisms to adjust quickly to such radical changes in their surroundings. As a result, the animal and plant populations in such disrupted situations generally die out or move elsewhere and the previously stable ecosystem collapses or, at a minimum, becomes less varied and less stable.

Limiting Factors

Why do corn plants thrive in central Illinois but not in Norway? Why don't ferns grow in the Mohave Desert? Why is the poison produced by the botulism bacterium (*Clostridium botulinum*) sometimes present in canned green beans but never in fresh ones? The reason why living things occur and thrive where they do depends upon a variety of conditions. Sometimes those conditions are quite obvious: summer temperatures in Norway are not hot enough nor is the growing season long enough to produce a bountiful corn harvest; lack of water and shade make survival of ferns impossible in a desert environment. In some cases the factors which control where a plant or animal lives are not quite so apparent: *Clostridium botulinum* can multiply and produce its deadly toxin only in an environment where oxygen is absent; hence it may present a threat in improperly canned foods, but seldom in fresh ones.

Environmental conditions that limit or control where an organism can live are called **limiting factors**. Obviously not every factor in an organism's environment is equally important in determining where that plant or animal can live. Components which are relatively constant in amount and moderately abundant are seldom limiting factors, particularly if the individual in question has a wide limit of tolerance. On the other hand, if an individual has a narrow limit of tolerance for a factor which exists in low or variable amounts, then that factor might indeed be the crucial determinant in where the organism can live. For example, most higher forms of life require a plentiful supply of oxygen to carry out their metabolic activities. Nevertheless, even though oxygen is essential, because it is so abundantly present and readily available to most land plants and animals (with the exception of some parasites and organisms living underground) it is almost never a limiting factor in terrestrial communities. On the other hand, lack of oxygen can definitely be a limiting factor for a number of aquatic organisms. The larvae of certain insects such as mayflies and caddisflies, as well as important game fish such as brook trout, simply die or move elsewhere when levels of dissolved oxygen in a waterway drop below a critical point.

Although the Massachusetts Indians who taught the Pilgrims to bury a dead fish in each hill of corn must have intuitively understood the concept, the idea of limiting factors was first formulated in 1840 by the German biochemist Justus Liebig while studying problems of fertility in agricultural soils. Liebig was experimenting with the use of inorganic chemical fertilizers in place of manures then currently in use and found that crop yields were affected not so much by the nutrients needed in large quantities—such as carbon dioxide and water, since these were generally present in plentiful supply—but by some mineral, such as copper, needed in minute amounts but lacking from particular soils. From this observation he proclaimed his famous "Law of the Minimum," stating that "the growth of a plant is dependent on the amount of foodstuff which is presented to it in a minimum quantity." Succeeding generations of ecologists have expanded Liebig's concept to include not only mineral nutrients but also such things as light, temperature, pH, water, oxygen supply, and soil type as possible limiting factors to the distribution of organisms.

Further investigations revealed a complicating fact: when some factor other than the minimum one is available in very high concentrations, this may moderate the rate at which the critical one is used. For example, plants growing in the shade require less zinc than those growing in the sun. Thus shade-grown plants are less affected by a zinc-deficient soil than are plants of the same species growing in full sunlight. Also, some organisms can substitute a chemically similar nutrient for one that is deficient, as can be seen in certain mollusks which partially substitute strontium for calcium in their shells when amounts of calcium are low.

To make matters more complex, by the early 20th century it became clear that the old adage, "If a little bit is good, then more must be better," was quite untrue so far as the needs of living things were concerned. The concept of the law of the minimum was broadened by the American ecologist Victor Shelford, who demonstrated that too much of a limiting factor can be just as harmful as not enough. Organisms have both an ecological maximum and minimum, the range in between these two extremes representing that organism's limits of tolerance.

Limits of Tolerance

Subsequent investigations in regard to tolerance ranges have revealed a great deal about why certain species live where they do. Not surprisingly, those plants and animals that have a wide range of tolerance for all factors are the ones that have the widest distribution. However, some organisms can have a wide tolerance range for some factors but a narrow range for others, and thus their distribution will be accordingly more limited. Not all stages of an animal's or plant's life cycle are equally sensitive to the effect of limiting factors. Among many spore-forming bacteria, for example, high temperatures that would be almost instantly fatal for actively growing cells have no effect on the spore stage unless the duration of exposure is fairly long. In general, the most critical period when environmental factors are most likely to be limiting (i.e. when the range of tolerance is narrowest) is during the reproductive period. Susceptibility of the young to conditions that adult organisms could tolerate with little difficulty is well established in regard to one of our major environmental problems at present, that of acid rainfall. The low pH levels that are blamed for the near-total

BOX 1-2

Where's Kermit?

Will Miss Piggy's sweetheart and his kin soon join the ranks of the dinosaurs, remembered only in children's stories and "Sesame Street" reruns? This is the nightmare of some biologists who watch in puzzlement and dismay as populations of once-abundant species of frogs, toads, and salamanders crash all over the world. Though never a dominant animal species, amphibians have been hardy enough to have survived and prospered for the past 350 million years as an evolutionary link between fish and reptiles, equally at home both in water and on land. Comprising almost 4000 known species, amphibians inhabit every continent except Antarctica—and everywhere they are rapidly disappearing.

The alarm was first raised in 1989 at an international conference in England where herpetologists (scientists specializing in the study of reptiles and amphibians) from 63 countries began comparing notes and were shocked to learn that the localized population declines each had observed were occurring all over the world. Admitting that amphibian populations naturally tend to exhibit wide fluctuations, they felt, nevertheless, that the simultaneous disappearance of frogs and toads in so many places was indicative of something new and disturbing. Like the caged canaries whose demise provided an advance warning to underground miners of the presence of toxic gases, vanishing frogs may be indicators of impending ecological catastrophe as human-generated pollutants continue to heap insults on land, air, and water. David Wake, a biology professor at Berkeley who heads a research task force trying to solve the mystery, remarked to a group of colleagues that "if frogs and salamanders are dying off in synchrony, there's a message there for us. They survived whatever wiped out the dinosaurs and they have thrived through the age of mammals. If they start to check out now, we'd better take it seriously."

In retrospect, it shouldn't be surprising that frogs and other amphibians are particularly susceptible to environmental contaminants. Laying their eggs in water, spending their early months as free-swimming tadpoles, and subsequently moving onto the land as adults, frogs and toads are exposed to a wide range of pollutants. Their thin, moist skins offer little protection against contaminants such as heavy metals or other pollutants that can easily pass into their bodies from surrounding soil or water. They also are at risk of exposure to toxins present in the smaller organisms they eat and readily accumulate these poisons in their systems. The search for a single, unifying explanation for the frogs' plight is likely to be unsuccessful, however; researchers suspect that a variety of forces are to blame.

In many areas, habitat destruction is the obvious culprit. When marshes are drained to construct shopping centers or when rice paddies are converted into golf courses, frogs disappear. Climatic conditions can also have an impact—several consecutive drought years can wreak havoc on amphibian populations. Over-harvesting as a food source can have a dramatic impact on numbers; in southern India, Bangladesh, and Malaysia there is widespread exploitation of these tasty amphibians as local workers try to meet foreign demand for frogs' legs as a gourmet food item. Some formerly fish-free mountain lakes have been stocked with sports fish for the enjoyment of anglers, resulting in precipitous declines of frog populations as the alien fish gobbled up tadpoles that had formerly been safe from predation.

While the cause of the frogs' demise in the situations just described is readily apparent, amphibians also are vanishing from many seemingly undisturbed areas of the world where the reasons for their disappearance are far more problematic. In Costa Rica's Monteverde Cloud Forest Reserve, for example, hordes of brilliant toads used to emerge from underground burrows during the breeding season, delighting naturalists who traveled from near and far to witness the spectacle. In 1987, thousands of toads participated in the age-old ritual; in 1988 only one adult male was spotted and since then none have been seen. In the 1970s a researcher from UCLA found ponds in California's High Sierras swarming with frogs; when he revisited 38 of them in 1989, he found frogs in only one. Around the world, from Australia to Canada to England, biologists sadly relate similar stories. In North America alone, almost one-third of the frog and toad species are in jeopardy.

Numerous theories, from acid rain to airborne pesticide fallout, have been advanced as possible explanations for the global extent of the problems buffeting amphibian populations. One of the ideas being intensively researched is the possibility that deterioration of the ozone layer is permitting excess amounts of damaging ultraviolet radiation to reach the earth's surface, with lethal effects on amphibian eggs. The fact that some of the most severely affected species are those living at high altitudes or in the Southern Hemisphere near the infamous Antarctic "ozone hole" makes this hypothesis especially provocative, but definitive evidence is still lacking.

Some biologists contest the idea that recent declines are indicative of anything more than normal, temporary population fluctuations, pointing out that many species continue to thrive and some regions remain unaffected. Others, however, unwilling to wait until the last bit of data is collected before sounding the alarm, are now hard at work on experiments aimed at elucidating the reasons for current trends while there are still frogs left to save. For skeptics who question all the fuss about small slimy creatures of little economic value and minimal emotional appeal, Dr. Wake responds: "Frogs are in essence a messenger. This is about biodiversity and disintegration, the destruction of our total environment."

References

Blakeslee, Sandra. 1990. "Scientists Confront an Alarming Mystery: The Vanishing Frog." *New York Times*, Feb. 20, B7.

Yoffe, Emily. 1992. "The Silence of the Frogs." *New York Times Magazine*, Dec. 13.

disappearance of many species of fish in lakes throughout eastern Canada, northeastern United States, and parts of Scandinavia have been shown to be lethal to fish eggs and fingerlings, but not to adult fish. Thus the effects of acid rain on aquatic life are much less dramatic than the effects of, for example, a chemical spill into a river. Rather than a massive, immediately visible (and smelly!) fish kill, the fish in an acidifying lake simply fail to reproduce and become less and less abundant, older and older, until they die out completely. Other examples of the vulnerability of the reproductive stage include the observations that while adult cypress trees can grow either on dry ground or with their bases continually submerged in water, cypress seedlings can only develop in moist, unflooded soil. Similarly, some adult marine animals such as blue crabs can tolerate fresh water that is slightly salty and so are frequently found in rivers some distance upstream from the sea. Their young, however, can thrive only in salt water, so reproduction and permanent establishment of these organisms in rivers cannot occur. Just as the very young of lower forms of life display less tolerance to environmental extremes than do adults, the same situation applies with humans. Many widespread environmental toxins have been shown, some in tragic ways, to have a much more devastating effect on developing fetuses and young children than on adults. The drug thalidomide and organic mercury are just two substances that have been ingested by pregnant women with no harmful effects on themselves but with disastrous results on their unborn children. Levels of air pollution that are largely ignored by the adult population can cause severe respiratory distress in infants and children. It's important for us to keep in mind the qualifications to the range of tolerance concept when we hear official assurances that exposure to this or that substance is "safe." What is safe for one segment of the population may be far from safe for others.

Energy Flow Through the Biosphere

Living things are dependent for their existence not only on proper soil and climate conditions but also on some form of energy; a basic understanding of the flow of energy through an ecosystem is fundamental to the study of how that system functions.

The ultimate source of all life activities, from the unfolding of a flower bud to the 100-meter dash of an Olympic athlete is, of course, the sun. Some 93 million miles (150 million km) from the earth, the sun emits vast amounts of electromagnetic radiation which, traveling through space at a rate of 186,000 miles (300,000 km) per second, takes about nine minutes to reach the earth's surface. There is no energy loss as the sun's radiation travels through space, but since its intensity decreases inversely as the square of the distance from the sun, the amount of solar radiation intercepted by the earth is but one two-billionth of the sun's total energy output. On this seemingly tiny portion all life on earth depends. More than half the incoming radiation is unusable by living things, however. Electromagnetic radiation consists of several different wavelengths. Of the total amount of energy received from the sun, 9% is in the form of short-wave, high-energy ultraviolet rays; 50% is in the form of long-wave, infrared waves (heat waves); and 41% is visible light. Only those wavelengths within the visible spectrum, particularly those in the red and blue range, can be absorbed and utilized by green plants. These, through the process of photosynthesis, convert solar energy into the energy of chemical bonds.

The complex and still not fully understood mechanism whereby plants harness certain wavelengths of sunlight and use this energy to join molecules of carbon dioxide and water to form the simple sugar glucose, releasing oxygen in the process, makes the existence of all higher forms of life possible. The transfer of this captured energy from organism to organism is basic to the functioning of ecosystems. Before examining the paths of energy flow, however, let us take a brief look at some physical laws that control and limit the amount of energy available to living things.

Laws of Thermodynamics

An understanding of many problems in both environmental science and energy technology depends on a basic conception of the principles that govern how energy is changed from one form into another. Known as the first and second laws of thermodynamics, these principles can be summarized as follows:

The First Law of Thermodynamics.   Sometimes called the Law of Conservation of Energy, it states that energy can neither be created nor destroyed, even though it may be changed from one form into another. **Solar energy** that is absorbed by rocks or soil or water on the earth's surface is converted into the **heat energy** which, because of temperature differentials and the earth's rotation, gives rise to winds and water currents that are a form of **kinetic energy**. When such kinetic energy accomplishes work such as the raising of water by wind, then it has been changed into **potential energy**, so-called because the latent energy of a water droplet in a cloud or at the top of a dam can be converted into some other kind of energy when it falls. In the same way, light energy absorbed by the chlorophyll molecules in a leaf is converted into the potential energy of chemical bonds within carbohydrates, proteins, and fats. As light energy passes from one form to another, it may appear that most of it is eventually lost or consumed (how often have we heard references to that misnomer, ''energy consumption''?). This is a misconception, however, for if one maintained a global balance sheet it would show that all the energy that enters the biosphere as light is reradiated and leaves the earth's surface in the form of invisible heat waves. The form of energy leaving the system is different from the incoming radiation, but no energy has been either created or destroyed during its passage through the biosphere.

The Second Law of Thermodynamics.   This law states that with every energy transformation there is a loss of *usable* energy (that is, energy that can be used to do work). Put another way, all physical processes proceed in such a way that the *availability* of the energy involved decreases (note that the availability, not the total amount, of energy is what decreases—the latter would be a violation of the First Law). The Second Law introduces the concept of **entropy**, the idea that all energy is moving toward an ever less available and more dispersed state. This process will continue until all energy has been transformed to heat distributed at a uniform temperature throughout the solar system—at which point the stable state will have been achieved.

The Second Law has some interesting implications concerning ecological relationships. Perhaps the most important of these is the fact that no type of energy transformation is ever 100% efficient—there will always be a significant loss of usable energy whenever energy is transferred from one organism to another. This explains why we need a continued input of energy to maintain ourselves and why we must consume substantially more than a pound of food in order to gain a pound of weight. In addition, because a given quantity of energy can be used only once, the ability to convert energy into useful work cannot be "recycled." Thus energy, unlike the essential minerals and gases, moves in a unidirectional way through ecosystems, becoming ever more dispersed and eventually being degraded to heat. Bearing these fundamental physical laws in mind, let's now take a more detailed look at the flow of energy through the biotic community.

Food Chains

Although overly simplistic, the concept of a **food chain** is useful for conveying a general understanding of how energy moves through ecosystems. Basically, a food chain involves the transfer of food energy from a given source through a series of organisms, each of which eats the next lower individual in the chain. In terms of energy flow, the living components of the ecosystem can be subdivided into three broad categories:

1. *Producers*—the green plants that convert the sun's energy into food energy. On land the major producers are the flowering plants and the conifers; in water they are mainly the diatoms, microflagellates, and green algae.
2. *Consumers*—animals; primary consumers are the herbivores and secondary consumers are the carnivores.
3. *Decomposers*—primarily bacteria and fungi, some insects. Decomposers are essential for recycling detritus back into the soil where it is once again available for use by producer organisms. No community could exist very long without decomposers.

There are basically three types of food chains. The most familiar of these, called a **grazing food chain** (or "predator chain"), may be typified by a grass-rabbit-fox association which starts with a plant base and proceeds from smaller to larger animals. Less conspicuous but equally important is the **detritus food chain**, where dead organic matter (detritus) is broken down by microorganisms, primarily bacteria. Small animals eat particles of this detritus, securing energy largely from assimilation of the energy-rich bacteria. The small animals, in turn, become a source of energy for larger consumers. A prime example of a detritus food chain accounting for a substantial portion of an ecosystem's energy flow can be found in the salt marsh habitat of many coastal areas. Here plants such as marsh grass die and are washed into estuaries where they are decomposed by microbes into finely divided particles which are then consumed by such primary consumers as fiddler crabs and mollusks. These, in turn, may be eaten by secondary consumers such as raccoons, water birds, or other crabs.

A variation on grazing food chains can be seen in certain **parasitic chains**, in which energy flows from larger to smaller animals (e.g. dogs which provide an energy source for fleas which in turn are fed upon by parasitic protozoans). In energy terms, however, there is no fundamental difference between a parasitic food chain and a grazing food chain, since a parasite is basically a "consumer."

Ecological Pyramids

Through the interactions of the community, a unidirectional flow of energy occurs from producers to primary consumers to secondary consumers, and so on. Each of these stages in a food chain is called a **trophic level**. It should be noted that placement of an organism into one trophic level or another depends on what that organism *does*, not to which species it belongs, since individuals of the same species may feed at different trophic levels, depending on factors such as age or sex. A male mosquito, for example, is an herbivore (primary consumer), dining on plant juices and nectar, while his mate would be classified as a carnivore (secondary consumer) when she takes the blood meal essential for egg laying. Similarly, while grazing animals such as cattle and horses are strict vegetarians as adults, their young thrive on a diet of mother's milk, making them, in effect, secondary consumers.

To describe the relationships among members of various trophic levels, ecologists frequently use the concept of **ecological pyramids**. If we examine a food chain in terms of the animals and plants which constitute it, it becomes apparent that these forms can be arranged into what is called a "pyramid of numbers." At the bottom of the pyramid are multitudes of energy-producing plants, then a smaller number of herbivores that feed upon them, then a still smaller number of primary carnivores, followed by an even smaller number of secondary carnivores. The animals at the top of the heap, the final consumers, are usually the largest in the community, while those organisms at the bottom of the pyramid, the producers, are usually the smallest, but much more abundant. In addition, the organisms at the lower trophic levels usually reproduce more rapidly and more prolifically than those higher up, so there is seldom danger of a predator eating itself out of its food supply. It should be noted, however, that in those cases where the size of the producer organisms is very large and the size of the primary consumers is small (e.g. a cherry tree being munched upon by hundreds of caterpillars), the shape of the pyramid of numbers may be inverted.

Just as the numbers of individual organisms in a community is generally greatest at the lower trophic levels, so the living weight, or **biomass** (measured as dry weight per unit area), is generally greatest at the producer trophic level. In the same way, biomass of the primary consumers will be greater than that of the secondary consumers, so the ecological biomass pyramids used to portray weight relationships among trophic levels will often look identical to numbers pyramids. Biomass, which in effect is an indicator of the amount of energy stored within an ecosystem, varies widely from one type of biotic community to another. For example, the amount of biomass in a tropical rain forest far exceeds that in a comparable area of abandoned field, while open ocean water is relatively poor in terms of biomass.

Although biomass pyramids, like numbers pyramids, usually have a broad base and tapered apex, in those situations where the organisms at the producer level are much smaller than the consumers, the shape of the biomass pyramid may be upside-down. This occurs because the "standing crop biomass" (the total dry weight of organisms present at any one moment in time) which can be maintained by a steady flow of energy in a food chain depends to a large extent on the size of the individual organisms. The smaller the organisms are, the greater is their metabolic rate per gram of biomass. Thus the smaller the organism, the smaller the biomass which can be supported at a given trophic level; in the same way, the larger the organism, the larger the amount of biomass at any one point in time. This is why in, say, an aquatic ecosystem the biomass of the blue whale would be far greater than the biomass of the microscopic diatoms and zooplankton on which it feeds. The biomass pyramid which illustrates the energy relationships in such a situation would be an inverted one. This doesn't mean that the producer organisms are defying the laws of nature; it simply reflects the fact that the tiny phytoplankton have very high metabolic rates and that they reproduce much more rapidly than do whales, having complete turnovers in their populations within very short time periods.

Whereas pyramids of numbers tend to exaggerate the importance of small organisms and pyramids of biomass often understate their role, pyramids of energy give the best picture of energy flow through a food chain, showing what actually is happening within the biotic community. As was mentioned earlier, light energy from the sun is captured by green plants and stored in the form of chemical bonds in the molecules of starch, glucose, fats, and so forth. However, as the Second Law of Thermodynamics states, only a portion of the energy stored by one trophic level is available to the next higher one, since a considerable amount is lost at every stage of transformation. Thus when cows graze in a pasture, some of the chemical bond energy in the grass is converted into the muscle tissue which represents stored food in the cow. The largest portion of energy derived from the grass, however, is lost in the form of waste heat during respiration. A lesser amount is lost as unassimilated food materials in feces or urine and as organic material which is not eaten by the next higher trophic level (i.e. just as people do not eat every part of a cow or pig, so many animals leave certain parts of their prey unconsumed; such "rejects" constitute an energy loss to the food chain).

At each transfer of energy within a food chain, approximately 90% (sometimes a bit more, sometimes less) of the chemical energy stored in organisms of the lower level is lost and therefore unavailable to the higher level. Since the total amount of energy entering the food chain is fixed by the photosynthetic activities of plants (and plants are less than 1% efficient, on the average, in converting solar energy into chemical energy), obviously more usable energy is available to organisms occupying lower positions in the food chain than to those at higher trophic levels. Expressing this concept in simpler terms, one might say, for example:

$$10,000 \text{ lbs. corn} \rightarrow 1,000 \text{ lbs. beef} \rightarrow 100 \text{ lbs. human}$$

By moving humans one step lower in the food chain, ten times more energy becomes directly available:

$$10,000 \text{ lbs. corn} \rightarrow 1,000 \text{ lbs. human}$$

In very simplified terms, this explains why countries like China and India are largely vegetarian. In order to produce enough food to sustain many millions of people, such nations cannot afford the luxury of wasting the amount of energy involved in raising animals for meat. Some people feel that at a time when massive food shortages are a fact of life in many parts of the world, Americans have a moral responsibility to abstain from our predilection for corn-fed beef and use midwestern farmlands to produce crops that humans can eat directly. From another viewpoint, the above equation indicates why populations which, because of their habitat, are almost exclusively dependent on meat as a food source cannot permit their numbers to grow very large. One important factor contributing to the small population size of Eskimo groups is that these people exist as top carnivores of a relatively long food chain:

$$\text{diatoms} \rightarrow \text{zooplankton} \rightarrow \text{fish} \rightarrow \text{seals} \rightarrow \text{Eskimos}$$

Such energy flow patterns indicate that if Americans want to retain meat as a major component of their diet, they cannot permit population levels to increase substantially.

The preceding observations should make it readily apparent that food chains are limited by energy considerations to no more than four or five trophic levels. A food chain of unlimited length is a physical impossibility, because the higher the feeding level, the less energy there is available within a given area. An animal that is a high level consumer must range over wide areas in order to find enough food to support itself. Eventually the point is reached where the energy required to secure the food is greater than the energy obtained by eating it. At such a point no more organisms can be supported and the upper limits of the food chain have been reached.

Of course in most real communities the actual structure of trophic levels is much more complex than the food chain concept portrays. A "food web" would be a more accurate depiction, since many organisms feed on many different species and in some cases on more than one trophic level. Humans, for example, can be quaternary or tertiary consumers by eating fish, secondary consumers when dining on roast turkey, or primary consumers when munching on peanut-butter sandwiches. The many interlocking food chains tend to promote stability for organisms at the higher levels, providing them with alternative food sources should one or more of the prey species become less abundant. In general, the more complex the food web, the more stable the ecosystem is likely to be.

Figure 1-2 Food Pyramid

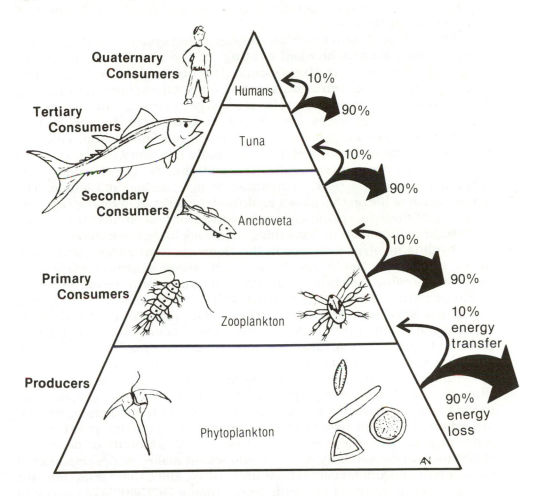

Biogeochemical Cycling

Every home gardener who maintains a compost pile in the backyard intuitively understands the basic principles of biogeochemical cycling. All living organisms are dependent not only on a source of energy, but also on a number of inorganic materials that are continuously being circulated throughout the ecosystem. These materials provide both the physical framework that supports life activities and the inorganic chemical building-blocks from which living molecules are formed. When such molecules are synthesized or broken down, changed from one form into another as they move through the ecosystem, the elements of which they are composed are not lost or degraded in the same way in which energy moving through a food chain becomes unusable. Indeed, the manner in which inorganic materials move through ecosystems differs fundamentally from the movement of energy through those same systems in that matter, unlike energy, is conserved within the ecosystem, its atoms and molecules being used and reused indefinitely.

The cycling of earth materials through living systems and back to the earth is called **biogeochemical cycling**. Of the 92 naturally occurring chemical elements, about 40 are essential to the existence of living organisms and hence are known as **nutrients**. Some of these nutrients are fairly abundant and are needed in relatively large quantities by plants and animals. Such substances are termed **macronutrients** and include carbon, hydrogen, oxygen, nitrogen, phosphorus, potassium, calcium, magnesium, and sulfur. Others that are equally necessary but are required in much smaller amounts are called **trace elements**. These include such substances as iron, copper, manganese, zinc, chlorine, and iodine. The perpetuation of life on this planet is ultimately dependent on the repeated recycling of these inorganic materials in more or less circular paths from the abiotic environment to living things and back to the environment again. Such cycling involves a change in the elements from an inorganic form to an organic molecule and back again. Biogeochemical cycles are important because they help retain vital nutrients in forms usable by plants and animals and because they help to maintain the stability of ecosystems.

Organisms have developed various adaptations to enable them to capture and retain nutrients. As we have seen in our discussion of biomes, plants in both the tropical rain forest and in desert regions have widespread, shallow root systems that permit them quickly to absorb water and the mineral nutrients that it carries in dissolved form before these can be lost through rapid run-off, competition from other organisms, or evaporation. In the tropical rain forest, for example, virtually all the mineral nutrients are retained in plant tissues and the topsoil of this biome is extremely nutrient-poor. If nutrient cycling did not occur, amounts of necessary elements would constantly decrease and would make the development of stable plant and animal populations impossible, since there is no constant addition to the source of nutrients from outside (as there is of energy in the form of sunlight).

There are basically two types of biogeochemical cycles—gaseous and sedimentary—depending on whether the primary source for the nutrient involved happens to be air and water (gaseous cycle) or soil and rocks (sedimentary cycle).

Gaseous Cycles

The elements moved about by gaseous cycles, primarily through the atmosphere but to a lesser degree in water, recycle much more quickly and efficiently than do those in the sedimentary cycle. Gaseous cycles pertain to only four elements: carbon, hydrogen, oxygen, and nitrogen. These four constitute about 97.2% of the bulk of protoplasm and so are of vital importance to life. An examination of two of these, the carbon and nitrogen cycles, give an idea of the complexity of gaseous cycles.

Carbon Cycle.   Carbon atoms are the basic units of all organic compounds and hence, along with water, could be considered the most important component of biological systems. The principal inorganic source of carbon is the carbon dioxide found in the atmosphere and dissolved in bodies of water (the concentration of carbon dioxide dissolved in water is about 100 times greater than the amount present in the atmosphere; for this reason, carbon dioxide is much more accessible to aquatic organisms than to species living on land). Another large source of inorganic carbon lies in storage within deposits of fossil fuels—coal, oil, gas—but the largest amount of all occurs in the form of carbonate sediments such as limestone, formed under the seas and gradually uplifted during slow geologic processes.

Carbon is made available to living organisms through the process of photosynthesis, whereby green plants utilize solar energy to combine carbon dioxide and water, ultimately producing carbon-containing simple sugars. These constitute the basic building blocks for the synthesis of all other organic molecules. Animals obtain the carbon they need by eating plants and resynthesizing these into new carbon-containing compounds. Completion of the cycle, the breakdown of organic molecules to release inorganic carbon dioxide, is accomplished by several different pathways: 1) through the processes of respiration, whereby plants and animals take in oxygen and release carbon dioxide as a waste product; 2) through the decay of dead organisms or of animal wastes, whereby bacteria and fungi decompose the carbon-containing organic molecules, releasing large amounts of carbon dioxide through their respiratory activities; 3) natural weathering of limestone; and 4) by the combustion of organic fuels (coal, oil, gas, wood). The last of these sources of inorganic carbon is causing growing concern among scientists who note that while the amount of atmospheric carbon remained relatively stable for millions of years, it has been increasing steadily since the onset of the Industrial Revolution and has particularly accelerated during the past century.

Nitrogen Cycle.   The major reservoirs of nitrogen in the ecosystem are the 78% of free nitrogen gas that makes up our atmosphere and the nitrogen stored in rock-forming minerals. Atmospheric nitrogen, however, is biologically inert and cannot be utilized as such by most green plants. Nitrogen in the air can be returned to the soil and converted to a form accessible to plants in one of two ways.

1. Lightning passing through the atmosphere can convert nitrogen to nitrogen oxide; when nitrogen oxide is dissolved in water it can be acted upon by certain bacteria in the soil which convert it into nitrate ions which can be absorbed by plant roots.

2. Fixation of atmospheric nitrogen by *Rhizobium* sp. bacteria which live in symbiotic association with leguminous plants inside root nodules, converting nitrogen to nitrates; certain species of free-living soil bacteria and some cyanobacteria also have the ability to fix free nitrogen into nitrates.

Of these two methods, fixation of atmospheric nitrogen by bacteria is by far the most significant way of making nitrogen available to other organisms. To complete the nitrogen cycle, nitrogenous wastes in the form of dead organisms, feces, urine, and so forth, are decomposed to ammonia by other types of soil bacteria; ammonia in turn is acted upon by nitrifying bacteria which form more nitrates. Such nitrates may be taken up again by plants or further broken down by another group of microorganisms called de-nitrifying bacteria, which act upon nitrates to produce free nitrogen which is once again returned to the atmosphere.

Sedimentary Cycles

Many of the elements that are essential for plant and animal life occur most commonly in the form of sedimentary rocks from which recycling takes place very slowly. Indeed, such sedimentary cycles may extend across long periods of geologic time and for all practical purposes constitute what are essentially one-way flows. In comparison with gaseous cycles, sedimentary cycles seem relatively simple in nature. Iron, calcium, and phosphorus are examples of nutrients whose cycling occurs via the basic sedimentary pattern. A brief look at the phosphorus cycle will give an idea of the transformations involved.

Phosphorus Cycle.   Phosphorus, a key element in the nucleic acids DNA and RNA, as well as a component of the organic molecules that govern energy transfer within living organisms, occurs principally in the form of phosphate rock deposits. Smaller, though locally significant, amounts occur where quantities of excrement from fish-eating birds accumulate (e.g. the guano deposits on islands off the coast of Peru) or in deposits of fossil bones. When such phosphate reservoirs are exposed to rainfall, phosphorus ions dissolve and can be absorbed by plant roots and incorporated into vegetative tissue. At the same time, much phosphorus is effectively lost from the ecosystem through run-off to the sea. Animals obtain the phosphorus they need by eating plants. When animals excrete waste products or when they die and decay, phosphates are returned to the soil where they once again become available for uptake by plants or are lost by downhill transport into the sea. Within the shallow coastal areas some of this phosphorus is taken up by the marine phytoplankton which constitute the ultimate source of phosphorus for fish and sea birds. However, much of the phosphorus entering the sea is carried by currents to the deeper marine sediments where it is inaccessible to living organisms and may remain locked up for millions of years until future geologic upheavals. The large amounts of phosphate being produced commercially today for use as fertilizers come from the mining of phosphate rock. Unfortunately, much as in the case of oil or coal, such phosphate deposits constitute an essentially nonrenewable resource, since the processes responsible for their creation occurred millions of years in the past.

The fact that the general pattern in sedimentary cycling is a downhill one, where materials tend to move through ecosystems into relatively inaccessible geologic pools, poses some interesting implications for the stability of ecosystems. The loss of soluble mineral nutrients from upland areas to the lowlands and oceans is curbed only by local biological recycling mechanisms which prevent downhill loss from outpacing the release of new materials from underlying rocks. Such local recycling depends upon the return of dead organic material to the soil where breakdown and reuse of materials can occur. Human disruption of this process through widescale removal of potential nutrients (e.g. by logging, which removes trees that would otherwise have died and decayed in place; grazing of livestock which consume local resources but whose flesh, wool, bones, and so on will be disposed of elsewhere) accelerates the impoverishment of certain ecosystems where essential mineral nutrients are already in short supply. In such situations the lowlands are not benefitted either, for the increased flow of materials they receive generally pass into the sea and out of biological circulation before they can be assimilated. Concern about the long-range stability of ecosystems demands that we begin to pay more careful attention to the biological recycling of inorganic materials that move in sedimentary cycles.

Change in Ecosystems

The fact that ecosystems undergo dramatic change over vast periods of time is now well accepted. Geologists have shown us how mountains are worn down and washed to the seas, forming thick layers of underwater sediments that eons later may be uplifted by immense tectonic pressures to form new mountains; deserts expand and retreat as rainfall patterns shift; and periodically great glacial ice sheets move southward, changing the face of the earth. As land forms and climate change, it is not surprising that the biotic communities within the affected ecosystems change also. It is now recognized that the biotic communities in past geologic eras differed greatly from those existing today. What is less well understood is that present ecosystems have a dynamic quality of their own, their component communities changing in an orderly sequence within a given area, a process known as **ecological succession**.

Succession

On May 18, 1980, Mount St. Helens volcano in southwestern Washington State exploded in a blast that obliterated the lush fir and hemlock forests that had blanketed its slopes for centuries. The collapse of the mountain's north face triggered an avalanche of mud and rocks that swept 15 miles down the Toutle River Valley, burying everything in its path under a 140-foot layer of volcanic debris. Observers surveying the scene at the time might understandably have wondered whether life could ever return to a scene of such devastation, yet within a year perennial wildflowers such as fireweed were blooming on the ash-laden mountainside. Year by year, the avalanche-affected area has become

BOX 1-3

Will Skiing Spoil the Alps?

If the 1994 Winter Olympics at Lillehammer, Norway, were indeed the first "green games" as their organizers claimed they would be, the credit may be due to the widespread dismay at the destruction caused by the 1992 extravaganza at Albertville in the French Alps. In order to provide facilities for athletes and accommodations for spectators during the two-week event, more than a million cubic yards of earth were gouged out of mountainsides, 60 acres of trees leveled, and Alpine pastures scraped smooth. Ambitious construction projects created new bridges, tunnels, hotel complexes, parking lots, garbage facilities, and 32 lanes of roadways for the streams of traffic entering and leaving this once-sleepy town. Whatever it contributed to the local economy and to the enjoyment of a worldwide television audience, the 1992 Winter Games constituted yet one more assault on an environment identified by some as "the most threatened mountain system in the world."

While the Olympics may have represented the most dramatic example of human interference with this ecologically fragile region, it certainly wasn't the first. Stretching from west to east in a 650-mile arc across central Europe, the Alps have experienced developmental pressures for millennia. Early farmers who settled the area at least 6000 years ago gradually created completely new ecosystems by cutting the forest to enlarge pasture lands and by cultivating crops in the valleys. Over the centuries these people learned essential techniques of sustainable land use and developed the traditional grazing and mowing practices that help prevent the avalanches and erosion to which mountain environments are so vulnerable. For the most part, traditional Alpine peoples recognized the necessity of living in harmony with nature; social norms ensured that the community's interest in sustainable resource use took precedence over short-term exploitation for individual gain.

The tranquil fabric of Alpine life began to unravel in the decades following the Industrial Revolution. First railroads and then highways opened up the region to contact with the outside world. Few aspects of the collision of cultures were more far-reaching, however, than the "discovery" of the Alps by tourists newly appreciative of lovely mountain vistas. The trickle of visitors who began arriving in the Alps' picturesque villages in the late 19th century assumed flood-like proportions after 1955, when mass tourism became an integral part of European life. By the mid-1960s the number of winter vacationers began to exceed those of the summer months, as the winter sports industry began transforming the region. Over 100 million visitors now throng the Alps each year; once-pristine tourist centers now experience levels of noise and air pollution comparable to those in Europe's largest cities. While thoughtless summer hikers may trample vegetation in ecologically sensitive highlands, many observers agree that no human activity in the Alps today is more environmentally disruptive than is downhill skiing. Since the advent of the winter sports boom in the early 1960s, more than 40,000 ski runs and 12,000 ski lifts have been constructed in the Alps. Frantic competition among Alpine communities for the tourist trade has resulted in chaotic, poorly planned development and over-construction of hotels, mountaintop restaurants, and other facilities catering to tourists. As one German critic remarked, "The Alps are being literally reconstructed because the good Lord was obviously not a skier."

Such development is now taking its toll on the Alpine environment: diminishing biodiversity as Alpine habitats are reduced into ever-smaller isolated segments; traffic congestion generated by the millions of vehicles regularly traversing what have become the busiest mountain roads in the world; and air pollution caused by truck and auto emissions, compounded by pollutants from the region's homes and manufacturing facilities. Observers fear that if air quality trends continue to worsen, one-third of Alpine forests could be destroyed within the next 50 years.

Protesting the growing despoliation of one of the world's most beautiful regions, European environmental groups are striving to raise public awareness of the inherent vulnerability of mountain ecosystems and to persuade governments to reconsider environmentally destructive development projects. Olympic officials might take a first step in this direction by heeding the appeal of the French group, Alp Action, to modify the Olympic Charter, combining a new commitment to environmental principles with the Games' traditional humanitarian ideals. By doing so, they suggest, the destruction at Albertville might yet be redeemed.

References

Denniston, Derek. 1992. "Alpine Slide." *World Watch* 5 (Sept./Oct.).

May, John. 1992. "World Class Destruction." *New York Times*, Feb. 17, A17.

Stone, Peter B., ed. 1992. *The State of the World's Mountains: A Global Report*. Zed Books, Ltd.

progressively greener. By the early 1990s, ecologists studying the area reported that 83 of the 256 plant species known to have been present prior to the eruption were once again thriving. While researchers concede that a return to anything resembling normal conditions will take more than a century (the area in the vicinity of the crater itself still remains virtually barren), the process of regeneration is well underway (Wilford, 1991).

The gradual replacement of one biotic community by another over time is termed **succession**. While the sequence of events following the Mount St. Helens eruption provides one of the most dramatic recent illustrations of the process, numerous examples of succession in action can be seen all around us. While a casual glance at the plants and animals living together on a vacant city lot or an abandoned pasture may suggest an environmentally stable situation, such an impression is deceptive. If one could observe the same scene over a period of many years, it would be obvious that the composition of the area's biotic community, as well as the physical environment itself, is slowly but surely changing in a directional manner toward a relatively stable, self-perpetuating stage called the **climax community**. Depending on the particular location involved, the changes might take thousands of years or be completed within decades, but in any case the process of change would follow a definite sequence.

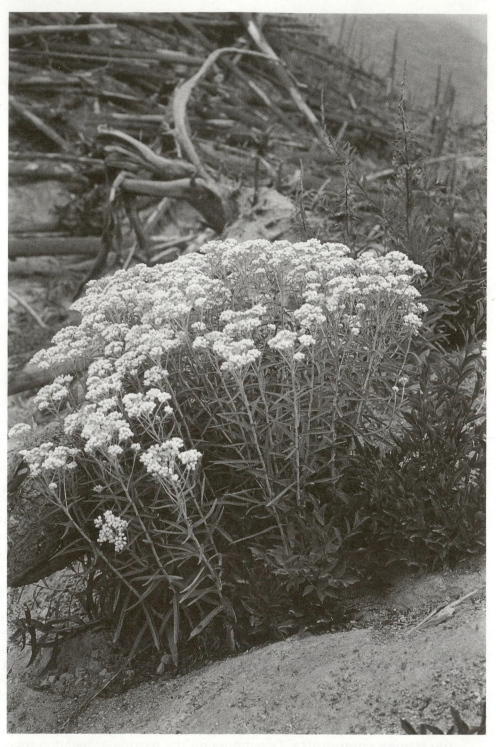

Wildflowers blooming against a backdrop of volcanic debris are indications of the regeneration that has occurred since Mt. St. Helens erupted in 1980. [Scott Shane]

The concept can be more easily understood by examining, step by step, the mechanisms of succession in a specific situation. Imagine that a retreating glacier has left behind a barren landscape of scoured bedrock or glacial till. Will the surface of the rock remain lifeless forever? Of course not; over a period of time, perhaps thousands of years if the climate is cold and dry, faster if it is warm and wet, changes in the biotic community occupying the surface of the rock will change it beyond recognition.

At first the only factors that can change the nature of the rock's surface are physical ones. Rain falls, combining with carbon dioxide in the air to form a dilute solution of carbonic acid. Bit by bit, this gradually begins to wear down the rocky surface. If the climate is a northern or temperate one, freezing and thawing may occur, helping to split the rock further. Wind erosion may also play a part. Algal and fungal spores or plant seeds will be carried to the site by air currents or by animals passing through the area, and colonies of lichens or other hardy plants establish themselves on the rock surface. The life processes of these organisms hasten the deterioration of the rock, and when the plants die, their dead organic matter contributes toward building up a thin layer of soil. These **pioneer plants** of the first stage of succession generally are small, low-growing species that can tolerate severe climatic conditions (e.g. intense sunlight, wide fluctuations in daily temperature, periodic wetting and drying), produce large numbers of spores or seeds annually, grow rapidly, and have short life cycles. While pioneer plants are quite tolerant of adverse physical conditions, they are generally intolerant of other organisms. For example, once lichens have helped to corrode rock, create a small amount of soil, and maintain better moisture conditions, mosses take over and crowd out the lichens. These may form a dense cover, attracting insects and other small invertebrates. The mosses continue to build up deposits of organic matter and soil as more rock is broken away and as the old mosses and lichens die. The most significant change these organisms can produce in an environment is that created by their own dead bodies. As decayed organic material accumulates, erosion of the rock slows down, but herbaceous plants move in and assume dominance. Insects and other arthropods will be the main form of animal life at this stage, but some small mammals and reptiles may be present also. Eventually shrubs and tree saplings will establish themselves, and since the taller plants furnish shade and act as a windbreak, the moisture conditions of the soil and near-soil atmosphere improve and temperature fluctuations at soil level become less extreme. Gradually the shrubs become the dominant plants, shading out many of the annual herbaceous species. Corresponding animal types change also, insects perhaps becoming fewer but bird species increasing in number. As the shrub stage matures, sapling trees begin to predominate. Shade-loving plants proliferate under the canopy. The large trees that characterize the late stages of succession in forest ecosystems are long-lived species that grow slowly and tend to persist for an indefinite period of time if environmental conditions of the area remain more or less constant. This relatively stable, self-perpetuating assemblage of species represents the climax community. Of course in reality a change in environmental conditions, especially climate, is not unusual and natural

Figure 1-3 Primary Succession

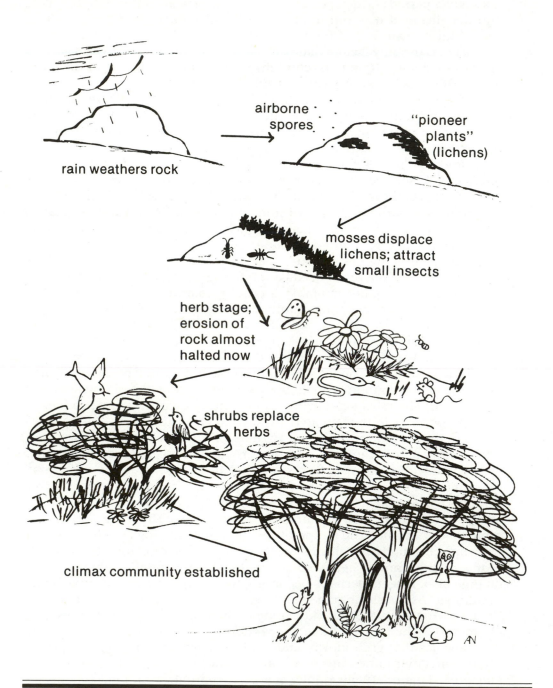

rain weathers rock

airborne spores

"pioneer plants" (lichens)

mosses displace lichens; attract small insects

herb stage; erosion of rock almost halted now

shrubs replace herbs

climax community established

Figure 1-4 Aquatic Succession

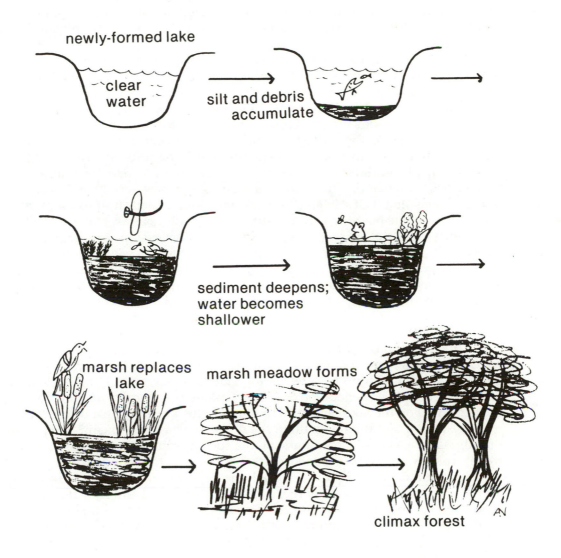

newly-formed lake

clear water

silt and debris accumulate

sediment deepens; water becomes shallower

marsh replaces lake

marsh meadow forms

climax forest

events such as fires, high winds, earthquakes, or pest outbreaks (or unnatural events such as lumbering or grazing) can create a mosaic of successional stages within a given region. It is important to note that during the successional process it is not only the composition of the biotic community that is constantly changing through time—the physical environment is being substantially altered as well. Thus succession represents a dynamic process in which abiotic factors influence the plants and animals of the community, and these, in turn, modify the physical habitat.

The preceding examples of succession beginning when pioneer organisms colonize an area formerly devoid of life is referred to as **primary succession**. A less extreme but far more common situation is that of **secondary succession**. In this case, succession proceeds from a state in which other organisms are still present; new life doesn't have to start from scratch, so to speak. Even in cases where the disturbed area may appear quite barren, roots, rhizomes, or dormant seeds lying underneath the soil surface quickly initiate the process of revegetation, joined by migrant species from outside the area taking advantage of the altered conditions. In the case of Mount St. Helens, for example, buried seeds and roots gave rise to new shoots pushing through the volcanic debris as erosion thinned the overlying ash. Examples of secondary succession are legion— abandoned Vermont farmland reverting to forest, revegetation of Yellowstone National Park after the devastating fires of 1988, untended suburban lawns growing up in weeds. In such cases succession begins at a more advanced stage but proceeds, like primary succession, in a directional, more or less predictable manner toward the climax community (Stiling, 1992).

Thus far we have only referred to terrestrial succession, but the same concept applies to most enclosed bodies of water as well. A newly formed lake (e.g. one left behind by a retreating glacier) will generally have clear water with little or no vegetation or debris. Gradually silt and dead materials are deposited on the lake bottom. The sides of the lake may also be eroded by wave action and thus help fill in the deeper parts of the basin. Around the edges of the lake rooted aquatic plants such as water lilies and pickerel weed, rushes, cattails, and so forth, become established. With the accumulation of dead organic material, the supply of nutrients necessary for the growth of algae and microorganisms is increased and they flourish accordingly, providing a food source for fish and other large animals. This process of nutrient enrichment is called **eutrophication**. The speed with which this phenomenon occurs is greatly accelerated when human-produced substances such as phosphate detergents, chemical fertilizers, or sewage is introduced. Eventually, as the lake becomes more completely filled with sediment, the whole area is converted into a marsh. Terrestrial grasses and moisture-tolerant plants subsequently move in, converting the marsh into a meadow, and finally the grasses are displaced by trees, resulting in a climax community. The length of time required for such succession to take place varies widely, depending on such variables as the original depth of the basin, the rate of sedimentation, and other physical conditions which affect the growth of organisms. It should be mentioned

BOX 1-4

Going, Going . . . Gone?

"Eco-catastrophe" is not an overly dramatic term for the environmental and human tragedy currently being played out in the not-so-long-ago fertile lands of Central Asia. Once a part of the Soviet empire, the now-independent republics of Uzbekistan and Kazakhstan are beset with declining harvests, powerful dust storms, climate change, and diminishing biodiversity—all consequences of misguided agricultural policies that are slowly destroying the region's key natural resource, the Aral Sea.

A vast inland body of fresh water fed by the Syr Darya and Amu Darya rivers, the Aral Sea was once the fourth largest lake in the world. For centuries the influx of river water was just sufficient to offset water losses from the lake due to high evaporation rates, and the size of the Aral remained relatively stable. However, in the early 1960s decisions made in Moscow led to the rapid expansion of irrigated agriculture throughout the Aral basin in an all-out effort to boost production of the region's "white gold"—cotton. As ever-increasing amounts of water from the Syr Darya, Amu Darya, and their tributaries were diverted to thirsty cotton fields, the amount of inflow available to replace water losses in this naturally arid region steadily declined. By 1989 parts of the sea had become so shallow that its basin divided into two separate parts; by the early 1990s the Aral had lost more than 60% of its former volume and 44% of its surface area.

The Aral's water quality, as well as its quantity, has steadily deteriorated over the past decades. Salt-laden runoff from improperly irrigated farmlands has increased the salinity of the lake to the point where most of its native fish species have disappeared and a once-thriving commercial fishing industry has collapsed. The lake's environment has now been so adversely altered that experts fear the damage may be irreversible. Even if diversions of water for irrigation were drastically reduced to permit flows into the sea to double, the Aral would continue to shrink to one-sixth of its size in 1960 and its salt content would rise to four times that of ocean waters.

Surrounding land areas have suffered as severely as the Aral itself. As the margins of the sea recede, the salt-encrusted exposed sea bottom has provided a seemingly inexhaustible source of toxic sand that is feeding dust storms so large and powerful that they are regularly tracked by Russian cosmonauts in orbit. Some of these storms may deposit their load as far as 1200 miles away, but the greatest amount falls on areas within the Aral basin where up to half a ton per acre of salts and sand poison farmlands—and farmers' lungs—each year.

The moderating effect the Aral has long exerted on regional climate is also diminishing as the sea shrinks ever smaller. Rainfall has become less frequent, temperature extremes more pronounced. The frost-free growing season in parts of the basin has now diminished to less than the minimum 200 days essential for cotton cultivation, threatening the region's economic viability. Irrigation diversions and faulty drainage practices have adversely impacted the Aral watershed far from the sea itself. Wetlands adjacent to the rivers, as well as floodplain forests, have dried up and vanished, as have many of the wildlife species which inhabited them. Salinization of soils, caused by excessive application of water without adequate drainage, has brought dissolved salts to the soil surface and significantly reduced crop yields.

The quality of the water remaining in the rivers has deteriorated to the point that it threatens the well-being of humans as well as wildlife. Run-off of phosphates, nitrates, and ammonia due to heavy fertilizer applications and contamination of drinking water supplies with toxic pesticides, chemical defoliants, and sewage is blamed in part for the scandalously high rates of infant mortality, maternal deaths, psychological disorders, and general poor state of health throughout the region. The incidence of hepatitis and typhoid fever has soared since the late 1970s, and some observers warn that unless immediate steps are taken to halt the use of dangerous pesticides, provide safe drinking water, and reverse the pollution of river water, the region may become uninhabitable.

Can the Aral be saved? In 1988 the USSR's top hydraulic engineer incautiously remarked that "it is time for all the wailing to stop. The case is closed, and the people here will have to learn to live without the sea." Not everyone is willing to surrender without a fight, however. In the late 1980s Uzbek nationalists demanded that certain Siberian rivers flowing into the Arctic Ocean be diverted southward to replenish the dwindling water reserves of the Aral. While such a massive water redistribution scheme was ultimately rejected, there has been growing awareness that a solution to the problems of the Aral basin will require developing new attitudes toward water use and reevaluating economic development policies. The breakup of the former Soviet Union has made implementation of programs to save the Aral even more problematic. The president of Kazakhstan has been especially bitter that the fledgling nations of the region have been left on their own to deal with the environmental deterioration of the Aral basin, while the cotton whose production is largely responsible for the current situation still is shipped to the European part of the former USSR where 10 million jobs are dependent on its use. Early in 1993, leaders of the newly independent republics of Central Asia met in Tashkent where they adopted a resolution to create an international fund to address the problems of the Aral Sea. Whether these struggling young nations are capable of implementing needed programs may determine the very survival of the region's inhabitants.

References

Feshbach, Murray, and Alfred Friendly, Jr. 1992. *Ecocide in the USSR*. Basic Books.

Frederick, Kenneth D. 1991. "The Disappearing Aral Sea." *Resources*, no. 102 (winter).

Kotlyakov, V. M. 1991. "The Aral Sea Basin: A Critical Environmental Zone." *Environment* 33, no. 1 (Jan./Feb.).

in passing, however, that not all aquatic succession results in the establishment of a terrestrial climax community. In cases where the body of water is very large and deep or where there is strong wave action, a stable aquatic community may form and undergo no further change.

Although the later stages of succession are characterized by biotic communities better able to withstand adverse environmental conditions and more stable in terms of species composition and population, humans have generally preferred to utilize the types of communities characterized by the earlier stages of succession. In aquatic ecosystems, for example, the desirable food and game fish such as trout, bass, and perch are all found in the clear, well-oxygenated water of deep, non-eutrophic lakes or in swiftly-flowing streams. The carp that thrive in waters at a more advanced successional stage are less highly regarded. In relation to land communities, the development of agriculture and pastoralism have resulted in humans exerting increasingly effective efforts to maintain succession at an early, simplified stage. By replacing natural biotic communities with large expanses of just a few species of crop plants and through the attempt to eliminate such competitors as insects, rodents, and birds, agricultural humans have further simplified biotic communities, often undermining the stability of ecosystems in the process.

The stresses that humans are today imposing upon natural ecosystems extend far beyond the biological simplification of agricultural communities, however. The toxic pollutants being discharged into the air and water in unprecedented amounts are subjecting biotic communities to pressures with which they are evolutionarily unequipped to cope. Perhaps even more serious, the sheer increase in numbers of humans and their domestic animals is creating physical pressures that in many parts of the world are changing ecosystems in ways which are severely detrimental not only to the biological communities which inhabit them but to human long-term interests as well ■

References

Ashworth, William. 1986. *The Late Great Lakes: An Environmental History.* Alfred A. Knopf.

Odum, Eugene P. 1959. *Fundamentals of Ecology.* W. B. Saunders.

Pianka, Eric R. 1988. *Evolutionary Ecology.* 4th ed. New York: Harper & Row.

Smith, Robert L. 1986. *Elements of Ecology.* 2d ed. New York: Harper & Row.

Stiling, Peter D. 1992. *Introductory Ecology.* Prentice Hall, Inc.

Wilford, John Noble. 1991. "The Gradual Greening of Mt. St. Helens." *New York Times*, Oct. 8, B9.

CHAPTER 2

Population Dynamics

Be fruitful and multiply and fill the earth and subdue it. . . .
—Genesis 1:28

Growth for the sake of growth is the ideology of the cancer cell.
—Edward Abbey

"Standing room only" is a phrase used only half in jest to describe the possible human predicament on this finite planet if present growth rates continue unchecked indefinitely into the future. Population projections for the year A.D. 3000, if growth rates hold steady at their present 1.6%, reveal that total world population at that time would be one billion billion people, a number that would squeeze 1700 humans onto every square yard of the earth's surface, including oceans, deserts, and polar ice caps. Obviously such figures represent an exercise in the absurd. Common sense observation of the world around us reveals that when populations of any organism explode, be they swarms of migratory locusts, tent caterpillars, or lemmings marching toward the sea, something, sooner or later, brings that population back into a state of relative equilibrium with its environment. There is no reason to suppose that humans, any more than locusts, caterpillars, or lemmings, can defy the laws of nature by multiplying indefinitely. Certain ecological principles govern the ways in which populations change in size. The study of such changes, or population dynamics, is of great practical importance to those who wish to predict or control the population size of other organisms or, even more important today, to forecast trends in human population growth and, if possible, guide such growth into ecologically sustainable patterns.

Population Attributes

As we saw in chapter 1, a biotic community is made up of populations of a number of different species that are bound together by an intricate web of relationships, interacting with each other and with the physical environment. Any population, be it leopard frogs in a farm pond, lions on the Serengeti Plain, or humans overcrowding Spaceship Earth, exhibits certain measurable group attributes which are unique to that population. Such group attributes include birth and death rate, age structure, population density, spatial distribution, and so forth. Knowing what these characteristics are for any given population is helpful in predicting how that population will change in response to changes in the environment.

Basically, assessing dynamic changes within a population largely revolves around keeping track of additions to that population from births and immigration and of losses from the same group due to deaths and emigration. Age structure of the population also must be taken into account in those species, such as *Homo sapiens*, where generations tend to overlap.

Limits to Growth

More than one hundred years ago Charles Darwin observed in his *Origin of Species* that all organisms have a tendency to produce many more offspring than will survive to maturity. Indeed, in nature a given population of organisms tends to maintain relatively stable numbers over a long period of time. Although a single oyster may produce up to 100 million eggs at one spawning, an orchid may release a million seeds, or one mushroom may be responsible for hundreds of thousands of fungal spores drifting through the air, nevertheless, the world has not yet been overwhelmed with oysters, orchids, or mushrooms. Even much less prolific species theoretically could give rise to staggering numbers of offspring. Darwin himself cited the example of the slow-breeding elephant (gestation period of 600–630 days), showing that the progeny from a single pair would number 19 million after 750 years, assuming that all survived to reproductive age.

Obviously the increase of populations as described above could only occur in a situation where no forces act to slow the growth rate—a scenario that is virtually nonexistent in the real world, at least for any extended period of time.

The maximum growth rate that a population could achieve in an unlimited environment is referred to as that population's **biotic potential**. In reality, of course, no organism ever reaches its biotic potential because of one or more factors which limit growth. Such limiting factors include food shortages, overcrowding, disease, predation, and accumulation of toxic wastes. Taken together, the environmental pressures that limit a population's inherent capacity for growth are termed **environmental resistance**. Environmental resistance is generally measured as the difference between the biotic potential of a population and the actual rate of increase as observed under laboratory or field conditions (Odum, 1959).

Population Growth Forms

Earlier in this century a number of population biologists were curious to discover what would happen to a population if most of the usual factors of environmental resistance were removed. They devised carefully controlled laboratory experiments to chart growth curves for populations where limitation of resources, predation, parasites, and other factors that normally contribute to high death rates would not come into play. Their findings revealed that populations exhibit characteristic patterns of increase that biologists call **population growth forms**. Experimentation with a wide variety of organisms has revealed two basic patterns, described as the S-curve and the J-curve.

S-Curve

A classic study in population dynamics was carried out by the Russian, G. F. Gause, in 1932 using a population of the protozoan,

Paramecium caudatum. Gause placed one paramecium into an aquarium with a broth of bacterial cells suspended in water to provide a food supply and then carefully observed the subsequent growth of that population. He found that numbers of paramecia increased rather slowly for the first few days, then increased very rapidly for a period; finally the rate of increase began to slow and gradually leveled off as the upper limits of growth were reached and a steady-state equilibrium was achieved. The growth pattern thus revealed is that of an S-curve (sigmoid curve). The upper limit of such a curve, called the **upper asymptote**, indicates that point at which increased mortality has brought birth and death rates into balance once again (in the case of Gause's paramecia, increased mortality was due to overcrowding in the culture and the inability of the constant food supply to support all the organisms). The population density at the upper asymptote thus represents an equilibrium level between the biotic potential of that population and the environmental resistance. Thus the upper asymptote of the S-curve is often referred to as the **carrying capacity** of that environment—the limit at which that environment can support a population.

J-Curve

The sigmoid growth pattern, typical of populations as diverse as microorganisms, plants, and many types of birds and mammals as well, results from the gradually increasing pressures of environmental resistance as the density of population increases. Another type of population growth form, more dramatic because it frequently results in the population "crashes" that attract journalistic attention, can be represented by a J-curve. In this type of situation population growth increases at rapid exponential rates up to or even beyond the carrying capacity of the environment. The environmental resistance becomes effective only at the last moment, so to speak, and as a result populations that have overshot the carrying capacity suffer severe die-backs. This pattern is frequently seen in many natural populations such as lemmings, algal blooms, and certain insects. It should be apparent that the early phases of growth represented by S- and J-curves are identical: a preliminary "lag" phase, during which time the rate of increase is relatively slow, followed by a logarithmic, or exponential, growth phase during which not only do the actual numbers grow rapidly, but the rate of increase also increases (in the manner of compound interest). Thus, a J-curve basically can be considered an incomplete S-curve since the sudden imposition of limiting effects halts growth before the self-limiting effects within a population become apparent.

Homeostatic Controls

Food shortage, excess predation, and disease are not the only factors which can cause populations to decline. Extensive research has shown that

Figure 2-1

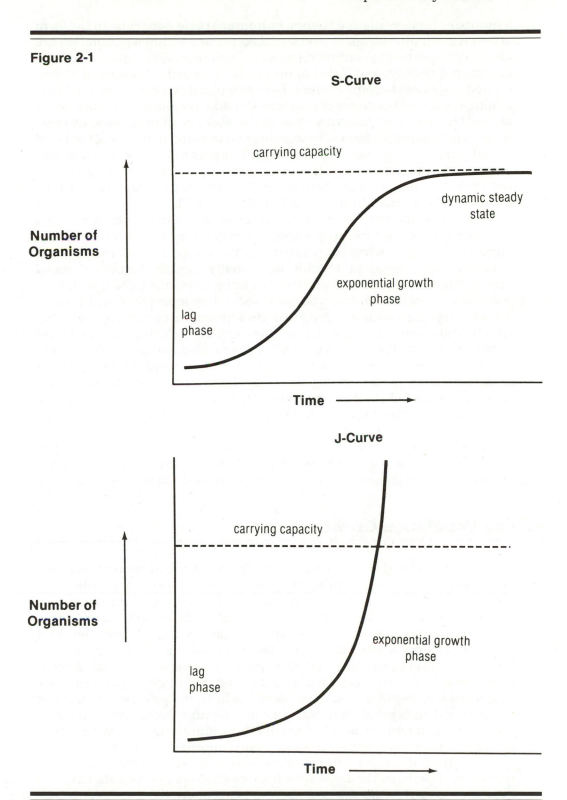

a number of self-regulating factors, or **homeostatic controls**, in the form of behavioral, physiological, and social responses within a population are also very important in controlling its size. Each population appears to have an optimal density, and if this optimum is exceeded a number of stress-related responses become evident. For example, it has been observed that among the snowshoe hares of northern Canada, population crashes occur at regular 9–10 year intervals even in the absence of predators, disease, or human hunting pressures. Researchers have found that during the rapid die-off phase of these oscillations, large numbers of hares suffer a stress-induced degeneration of their livers, resulting in inadequate glycogen reserves. The animals may then exhibit "shock disease," lapsing into convulsions, coma, and ultimately death (Farb, 1963).

Classic studies on the effects of overcrowding in rats have shown that even when abundant food is present, self-regulating mechanisms induce population crashes when rat populations exceed a certain density. When crowded, rats begin to exhibit abnormally hostile behavior; social interactions become pathological and fighting intensifies, often with fatal results to one of the combatants. Some individual males become hyperactive and hypersexual, attempting to mate without the customary courtship rituals and often mounting males, nonreceptive females, and juveniles indiscriminately. Pregnant females under crowded conditions frequently abort; if the young are born alive they are frequently killed by the mother or die as a consequence of neglect. It has been suggested that the cause of such deviant behavior can be traced to the effects of crowding-induced stress on the functioning of the endocrine system, which regulates hormone levels in animals. Whether the rats' response to crowding is indicative of what we can expect among human populations as our species continues to increase is open to question, but there are those who point to rising levels of violence and aggression in many parts of the world as ominous portents.

Human Population Growth

Insights gained from laboratory studies of microbial populations have an importance far transcending mere academic interest. The exponential curves tracking the growth of paramecia in biologists' aquaria or of migratory locusts in the Sahel have a parallel in the growth patterns that typify many human societies today. The fact is that during the 20th century—and particularly during the last 50 years—the human species has been experiencing an unprecedented population explosion, with growth rates resembling those depicted on a J-curve. Although the average *rate* of growth has begun to decrease slightly within the past two decades or so (perhaps indicating that humans are S-curve rather than J-curve organisms?), in terms of absolute numbers the annual increment continues to grow inexorably year after year. Many informed observers strongly contend that the most critical environmental issue facing humanity today—and perhaps the most difficult to tackle—is overpopulation. The explosive growth of the human species is arguably the most significant development of the past million years. No other event, geological or biological, has posed a threat to earthly life comparable to that of human overpopulation. We have little hope of significantly reducing other types of environmental degradation if present rates of population increase are not reversed.

Until very recently, people who warned of an impending population-resource crunch or advocated even the mildest measures to restrain birth rates were either ridiculed, castigated, or ignored. One of the earliest to voice alarm as human numbers began their dramatic climb was British clergyman-economist Thomas Malthus who, almost two hundred years ago, argued that the rapid population growth his country was then experiencing was a prelude to mass misery. Demonstrating that population grows geometrically (2, 4, 8, 16, 32) while agricultural production increases only arithmetically (1, 2, 3, 4, 5), Malthus contended that population would always tend to outpace additions to the food supply, thereby condemning the bulk of humanity to a marginal standard of living and frequent bouts of famine, war, and disease. Although Malthus' "dismal theorem" stimulated a great deal of discussion at the time, his views were soon discounted when improvements in British agricultural technology and the opening of the American prairies to grain production resulted in food supply increases far exceeding the number of new mouths to be fed. As a result, Malthus' warnings were largely dismissed and forgotten. The prevailing attitude throughout the 19th century and well into the 20th viewed population growth as a desirable phenomenon, enhancing a nation's productivity, wealth, and power—an opinion still held in some quarters (see Box 2-1). Indeed, as late as the 1930s, the main population concern in the United States was that the temporary dip in the American birth rate experienced during the Depression years might indicate a worrisome *shrinking* of United States population size!

BOX 2-1

Population Growth: Boon or Bane?

The debate has been raging ever since Thomas Malthus penned his 1798 polemic, *Essay on the Principle of Population* (see text). Malthus' pessimistic outlook was sharply at odds with the views of many of his contemporaries who espoused the perfectibility of society and the desirability of a steadily growing population. His thesis provoked a heated rebuttal by a number of 19th century reformers and socialists—among them Karl Marx—who derided the *Essay* as a "libel on the human race" and blamed capital-

ism, not overpopulation, for the world's woes. Across the Atlantic, American land reformer Henry George also took issue with Malthus' contention that population growth could pose problems. Quite the contrary, George argued, the U.S. experience with mass immigration proved that a large increase in population enhances overall prosperity; the true cause of poverty is not overpopulation, declared George, but social injustice and war. Poverty causes overpopulation, not vice-versa. While socialists attacked Malthusian doctrine from the left, conservatives of the far right were equally hostile. Population growth, in their opinion, created wealth—"The increase of man results in the increase of his food."

The intensity of the population debate waned as mid-19th century improvements in agricultural technology boosted harvests and temporarily discredited Malthus' ideas. Not until the "population explosion" of the post-World War II years sent growth rates soaring were the old arguments revived. So-called "neo-Malthusians" insisted that Malthus was right all along—a prophet ahead of his times. Paul Ehrlich, one of the most persuasive proponents of the neo-Malthusian message, set the stage for the modern debate with his 1967 best-seller, *The Population Bomb*. Contending that overpopulation is the single most serious threat to the continued habitability of the planet, Ehrlich argued for urgent action to slow growth rates, proclaiming that "Whatever your cause, it's a lost cause without population control." Publication in 1972 of the Club of Rome study, *Limits to Growth*, reinforced the neo-Malthusian arguments, utilizing simple computer models to predict a population crash early in the next century due to human numbers overshooting the earth's long-term carrying capacity. The counterattack to these gloom-and-doom pronouncements was not long in coming. From the left, writers like Frances Moore Lappe (of *Diet for a Small Planet* fame) argued that overpopulation is not the *cause* of environmental degradation, but rather a symptom of other, more profound problems such as poverty, brought about by exploitation and inequality. Social justice, not birth control, was the answer to relieving human misery. Others, most notably biologist Barry Commoner, contended that the prime villain responsible for our environmental dilemmas is modern technology run amok, churning out ever-increasing volumes of nondegradable waste by-products which are overwhelming and poisoning the natural world. To these critics on the left, high rates of population growth may be unfortunate, but they aren't the major cause of environmental degradation as the neo-Malthusians insist. "Hogwash!" reply groups to the right of the political spectrum. These so-called "Cornucopians" not only deny that population growth is our number one environmental problem—they deny that it's a problem at all. In fact, Cornucopians such as economist Julian Simon passionately argue that continued population growth is both desirable and beneficial. Contending that throughout history standards of living have risen as population size increased, Simon asserts that people are *The Ultimate Resource*, as the title of his book on the subject proclaims. The more people born into the world, the more brains there will be to solve the problems humanity creates. Growing populations may provoke temporary resource shortages, but human inventiveness will quickly rise to meet the challenge, devising better and cheaper substitutes for the original—no need to worry in this best of all possible worlds!

So who's right? Should efforts to halt or reverse population growth be a top priority for preventing environmental calamity or is the issue of minor importance? Surprisingly, while an extensive amount of research has been done on the *causes* of population growth, very little work has focused on the environmental *consequences* of escalating human numbers. Opinions are plentiful and fiercely defended, but hard data is largely lacking. Paul Harrison, in his 1992 book, *The Third Revolution*, contends that all parties engaged in the population debate are right—to a point—but all oversimplify the issues. For example, Harrison points out, the Cornucopians are correct in their assertion that pressures generated by growing populations are a major force propelling social and technological change. Similarly, problems of scarcity or pollution, once they're perceived as sufficiently serious, are usually tackled and resolved. Where the Cornucopians err, says Harrison, is in their *complacency*—their assumption that necessary adjustments will always be made in time. To the contrary, such is the momentum of current rates of increase that very severe damage—sometimes *irreversible* damage—may be done before the problem is resolved or even recognized. Cornucopians also overlook the fact that, in some cases, existing social or political realities render the necessary adaptations impossible. Likewise, those who contend, like Commoner, that modern technology is the cause of many environmental problems can accurately bolster their argument by pointing to situations like the CFC-provoked depletion of the ozone layer, radioactive fallout from weapons testing, or pesticide contamination of well water. Population growth had little or nothing to do with such problems. On the other hand, they overlook the fact that modern technology often has a beneficial environmental impact in reversing damage caused by human activities: witness the catalytic converter that has significantly lowered levels of automotive pollutants in urban air. Neo-Malthusians are quite correct in pointing out that population growth *does* have a significant impact on many types of environmental destruction—tropical deforestation, species loss, and CO_2 emissions are obvious examples—but consumption levels and technology are pivotal determinants also. The fact that the 16% of humanity living in rich nations amass 73% of the world's Gross Domestic Product, consume the bulk of the planet's nonrenewable resources, and generate more than 90% of its industrial waste means that every baby born into a low-growth affluent country like Japan or Switzerland has a far greater environmental impact today in terms of pollution and resource depletion than a baby born to peasant farmers in densely populated Bangladesh. Affluence = excessive consumption = environmental impact. The prospects for pollution in a world where rising incomes would permit every family in China and India to possess a refrigerator and a car are frightening to contemplate.

Reversing environmental degradation, argues Harrison, will require a strategy that tackles all the interrelated elements of the problem simultaneously. Overconsumption in the rich nations of the North must be reduced, more environmentally benign technologies adopted, *and* a stabilization of world population size must be vigorously pursued if humanity is to achieve a sustainable balance with the natural environment. The times demand a holistic view of the world and across-the-board changes to counter the pace of environmental degradation, for such is the current momentum of growth that the decade of the 1990s may be humanity's last chance for effective action.

Reference

Harrison, Paul. 1992. *The Third Revolution: Environment, Population, and a Sustainable World*. I. B. Tauris & Co., Ltd.

However, after World War II, and especially since the 1960s, concerns that population growth rates were excessive began to be expressed, first by a handful of far-sighted individuals and private organizations, later by national governments and international agencies. Such concern was precipitated by the awareness that intensive efforts to improve living standards and ensure national stability in the newly independent developing nations were largely being nullified by the rapid population growth they were experiencing. Today the vast majority of Third World governments regard their rate of population increase as too high and have adopted policies aimed at stabilizing numbers as quickly as possible. Unfortunately, such efforts should have been launched decades earlier; the momentum of growth is now so enormous and the existing population base so large, that the ability of some countries to curb growth before national carrying capacity is surpassed is very much in doubt. In order to understand why the seriousness of our current population crisis was recognized so belatedly and why there's such a sense of urgency now, we need to look at some demographic facts.

Historical Trends in Human Population Growth

Assuming that the first humans appeared on earth between 1.5 million and 600,000 years ago, we can estimate that somewhere between 60 and 100 billion people have inhabited the planet at some time. Today the earth supports about 5.6 billion human inhabitants—close to 5% of all who have ever lived. We don't have enough information to estimate accurately what populations were before A.D. 1650, but we can make some educated guesses based on circumstantial evidence (e.g. number of people who could be supported on X square miles by hunting and gathering, by primitive agriculture, and so on). On this basis, it's been calculated that the total human population at 8000 B.C. was about five million people. By the beginning of the Christian Era, when agricultural settlements had become widespread, world population is estimated to have risen to about 200–300 million, and increased to about 500 million by 1650. It then doubled to one billion by 1850, to two billion by 1930, and to four billion by 1975; by the late 1980s, world population passed the five billion mark and continues to climb. Thus not only has world population been increasing steadily (with minor irregularities) for the past million years, but the rate of growth has also increased.

Doubling Time

Perhaps the best way to describe growth rate is in terms of **doubling time**—the time required for a population to double in size. During the period from 8000 B.C. to A.D. 1650, the population doubled about every 1500 years. The next doubling took 200 years, the next 80 years, and the next, 45 years.

Historical evidence indicates that the increase in human numbers did not occur at a steady, even pace but rather that three main surges occurred.

Figure 2-2 Trends and Projections in World Population Growth, 1750–2050

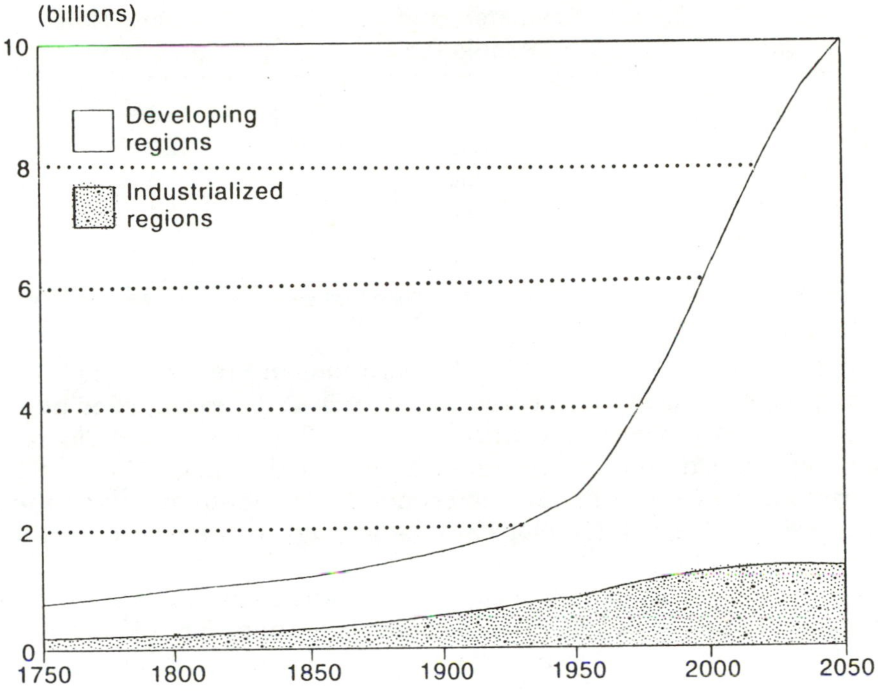

(billions)

Source: World Resources Institute, based on data from United Nations Population Division, *Long-range World Population Projections: Two Centuries of World Population Growth, 1950–2150* (1992).

The first took place about 600,000 years ago with the evolution of culture (developing and learning techniques of social organization and group and individual survival); the next occurred about 8000 B.C. with the agricultural revolution; and the most recent began about 200 years ago with the onset of the industrial-medical-scientific revolution (Ehrlich, Ehrlich, and Holdren, 1977). Bearing in mind that changes in the size of populations occur when birth and death rates are out of balance, one can reasonably conclude that each of these spurts indicates that the story of human population growth is not primarily a story of changes in birth rates, but of changes in death rates. Let's now take a closer look at some of the demographic facts that help to explain our current population dilemma.

Birth Rates, Death Rates, and Fertility Rates

Birth rates are generally expressed as the number of babies born per 1000 people per year. Prior to the Industrial Revolution, birth rates in every

Figure 2-3 Doubling Time of World Population

Date	Estimated Human Population	Doubling Time (in years)
8000 B.C.	5 million	1500
A.D. 1650	500 million	200
A.D. 1850	1 billion	80
A.D. 1930	2 billion	45
1975	4 billion	36

society typically were in the 40–50 per thousand range. Today the birth rate gap between nations has widened dramatically, exemplified by Spain's 10, the world's lowest, and with a high of 53 in the West African nation of Niger. Indeed, in recent years a nation's birth rate can be looked at as a crude barometer of its level of economic development, since the most prosperous, most technologically advanced countries generally are characterized by low birth rates.

Death rates are calculated in the same way as birth rates, representing the annual number of deaths per 1000 population. Birth and death rates are frequently referred to as "crude" rates because they don't reflect the wide variations in age distribution within a population—a fact that might result in misleading conclusions when comparing statistics from different countries. For example, the fact that Jordan has a death rate of 5 per thousand population while the death rate in Germany is 11 might lead one to assume that Jordanians enjoy better health care and a higher standard of living than do Germans. Such an assumption would be erroneous, however, since the reason for Jordan's apparent advantage is that nearly half the Jordanian population (41%) is under the age of 15—an age cohort everywhere typified by a low likelihood of death. Germany, on the other hand, is characterized by an aging population; only 16% of Germans are under 15, while 15% are over age 65 (compared to just 3% in Jordan). Even with excellent medical care, death rates are bound to be higher in a predominantly middle-aged to elderly population than in one primarily composed of the very young.

Total fertility rates (TFR), representing the average number of children each woman within a given population is likely to bear during her reproductive lifetime (assuming that current age-specific birth rates remain constant), perhaps give a clearer picture of reproductive behavior than do crude birth rates. Although *world* TFR has been gradually falling in recent decades to its present level of 3.2, the wide discrepancies in national fertility rates are illustrated by countries such as Yemen whose TFR of 7.6 is currently the world's highest, and by Hong Kong, whose TFR of 1.2 suggests a preference for one-child families on that crowded island (Population Reference Bureau, 1994).

BOX 2-2
Will AIDS Defuse the Population Bomb?

Current statistics are horrifying enough: by 1994 approximately 17 million people worldwide had been infected with the human immuno-deficiency virus (HIV); over 3 million had developed full-blown AIDS, and of these 2.5 million had already died. Nevertheless, public health officials fear that the grim toll exacted since HIV/AIDS was first described in 1981 represents but the "tip of the iceberg" in terms of future disease and death. In spite of extensive public information efforts and millions of dollars poured into medical research, the epidemic shows no signs of abating. To the contrary, HIV/AIDS has become a **pandemic**—global in scope—affecting virtually every country in the world. In regions such as central Africa, the Caribbean, and North America where the disease has been well-established since the early 1980s, the infection continues to expand and intensify; in areas previously spared, HIV/AIDS is now spreading rapidly. In Africa, rural hinterlands where the majority of the population lives are now experiencing rates of HIV infection nearly as high as those characterizing urban centers for more than a decade. HIV/AIDS is pro-liferating in eastern Europe and has been reported from areas as far-flung as Greenland and tiny island nations in the Pacific. No place, apparently, is remote enough to escape the on-slaught. Particularly threatened are the nations of southern and southeast Asia, especially India, Burma, and Thailand, where more than a million people are estimated to have become infected within the last few years. Health officials predict that in the decades ahead there will be more AIDS cases in this region than anywhere else in the world.

Just as the geography of HIV/AIDS is expanding, the sociology of the pandemic is volatile and dynamic as well. Population subgroups formerly thought to be at low risk of infection are now experiencing an alarming increase in disease rates. Once confined pri-marily to homosexual men and intra-venous drug abusers, HIV/AIDS prevalence is rising dramatically among women and infants as hetero-sexual contact becomes the main route of transmission in many countries.

These realities lead many re-searchers to conclude that the present AIDS drama is but the preview of a much greater tragedy yet to be played out. Some health experts anticipate that by the year 2000, as many as 110 million people worldwide will be HIV-positive and nearly 25 million will have developed AIDS. Significantly, the overwhelming majority of victims will live in the densely populated nations of the Third World: 42% in Asia and Oceania, 31% in sub-Saharan Africa, 14% in Latin America and the Caribbean. In the context of such an exponential rate of increase in the incidence of an inevitably fatal disease, it seems logical to question whether AIDS may serve as an example of one of those forces of environmental resistance acting to bring a halt to population growth.

In regions such as North America and western Europe where the chief means of HIV transmission to date has been homosexual contact, AIDS will have some impact on adult male death rates, but little overall influence on population growth. However, in regions such as Africa, the Caribbean, and southern Asia where heterosexual relations constitute the major route by which the infection is spread, AIDS' demographic implications are a subject of considerable speculation. The question looms largest in terms of AIDS' impact on Africa's population explosion, since it is in this region where HIV infection rates are currently among the highest in the world—up to 30% of young adults in some urban areas. If women of childbearing age sicken and die while still relatively young, total fertility rates obviously will be lower than they would have been in the absence of AIDS. Similarly, if child mortality rates rise because pregnant HIV-positive mothers are infecting their unborn babies, overall growth rates will be affected.

Whether AIDS-influenced declines in growth rates will be large enough to cause an actual decrease in population size—or even a leveling off—in rapidly growing African countries is doubtful, however. Data from Uganda and Malawi, where AIDS cases have been soaring in recent years, yield no evidence that the disease is having any noticeable influence yet on high fertility rates. This situation can be explained, at least in part, by the fact that death due to AIDS generally doesn't occur until 8–10 years after infection with HIV. If a woman acquired her infection soon after becoming sexually active in her late teens or early twenties, she could still live long enough to bear a number of children before dying. Thus,

while AIDS may reduce fertility to some extent (i.e. AIDS may prevent the additional births which would have occurred were the woman to live a normal lifespan), researchers predict that the impact of such a decline will simply be to lower the present 3% African population growth rate to somewhere between 1–2% annually early in the next century—a rate that still represents relatively rapid growth. A few observers have even suggested that Africa's AIDS epidemic might actually lead to *higher* fertility if it encourages women to marry at an earlier age when the likelihood of HIV infection presumably is less (in general, the younger a woman is at the time of marriage, the more children she is likely to bear during her lifetime). While much remains to be learned about the association between HIV/AIDS and fertility, there seems to be a general consensus among demographers that in spite of the human tragedy that the disease represents for the foreseeable future, African populations will continue to grow—not quite as rapidly as they would in the absence of AIDS, but grow nevertheless.

Reference

Mann, Jonathan, Daniel J. M. Tarantola, and Thomas W. Netter, eds. 1992. *A Global Report: Aids in the World.* The Global AIDS Policy Coalition, Harvard University Press.

Growth Rates

Since birth rates represent additions to a population and death rates represent subtractions, a change in population size is represented by the difference between the two, i.e. by the **growth rate** (sometimes called the **rate of natural increase**). Growth rates, which do not take migration into account, can be calculated quite simply by subtracting the death rate from the birth rate. Take the case of Iran, for example: with a 1994 birth rate of 44 and a death rate of 9, the growth rate of Iran's population will be 44

Figure 2-4 1994 Population Data for Selected Countries

Region or Country	Population (millions)	Birth Rate	Death Rate	Growth Rate	Doubling Time-yrs.
WORLD	5,607	25	9	1.6	43
AFRICA	700	42	13	2.9	24
Egypt	58.9	30	8	2.3	31
Ethiopia	55.2	46	15	3.1	22
Ghana	16.9	42	12	3.0	23
Nigeria	98.1	44	13	3.1	23
South Africa	41.2	34	8	2.6	26
Uganda	19.8	51	21	3.0	23
Zaire	42.5	48	15	3.3	21
ASIA	3,392	25	8	1.7	41
Bangladesh	116.6	37	13	2.4	29
China	1,192.0	18	7	1.1	61
India	911.6	29	10	1.9	36
Iraq	19.9	45	8	3.7	19
Japan	125.0	10	7	0.3	267
Philippines	68.7	30	7	2.4	29
Thailand	59.4	20	6	1.4	50
Turkey	61.8	29	7	2.2	32
Vietnam	73.1	30	7	2.3	30
LATIN AMERICA	470	27	7	2.0	35
Argentina	33.9	21	8	1.3	53
Brazil	155.3	25	8	1.7	40
Colombia	35.6	25	5	2.0	35
Cuba	11.1	15	7	0.8	91
Mexico	91.8	28	6	2.2	31
Nicaragua	4.3	37	7	2.9	24
Peru	22.9	28	8	2.0	34
Venezuela	21.3	30	5	2.6	27
NORTH AMERICA	290	16	9	0.7	98
Canada	29.1	14	7	0.7	98
United States	260.8	16	9	0.7	98
EUROPE	728	12	11	0.1	1,025
France	58.0	13	9	0.4	182
Germany	81.2	10	11	-0.1	—
Hungary	10.3	11	14	-0.3	—
Italy	57.2	10	10	0.0	2,310
Poland	38.6	13	10	0.3	257
Russia	147.8	11	12	-0.2	—
Spain	39.2	10	9	0.1	630
Sweden	8.8	14	11	0.3	255
United Kingdom	58.4	13	11	0.2	281

Source: Population Reference Bureau, 1994 World Population Data Sheet

minus 9 or 35 per 1000 population. However, because growth rate is expressed as a percentage (i.e. per 100), not per 1000 as in birth and death rates, Iran has a growth rate of 3.5% annually.

Growth rate is the critical factor to look at to get a quick impression of what is happening to a particular population. It is entirely possible that a country could have a traditionally high birth rate and still have a relatively low growth rate if the death rate is high also. In fact, just such a situation was characteristic of most human societies until only a few hundred years ago.

BOX 2-3

Riddle of the Magic Lily Pond

In his book, *The Twenty-Ninth Day,* Lester Brown recounts a simple yet vivid illustration of the doubling time concept, one which very effectively dramatizes how quickly a given scenario can shift from a condition of abundance to one of scarcity when growth rates are increasing exponentially.

Recalling a French childhood riddle, Brown describes a mythical lily pond containing but one lily pad. Each day, however, the number of leaves doubles, so that on the second day there are two lily pads, on the third day four, on the fourth day eight, and so on. The question posed is: If the lily pond is completely full on the 30th day, when is it half-full? The answer, of course: the 29th day.

The relevance of this riddle to the present world situation is that in terms of the earth's carrying capacity, many authorities consider our global lily pond to be half full already. The implications for tomorrow should be clear.

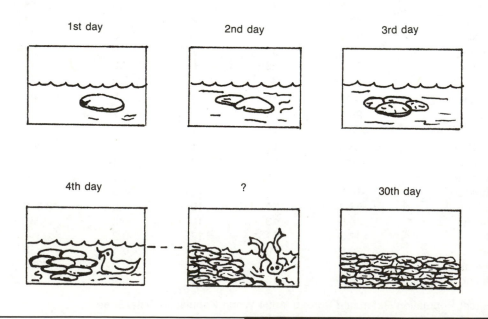

1st day   2nd day   3rd day

4th day   ?   30th day

When the average person hears that Iran has a population growth rate of 3.5% (or that Syria's numbers are increasing by 3.7% annually, or Sudan's by 3.1%), the number in question may fail to make an appropriate impact, since most of us find it difficult to conceptualize what a 3.5% growth rate means in human terms. Besides, 3.5% really doesn't sound like very much! However, when expressed in terms of doubling time, the importance of growth rates takes on a new perspective. By calculating the annual growth rate of a population and then referring to a conversion table, we can learn what the doubling time of that population will be:

GROWTH RATE	DOUBLING TIME
0.5%	140 years
0.8%	87 years
1.0%	70 years
2.0%	35 years
3.0%	24 years
4.0%	17 years

Thus, with an annual growth rate of 3.5%, the population of Iran will double in just 20 years. In human terms this means that *just to maintain present standards of living* (which for the bulk of the population are none too high, though better than those of many other developing countries), *everything* in Iran needs to be doubled in 20 years—food production, provision of jobs, educational facilities, medical personnel, public services, and so forth. Whether such a herculean task can be accomplished remains

Figure 2-5 World Population Growth: Rates and Numbers Tell a Different Story

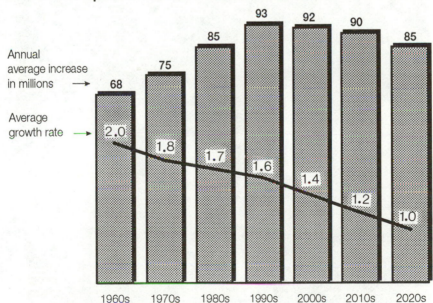

Source: Population Reference Bureau, based on United Nations data.

to be seen; certainly the leaders of Iran (and of a great many other nations whose doubling times are similarly brief) face a formidable challenge in the decades ahead, especially at a time when the "revolution of rising expectations" has created a grassroots demand for improved living standards, not just maintenance of the status quo.

Population Explosion

With a basic understanding of what birth, death, and growth rates imply, let us now turn our attention to the crucial question of why growth rates have so accelerated during the past several generations. Surveying the history of human population growth (an admittedly risky enterprise, particularly for the prehistoric period), we can say with a fair degree of certainty that birth rates throughout the world were uniformly high until relatively modern times. (Recently some anthropologists doing research among contemporary hunter-gatherer societies have forwarded the idea that, prior to the agricultural revolution, birth rates among primitive peoples were lower than among subsequent agricultural societies. This they attribute to environmental restraints causing such groups to attempt to space the births of their children). That women in many societies continue to bear children at traditionally high levels can be readily perceived by glancing at the current birth rates of most of the nations of Africa and many in Asia and Latin America as well.

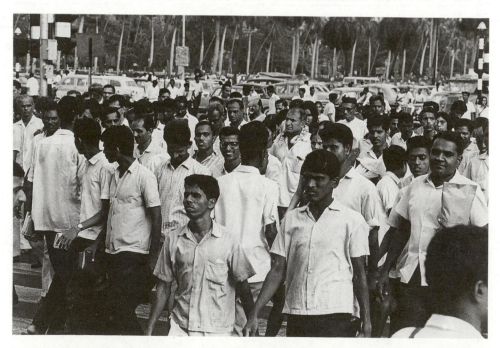

India's population crisis is fueled by a growth rate that could lead to a doubling of its current size in just 36 years. [Agency for International Development]

With birth rates having apparently held steady during most of human history, we must look then to changes in death rates to explain why growth rates have shot upwards. Each of the three major changes in human life-style mentioned earlier effected a decline in the death rate. Cultural advances among prehistoric humans probably reduced the death rate to some slight degree, but the consequences of this cultural evolution were minor compared with the changes wrought by the agricultural revolution. The increase in food supply, the more settled mode of existence, and the general rise in living standards are thought to have reduced mortality rates and increased life expectancy to some degree over that of primitive peoples.

Even so, the gains were gradual until about 200–300 years ago when improvements in public sanitation, advances in agriculture, and the control of infectious disease resulted in a precipitous decline in death rates, particularly in regard to infant and child mortality.

The growth in human numbers that resulted from these improved conditions was not, of course, a steady, uninterrupted rise. Wars, famine, and disease provoked periods of sharp population declines among localized groups. Certainly the most spectacular reversal of the overall growth trend was the impact of bubonic plague (the notorious "Black Death" of the Middle Ages) on the societies of Europe. Plague first reached the Continent in A.D. 1348 and within two years had killed approximately 25% of the total population. Successive outbreaks of the disease continued to sweep across Europe during the next several decades, during which time the population of England dropped by nearly one-half (two-thirds of the student body at Oxford University died during one episode of plague), and many regions in both Europe and Asia were similarly decimated. Nearly constant warfare and the disease and famine that frequently accompanied such conflict also had a negative influence on population growth. Particularly devastating in terms of civilian suffering was the Thirty Years' War (1618–1648), during which time it is estimated that as many as one-third of the inhabitants of Germany and Bohemia died as a direct result of the war. Outside of Europe, warfare, even prior to the World Wars of the 20th century, resulted in enormous loss of life. Conquest and subjugation of Native American civilizations by European colonizers, tribal warfare in Africa, the Moghul invasion of Hindu India, and centuries of internal strife in China resulted in high death rates and sometimes severe depopulation within the affected groups. Perhaps the most extreme example of a population being decimated by warfare involves the most bloody, savage war ever fought in South America. This five-year conflict, which ended in 1870, pitted the combined forces of Brazil, Uruguay, and Argentina against those of Paraguay. The result was virtual extinction for the Paraguayans, whose army was outnumbered 10 to 1 and included 12-year-old boys fighting alongside their grandfathers. Within a five-year period, the population of Paraguay dropped from an estimated 525,000 to 221,000, of whom slightly less than 29,000 were men. A new generation of Paraguayans was sired courtesy of the Brazilian army of occupation (Herring, 1960).

Such examples, while tragic in terms of individual suffering, and occasionally disastrous to certain ethnic groups or nationalities (e.g. the total extermination of native Tasmanians by white settlers), nevertheless represented only minor aberrations from the general upward trend. In general, world population has increased more or less steadily, at first quite slowly but subsequently faster and faster from ancient times right up to the present.

Demographic Transition

By the latter half of the 19th century, Western Europe began to witness a demographic phenomenon unlike any that had occurred previously anywhere in the world. Toward the end of the 1700s and early in the 1800s, as the Industrial Revolution began transforming an entire way of life, death rates started to fall gradually in response to a more adequate food supply, improved medical knowledge, better public sanitation, and so forth. As a result, growth rates predictably accelerated, and during the early years of the 19th century Western Europe experienced a population boom. This led, among other things, to massive emigration to the Western Hemisphere. By approximately 1850 another rather surprising trend became apparent—throughout the industrializing nations of that era, birth rates began to fall for the first time since the agricultural revolution. The Scandinavian countries (which were among the first to compile accurate demographic records) provide a good example of the changes that were occurring. In Denmark, Norway, and Sweden the combined birth rate was about 32 in 1850; by 1900 it had dropped to 28 and today stands at 14, among the lowest in the world. Elsewhere in Western Europe similar declines were becoming apparent. This phenomenon—the falling of both birth and death rates that has characteristically followed industrialization—marked the onset of the **demographic transition**, a trend that has carried on and accelerated into the 20th century. By the 1930s, decreases in the birth rates in some countries had outpaced decreases in death rates, though actual birth rates remained somewhat higher than death rates. Reasons for the demographic transition are still being debated, but the cause for declining birth rates probably centers on the realization by married couples that in an industrial society children are an economic liability; they are expensive to feed, clothe, and educate; they reduce family mobility and make capital accumulation more difficult. In rural areas of Europe, population pressures on a finite amount of land and the modernization and mechanization of farming techniques, which reduced the amount of manual labor needed, combined to bring about a reduction in rural birth rates also. In addition, during the late 1800s and into the 20th century, a trend toward marrying at a later age undoubtedly contributed to the decreasing birth rates.

The decline in both birth and death rates that marked the demographic transition in Western Europe became noticeable in both Eastern Europe and North America several decades later. Although birth rates in the latter have still not fallen as low as those in the nations where the demographic transition began, the trends are quite clearly in the same direction.

Incomplete Demographic Transition

In the nations of Asia, Africa, and Latin America where traditional societies were only marginally influenced by the dynamic economic and social changes occurring in Europe and North America, demographic patterns changed very little until early in the present century. In the areas under the control of imperial powers, improvements in public sanitation and an imposed peace between formerly warring factions within the subject nations permitted a gradual increase in population levels. This gradual decline in death rates in the underdeveloped countries took a quantum leap in the years immediately following World War II as modern drugs and public health measures were exported from the industrialized nations to the Third World countries. Virtually overnight, the widely applauded introduction of "death control" into traditional cultures produced the most rapid, widespread change known in the history of population dynamics. The situation in Sri Lanka (formerly Ceylon) is a good case in point.

Prior to World War II, a major killer in many tropical countries was the mosquito-borne parasitic disease, malaria. In Sri Lanka a malaria epidemic during 1934–1935 may have been responsible for half the deaths occurring in the country that year (Sri Lanka had a death rate of 34 during that time period). Not only did many victims die outright, but many others were so debilitated by their bouts with the recurring cycles of chills and fever that they became more susceptible to other illnesses. Thus malaria was a contributory cause of death in some cases and a primary cause in others. In 1945, at the end of the Second World War, the death rate in Sri Lanka stood at 22. One of the great technological innovations to rise out of the global conflict was introduced into Sri Lanka—the synthetic chemical insecticide DDT. Widescale spraying with DDT brought rapid control over the mosquitoes, with a corresponding plunge in the incidence of malaria. As a result, the death rate on the island was cut by more than half within a decade and has continued to drop since then to its present low of 6. As a consequence, the number of Sri Lankans has soared upwards.

Victory over malaria, yellow fever, smallpox, cholera, and other infectious diseases has been responsible for similar decreases in death rates throughout most of the underdeveloped world. This trend has been most pronounced among children and young adults. Since 1960, according to a World Bank report, the number of children who die before reaching their fifth birthday has declined by two-thirds, thanks to greater public access to standard immunizations and oral rehydration therapy for treating diarrheal diseases (Altman, 1993).

A typical example is Tunisia, where the child mortality rate (deaths of children under age five per thousand live births) plummeted from 210 to 99 in the brief five-year period between 1965–1970. The child mortality rate in Tunisia has continued to drop, albeit not quite so dramatically as during the 1960s, and now stands at 43, one-fifth the level of just a generation ago. Not surprisingly, the population size of Tunisia doubled between 1960 and 1990 (Kennedy, 1993).

This decline in death rates is different in kind from the long-term slow decline that occurred throughout most of the world following the agricultural revolution. It is also different in kind from the comparatively more rapid decline in death rates in the Western world over the past century. The difference is that it is a response to a spectacular environmental change in the underdeveloped countries largely through control of infectious diseases, not a fundamental change in their institutions or general way of life. Furthermore, the change did not originate within these countries, but was brought about from the outside. The factors that led to a demographic transition in the West were not and are not present in the underdeveloped nations. Instead, a large proportion of the world's people have moved rapidly from a situation of high birth and death rates to one of high birth and low death rates, a situation referred to as an **incomplete demographic transition**. This, in essence, is the cause of what biologist Paul Ehrlich refers to as the "population bomb."

Thus have we arrived at the present situation where the bulk of world population growth is occurring in Third World countries that are already finding it difficult to support their existing populations.

Until recently, demographers assumed that societies currently experiencing rapid rates of population increase would, like Europe and North America, witness a significant decline in birth rates as rising incomes and better living conditions resulted in a general desire for smaller families. However, after nearly 40 years of explosive population growth, many Third World nations appear to be trapped in the mid-stage of their demographic transition, unable to attain the social and economic progress essential to reducing birth rates. The world is today witnessing a sharp demographic polarization between nations where population growth is slow (1.0% or less) and living standards are improving, and countries where rapid population growth rates (2.2% or higher) continue to prevail and living conditions are deteriorating. The demographic middle ground has all but vanished, with slightly less than half the world's people living in low-growth regions, the remainder in rapid-growth areas. The concern among population experts, who agree that an incomplete demographic transition cannot continue indefinitely, is that the pressure of human numbers is overwhelming the natural life-support systems in high-growth countries. As demands for food, water, fuel, and living space continue to escalate, the resource base itself is being consumed. The decline in incomes and living standards anticipated as a consequence of exceeding the local environment's carrying capacity may well trigger a rise in death rates and thrust such nations backward into the high birth/high death rate situation characteristic of the pre-demographic transition era.

Age Structure

It's relatively easy to comprehend the significance of birth and death rates so far as population growth is concerned, but there are other characteristics of a population that are important also.

Age structure refers to the number of people in different age categories within a given population. In countries where populations are growing rapidly because of high birth rates and declining death rates, a large

Figure 2-6

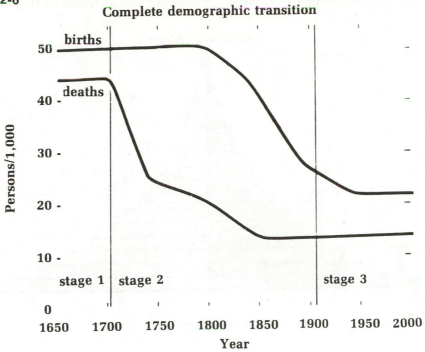

Complete demographic transition

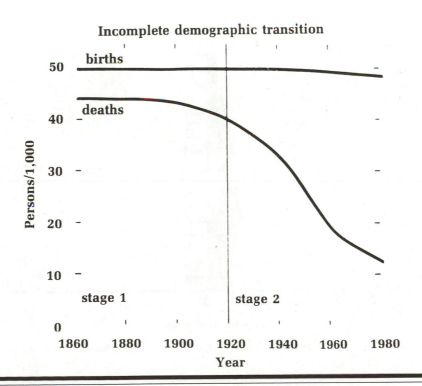

Incomplete demographic transition

Figure 2-7 Age Structure Pyramids of Developing and Developed Regions

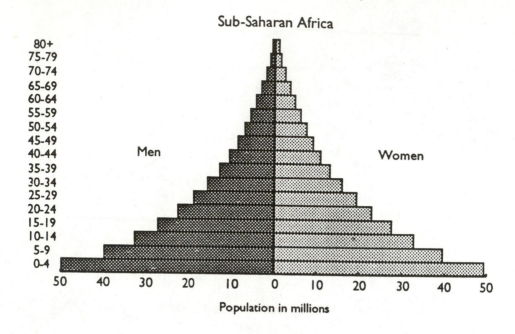

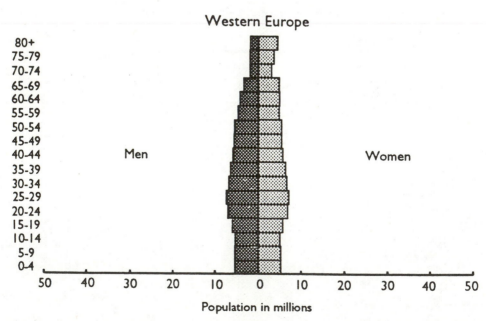

Source: Population Reference Bureau, *Population Today* 49, no. 1, 1994, based on U.N. data.

percentage of the population is made up of young people; in many Third World countries nearly half the population is under the age of 15. In Western Europe, by contrast, there are proportionately many more people in the middle and older age groups. In countries where children comprise a large segment of the population, there hasn't been time yet for individuals born during the period of "death control" to reach the older age groups where death rates are higher than those of the younger age categories. In most of these countries the greatest decreases in death rates among infants and children occurred in the late 1940s and the large numbers of children born in that period reached their peak reproductive years in the 1970s. Their children, in turn, will further inflate the lower tiers of the population structure. Eventually either population control will lower birth rates in these countries or famine, disease, or other factors will once again increase mortality rates. In the absence of such calamities, death rates in the extraordinarily young populations of the underdeveloped nations may temporarily fall below those of the industrialized countries.

One of the most significant features of age structure in a population is the proportion of people who are economically productive (arbitrarily considered to be those persons between 15 and 59) in relation to those who are dependent on them. The proportion of dependents in the under-developed countries is much higher than in the developed nations, presenting an additional heavy burden to those countries as they struggle for economic development. The high percentage of people under 15 is also indicative of the explosive growth potential of their populations. In most developing nations this percentage is 40–45%, while in Libya children comprise fully 50% of the population! By contrast, the percentage under 15 in most industrialized countries is 16–25%. In the United States, for example, there are two people of working age for every one who is too young or too old to work; in Mexico and Nigeria there is only one. Thus, underdeveloped countries have a much greater proportion of people in their pre-reproductive years. As they grow up and marry, the size of the child-bearing faction of the population will increase tremendously and their children will further inflate the size of the youngest age groups. The existence of such large numbers of young people means that even if great progress were made immediately in reducing the number of births per female in those countries, it would still be some 30 years before such birth control could significantly slow down population growth.

Population Density

Humans quite obviously are not evenly distributed over the face of the earth. Population density is usually expressed in terms of numbers of individuals per square mile or kilometer. Assessing how crowded or uncrowded a country is on the basis of density figures can be quite misleading, because such statistics take no account of areas which are uninhabited or uninhabitable. Thus a nation like Egypt has 99% of its people squeezed into 3.5% of its area. Overpopulation is usually not thought of in terms of the absolute size of the population, but rather in terms of

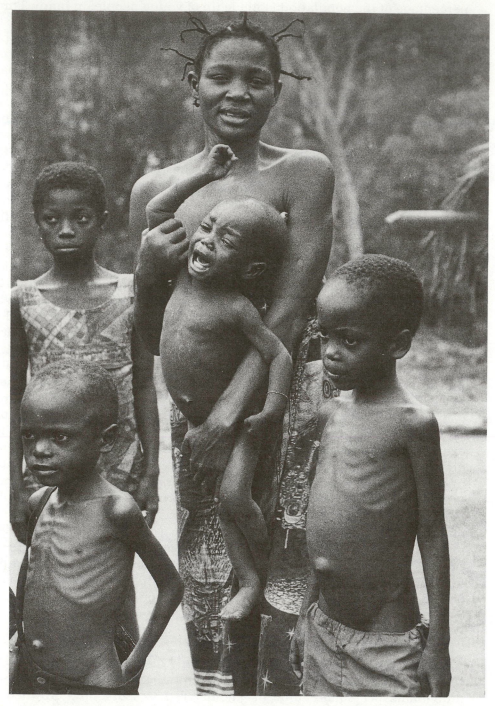

In many Third World countries children make up nearly 50% of the population, indicative of the explosive growth potential in those nations least able to provide for a rapidly growing population. [Agency for International Development]

BOX 2-4

Are Europeans an Endangered Species?

In demographic terms, Europe is vanishing. Twenty years or so from now, our countries will be empty, and no matter what our technological strength, we shall be incapable of putting it to use.

—Jacques Chirac, 1984

The above lament by the then-Prime Minister of France reflected a century of national concern about the population stagnation inherent in his country's low birth rate. Few demographers would echo Chirac's alarmist pronouncements, correctly pointing out the slowness and momentum of any significant change in population size, as well as the notorious inability of demographers to predict future childbearing patterns. Nevertheless, current fertility trends portend inevitable population decline in Europe, as birth rates continue to drop in nations all across the continent. After reaching a post-World War II peak exceeding 2.5 children per woman in 1965, fertility rates have fallen below replacement level in all European countries except Albania, Iceland, and Ireland. In Bulgaria, Estonia, Germany, Hungary, and Latvia deaths already exceed births, resulting in a slow but steady decline in the size of their populations—a trend that will soon be evident in Russia, Italy, Romania, the Czech Republic, Denmark, Spain, and Portugal (concerns about these trends should be allayed somewhat by the realization that even if unusually low fertility rates continue to prevail, it will be from 42 to 131 years, depending on the country in question, before population size falls to the level prevailing in those nations at the beginning of World War II). According to the most recent U.N. projections, the population of Europe as a whole will rise only marginally from its present 513 million, reaching a peak of 523 million around 2010, after which it will slowly decline. As birth rates fall, the age structure of European societies will shift upward. The United Nations estimates that by 2025 one out of every five Europeans will be 65 or older and that the working age population that must support these senior citizens will be steadily shrinking.

The consequences of an aging and dwindling population have been the subject of heated debate between European pronatalists and antinatalists for nearly two decades and raise issues that may be of relevance in North America as well, since similar demographic trends loom on our horizon. Proponents of the pronatalist viewpoint, such as former Prime Minister Chirac, raise the cry, "No children, no future." They view the emerging female preference for personal development and a profession as destructive to family life and a form of collective suicide. They fear loss of world influence and European cultural identity as non-European populations continue rapid growth. They warn that with too few young men being produced for military service, young women may have to be recruited and they foresee the possible collapse of Europe's elaborate social welfare system as the demands of swelling numbers of the elderly overwhelm the ability of a proportionally smaller workforce to support them.

Discounting such worries as grossly exaggerated, opponents of the pronatalist position insist that Europe need never fear for lack of leadership and innovation as long as it ensures that a substantial fraction of its young people receive a good education—something that is easier to accomplish when the population is not growing rapidly. They charge that talk of maintaining national military strength is reminiscent of a fascist past and a hindrance to greater European solidarity. Welcoming the greater individual freedom that lower fertility rates provide, they oppose any measures aimed at encouraging increased childbearing. Reflective of such attitudes was a polemic in the German feminist journal *EMMA* which proclaimed, "All attempts to influence the decision of women for motherhood must again and again be confronted with the demand for self-determination; in concrete terms: my belly is mine!" Philosophically, antinatalists feel it would be wrong to encourage national population growth at a time when global overpopulation is perceived as a serious problem. Pointing out that economic strength is more important than population size or military might in determining a country's international standing, they stress that economic integration, rather than an attempt to boost fertility, is the way to safeguard Europe's position in the world. They point to technological advances in the workplace as reducing the need for an expanding human workforce, and insist that as long as productivity increases,

funding social security systems will pose no problem.

For the most part, European politicians have been hesitant to choose sides in this debate, knowing that any position they might take would offend large blocs of voters. Several nations, most notably France and several East European countries, have implemented economically costly incentives to encourage childbearing, but for the most part such programs have had minimal long-term effects on fertility. Regardless of the rantings of political leaders, the emphasis of young Europeans on individual rights and self-fulfillment makes it highly unlikely that fertility rates will rebound anytime soon. Thus although Europeans are certainly not about to join the Siberian tiger or the black-footed ferret on the "endangered" list, a long-term population decline for most of the continent's nations appears irrevocable and is now well underway.

Reference

van da Kaa, Dirk J. 1987. "Europe's Second Demographic Transition." *Population Bulletin* 42, no. 1 (March).

its density and the extent of the resource base on which that population is dependent. Until fairly recent times, pressures caused by increasing population densities were generally eased by migration from more crowded to less crowded regions. The massive 19th century migration of Europeans to sparsely settled lands in the New World and Australia reflected increasing population densities in the emigrants' homelands during the mini-population explosion that characterized the initial phase of the demographic transition. Emigration thus served as an effective "safety valve" that helped prevent Malthus' dire predictions from becoming reality. In today's crowded world, international migration threatens to cause more problems than it solves. Unfortunately, there are few, if any, places left which have the capacity—or the desire—to sustain a large influx of new arrivals. In recent years millions of economic refugees from the Third World have sought a better life elsewhere only to find fear, anger, and sometimes overt hostility in the more affluent regions they seek to enter. Immigration laws have recently been tightened in a number of European countries and everywhere the "welcome" mat is conspicuously absent. The sad spectacle of today's Haitian "boat people" and Bosnia's victims of "ethnic cleansing" may be but harbingers of an ever-increasing number of asylum-seekers doomed to drifting from one temporary shelter to another, with no nation willing to provide a permanent haven.

Urbanization

The "urban explosion," referring to the tremendous population increase in metropolitan areas, has been one of the most marked phenomena related to the overall growth of human populations during the 20th century. Urbanization is, of course, one of the oldest of demographic trends, having its roots in the small settled communities made possible by an agricultural way of life. The first true cities are believed to have arisen in Mesopotamia about five or six thousand years ago, but growth of urban areas proceeded rather slowly during the millennia that followed. Increase in urban populations depended almost entirely on an influx of new residents from the surrounding countryside. Due to extremely poor sanitary conditions and crowded living conditions, mortality rates in these urban centers were higher than birth rates, and not until recent times have urban centers become self-sustaining in terms of population growth.

The advent of the Industrial Revolution gave a tremendous impetus to the growth of cities, and the rate of increase has continued to accelerate ever since. As an example of the great population shift that has occurred, consider the change in rural-urban ratios in the United States: in 1800 a mere 6% of all Americans lived in an urban area; the number of city dwellers increased to 15% by 1850 and to 40% by 1900. In 1993, 75% of the U.S. population lived in cities. [Note: in the United States, "urban" is defined as any community with a population of 2,500 or more. Different countries use different cutoff points to distinguish "urban" from "rural" populations, complicating the comparison of urbanization statistics from various parts of the world. For example, while American demographers utilize the 2,500 figure, their colleagues in Iceland consider a village of 200 as "urban"; in Italy the corresponding number is 10,000, while in densely populated Japan, a community is considered "urban" only when its population surpasses 50,000! (Haub, 1993)].

In the world as a whole, population increased by a factor of 2.6 during the years between 1800 and 1950; during that same time period the number of people living in cities over 20,000 population grew from 22 million to over half a billion—a factor of 23. In the largest cities (100,000 or more) of the industrialized countries, the growth was even more rapid, increasing by a factor of 35. By 1950, 29% of the world's people lived in cities; by 1990 the percentage of urban dwellers in the world as a whole had risen to 43 and is expected to surpass 50% by 2005 (U.N. Population Division, 1992).

In recent years this urban expansion in the developed world has slowed somewhat, but since 1900 has accelerated at a great rate in the nations of Asia, Africa, and Latin America. United Nations projections indicate no slowdown in the mass movement to the cities in the poorer countries; according to the World Bank, some of Africa's cities are growing at the phenomenal rate of 10% a year—the fastest rate of urbanization ever documented. The current 35% urban component of Third World population is expected to rise to 40% by the turn of the century and to 57% by 2025. In terms of actual numbers, cities of the developing world can be expected to mushroom from their current 1.5 billion to over 4 billion in 2025. By the end of the current decade, the developing nations will boast 17 of the world's 21 largest cities, each with a population of 10 million or more (Kennedy, 1993). Such growth is already having a staggering impact on the ability of those municipalities to provide even the rudiments of a decent standard of living. Much of the population growth in Third World cities occurs in the euphemistically labelled "uncontrolled settlements"—slum areas and shantytowns spreading like ugly cancerous growths around the periphery of almost every large city in the developing world. These uncontrolled settlements are growing even faster than the urban areas as a whole, with the consequence that in the years ahead an ever-larger segment of Third World urban populations will be living in the squalor and hopelessness that characterize these shantytowns.

In most cases the trend to the cities seems to be caused by the hope for a better, more comfortable life, and though most migrants continue to live in abject poverty, nearly all seem to prefer to remain there rather than return to the deprivation of their rural home villages. Historically, urbanization seems to have the universal effect of breaking down the traditional cultures of those who migrate to the cities, where anonymity is the main feature. The overwhelming majority of urban dwellers in the Third World are migrants who have brought their peasant culture with them. They generally lack the specialized education and skills required to penetrate the city's complex social web. Migrants inevitably find that their limited skills make them incapable of contributing to the economy and consequently they are scarcely any better off than before. Many migrants form modified village societies within the city and thus tend to transfer aspects of village culture to the city. This may explain why the reproductive rates and attitudes of these city dwellers closely resemble those of their rural relatives.

The rapid increase in the populations of Third World cities presents a number of very serious problems that government officials are going to find extremely difficult to manage. Two of the most pressing needs, if disease outbreaks are to be prevented, will be the provision of safe drinking water and sewage disposal. During the decade of the 1980s impressive gains were made in bringing water and sanitation services to urban residents in the developing nations. By 1990, approximately 500 million more city dwellers worldwide had access to adequate drinking water than was the case in 1980; similarly, those served by sewerage projects increased

Figure 2-8 World's Largest Cities in A.D. 2000

Rank	Population (in millions)
1. Tokyo, Japan	28.0
2. Sao Paulo, Brazil	22.6
3. Bombay, India	18.1
4. Shanghai, China	17.4
5. New York City, U.S.A.	16.6
6. Mexico City, Mexico	16.2
7. Beijing, China	14.4
8. Lagos, Nigeria	13.5
9. Jakarta, Indonesia	13.4
10. Los Angeles, U.S.A.	13.2
11. Seoul, Korea	13.0
12. Buenos Aires, Argentina	12.8
13. Calcutta, India	12.7
14. Metro Manila, Philippines	12.6
15. Tianjin, China	12.5
16. Rio de Janeiro, Brazil	12.2
17. Karachi, Pakistan	11.9
18. New Delhi, India	11.7
19. Dacca, Bangladesh	11.5
20. Cairo, Egypt	10.8

Source: United Nations Population Division.

by close to 300 million. Nevertheless, because of the huge influx of rural migrants into the cities during those years, the number of urban residents *lacking* such services remained constant in terms of water supply and actually increased by 70 million so far as sanitation services were concerned (Briscoe, 1993). Municipal officials might be forgiven for wondering if they were on a treadmill—having to run faster and faster just to remain in place!

As urban populations continue to expand, provision of such basic services will undoubtedly lag even further behind, increasing the threat of epidemic disease and worsening already serious problems of water pollution. Air quality, already at critical levels in many Third World cities, will continue to deteriorate as the number of old, poorly maintained automobiles and pollutant-emitting motorbikes, scooters, and motorcycles continue to rise. Pressures on municipal authorities to provide jobs, housing, transportation, and social facilities will mount inexorably within the coming years and will present those societies with economic and environmental challenges which may prove impossible to meet.

Population Projections

The obvious question to anyone looking at a graphic representation of human numbers soaring toward infinity on the upswing of a J-curve is, "How long can this continue?" and "Where will population stabilize?" The inherent assumption, and one which is validated by the results of numerous animal experiments in population dynamics, is that such growth rates cannot continue forever. Statistical evidence indicates, in fact, that human population growth rates peaked in the early 1970s, declining slightly since then and remaining relatively stable at 1.7–1.6% since the mid-1980s. Nevertheless, although a growth rate decrease is heartening, in terms of absolute numbers population will be growing faster during the remainder of this century than it is right now, due to the enormous size of the present population base. By the year 2000, world population will be increasing by 100 million people each year (95 million of whom will be residents of Third World countries) compared with 87 million a year in the late 1980s.

The United Nations, an organization logically quite interested in future world growth patterns, regularly publishes projections of population size for the next several decades. Such projections are not just extrapolations of present trends, but take into consideration trends in fertility, mortality, migration, and so on (they do not consider the possibility of major disasters such as a nuclear war, however). The United Nations presents several sets of projections, all of which assume that there will be some lowering of fertility rates (a substantial drop in fertility is assumed for the low projection, a less significant decline for the high projection) in regions where these are currently quite high. The most widely used medium range projection presupposes a continued steady decline in death rates, with an ultimate worldwide life expectancy of 85 years and a total fertility rate of 2.06 (i.e. average family size throughout the world of 2 children per couple). Given these assumptions, the United Nations' "best guess" for ultimate world population size is 11.5 billion, to be reached sometime around the year 2150. However, if fertility rates deviate even slightly from the replacement level figure presumed for the medium-range estimate, world population totals in 2150 could differ dramatically from the 11.5 billion figure cited above. If TFR were to drop slightly below replacement level to 1.7 children per woman, world population in 2150 would be 4 billion— lower than it is today. By contrast, if TFR falls only to 2.5 instead of 2.06, world population in 2150 will reach 28 billion and continue climbing. As mentioned before, the five U.N. projections displayed in Figure 2-9 all assume some reduction in current fertility rates. Not represented, because U.N. demographers are convinced that human reproductive behavior *will* change, is a "constant fertility" projection that assumes no drop in the current world TFR of 3.3. Under that scenario, the earth's human population by 2150 would reach an incredible *694 billion*, 692.5 billion of whom would be living in Asia, Africa, and Latin America (McNicoll, 1992).

Figure 2-9 Long-Range Population Projections, 1990–2150

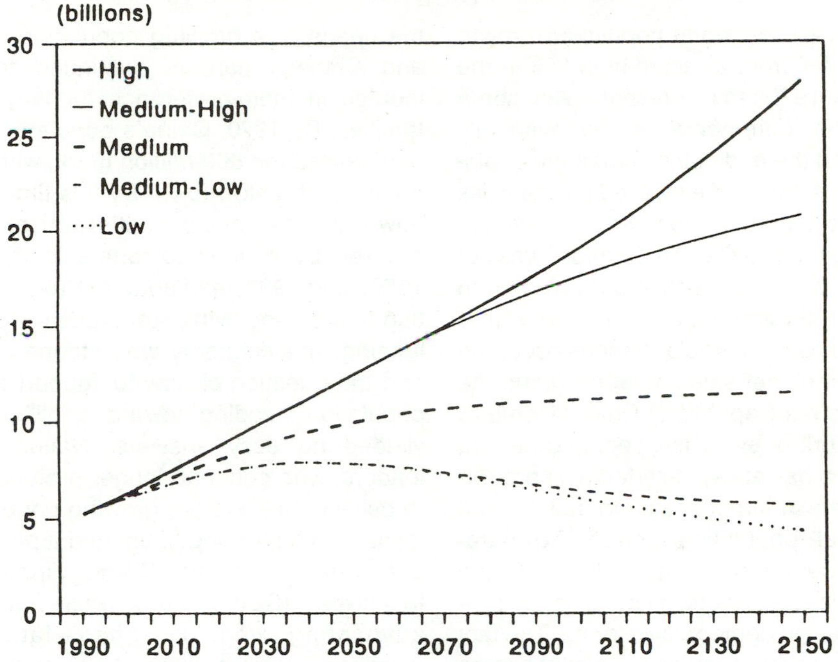

(billions)

Variations in population projections depend primarily on different assumptions about fertility trends. The low projection assumes fertility will stabilize at 1.7 children, the medium projection assumes stabilization at 2.06, and the high projection assumes stabilization at 2.5 children.

Source: World Resources Institute, based on data from United Nations Population Division, *Long-Range World Population Projections: Two Centuries of Population Growth, 1950–2150* (1992).

While both the United Nations and the World Bank are proceeding on the debatable assumption that world population growth will stabilize approximately a century and a half from now, widely divergent fertility patterns in different areas of the world guarantee that some regions will achieve population stability long before others do. As can be seen in the Population Data Chart (Figure 2-4), Italy has already reached zero population growth (ZPG), while several countries, including Germany, Hungary, Bulgaria, and Latvia, actually have negative growth rates. Similarly, in Japan, where the average number of children born during a woman's lifetime is now just 1.5, population size will soon peak at a level only slightly higher than present numbers and then begin a slow decline as deaths among the large cohorts of elderly Japanese outnumber births (Yanagashita, 1993).

Looking at population projections on a regional basis, the countries of South Asia (India, Pakistan, Bangladesh) will experience the largest population increase, adding almost 3 billion people to their present 1.3

Box 2-5

China: Demographic Billionaire

When the world population growth rate fell from a record-high 2% in the early 1970s to its present 1.7%, some media commentators optimistically hailed the end of the population explosion. If they had examined the statistics more carefully, however, they would have noticed that the downturn was not due to an across-the-board decline in births throughout the world, but rather to some remarkable changes occurring in the planet's demographic giant, the People's Republic of China. Home to one out of every five people on earth, China has always exerted a disproportionate influence among nations on global population trends. To paraphrase an old adage "when China sneezes, the world gets pneumonia"— at least in demographic terms. The fact that world population growth rates today hover between 1.6–1.7% rather than close to 2% as they did 20 years ago is almost entirely due to the rapid decline in Chinese birth rates; elsewhere in the developing world, annual population growth still averages 2.3%.

Since 1970 China has undergone a demographic transition unprecedented for the speed with which it was carried out. During the years immediately following the 1949 revolution, Chinese mortality rates plummeted as peace was restored and improvements in health and living standards became widespread. As a result, population growth rates rose sharply, averaging more than 2% annually for the next 25 years. Although China's population was already well in excess of 600 million by this time, there was little official concern about overpopulation. Voicing orthodox Communist doctrine, Chairman Mao Zedong proclaimed that "revolution plus production" would enable China to provide adequately for the needs of a growing population— and Chinese parents continued to indulge in their preference for large families. By 1970, China's population had passed the 800-million mark, with no signs of a slowdown. By this time, however, the heady optimism expressed by national planners in the 1950s and 1960s had abated. Production figures and living standards were lagging, the economy was stagnant, and the question of how to support a population heading toward 1 billion yielded no easy answers. National leaders, who could no longer pretend to believe that a large, growing population was a blessing, launched a program of "Strategic Demographic Initiatives" (SDI) to curb fertility. By advocating *wan, xi, shao*—later marriage, longer interval between pregnancies, and fewer children per mother—Chinese leaders pursued a goal of slowing the growth rate sufficiently to enable the nation to deal with existing population-related problems more effectively. At the time SDI was introduced in the early 1970s, there was no intention of halting growth or reducing population size—the idea was merely to slow the pace of increase. By the late 1970s, however, Communist Party officials had formulated new economic targets that would be unattainable so long as the country's population size continued to grow. Accordingly, the Chinese government developed an official policy position stating that China should not exceed a population maximum of 1.2 billion by the end of the century and should then strive to reduce total numbers to an ultimate population size more appropriate to the nation's carrying capacity— around 700 million. To achieve this goal, Chinese planners in 1978 adopted the now-famous one-child-per-family policy, an idea which, ironically, they seem to have picked up from Zero Population Growth (ZPG) advocates in the United States. Interestingly, by the time the one-child policy was adopted, Chinese birth rates had already fallen to the lowest levels ever recorded in that country; by promoting the concept that "One is not wanting, two are good, and three are excessive," China succeeded in lowering the national fertility rate from six in 1950 to three in 1979. Implementation of the more stringent one-child policy had only a limited additional impact on China's demographic statistics until quite recently. By the mid-1980s, less than 16% of Chinese couples had signed "Only Child Glory Certificates"—contracts guaranteeing preferences in housing, education, and employment so long as the couple had only one child. Desire among Chinese parents to have at least two children remained strong, particularly if the first child was a girl; in the rural areas where most Chinese still live, fertility levels never dropped below 2.5, although in cities one-child families became increasingly common.

The rapid decline in birth rates which China witnessed during the 1970s leveled off during the decade of the 1980s and, in fact, inched upward slightly, thanks to a relaxation in the marriage age laws and a shift in the age structure (women born during the "baby boom" of the 1960s entered their prime reproductive years during the 1980s). By 1982, Chinese population passed the 1 billion mark and hopes for stabilizing growth at 1.2 billion quickly faded. The impact of trends in China on overall world growth prospects was reflected a few years later when U.N. demographers, noting that Chinese fertility hadn't fallen quite as much as anticipated, raised its estimates for ultimate world population size from 10.5 billion to 14.2 billion. In a nation as large as China, even relatively minor up or down fluctuations in fertility rates can have major implications in terms of actual numbers.

By the 1990s, Chinese officials, eyeing projections that the country's population would shoot past the two billion mark by 2050 if fertility were not quickly reduced from the present 2.3 children per family, once again began tightening enforcement of its family limitation policies, much to the consternation of United Nations officials who have been providing funds to support family planning activities in China. Recent reports that Chinese authorities were forcibly sterilizing peasant women who had already borne their quota of one or two babies caused international donors to consider withdrawing population assistance programs as a protest against China's coercive policies. Nevertheless, such policies seem to be having the desired demographic impact; in 1993, for the first time ever, China's fertility rate dropped below replacement level to 1.9 lifetime births per woman—and the total world growth rate correspondingly fell to its lowest level in more than 30 years.

While China has made enormous progress in lowering birth rates to levels approximating those of the industrialized nations within an amazingly brief time span, these efforts will not be sufficient to achieve the country's population goals. Since the number of Chinese women in their peak child-bearing years will be steadily increasing during the present decade, China's population is likely to reach 1.3 billion by 2000, even if the government's population policies are strictly implemented. Although China has largely completed its demographic transition, with few children per family the national norm, moving on to what some call a "second demographic transition," typified by one-child or childless families, will be much more difficult, given the current socio-economic conditions and cultural values in that country. Nevertheless, the historic experiment being played out in China will be followed with extreme interest by all who realize that the ultimate size of world population will be determined to a considerable extent by the success or failure of China's attempt to tame the population monster.

References

Haub, Carl. 1993. "China's Fertility Drop Lowers World Growth Rate." *Population Today* 21, no. 6 (June).

Kristof, Nicholas D. 1993. "U.N. Unit May Quit China Over Coercive Birth Curbs." *New York Times*, May 15.

Tien, H. Yuan, with Zhang Tianlu, Ping Yu, Li Jingneng, and Liang Zhongtang. "China's Demographic Dilemmas." *Population Bulletin* 47, no. 1 (June).

billion before numbers stabilize. India alone, growing by 18 million annually, will likely surpass China to become the world's most populous nation by 2025. At the other extreme, European populations should peak around 2010 with a total of 523 million people, and then begin a gradual decline. Africa, currently boasting the world's highest growth rate and with no indication yet of a trend toward declining fertility, will have a population in 2150 almost five times larger than at present and will be second only to Asia in total numbers. Together, Africa and Asia will account for fully 80% of the world's total population at the time of stabilization. Latin America is currently growing at a rate second only to Africa. In 1960 there were approximately equal numbers of Latin Americans and North Americans. By 2025 there will be twice as many inhabitants south of the Rio Grande as there are in Canada and the United States. By the time of stabilization, the United Nations estimates the population of Latin America will exceed one billion, more than three times that of North America. The United States, unlike other industrialized countries, has experienced an unanticipated increase in fertility rates within the past several years; earlier Census Bureau estimates that the U.S. population would stabilize at about 300 million early in the 21st century have recently been revised upward. As a result of increased childbearing and a major surge in immigration, U.S. population will continue to grow fairly rapidly for the foreseeable future, reaching 275 million by the year 2000 and surpassing 350 million by 2050 (Pear, 1992).

Obviously, making global population projections is a risky business, with accuracy of forecasts depending not only on the childbearing decisions of millions of individual couples but also on trends in mortality rates. A number of demographers fear that an increase in death rates may be as influential in curbing growth as a decrease in birth rates. Already there is evidence that in widely scattered areas of the developing world child mortality rates are rising due to increasing levels of malnutrition. There is a real danger that mounting human pressures on already overtaxed ecosystems may cause a collapse in the food-producing capabilities of many regions. While most long-range projections show global population growth halting around the year 2150, the ability of natural ecosystems to support

Figure 2-10 Regional Population Growth into the 22nd Century

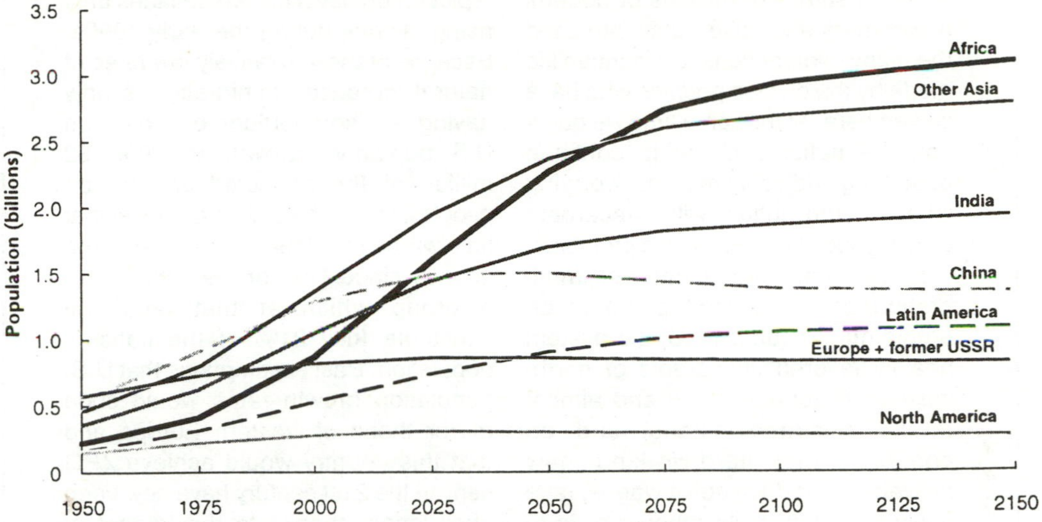

Source: Population Reference Bureau, based on U.N. data.

BOX 2-6

U.S. Prospects for ZPG: The Impact of Immigration

Give me your tired, your poor
Your huddled masses, yearning to breathe free,
The wretched refuse of your teeming shore,
Send these, the homeless, tempest-tossed to me:
I lift my lamp beside the golden door.

The inspirational words of Emma Lazarus inscribed on the Statue of Liberty have greeted successive waves of immigrants to American shores and extend a national welcome to newcomers from a country which has long been proud of its "melting pot" tradition. In recent years, however, a rising tide of sentiment to "bar the door" against additional would-be immigrants is gaining force as the number of new arrivals soars to record highs. Current levels of immigration to the United States substantially exceed those of any other country and come close to equalling the number of new arrivals in 1907 and 1914, the previous peak years of immigration, when more than 1.2 million newcomers streamed through the "Golden Door." Today, according to U.S. Census Bureau figures, approximately 880,000 to 1.4 million immigrants, including an estimated 200,000 illegal entrants, are arriving in the country each year—and barring changes in federal immigration policies, will continue to do so for the next 60 years.

Although we are truly a "nation of immigrants," Americans historically have exhibited an ambivalent attitude toward immigration policy. We have congratulated ourselves for providing a place of refuge and an opportunity for a "fresh start" for millions of hopeful newcomers and have rightly stressed the many contributions to American life made by the diverse peoples who have settled here. At the same time we question the nation's ability to continue absorbing additional millions, worrying whether the influx will exacerbate existing social and economic problems.

In the past, controversy over immigration policy focused primarily on ethnic quotas (until 1965, the system heavily favored immigrants of northwestern European origin and almost totally excluded Asians) and on concerns that hard-working new arrivals would drive down wages, take away jobs that might otherwise go to citizens, or, conversely, that unskilled immigrants would go on welfare and become a burden to taxpayers. More recently, however, a new element has been added to the policy debate pertaining to immigration law reform. Immigration's impact on American population growth is now being recognized as the single most important variable in our country's demographic future—the factor that will largely determine the ultimate population size of this country and the date at which population stabilization occurs.

Changes in population size occur only through fluctuations in the ratio between birth and death rates or as a result of changes in net migration (the difference between emigration and immigration). In the vast majority of countries today, with the possible exception of Israel and several European nations, immigration's impact on total population size is negligible. Such is not the case in the United States, however. While numbers of new arrivals rose significantly throughout the 1980s, American fertility rates remained stable at below-replacement level for two decades until rising slightly during the early 1990s. Because of these relatively low rates of natural increase, immigration is now having a disproportionate impact on U.S. population growth. By 2050, 82 million of the projected 383 million people living in the United States at that time will be individuals who entered the country since 1991 or their children—a group which at that time will constitute fully 21% of the nation's population. Past assumptions that U.S. population growth rates would soon mirror those of western Europe and that this country would achieve ZPG early in the 21st century have now been abandoned, thanks to the impact of immigration.

Although the nation has yet to adopt a national population policy, as long ago as 1972 the President's Commission on Population Growth and the American Future concluded: "Recognizing that our population cannot grow indefinitely and appreciating the advantages of moving now towards the stabilization of population, the Commission recommends that the nation welcome and plan for a stabilized population." Do Americans agree with the President's Commission that at some time, preferably sooner rather than later, zero population growth is desirable? If so, policymakers must seriously consider lowering the ceiling on annual immigration, taking U.S. fertility trends into account, in order to attain the agreed upon goal.

Reference

Bouvier, Leon F., and Robert W. Gardner. 1986. "Immigration to the U.S.: The Unfinished Story." *Population Bulletin* 41, no. 4 (Nov.).

a substantial rise in human numbers for another century and a half has been questioned. Since 95% of the expected increase will occur in the poorest countries, many observers insist that population growth needs to be stabilized long before it reaches the theoretical levels projected by the United Nations. Reflecting the sentiments of a growing number of his colleagues throughout the developing world, a Kenyan official several years ago remarked:

> If more and more people keep pouring into a country that can only deliver so much, you can expect political unrest, serious shortage of food and everything else that people need to live, and in general, chaos■

References

Altman, Lawrence K. 1993. "Big Health Gains Found in Developing Countries." *New York Times*, July 7.

Briscoe, John. 1993. "When the Cup is Half Full: Improving Water and Sanitation Services in the Developing World." *Environment* 35, no. 4 (May).

Ehrlich, Paul R., Anne H. Ehrlich, and John P. Holdren. 1977. *Ecoscience: Population, Resources, Environment*. W. H. Freeman and Co.

Farb, Peter. 1963. *Ecology, Life Nature Library*. Time Inc.

Haub, Carl. 1993. "Tokyo Now Recognized as World's Largest City." *Population Today* 21, no. 3 (March).

Herring, Herbert. 1960. *A History of Latin America*. Alfred A. Knopf.

Kennedy, Paul. 1993. *Preparing for the Twenty-First Century*. Random House.

McNicoll, Geoffrey. 1992. "The United Nations' Long-Range Population Projections." *Population and Development Review* 18, no. 2 (June).

Odum, Eugene P. 1959. *Fundamentals of Ecology*. W. B. Saunders Company.

Pear, Robert. 1992. "New Look at the U.S. in 2050: Bigger, Older, and Less White." *New York Times*, Dec. 4.

World Urbanization Prospects. 1992. U.N. Population Division.

Yanagashita, Machiko. 1993. "Slow Growth Will Turn to Decline of the Japanese Population." *Population Today* 21, no. 5 (May).

CHAPTER 3

Population Control

> *We need to make a world in which fewer children are born, and in which we take better care of them.*
>
> —Dr. George Wald

Studies of population dynamics clearly indicate that no population can sustain limitless growth, raising the as-yet unanswered question: what will eventually bring a halt to still-climbing human numbers? Basically, one of two factors could effect a drop in growth rates: a decrease in birth rates or an increase in death rates. Either change would result in a narrowing of the gap between births and deaths that has been responsible for the unprecedented growth in human population during the past century. A decrease in the death rate caused the population explosion, and a number of demographic experts gloomily predict that a reversal of this trend in the future will bring a halt to further growth. They point to an observable rise in infant mortality rates due to the increasing frequency of malnutrition; to the possibility of global pandemics as population densities increase; and to the growing likelihood of military confrontations as nations compete for dwindling resources.

However, no rational individual would advocate starvation, epidemics, or war as a means of ending the population explosion. The humane approach to a very real problem lies instead in attempts to reduce growth by lowering birth rates to the point at which they will be in approximate equilibrium with death rates, thereby achieving a stabilization of population size, popularly referred to as ZPG ("zero population growth").

Early Attempts at Family Limitation

Although most traditional cultures have consistently encouraged prolific childbearing, records indicate that during stressful periods of famine, war, or civil upheaval many couples throughout history have attempted in various ways to prevent unwanted births. While some of the methods employed were based on nothing more than superstition, others were moderately effective and continue to be used today.

One of the oldest documented means of contraception, referred to in the Old Testament story of Onan (Genesis 38:9), is that of withdrawal (*coitus interruptus*), whereby the man withdraws his penis from the vagina prior to ejaculation. Since a keen sense of timing is essential to the success of this method, withdrawal has the highest failure rate of any major method of birth control, but it does have the advantage of requiring no drugs or devices nor access to medical personnel for its use—and it costs nothing. Where couples are highly motivated not to have children, it can be fairly successful and, in fact, is believed to be the method by which European couples substantially reduced birth rates in that part of the world during the early years of the demographic transition. The popularity of withdrawal prompted numerous attacks on the method by certain disapproving segments of society. Some doctors declared that the practice would lead to both physical and mental illness, but such admonitions fell largely on deaf ears. One 40-year-old German farmer, warned of the dire consequences of indulging in coitus interruptus, calmly retorted, "I don't believe that. Otherwise everybody would be sick."

Crude barriers to the cervix, similar in concept to the modern diaphragm or cervical cap, were used by women in ancient Egypt who fashioned such devices out of leaves, cloth, wads of cotton fibers, or even crocodile dung!

Herbal concoctions have been used for both contraceptive and abortive purposes for thousands of years. The modern era's contraceptive pill, along with hormonal implants and injectables, are but the most recent in a venerable line of antifertility drugs widely employed in ancient and medieval societies as well as in folk cultures right up to the present time. Although it long was fashionable to dismiss such brews as totally useless, recent research has found that some of the plants used are, in fact, remarkably effective in preventing pregnancy, while others are powerful abortifacients. The contraceptive properties of drugs extracted from such plant materials as pomegranate rind, black pepper, ivy, cabbage flowers, and willow bark were described in Greek and Roman medical literature almost two thousand years ago. Pennyroyal (*Mentha pulegium*), a member of the mint family, was widely used for centuries to induce abortions, as was rue (*Ruta graveolans*), which has both abortifacient and contraceptive properties. In recent decades the results of a number of studies and field observations confirm that certain plant substances do indeed exert an antifertility effect (a phenomenon first noticed in relation to spontaneous abortions or a failure of ovulation among grazing animals when feeding on certain plants). Preliminary research has confirmed many of the claims made by ancient medical authorities and efforts are now on-going in a number of countries, especially India and China, to conduct clinical and laboratory tests of traditional drugs believed to possess contraceptive properties (McLaren, 1990; Riddle, 1992).

The use of condoms dates back at least to the 16th century when a fine linen sheath worn on the penis during intercourse was recommended as a means of preventing the spread of venereal disease. By the 17th century condoms made of lamb intestines, tied shut at the end with a ribbon, were introduced for the express purpose of preventing conception and by the 18th century were reportedly available for use by patrons at all the finer houses of prostitution in Europe (some versions were also made of silk!). With the advent of vulcanized rubber in 1844, a truly effective and relatively cheap (advertised at $5 per dozen in 1850) male contraceptive became available for the masses. Nevertheless, rubber condoms were not widely used until World War I when they were distributed among the troops as protection against venereal disease (Stokes, 1980; McLaren, 1990).

Other birth-control practices with a similarly long history include douching (flushing out the vagina with a water solution immediately after intercourse), almost totally ineffective in spite of its popularity; and breast-feeding of infants, quite an effective means of suppressing the onset of ovulation following childbirth and thereby helpful in spacing pregnancies.

In fact, prior to the advent of modern contraceptives, breast-feeding was the chief tactic employed by women to prevent an unwanted second pregnancy soon after childbirth. A recent survey conducted in Bangladesh revealed that, on average, each month of breast-feeding increases the birth interval between babies by about 0.4 months (Weiss, 1993; Kleinman and Senanayake, 1984).

When such birth-control methods failed, as they frequently did, women commonly resorted to abortion, a very ancient practice believed to have been the most prevalent method of family limitation throughout history.

As a last resort, unwanted children in past centuries frequently fell victim to infanticide—the deliberate killing of babies, particularly girl babies, immediately after birth. This practice was quite common in ancient Greece and in several Asian countries up until fairly recent times, especially during periods of famine or civil upheaval.

Modern Family Planning Movement

The origins of the modern family planning movement in the United States can be traced to the publication in 1832 of a contraceptive textbook, *Fruits of Philosophy*, written by Dr. Charles Knowlton. Dr. Knowlton won renown as the first person in this country to be jailed for advocating birth control. The development of the diaphragm in the 1840s further stimulated public interest in contraceptive techniques and although proponents of birth control were viciously persecuted by so-called "societies for the suppression of vice," the resultant notoriety only enhanced sales of birth-control literature. Open discussion of sex or reproductive matters was still taboo during those years of Victorian morality, however, and an "establishment" backlash against the growing birth-control movement was reflected in the passage in 1873 of the Comstock Law, a federal mandate that prohibited sending birth-control information or devices through the mail, such items being defined as "obscene."

Toward the end of the 19th century, the burgeoning feminist movement lent support to the concept of family planning, stressing the health burdens imposed on women by too many children born too close together. An outstanding pioneer of family planning in America was Margaret Sanger, a nurse in New York City who was appalled by the extent of poverty due to over-large families and the rate of maternal death due to abortion among the people with whom she worked. Recognizing that the Comstock Law prevented such people from obtaining the contraceptive information they so badly needed, she launched a personal crusade to overturn that legislation. In 1914 Sanger founded the National Birth Control League and began publishing a monthly magazine, *The Woman Rebel*, containing birth-control information—which the Post Office therefore refused to distribute. The following year she circulated a more comprehensive birth-control pamphlet, *Family Limitation*, which also violated the Comstock Law. Sanger was indicted for this action, but the

BOX 3-1

Abortion

Regarded as the most widely practiced method of family limitation throughout history, abortion remains today a method of last resort when contraceptives are unavailable, unused, or fail. On a worldwide basis, rough estimates suggest there are between 40 to 60 million abortions annually. In the United States, the number of legal abortions each year has remained relatively stable at 1.6 million since the mid-1980s; added to these, Planned Parenthood reports an additional 20,000 illegal abortions per year. Currently the subject of intense controversy, abortion was not always legally prohibited. Among ancient Greeks and Romans no social or criminal stigma was attached to abortion; during the early Christian era abortion was viewed as murder only after the soul became "animated"—a time established as 40 days after conception for males and 80 days for females. Under English common law, which prevailed in the United States as well as in England, life was regarded as beginning with "quickening," or the first perception of fetal movement by the mother, generally occurring around the beginning of the fifth month. Prior to that time, no penalties accrued to abortion; even after quickening, abortion was not regarded as serious a crime as murder.

For the first quarter of the 19th century, no U.S. laws—federal or state—addressed the issue of abortion. This situation gradually changed as the century progressed; physicians lobbied vigorously to outlaw abortion, motivated in part by a desire to put "quack" doctors out of business, by a belief that abortion was morally wrong, and by opposition to new social roles for women.

By 1900 abortions were illegal everywhere in the United States, a situation that prevailed until the 1960s when public attitudes toward abortion began to liberalize. Concerns about the "quality of life," as opposed to mere biological existence, were voiced, as was the view that antiabortion statutes discriminated against poor women since the wealthy could, and did, travel abroad to obtain a desired abortion. At the recommendation of the American Law Institute, about one-third of the states by the late 1960s had amended their statutes to permit abortion in cases where 1) continuation of pregnancy would endanger the physical or mental health of the mother, 2) when the child might be born severely deformed or mentally retarded, or 3) when rape or incest resulted in pregnancy or when an unmarried girl under 16 became pregnant. By 1970 the states of Alaska, Hawaii, New York, and Washington had completely legalized first-trimester abortions.

In 1973 the U.S. Supreme Court invalidated all remaining state antiabortion laws when, in the historic *Roe vs. Wade* decision, it ruled that states cannot place any restrictions on abortions during the first trimester other than to require that the procedure be performed by a physician. During the second trimester the state can regulate abortion only in ways to protect maternal health; only during the last trimester, said the Court, may the state prohibit abortion unless the life of the mother is in danger.

Today Americans are among the 76% of the world's people who live in countries where induced abortion is legal. In such nations, where an abortion can be performed early in pregnancy by trained medical personnel, abortion is 11 times less dangerous for the mother than is carrying a baby full term (less than one woman in 100,000 in the United States dies of legal abortion, while eight out of every 100,000 die from complications of pregnancy or childbirth). However, in societies where abortion is illegal or difficult to obtain due to cost or lack of facilities, many women resort to unskilled practitioners or try to self-abort. In such cases, lack of hygienic conditions and inexpert techniques entail a high risk of complications or even death. In fact, Planned Parenthood estimates the risk of death from illegal abortion as 30 times higher than that of a legal abortion. While accurate figures on such a delicate subject are difficult to obtain, the World Health Organization estimates that approximately 200,000 women worldwide die of illegal abortions each year, most of them in Third World countries where access to legal abortion is still largely unavailable. In some Latin American nations, a large proportion of all maternal deaths result from botched illegal abortions, and complications due to such back-alley procedures are responsible for approximately half of all admissions to hospital obstetric units in that part of the world.

The impact that abortion's legal status has on maternal health was most dramatically illustrated by the situation in the eastern European nation of Romania during the repressive regime of Nicolae Ceaucescu. Spurred by concerns about a declining national birth rate, the Romanian dictator in 1966 reversed the country's previously liberal abortion laws, declaring the procedure illegal and threatening doctors who performed such operations with lengthy imprisonment or, in a few cases, execution. Subsequently, the pronatalist government outlawed contraceptives as well. Predictably, the number of illegal abortions in Romania soared, with an estimated 200,000 occurring annually during the 1980s, and maternal deaths due to abortion jumped sevenfold. Quite obviously, prohibitions against abortion don't end the practice—they simply make it more dangerous. So devastating were the consequences of government policy that, following the overthrow and execution of Ceaucescu during the December 1989 Romanian revolution, one of the first acts taken by the country's new leaders was the legalization of abortion.

Ironically, just as Romanians were once again opening the doors to abortion services, another country in the region was moving in the opposite direction. After nearly 40 years of providing abortion on demand, Poland in 1993 bowed to pressure from the Roman Catholic Church and imposed the most restrictive abortion laws in eastern Europe. The new prohibitions permit abortion only in cases of rape, incest, severe malformation of the fetus, or when the life or health of the mother is seriously threatened; physicians who are convicted of performing an abortion can receive a two-year prison sentence. Although 95% of Poles identify themselves as Catholics, public opinion polls reveal that a large majority favor keeping abortion legal and are dismayed by the loss of a right they had long taken for granted. The predictable results have already begun to occur—abortions are going underground, affluent women are traveling to the Ukraine or the Czech Republic to obtain the desired procedure, and poor women are risking their health and their lives by resorting to back-alley practitioners or self-induced abortions.

From the perspective of slowing population growth, the legalization of abortion in itself does not greatly reduce birth rates because most legal abortions simply replace illegal operations. However, as a means of enhancing maternal health, access to legal abortion is an important part of a national health care program.

References

Darnton, John. 1993. "Tough Abortion Law Provokes Dismay in Poland." *New York Times*, March 11.

Henshaw, Stanley. 1986. "Induced Abortion: A Worldwide Perspective." *Family Planning Perspectives* 18, no. 6 (Nov/Dec).

League of Women Voters Education Fund. 1982. *Public Policy on Reproductive Choice*, no. 286 (July).

indictment was subsequently dropped. In 1916 Mrs. Sanger opened the first birth-control clinic in America, in a section of Brooklyn, New York. For this offense she was arrested and served 30 days in prison, but the resulting public outcry led to a gradual easing of legal restrictions against the family planning movement. Mrs. Sanger traveled extensively throughout the country, seeking to persuade both the medical profession and the public at large of the importance of facilitating access to birth control. By 1932 the Birth Control League had established 80 clinics throughout the United States; in 1937 the American Medical Association officially endorsed birth control; finally, by 1938, two major court cases resulted in the overthrow of the Comstock Law and, in effect, made it possible for doctors to prescribe contraceptives to patients (except in Connecticut and Massachusetts where contraceptives remained illegal under state law until the 1960s). In 1942 the National Birth Control League and its affiliated clinics became Planned Parenthood Federation, with Margaret Sanger as honorary chairperson (League of Women Voters Education Fund, 1982).

Birth Control—Its Health Impact

Over the years the services offered by Planned Parenthood have expanded to include premarital counseling and fertility assistance in addition to the original intent of providing birth-control information to married women. However, the basic rationale of all family planning work in America—today as in 1916 when the first clinic opened its doors—is to promote the health and well-being of mothers and children by preventing unwanted births. Because of the threat which uncontrolled fertility poses, both to maternal health and to that of infants, it is generally accepted today that no community health program can be considered complete if it fails to provide ready access to birth-control devices and information.

Enhancement of maternal and child health through family planning is largely related to one of three basic parameters: 1) age of the mother, 2) interval between births, and 3) total number of births during a woman's reproductive lifetime. A brief examination of each of these factors reveals how uncontrolled fertility has a major impact on mortality and morbidity rates among both women and infants.

Age of Mother

Although the average woman is fertile from her early teens until her late 40s, the biologically optimum period for childbearing is much shorter, extending from approximately 20 years of age to age 30. In fact, research results suggest that simply becoming pregnant is increasingly difficult as women approach middle age. The ability to conceive appears to peak at age 31 and declines steadily every year thereafter. From a safety standpoint, mothers either younger or older than this optimum age span run an increased risk of difficulties or death during pregnancy and childbirth, and their infants are statistically more likely to die than are babies of mothers in their 20s.

Teenage mothers, whose reproductive organs are not yet fully developed, are more likely to die during childbirth than are women in their prime reproductive years. In addition, babies of young mothers have a tendency to be born premature or underweight, factors which greatly increase their susceptibility to infectious diseases and malnutrition. Studies have revealed consistently higher infant mortality rates among babies born to mothers under age 20 as compared to those born to mothers in their late 20s.

Among women over 35, pregnancy poses an increased risk of complications during childbirth; after age 45, statistics show a significant rise in maternal death rates. Mothers over 35 are more likely than younger women to bear a child with congenital disorders such as Down's Syndrome (however, a recent Canadian study of more than half a million births revealed no greater risk of nonchromosomal birth defects among babies born to older mothers than among infants whose mothers were younger). In addition to concerns regarding birth abnormalities, mothers in their 30s and 40s have reason to worry about the general health of their babies. Up to age 30, a pregnant woman has an 89% likelihood of delivering a healthy baby; this level of assurance diminishes by 3.5% for each additional year of maternal age (Baird, Sadnovnick, and Yee, 1991; van Noord-Zaadstra, 1991). Research has shown that babies of women in their 30s and 40s are twice as likely to be born underweight (less than 5.5 pounds) and that, in general, the older a woman is, the greater the potential for reduced fetal growth. Since there is a direct correlation between low birthweight and death during infancy, it is not surprising that these studies found that babies born to mothers aged 40 or older are at much higher risk of dying before their first birthday than are infants born to women in their 20s and 30s (Lee et al., 1988; Friede et al., 1988).

Interval Between Births

Since a developing fetus draws on its mother's nutritional reserves, it should not be surprising that when the interval between successive pregnancies is short, time is insufficient for adequate replenishment of these reserves and serious health problems can be manifested in both woman and infant. Such effects are particularly noticeable among poorly-nourished individuals. While pregnant, a moderately active woman needs about 300 more calories per day than usual; if she is unable to secure this extra amount, her body draws upon its own reserves, with resulting harm both to herself and to her unborn baby. A condition called "maternal depletion syndrome," characterized by premature aging, weakness, and anemia is frequently observed among undernourished women in poor societies, where teenage marriage is typically followed by about 20 years of uninterrupted pregnancy. Such women are particularly likely to die of complications during childbirth or to fall victim to infectious diseases at any time. Their infants, too, face heightened risk. Studies done in rural India revealed that babies born less than two years after a previous birth were 50% more likely to die before their first birthday than were babies born after a birth interval of more than two years. Researchers working with the U.S. Agency for International Development in Bangladesh report that efforts to encourage women to space their pregnancies had a greater impact on reducing infant mortality than did childhood immunization campaigns or oral rehydration therapy.

Total Number of Births

Contrary to the popular notion that mothers with large numbers of children give birth "as easy as rolling off a log," statistics reveal that such women are especially prone to problem pregnancies and death during childbirth. Indeed, the total number of babies born to a woman during her lifetime can have a significant impact on her general state of health.

Generally speaking, a woman's second and third births are the safest; the first birth carries slightly greater risk statistically because it will reveal any physical or genetic abnormalities in the parents that could cause problems. With the fourth pregnancy, risk of maternal death, stillbirth, and infant death begins to rise, increasing sharply with the birth of the fifth and every succeeding child. Health workers in Bangladesh report triple the number of deaths among women giving birth to their eighth child as among those bearing their third. Degree of risk depends to a considerable extent on the socioeconomic status of the mother, the greatest hazards being faced by women from the lowest income groups. However, even among well-fed, affluent women, every birth after the fourth involves an increased degree of danger for both mother and child.

Significantly higher rates of infant and child mortality among higher-order births in poor families seem to be due primarily to poor nutrition, as the limited amount of food available must be divided among many mouths. Unlike their older siblings, the latest born children must survive on reduced average portions during those early years when they are most susceptible to the effects of nutritional deficiency (Eckholm and Newland, 1977).

Thus a family-planning program that provides contraceptive protection for teenage women, women over 35, mothers who have already borne three or more children, and women who have recently given birth can make a very positive contribution to improving public health.

Contraceptive Safety

In assessing the health impact of family planning, one must of course take into account possible risks posed by contraceptive use. There has been considerable controversy in recent years regarding the safety of the birth-control pill and the intrauterine device (IUD), raising public concerns and causing potential contraceptors to turn to less reliable methods or to abandon attempts at birth control altogether. What indeed are the risks and benefits of the most commonly used contraceptives? A brief summary of the most popular methods used in the United States indicates that although various adverse side effects may accompany the use of contraceptives for some women, all common means of contraception entail fewer risks than do pregnancy and childbirth.

Hormonal Contraceptives

Such contraceptives are made of synthetic substances similar to the hormones that occur naturally in women's bodies. They prevent pregnancy by inhibiting ovulation.

Birth-Control Pill.   The most popular method of birth control in the United States, ''the Pill'' is used by approximately 39% of women at risk of an unwanted pregnancy. Available either as a combination pill (containing both estrogen and a progestin) or as a ''mini-pill'' containing progestin only, oral contraceptives, when used correctly, are 97–99% effective in preventing pregnancy. Since the early 1960s when the birth-control pill first became available, safety concerns centered around a possible increased risk of cardiovascular disorders such as blood clots, which could lead to a stroke or heart attack. For this reason medical authorities feel that a decision to use oral contraceptives should be made only after consultation with a health professional, and currently in all Western nations a doctor's prescription is required for the purchase of birth-control pills. Nevertheless, the results of extensive epidemiological research on oral contraceptive safety over more than three decades of pill use indicate that women over 40 are the only group for whom pill use poses a greater health threat than does childbearing; among this group an increase in cardiovascular problems suggests the advisability of discontinuing pill use in favor of other contraceptive methods. However, for younger women, with the exception of those who smoke or have certain medical conditions (e.g. a history of blood clots, heart problems, cancer of the breast or female organs), medical evidence supports the view that the Pill is quite safe. Moreover, contraceptive pills offer users some unexpected health benefits, including significant protection against ovarian and endometrial cancer, pelvic inflammatory disease, iron-deficiency anemia, and fibrocystic breast disease. In addition, women who use oral contraceptives have a lower risk of developing ovarian cysts. Research results to date do not support claims that pill use may increase a woman's risk of breast cancer, though investigation into the possibility continues. Despite some lingering uncertainties regarding breast cancer, the Alan

BOX 3-2

RU-486: Debate Over the French Pill

Will the angry confrontations and violent clashes outside abortion clinics currently polarizing communities from Omaha to Buffalo soon be relegated to the history books? Will the bitter epithets hurled back and forth by placard-wielding supporters and opponents of legalized abortion be supplanted by rational, private discourse between a pregnant woman and her doctor? Answers to these questions, in all likelihood, will hinge on the outcome of negotiations now underway to bring the French antifertility pill, RU-486, to market in the United States.

Approved for use by the French Ministry of Health in the fall of 1988, RU-486 is now available in France, Sweden, and the United Kingdom where more than 120,000 women have taken the drug, proving its effectiveness in 96% of all cases. Nevertheless, its manufacturer, Roussel-Uclaf, until recently expressed no interest in trying to secure FDA approval for marketing the product in the United States, largely due to fears that right-to-life groups would retaliate by launching a boycott against the company's other products.

Why all the fuss over a birth-control pill? Because RU-486 (mifepristone), an antiprogestin, essentially acts as an abortifacient, blocking the action of progesterone, the hormone that prepares the lining of the uterus for embryo implantation. Taken within 7–9 weeks of a missed menstrual period, RU-486 causes the onset of menstruation, flushing the embryo from the uterus and, in effect, terminating the pregnancy.

Experts consider RU-486 to be safer, cheaper, and easier than surgical abortion. Since 1988 when RU-486 became commercially available, complications following use of the drug have been extremely rare. The most common side effect of the abortion pill is heavy menstruation-like bleeding; in addition, some women experience a brief period of light nausea and diarrhea. Most women who have taken RU-496 report having no pain at all, although a small percentage had enough discomfort to require aspirin or some other pain killer. Due to concerns about misuse of the drug, where RU-486 is now legal, Roussel-Uclaf requires at least three visits to a physician. On the first visit the pill will be administered and the patient will then go home, since RU-486 takes at least 36 hours to act on the fetus. Two days later the woman must return to receive an injection of contraction-inducing prostaglandin; generally she will remain at the clinic until the fetus is expelled, usually within three hours of the injection. A follow-up medical exam is subsequently given a week or so later to confirm that the abortion was successful. Careful medical supervision of each RU-486 abortion is deemed essential because improper use of the drug could conceivably result in a damaged fetus being brought to term. The possibility of a black market for RU-486 developing in countries where the drug is not legally available is particularly worrisome because a woman who surreptitiously takes the pill but fails to follow this with the dose of prostaglandin runs the risk of an incomplete abortion with subsequent infection or dangerous bleeding.

Although RU-486 was developed specifically as an abortifacient, its antiprogesterone qualities suggest its usefulness for treating a number of other medical conditions. The drug is already being used in Europe for facilitating difficult childbirth, stimulating uterine contractions and speeding dilation of the cervix; experimental research suggests that it also has potential to block ovulation and serve as an effective late "morning after" pill, acting as a contraceptive when taken between the 14th and 28th day of the menstrual cycle. Cushing's Syndrome, a potentially fatal condition caused by excess production of the hormone cortisol, can be managed more successfully when RU-486 is administered prior to surgery and the growth of inoperable meningioma brain tumors similarly can be halted or reversed with RU-486 treatments. Studies have also shown the drug to be effective against endometrial cancer and endometriosis, the latter a leading cause of infertility among American women. Unfortunately, political opposition to abortion has stymied research on these and other potential medical benefits of RU-486 just as it has denied access for American women to a safer, noninvasive method of abortion.

With the advent of the Clinton Administration to the White House, the chances for RU-486 receiving FDA approval brightened considerably. In the spring of 1994 Roussel-Uclaf donated its U.S. patent rights to the nonprofit Population Council which launched clinical trials of the drug in the fall of that year—a first step in the lengthy process of legalizing the use of RU-486 in the United States. At a time when nearly 90% of U.S. abortions are performed in neighborhood clinics increasingly harassed by disruptive demonstrators, access to the French pill could radically alter the national abortion debate. RU-486, as pro-choice advocates know and antiabortion forces fear, could render the entire issue moot since its availability will make it possible for a woman desiring an abortion to induce fetal loss in the privacy of her doctor's office without acquaintances or protest marchers being any the wiser.

References

Lader, Lawrence. 1991. *RU-486*. Addison Wesley.

Hilts, Philip J. 1993. "Door May Be Open for Abortion Pill to be Sold in U.S." *New York Times,* Feb. 25.

Guttmacher Institute, a private, nonprofit organization specializing in research on contraception, categorically states that "the average woman who has ever used the Pill is less likely to get cancer and die as a result before age 55 than a woman who has never used the Pill."

Norplant.   First approved for use in the United States in December, 1990, Norplant has been hailed as the most radical new form of birth control since the Pill—an extremely safe, nearly 100% effective contraceptive for women weighing less than 150 pounds. Consisting of six small progestin-containing capsules inserted by a health care professional just below the skin of the upper arm, Norplant continuously releases a small amount of contraceptive hormone into a woman's body over a five-year period, providing a consistently high level of protection without any further action on the part of the woman or her partner. A completely reversible method, Norplant begins providing protection within 24 hours after insertion; if at any time during the five-year period of use a woman decides she would like to have a baby, the capsules can be removed in a minor surgical procedure and fertility is immediately restored. Norplant has an excellent safety record, although during the first year after implantation some users experience minor side effects such as irregular menstrual bleeding, weight gain, acne, or rashes. In general, women whose medical condition precludes pill use should avoid Norplant also. Since Norplant is a relatively new contraceptive option, the percentage of women relying on this method is still relatively small. Nevertheless, early indications suggest that potential demand is high, the main limitation being the high up-front cost ($500–800 for the Norplant kit and doctor fee for insertion). Among women who are using Norplant, 98% report satisfaction with the method—the highest favorable opinion rating for any contraceptive currently available.

Depo-Provera.   A relatively new birth-control option for American women, this injectable contraceptive was approved by the FDA in 1992 after more than 20 years of use in over 90 countries worldwide. Administered as an injection in the arm or buttocks every 3 months, Depo-Provera fills a need for women who want the reliability of hormonal contraceptives without having to worry about forgetting to take a daily pill. Depo-Provera is a synthetic form of progesterone that works by inhibiting ovulation, and it is 99% effective in preventing pregnancy. Worldwide, more than 30 million women have taken the drug since it was first introduced in 1969 and its overall safety record is good. Side effects among women receiving a Depo-Provera injection are similar to those experienced by Norplant recipients or users of the progestin-only "mini-pill"; in addition, about half the women who use Depo-Provera for a year or more experience **amenorrhea** (no menstrual period).

Surgical Sterilization

The second most popular method of family limitation in the United States (and the top choice among married women), sterilization is a logical alternative for those who have already attained their desired family size. Currently, sterilization is the contraceptive method of choice for 31% of all sexually active women and for almost half of all married couples. Vasectomy, or male sterilization, is a simple operation involving an incision in the scrotum to cut or block the vas deferens (tubes which carry semen from the testes to the penis) and accounts for slightly more than a third of the sterilizations performed in the United States each year. Vasectomy most often is performed under local anesthesia in a doctor's office, the entire procedure generally taking less than 30 minutes. In rare cases minor post-operative infections may develop, but in general male sterilization is among the safest of all birth-control methods. Female sterilization, or tubal ligation, entails a slightly higher degree of risk since it involves sealing off the fallopian tubes—an operating room procedure done under general anesthesia. Although major complications are rare, they occur in an estimated 1.7% of cases. Sterilization, both male and female, is more than

Figure 3-1 Preferred Contraceptive Methods by U.S. Women Aged 15–44 at Risk of Unwanted Pregnancy

Method	% Total	% Married	% Unmarried
All users	94	97	92
Pill	39	28	52
Sterilization	31	48	11
Female	19	27	10
Male	12	21	1
Condom	25	19	33
Withdrawal	8	6	11
Rhythm method	4	5	4
Diaphragm	4	4	4
Sponge	3	3	3
Suppository	3	1	3
Douche	3	*	1
IUD	1	1	1
Foam	1	1	1
Cream/jelly	1	1	1
Implant	1	*	1
Cervical cap	*	*	*
Nonusers	6	3	8
Total	100	100	100

*Less than 0.5%

Note: The sum of the proportions using each method exceeds the total proportion of users because some respondents used more than one method.

Source: 1992 Ortho Birth Control Study

99% effective in preventing pregnancy and ends any further expense, fuss, or bother related to contraceptive use. However, sterilization is a permanent method of birth control and such a decision should not be made lightly. Efforts to date at reopening the vas deferens or fallopian tubes have met with minimal success, so sterilization should be regarded as irreversible.

Intra-uterine Device (IUD)

Once among the most popular forms of contraception in the United States and still widely relied upon by women in other countries (particularly in China where it is the most common method of birth control), the IUD today is the method of choice for only 1% of contracepting American women. Indeed, by the mid-1980s IUDs had nearly disappeared from the marketplace, withdrawn by manufacturers fearing legal liability for alleged harmful side effects of the device (a situation brought about by thousands of lawsuits against the A.H. Robins pharmaceutical firm, charging that the company's Dalkon Shield had caused numerous cases of bleeding, pelvic infections, and resultant infertility among users). Nevertheless, physicians and manufacturers consider most IUDs both safe and reliable. Recently the Paragard T 380 A, effective for eight years, was introduced into the marketplace, joining the only other American IUD, Progestasert, a hormone-releasing IUD that must be replaced yearly. Among malnourished, anemic women IUD use has sometimes been correlated with increased blood loss during menstruation. For healthy, well-fed women, however, IUDs are as safe as the Pill and nearly as dependable. The major problem associated with IUD use is an increased risk of pelvic inflammatory disease (PID) which, if severe, can result in permanent infertility. IUDs are not recommended for women who have never been pregnant and in general are considered most suitable for young women in mutually monogamous relationships (PID incidence is highest among women with several sex partners) who want no more children but are not yet ready for an irreversible surgical sterilization.

Spermicides

Spermicidal foams, creams, suppositories, or gels must be inserted into the vagina within an hour before having intercourse and must be replenished if intercourse is repeated. They act to form both a physical and chemical barrier to sperm and are available without a prescription. While few problems are associated with spermicides (those who experience a burning sensation or irritation should avoid their use), their effectiveness when used alone is only 70–80%.

Barrier Methods

Barrier methods employ some device that prevents the egg and sperm from uniting, thus preventing fertilization.

Vaginal Contraceptives.   Diaphragms, cervical caps, sponges, and the recently introduced female condom all work by keeping egg and sperm apart. (The polyurethane female condom is also intended to provide some protection against sexually transmitted disease, but medical authorities caution that for best protection, male latex condoms are preferable.) When used in conjunction with spermicides, vaginal contraceptives have few, if any, adverse physiological effects and are moderately effective at preventing pregnancy. Both the sponge and the female condom have an estimated failure rate of about 1 in 4; the cervical cap and diaphragm are somewhat more trustworthy, with failure rates ranging from 6% for a diaphragm used with spermicide to 18% for the cervical cap.

Condoms.   Like the vaginal contraceptives, condoms cause no adverse health effects other than an occasional allergic reaction to rubber among some individuals. Used alone, their reliability is significantly less than pills or IUDs, but in combination with vaginal contraceptives and in situations where legal, early abortion is available, they offer the safest means, other than sterilization, of totally effective fertility control. The third most commonly used contraceptive method in the United States today, the condom is being actively promoted by health agencies not only for birth-control reasons but also as an effective prophylactic against the spread of AIDS and other sexually transmitted diseases. Concerns about HIV transmission were pivotal in a 1992 decision by the Japanese Health Ministry not to reverse that country's longstanding prohibition against the sale of oral contraceptives (while Japanese women can obtain the Pill for purposes of regulating their menstrual cycle, Japan is unique in banning the use of oral contraceptives for family-planning purposes). Currently condoms are the principal method of birth control in Japan, used by over 80% of married couples, and the government feared that legalization of the Pill would contribute to a decline in condom use, thereby contributing to the spread of AIDS!

Natural Family Planning

Frequently referred to as the "rhythm method" or "periodic abstinence," this approach to birth control carries no health risk but has a consistently high failure rate. To utilize this method, a woman attempts to determine when she is ovulating by charting daily bodily functions such as basal temperature (i.e. temperature when the body is at its lowest level of metabolic activity, usually measured before getting out of bed in the morning) and by examining her cervical mucus. The problem is that many women experience monthly variations in their menstrual cycle, making accurate calculation of the fertile period problematic. In addition, the abstinence from sexual activity during fertile periods which must be rigorously observed by couples using natural family planning requires a high degree of motivation and cooperation between partners and can significantly limit the number of days each month when couples can have intercourse free from fear of unwanted pregnancy.

The success of the family planning movement in the United States is evident from surveys which reveal that among sexually active women at risk of an unwanted pregnancy, fully 94% are using some method of birth control. Among married women the figure is even higher—97%. In an age when sexual activity seems to be as popular a pastime as it ever was, an even more convincing indicator of contraceptive usage is the fact that the average number of children per U.S. couple is now just two, one of the lowest figures in our history. Apparently most Americans now agree with the family planning sloganeers who affirm that "A small family is a happy family" (Goldberg, 1993; Forrest and Fordyce, 1993).

Family Planning in the Third World

Whereas the birth-control movement in the United States and Europe grew out of the conviction that health and social considerations demanded that women receive help in regulating their fertility, the impetus for family planning in most Third World countries grew directly out of concerns over the high rates of post-World War II population growth and the awareness that this "population explosion" would impede their rate of economic development. Only after family-planning programs had been launched did Third World governments attempt to justify their support for such efforts on the basis of protecting maternal and child health and of guaranteeing couples the means for regulating the spacing and number of their children. This superficial shift in emphasis constituted a publicly acceptable rationale for reconciling the interests of the nation with those of individuals.

In most cases, the initial promoters of family planning in the Third World were private organizations such as International Planned Parenthood Federation, the Ford and Rockefeller Foundations, and the Population Council. By the 1960s, however, even earlier in some countries, national governments were becoming increasingly active in establishing their own family-planning programs, usually in conjunction with their ministries of health. Generally they were assisted by the private organizations mentioned above and, in later years, by the U.S. Agency for International Development and various United Nations agencies such as the World Bank and the United Nations Fund for Population Activities (UNFPA). Funds, both governmental and private, allocated for family-planning work increased sharply after the mid-1960s, but even today constitute a very small percentage of most national budgets. Today the vast majority of developing countries have some sort of family-planning program in operation. How effective those programs are in achieving their goal of reducing national birth rates will in large part determine the success of such countries in raising living standards and ensuring a bright future for their people.

Spreading the Word

Since the main impetus for implementing family planning came from central governments or outside agencies rather than reflecting grassroots interest, as was the case in North America and Europe, success required intensive efforts to reach all elements of society, the majority of whom lived at subsistence level in rural areas, often isolated from adequate medical care and frequently illiterate. Such people had to be made aware of the existence of fertility-regulating methods, provided with regular access to the same, and convinced that it was in their own best interest to use them.

In pursuing this goal, family-planning workers in Third World countries adopted methods radically different from those used in Western nations. Mobile units in the form of specially equipped vans or buses have been essential in carrying health workers and equipment into villages far from any hospital. Trained field workers actively attempt to recruit

Figure 3-2 Birth Control Guide

Efficacy rates given in this chart are estimates based on a number of different studies. They should be understood as yearly estimates, with those dependent on conscientious use subject to a greater chance of human error and reduced effectiveness. For comparison, 60 to 85 percent of sexually active women using no contraception would be expected to become pregnant in a year.

Type	Estimated Effectivenes	Risks	STD Protection	Convenience	Availability
Male Condom	About 85%	Rarely, irritation and allergic reactions	Latex condoms help protect against sexually transmitted diseases, including herpes and AIDS	Applied immediately before intercourse	Nonprescription
Female Condom	An estimated 74–79%	Rarely, irritation and allergic reactions	May give some protection against sexually transmitted diseases, including herpes and AIDS; not as effective as male latex condom	Applied immediately before intercourse; used only once and discarded	Nonprescription
Spermicides Used Alone	70–80%	Rarely, irritation and allergic reactions	Unknown	Applied no more than one hour before intercourse	Nonprescription
Sponge	72–82%	Rarely, irritation and allergic reactions; difficulty in removal; very rarely, toxic shock syndrome	None	Can be inserted hours before intercourse and left in place up to 24 hours; used only once and discarded	Nonprescription
Diaphragm with Spermicide	82–94%	Rarely, irritation and allergic reactions; bladder infection; very rarely, toxic shock syndrome	None	Inserted before intercourse; can be left in place 24 hours, but additional spermicide must be inserted if intercourse is repeated	Rx
Cervical Cap with Spermicide	At least 82%	Abnormal Pap test; vaginal or cervical infections; very rarely, toxic shock syndrome	None	Can remain in place for 48 hours, not necessary to re-apply spermicide upon repeated intercourse; may be difficult to insert	Rx

Source: *FDA Consumer*, September 1993.

Type	Estimated Effectivenes	Risks	STD Protection	Convenience	Availability
Pills	97%–99%	Blood clots, heart attacks and strokes, gall-bladder disease, liver tumors, water retention, hypertension, mood changes, dizziness and nausea; not for smokers	None	Pill must be taken on daily schedule, regardless of the frequency of intercourse	Rx
Implant (Norplant)	99%	Menstrual cycle irregularity; head-aches, nervous-ness, depression, nausea, dizzi-ness, change of appetite, breast tenderness, weight gain, en-largement of ovaries and/or fallopian tubes, excessive growth of body and facial hair; may subside after first year	None	Effective 24 hours after implantation for approximately 5 years; can be removed by physician at any time	Rx; minor outpatient surgical procedure
Injection (Depo-Provera)	99%	Amenorrhea, weight gain, and other side effects similar to those with Norplant	None	One injection every three months	Rx
IUD	95–96%	Cramps, bleed-ing, pelvic inflam-matory disease, infertility; rarely, perforation of the uterus	None	After insertion, stays in place until physician removes it	Rx
Periodic Abstinence (NFP)	Very variable, perhaps 53–86%	None	None	Requires frequent monitoring of body functions and periods of abstinence	Instructions from physician or clinic
Surgical Sterilization	Over 99%	Pain, infection, and, for female tubal ligation, possible surgical complications	None	Vasectomy is a one-time procedure usually performed in a doctor's office; tubal ligation is a one-time procedure performed in an operating room	Surgery

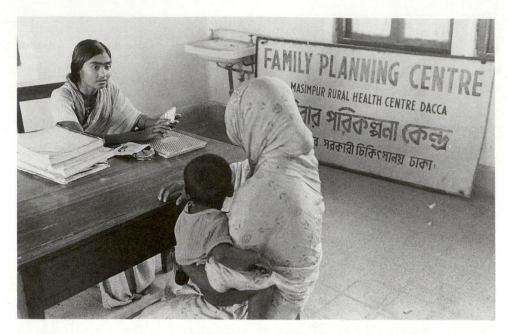

A family-planning worker in Bangladesh advises the wife of a rickshaw driver on spacing her children. Such counselors often divide their time between working at health centers and visiting nearby villages. [Agency for International Development]

contraceptive acceptors, meeting with women's groups, farmers, and so on, to persuade them of the advantages inherent in limiting family size. Considerable reliance has been placed on mass media communications. Advertisements in newspapers, on radio, and in cinemas regularly stress the benefits of small families while roadside billboards or posters on buses, in train stations—even painted on the hides of farm animals—proclaim such messages as "Two or Three—Enough!" Some governments have attracted participation by offering gifts to contraceptive acceptors. In India thousands of men agreed to vasectomies in order to receive a free transistor radio; in Thailand the government has sponsored free distribution of condoms at sporting events or all-expense paid tours of Bangkok's temples for rural men agreeing to sterilization!

Most Third World programs, like those in the West, offer a choice of birth-control methods and generally include information on child-spacing, nutrition, and child-care along with contraceptive services. Some also enlist the services of midwives, teachers, or other respected community leaders to act as distributors of contraceptives, particularly pills and condoms, thereby giving these influential individuals a vested interest in the success of such programs.

Motivation—The Key to Success

Efforts to reduce significantly birth rates in developing nations have had mixed results. The World Fertility Survey, conducted under United

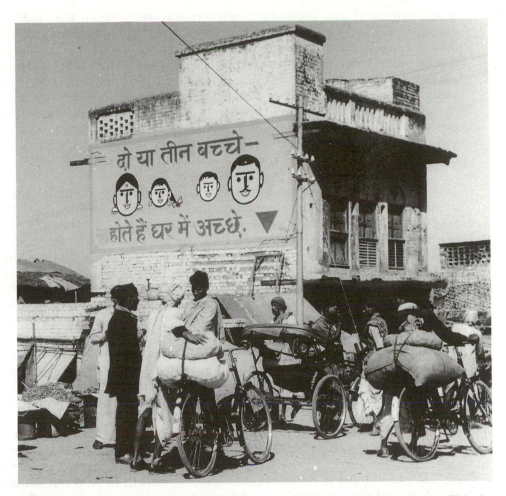

Wall paintings and billboards throughout India carry the family-planning message. This sign with the symbolic family of four bears the slogan, ''Two are enough!'' [Agency for International Development]

Nations auspices during the late 1970s and early 1980s, revealed that fertility has been declining in all major regions of the world except Africa, but that none of the Third World countries has yet achieved a birth rate under 20, the average for developed nations. The survey made it clear that the vast majority of women in such countries knew of the existence of at least one modern method of contraception, yet only 32% of such women, or their husbands, were using some form of birth control, compared to 72% in developed countries (Lightbourne and Singh, 1982). To some extent, failure to use contraceptives is related to easy access; not surprisingly, contraceptive use was higher in communities where a family-planning clinic or other source of contraceptive supplies was close by—a particularly important factor among people using either pills or condoms. A far more important determinant in contraceptive practice, however, is motivation—the desire of couples to limit family size. In many parts of the developing world economic and social factors interact to perpetuate the traditional attitudes toward childbearing. For very practical reasons, many Third World couples have concluded that although two or three children per family might be in the best interest of society, they want and feel they need a significantly larger number themselves. In the absence of coercion, when individual and societal needs conflict, personal desires generally prevail.

Factors contributing to this continued preference for large families among many Third World couples include high infant mortality rates, the view of children as "social security," the desire for sons, and the low educational and economic status of women.

High Infant Mortality Rates. Although the drop in infant and child death rates was a major factor in fueling the explosive growth of Third World populations, such rates are still substantially above the levels prevailing in developed countries. In many parts of Africa, for example, infant death rates are over 100, as compared to about 9 in the United States. The World Fertility Survey found that at the personal level, fertility consistently increased as the number of child deaths increased. Where childhood deaths are common, it is difficult to convince parents to limit themselves to two births.

Children as "Social Security". In most Third World countries, lack of extensive social welfare programs means that most parents are dependent on their grown children for financial support in their post-retirement years. In such cultures, responsibility for elderly parents falls primarily on the sons; thus a couple may feel the need to produce at least two or three boys to ensure their being adequately provided for in old age. In addition, even young children may be regarded as financial assets, since their labor is needed on the farm or around the home. In such situations an additional baby is not viewed as another mouth to feed but rather as an additional pair of hands to gather wood, tend livestock, haul water, and so forth.

Desire for Sons. Many family-planning program administrators fear that the preference for sons rather than daughters will keep fertility rates high in many developing countries. Son preference is apparent in surveys of American couples but is even more pronounced among parents in most Third World nations. In such cultures, doubt about whether they will have enough boys concerns parents who are asked to produce no more than two or three offspring. A woman's status, even the stability of her marriage, is dependent on her having sons. To some extent, such preferences are based on economic concerns: sons can support parents in old age while daughters are a financial liability, often requiring an expensive dowry at time of marriage. In some societies daughters are considered expensive luxuries. Wherever such views are strongly held it is unlikely that couples will voluntarily limit their families to two children if the first two happen to be daughters. If a couple desires two or three boys, it is quite likely that they will ultimately have four to six children, since the male-female sex ratio at birth is almost equal (Williamson, 1978).

The bias in favor of sons has taken a tragic twist in recent years, with a noticeable rise in female infanticide in several countries. After promulgation of the one-child policy in China—where the age-old view that "more sons mean more happiness" still prevails—numerous cases were reported of newborn girls being murdered by parents who hoped that a second try would produce a boy. More recently, parents' efforts to ensure the birth of male offspring have been given a major boost by the advent of a modern device whose impact is revolutionizing Asian societies—the ultrasound scanner. In Korea, China, India—indeed throughout Asia—ultrasound and other medical technologies like amniocentesis are being used not to detect developmental abnormalities but to learn the sex of the fetus. And if it's a girl, abortion provides a quick solution to the problem. By the early 1990s, more than 100,000 ultrasound scanners were in use in China; even illiterate peasants in remote villages are now aware of the existence of machines that can tell the sex of an unborn child. In India, the widespread practice of aborting female fetuses led authorities in Bombay to prohibit prenatal tests for women under age 35 unless they had a family history of birth defects (an earlier survey conducted in that city's hospitals revealed that of 8000 abortions performed, all but one were of female fetuses). While the use of medical procedures for sex selection has generated sharp criticism among some commentators in India, others defend the practice on the grounds that it is preferable for a woman to have abortions rather than produce six or seven children in hopes of having one or two boys. Citing the abuse often directed at Indian wives who bear too many daughters, one physician defended the practice of sex selection as a "lesser evil," declaring that "it is better to have feticide than matricide." Ironically, with the exception of a few vague warnings in the official press about future "bachelor villages" where wives will be a scarce commodity, few Asian parents today seem concerned about the social consequences of a population where young women are vastly outnumbered by young men. While some government officials recognize the problem and are trying to curtail use of ultrasound scanners, the devices are now so widespread, corruption so rampant, and the desire for sons so strong that curbing the abuse of medical technology is likely to prove impossible (Kristof, 1993; Green, 1986).

Low Educational and Economic Status of Women.   Birth rates today are highest in those parts of the world where women have little schooling and where opportunities for paid employment outside the home are few. In such societies, a woman's worth is measured in terms of her childbearing abilities. Such women, striving to maintain favor with their husbands and in-laws, are unlikely to respond favorably to the idea of family limitation. In addition, illiterate women or women with only an elementary education are less likely than their better educated sisters to have heard about modern contraceptive techniques or to know how to use them. Surveys indicate that providing women with at least a secondary school education is one of the most effective ways of reducing the birth rate in developing countries. In general, fertility drops noticeably as the level of female education increases, primarily because educated women tend to

BOX 3-3

The Elusive Quest for ZPG: India's Family-Planning Program

According to the *Guiness Book of World Records*, the most common family name on the face of the planet is **Chang**—not particularly surprising in light of the fact that every fifth person in the world today is Chinese. However, a generation or so hence the Changs may cede their preeminence to the **Patels** or **Singhs** or **Mehtas** as India overtakes China as the world's most populous nation. Indeed, with an annual growth rate hovering around 2% and with 36% of its people still in their pre-reproductive years, India could well surpass the two billion mark before population growth halts.

India's continued rapid pace of growth is ironic in light of the fact that it was one of the first countries in the world to concede that high rates of population increase were hindering national development. Soon after independence from colonial rule in 1947 the Indian government adopted an official policy goal of lowering fertility rates to replacement level in order to achieve a stable population size. At that time India's population was under 400 million, increasing by about 7 million a year. By the early 1990s, the annual increment of growth approximated 18 million, with total population size projected to reach one billion before the end of the decade. How is it that after more than 40 years of trying to stabilize growth, Indian leaders see their country poised to become the world's demographic giant? A look at the strengths and weaknesses of the Indian family-planning program illustrates the challenges inherent in an effort to bring about behavioral change in a traditional Third World society.

Although officially launched in 1951, India's family-planning program got off to a slow and unimpressive start. Vastly underfunded during its early years, the new program was confined to providing services at urban clinics and relied exclusively on the promotion of periodic abstinence (rhythm method)—an unreliable form of birth control and particularly inappropriate in a culture where high levels of illiteracy rendered the concept of "safe" and "unsafe" periods mysterious indeed. The government's efforts floundered along, making little headway and receiving only perfunctory attention from national leaders until the results of the 1961 census revealed an unexpected surge in the population growth rate from a relatively moderate 1.5% during the 1940s to almost 2% during the 1950s. Alarmed, national leaders increased funding to permit expansion of program activities into the previously unserved rural areas where three-fourths of India's people live. They also initiated a mass media effort, employing catchy slogans and billboard advertising to promote the small family ideal. Throughout the 1960s, IUD insertions were the focus of government family-planning efforts. Unfortunately, widespread reports of complications (not uncommon among anemic or malnourished women) and lack of adequate follow-up care led to a sharp decline in IUD acceptance by the end of the decade.

When the 1971 census results revealed still-rising rates of population growth, the government responded with additional measures, prohibiting the marriage of girls under 18 (a law that has been nearly impossible to enforce) and enacting one of the Third World's most liberal abortion laws (interestingly, there has been virtually no public controversy in India over the issue of legalized abortion; however, the practice is not very common.

With the failure of the IUD effort,

family-planning strategies shifted to an emphasis on male sterilization. Prizes or cash awards were offered to men who agreed to undergo vasectomy and early statistics appeared impressive (however, a closer look at sterilization figures revealed that a significant percentage of vasectomy clients were men whose wives were in their forties or older—well beyond their prime reproductive years). In 1975 the vasectomy campaign took a fateful (and fatal) turn when the powerful and politically ambitious son of then-Prime Minister Indira Gandhi decided to espouse population control as a high-priority personal commitment. During a two-year period of emergency rule, when usual democratic procedures were suspended, lower-level officials attempted to curry favor with Gandhi by harassing and sometimes coercing thousands of men to submit to vasectomy in an effort to achieve regional sterilization quotas. During these months male government employees frequently were denied promotions, desired transfers, food ration cards, and various other benefits unless they could produce a vasectomy certificate. Rumors spread of men being rounded up in railway stations and forcibly sterilized. In some rural areas, wary villagers slept in their fields at night, fearing police raids during which all men captured would be vasectomized. Some Indian states at this time seriously debated legislation that would have made sterilization mandatory for any couple with three or more children. From 1976–1977 the number of men with vasectomies jumped from 2.7 million to 8.3 million, but at the grass-roots level opposition to the campaign of forced sterilization was mounting, occasionally erupting into riots and demonstrations. When general elections were held in 1977, the Gandhi government was decisively defeated, largely as a result of public anger at the excesses committed in the name of family planning.

The debacle of the coerced sterilization effort represented a devastating setback to India's family-planning program. For years afterwards, government officials for the most part distanced themselves from any active association with birth-control efforts, seldom going further than to support maternal and child health services. In a semantic break with the past, the name of the program was changed in the 1980s to "family welfare program," and in yet another about-face, the contraceptive strategy emphasis shifted from male to *female* sterilization. In spite of a conspicuous absence of strong public support, India's leaders significantly increased government funding for family-planning activities. Only since the mid-1991 election of Prime Minister Narasimha Rao has the Indian government once again assumed an active leadership role in promoting the family welfare program—but doubts remain that the overdue renewal of interest will be translated into the fundamental changes necessary if the effort is to achieve its desired impact.

While Indian family-planning initiatives have the advantage today of strong political support and steadily increasing (though still inadequate) funding, the program nevertheless is characterized by several glaring weaknesses that must be resolved if national goals are ever to be attained.

Overreliance on sterilization as the chief means of limiting fertility is the main reason for the program's negative public image. Family-planning workers spend an inordinate amount of time recruiting clients in order to meet sterilization targets set by the central bureaucracy, and the fact that they receive a cash bonus for each client recruited provides temptation for abuse.

The near-absence of alternative reversible contraceptive options essentially means that the needs of young couples who would like to postpone childbearing or to space intended births are largely neglected. While in theory the government program provides four contraceptive choices—sterilization, IUDs, condoms, and pills—in fact only sterilization and IUDs have been routinely available throughout the country. Birth-control pills and condoms can be readily obtained in urban areas but are difficult to find in many regions in the countryside. Realizing that a much wider range of fertility control options is needed in order to increase contraceptive use, the Indian government recently announced plans to introduce, on a limited basis, both Norplant and a new injectable contraceptive.

Another serious deterrent to public acceptance of family-planning services is the widespread perception that clinic staff are discourteous to clients and unwilling to provide follow-up care to the patients they so eagerly recruit for sterilization. At some clinics, women giving birth to a second or subsequent child report considerable pressure to agree to sterilization before returning home; in a few cases, new mothers have had IUDs inserted without their knowledge or consent. While the quality of health care providers in India is generally quite high, many rural clinics are staffed by inexperienced doctors fresh out of medical school, most of whom received minimal training in family planning or public health. Physicians' lack of knowledge regarding correct use and possible side effects of reversible birth-control methods, particularly the contraceptive pill and new hormonal implants and injectables, is a major deterrent to increasing contraceptive use.

The virtual absence of an effective public education effort geared to the special informational needs of a semi-literate or illiterate audience is another glaring weakness of the Indian program. Although mass media advertising has created nationwide awareness of the concept of family limitation, there is an enormous unmet need for educational materials on specific contraceptive methods and for trained workers who can convey such information in language clients can understand.

Finally, perhaps the most essential element in achieving India's population goals is improving the status of Indian women. By expanding girls' access to education (only 39% of females in India are literate, compared to 64% of males), supporting programs to encourage later marriage, and increasing opportunities for female employment, the government could help to create a cultural climate conducive to fertility reduction. Evidence that such a transition is possible even in the absence of marked economic development can be seen in the case of Kerala, a state at the southwestern tip of India where 87% of women are literate, contraception is practiced by 80% of couples, and the two-child family is the norm. It will require a major restructuring of India's family-planning program and a major commitment of additional funding to extend the fertility reduction achievements of Kerala to the rest of the country. However, given the mounting social and environmental pressures posed by the demographic nightmare, India's leaders have no choice but to redouble their efforts to reach the stabilization goal proclaimed nearly a half century ago.

Reference

Conly, Shanti R., and Sharon L. Camp. 1992. *India's Family-Planning Challenge: From Rhetoric to Action.* Country Study Series #2, The Population Crisis Committee.

marry later, have greater opportunity for employment outside the home, are more aware of the advantages of smaller family size, and understand how to practice contraception more effectively (Lightbourne, 1982).

Such factors support the contention of many demographers that broad-based social and economic changes must precede or accompany population programs in developing nations if population growth is ever to be stabilized; simply making contraceptives more widely available will not be enough to overcome traditional biases that favor large families.

Family Planning versus Population Control

With few exceptions, the family-planning programs currently operating in most countries, the United States included, are aimed at helping couples to have the number of children they want. An implicit assumption in such programs is that most modern couples desire to control their fertility, but theoretically if a childless couple came to a clinic wanting assistance in producing 12 offspring, they would be helped to do so. The primary goal of such programs is to reduce birth rates by ensuring that "every child is a wanted child" through the prevention of unplanned pregnancies. Such a program, accurately designated as "family planning," makes no attempt to look at the implications of population growth from a societal standpoint, but rather from a purely individual one. In light of the impact that population growth has on depletion of natural resources and on environmental quality in general, many people today question whether reliance on family planning to curb population growth will be sufficient.

Obviously, the crucial consideration in family planning is the number of children the average couple says it wants. For population growth to stabilize (i.e. to attain ZPG), couples must just reproduce themselves. In developed countries, where infant mortality rates are relatively low, this means that an average of 2.1 children per family would maintain a stable population size. In the United States, with average family size currently standing at 2 children each, family planning alone will provide the means to achieve ZPG, assuming a continuation of present reproductive behavior (always a risky assumption!). In most of the developing world, by contrast, simply helping couples to prevent unwanted births cannot stabilize population growth because the majority of couples want more than the number necessary to achieve stabilization. Since infant mortality rates are slightly higher in Third World countries than in the West, an average family size of 2.3 children (rather than 2.1) would be required to attain ZPG. However, in every one of these nations, the preferred number of children per family is greater than this, averaging 4.7 in the Third World as a whole, but as high as 7 or 8 in some African countries and 6 in parts of the Middle East. A family-planning program that assists a Kenyan woman in having "only" 7 babies when she probably would have had 10 without contraceptives is certainly of benefit to the woman involved, but it does little to help stabilize population growth in Kenya.

In such cases, critics contend, what is needed is not family planning, but rather programs aimed at population control. A true population control policy would represent a conscious decision on the part of society (or the government) to establish an optimum population size for that society given the availability of natural resources, the carrying capacity of that society's environment, and other such considerations. Once such a decision is made, policies would be implemented to achieve that population size. For example, if a government decides that its population is too small, it might promote childbearing by giving cash allowances or tax deductions for each additional child, special bonuses for "Hero Mothers," or by encouraging immigration. A case in point is that of the former East Germany where, prior to unification, the Communist government pursued a pronatalist policy that had a demonstrable impact on declining national fertility rates. To encourage couples to produce more children, the East German authorities increased paid maternity leave from 18 to 26 weeks for the first baby—a benefit that was extended to a full year for mothers with two or more children. In a nation where virtually all women were employed outside the home, this policy was perceived as a major improvement in the well-being of women with children and led to a fertility increase of about 20% (Heilig, Buttner, and Lutz, 1990).

A population control policy to halt growth would undoubtedly involve less popular moves; the world's most ambitious and widely discussed population control policy is the one currently being pursued in the People's Republic of China. The Chinese government has implemented a program aimed at rapidly stabilizing growth at a level only slightly higher than its present population size by urging couples to have no more than one child. Though such a program would be extremely controversial in a democratic nation (indeed, reports out of China indicate a certain amount of resistance even in that tightly controlled society), the idea of striving to maintain human numbers at or below the carrying capacity of their environment makes eminently good sense. Demographers and environmentalists alike will be viewing the Chinese experiment with great interest to see what lessons it has to offer for an increasingly crowded world■

References

Baird, P. A., A. D. Sadovnick, and I. M. L. Yee. 1991. "Maternal Age and Birth Defects: A Popluation Study." *Lancet* 337:527.

Eckholm, Erik, and Kathleen Newland. 1977. "Health: The Family Planning Factor." *Worldwatch Paper 10*, Worldwatch Institute.

Forrest, Jacqueline Darroch, and Richard R. Fordyce. 1993. "Women's Contraceptive Attitudes and Use in 1992." *Family Planning Perspectives* 25, no. 4 (July/Aug.).

Friede, A. et al. 1988. "Older Maternal Age and Infant Mortality in the United States." *Obstetrics and Gynecology* 72:152.

Goldberg, Merle S. 1993. "Choosing a Contraceptive." *FDA Consumer* (Sept.).

Green, Laura. 1986. "Amniocentesis as a Weapon." *Chicago Tribune*, Sept. 9.

Heilig, Gerhard, Thomas Buttner, and Wolfgang Lutz. 1990. "Germany's Population: Turbulent Past, Uncertain Future." *Population Bulletin* 45, no. 4 (Dec.).

Kleinman, R. L., and P. Senanayake. 1984. *Breastfeeding, Fertility, and Contraception*. IPPF Medical Publications.

Kristof, Nicholas D. 1993. "Peasants in China Discover New Way to Weed Out Girls." *New York Times*, July 21.

League of Women Voters Education Fund. 1982. *Public Policy on Reproductive Choice*. No. 286 (July).

Lee, K. S. et al. 1988. "Maternal Age and Incidence of Low Birth Weight at Term: A Population Study." *American Journal of Obstetrics and Gynecology* 158:84.

Lightbourne, Robert Jr., and Susheela Singh, with Cynthia P. Green. 1982. "The World Fertility Survey: Charting Global Childbearing." *Population Bulletin* 37, no. 1. Population Reference Bureau.

McLaren, Angus A. 1990. *A History of Contraception*. Basil Blackwell, Ltd.

Riddle, John M. 1992. *Contraception and Abortion from the Ancient World to the Renaissance*. Harvard University Press.

Stokes, Bruce. 1980. "Men and Family Planning." *Worldwatch Paper 41*. Worldwatch Institute.

Van Noord-Zaadstra, B. M. et al. 1991. "Delaying Childbearing: Effect of Age on Fecundity and Outcome of Pregnancy." *British Medical Journal* 302:1361.

Weiss, Peter. 1993. "The Contraceptive Potential of Breastfeeding in Bangladesh." *Studies in Family Planning* 24, no. 2 (March/April).

Williamson, Nancy E. 1978. "Boys or Girls? Parents' Preferences and Sex Control." *Population Bulletin* 33, no. 1. Population Reference Bureau.

The People-Food Predicament

One man's hunger is every man's hunger. One man's need is everyman's need.

—Binay Ranjan Sen (former Director General, FAO)

Today we must proclaim a bold objective—that within a decade no child will go to bed hungry, that no family will fear for its next day's bread, and that no human being's future and capacities will be stunted by malnutrition.

—Secretary of State Henry Kissinger

In the early post-World War II years, attainment of the lofty goals proclaimed by Secretary of State Kissinger at the 1974 U.N.-sponsored World Food Conference appeared within reach. From 1950 until 1984 the world's farmers were successful in producing increased quantities of food more rapidly than the world's parents were producing babies. The global grain harvest more than doubled, rising from 624 million tons in 1950 to 1.6 billion tons in 1984. In spite of spiralling population figures, per capita availability of food also increased steadily during the period, resulting in impressive nutrition gains in many Third World countries. This favorable overall trend was somewhat deceptive, however, for global food production averages were largely reflective of the massive increase in North American crop yields during those years and masked the gloomier statistics which showed that in many of the poorer nations per capita increase in food production had halted by the late 1950s due to high rates of population growth. A decade later, a reverse trend became evident in some Third World regions, even while global averages conveyed the impression that all was well on the food front. Since 1967 Africa's baby boom has resulted in a 15% drop in food output per person on that continent; since 1981 Latin America has experienced a similar decline.

General optimism about world food security was given a jolt in the early 1970s when a combination of factors caused an abrupt, though temporary, halt to the steady increase in per capita food supply that the world's people had come to take for granted. Several years of bad weather (floods in some areas, droughts in others) sharply reduced harvests in several of the world's major grain-growing areas. Huge purchases of American wheat by the Soviet Union in 1972, the largest food import deal in history up to that time, initiated the upward surge in food prices that has continued to the present. Food price stability, which had characterized the preceding two decades, suddenly vanished as the world price of grain doubled within months. While sharply escalating farm prices undoubtedly had a devastating impact on nutritional levels among the world's poor, it provided agriculturalists with a financial incentive to expand production, which they promptly did. In the United States, all the cropland idled under the Soil Bank program was returned to cultivation; elsewhere in the developing world, the resource-intensive technologies of the Green Revolution became profitable and once again overall production increased. Until as recently as the mid-1980s, news of huge crop surpluses dominated the farm pages of newspapers and laments of a worldwide "grain glut" were heard from Chicago to Melbourne. Even Western Europe, reliant on food imports for the past two hundred years, became a major grain exporter during those golden years.

Behind the encouraging figures, however, some worrisome trends were becoming evident. After nearly 40 years of steady growth in world food output, a significant slowdown became apparent in many of the world's most populous countries. In India, grain production has been stagnant since 1983—at a time when India's population continues to increase by 18 million yearly; in China, agricultural output has dropped since 1984's peak harvest; Indonesia and Mexico have witnessed a leveling-off of their production, while in Japan, Taiwan, and South Korea grain output has been declining for years. In contrast to the 3% annual increases in grain harvests that characterized the period between 1950 and 1984, during the past decade world grain output has grown by just 1% a year—while world population figures continue to climb at a 1.6% annual rate. This gap between grain production and people production means that food availability *per capita* has actually declined by about 11% since the mid-1980s, even though the annual global grain harvest continues to grow in absolute terms, albeit at an ever-slower pace.

Of course "man does not live by bread alone"—livestock production and fisheries also contribute significantly to human diets. Here too, however, recent trends give cause for concern. While beef and mutton production worldwide rose from 24 million tons in 1950 to 62 million tons in 1990, production has leveled off since then and is unlikely to show further gains in the foreseeable future. Given the deteriorating condition of overgrazed rangelands, simply maintaining *present* levels of meat production poses major challenges; as population continues to grow, stagnation of livestock production inevitably will mean less meat per person in the years ahead. Nor can fisheries be expected to fill a widening protein gap; as will be discussed in greater detail in a subsequent section, global fish catch, which soared from 22 million tons in the early 1950s to the record 1989 catch of 100 million tons, is now declining amid fears that we may already have exceeded the carrying capacity of the world's oceans (Brown, 1994).

While many national leaders tend to blame adverse weather conditions for food shortfalls, the true causes are more complex: loss of good cropland to erosion and non-farm uses, inefficient agrarian structures, lack of investment in agriculture by city-oriented government officials, rising energy costs, and *too many people*.

Factors Influencing Food Demand

While it is obvious that the total yield of the world's croplands, pasturelands, and fisheries constitutes the world's food *supply*, assessing food *demand* is slightly more complicated. **Population growth**, not surprisingly, is the single largest factor in determining food demand. Since 90% of the world's population increase is occurring in the countries of Asia, Africa, and Latin America, food supply problems currently are most acute in these regions. An additional factor must be considered in assessing food demand, however. **Rising personal incomes** that have characterized the economic development of most industrialized countries since the Second World War have greatly added to world food demand. This is not because the typical American, Swede, or Japanese eats tremendously greater quantities than the average Peruvian, Pakistani, or Sudanese, but because higher incomes generally translate into an increased demand for high-quality foods, particularly meat and dairy products. As you will recall from our discussion of trophic levels and energy transfer (chapter 1), it requires approximately 10 times as much grain to produce a pound of human flesh from beef as it would if that same grain were eaten directly, due to inescapable inefficiencies of energy conversion. Thus the shift to a greater reliance on animal products in the diets of citizens of the more affluent countries is having a marked impact on increasing food demand in those areas. Perhaps nowhere does the pent-up consumer craving for animal protein have more explosive potential than in the People's Republic of China, where rapid economic growth is bringing hitherto undreamed-of prosperity to the world's most populous nation. Visiting China in the late summer of 1993, a *New York Times* reporter questioned a villager on how changing conditions were affecting him personally. Offering a revealing insight on how newfound wealth can boost food demand, the farmer replied, "Overall life has gotten much better. My family eats meat maybe four or five times a week now. Ten years ago we never had meat" (Kristof, 1993). As the people of China—and elsewhere—shift from primarily vegetarian to more heavily meat-based diets, world grain demand will grow even faster than mere population figures would suggest.

Extent of Hunger

Determining the number of hungry people in the world today is a rather tricky business. Certainly there is a quantum difference between the teenager coming home from school complaining, "When's dinner, Mom? I'm starving!" and a Somali child with stick-like limbs and protruding abdomen, dying of acute malnutrition. In an attempt to establish some basis for comparison, the Food and Agriculture Organization (FAO) of the United Nations has devised a concept called the **basal metabolic rate** (BMR). The BMR is defined as the minimum amount of energy required to power human body maintenance, not including energy required for activity. On this basis, the FAO considers anyone receiving less than 1.2 BMR food intake daily to be undernourished. Using this rather conservative figure (some authorities feel the cut-off point should be raised to 1.5 BMR), the FAO estimates that today approximately 500 million people—one-tenth of humanity—are undernourished. Hunger, of course, is not equally shared among nations or even within nations. The vast majority of the world's hungry people inhabit the South Asian countries of India, Pakistan, and Bangladesh, parts of Southeast Asia, Africa south of the Sahara, and the Andean region of South America—all regions where rates of population growth continue to be high. Nevertheless, pockets of hunger can be found even within many affluent societies. In the United States malnutrition is distressingly common among the poor, the elderly, migrant farm workers, and Native Americans. More than half of the world's undernourished people are children under the age of five, and a significantly higher percentage of women than men are affected (Presidential Commission on World Hunger, 1980). This situation exists because within households in many cultures men, being the primary workers and providers, are served the best food before the rest of the family eats. Children and women, including both pregnant and nursing mothers, whose nutritional needs in proportion to their size exceed those of men, subsist on whatever remains. In such situations, girl children frequently receive less than boys, since males are more highly regarded. While landless laborers are often fed on the job by their employers, their families are not, thus increasing the disparity in nutritional levels within families (Ehrlich, Ehrlich, and Holdren, 1977).

The hunger issue most frequently impinges on the public consciousness during periods of severe famine, generally caused by prolonged droughts, floods, or wartime upheavals. During recent years, media coverage of starving children and anguished parents in Somalia, Angola, Sudan, and Ethiopia have kept us grimly aware of human suffering during times of calamity elsewhere in the world. Such periodic episodes of famine, tragic though they are, do not represent the world's major hunger problem at present, however. Rather, the chronic, undramatic, day-after-day undernutrition of those who know that, good harvest or poor, their bellies will never be full constitutes today's most serious food supply dilemma.

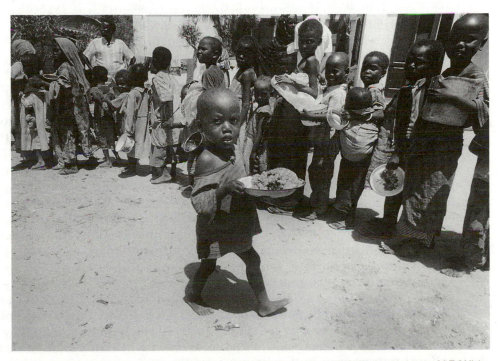

Orphaned children in war-torn Somalia wait in line for a bowl of rice and beans. [AP/Wide World Photos]

Causes of Hunger

The existence of nearly half a billion undernourished people seems paradoxical when one considers the World Bank's report that if the global grain harvest were equally distributed, each person would receive 3000 calories and 65 grams of protein per day—more than enough for good health. A number of commentators have similarly concluded that resources exist to meet the food demands of the projected world population at the turn of the century. If this is so, why are so many people today suffering from inadequate diets? The current situation is caused largely by two factors: **uneven distribution** of food and **poverty**.

Although global averages suggest that there should be enough food for everyone, as was stated earlier many of the areas where hunger is endemic are regions where there is a widening gap between food production and population growth; only imports from food-surplus areas prevent the problem from worsening further. However, as human numbers continue to climb, more equitable distribution of existing resources may not suffice—particularly if a high-quality diet rather than caloric content alone is the goal. Researchers at Brown University calculate that an even apportioning of the current world harvest, without any diversion of grain for livestock fodder, would provide an adequate vegetarian diet to a world population of six billion people—just slightly above the world's present numbers. A diet comparable to that currently consumed by South Americans, consisting of about 15% animal products, could be evenly distributed to four billion. To provide everyone with a typical North American or European-style diet (about 30% of calories derived from animal products), world population could barely exceed two billion—less than half the numbers currently dwelling on Planet Earth (Chen, 1990).

On a more practical level, however, the most basic explanation for the prevalence of hunger is poverty. Even in chronically food-short countries, the rich eat quite well. By contrast, even in the wealthiest nations, where markets bulge with a veritable cornucopia of foods, people who lack money to purchase groceries go hungry. In Third World countries almost 40% of the people are too poor to afford a minimally adequate diet. For these hungry people, an increase in world food production will mean little unless corresponding social and economic changes increase their purchasing power. In this context, statistics indicating a 2% income decline per capita on a worldwide basis between 1990 and 1993 represent a worrisome drop in living standards. While this trend may simply reflect a temporary economic downturn in several of the major industrial nations, in more than 40 developing countries, including many of the poorest in the world, average personal incomes have been falling ever since 1980 (Brown, 1994).

Poverty's role as a determinant of hunger was clearly evident during the 1967 drought in Bihar, a state in eastern India threatened with severe famine due to near-total crop failure. Food aid rushed into the area by the United States and other donors was credited with averting large-scale loss of life and interviews with villagers after the crisis was over revealed that many of them ate better during this period of natural disaster than at any other time in their lives. Why? Because the donated wheat was distributed to the needy free of charge and all received a share. During normal times the poorer segments of society lacked money to buy sufficient food in the marketplace and so went hungry. As George Verghese, editor of the *Hindustan Times* and information advisor to Prime Minister Gandhi during the famine eloquently described:

> For the poorest sections of the society, 1967, the Year of the Famine, will long be remembered as a bonus year when millions of people, especially the children, probably for the first time were assured of a decent meal a day . . . in a "normal year," these people hover on the bread line. They are beyond the pale, nobody's concern, they starve. In a famine year, they eat. Their health is better and the children are gaining weight. For them this is a year of great blessing. This is the deep irony, the grim tragedy of the situation.

Ironically, some of the improvements in agricultural technology much-heralded in recent years (i.e. "The Green Revolution") have actually worsened the nutritional status of landless laborers who found themselves displaced by machines, hence without any income to purchase food. The inflation of food prices that began with the Russian grain purchase of 1972 and has continued steadily in the years since has probably been more instrumental than any other single factor in reversing the nutritional gains witnessed during the 1950s and 1960s. The sharp increase in energy costs (e.g. gasoline to power farm machinery, natural gas for making nitrogen fertilizer and for drying grain) heightened demand for livestock feed in the developed countries, and continued rapid increase in population size in the less-developed nations all assure a continued escalation in food prices during the years ahead. Unless world economic conditions improve, with a more equitable distribution of resources and income, and unless there are improvements in productivity and a slowing of population growth rates, it is unlikely that world poverty, which is the principal cause of hunger, can be substantially ameliorated.

Health Impact of Hunger

Stressing the national security aspect of world hunger issues, the Presidential Commission on World Hunger issued a report several years ago stating that:

> Hunger has been internationalized and turned into a continuing global issue, transformed from a low-profile moral imperative to a divisive and disruptive factor in international relations. The most potentially explosive force in the world today is the frustrated desire of poor people to attain a decent standard of living. The anger, despair, and often hatred that result represent a real and persistent threat to international order.

Malnutrition

Political instability may be a worrisome consequence of hunger, true enough, but an even more fundamental reason for trying to eliminate hunger is its adverse impact on public health and well-being. Even during years when acute famine is absent, inadequate caloric intake has a significant impact on death rates. Among the poor in Third World countries, malnutrition is the number one health problem and is the major factor responsible for the wide gap in infant mortality rates between developed and less-developed societies. Chronic undernourishment, harmful at any age, is particularly devastating to young children. If children receive less than 70% of the daily standard food requirement, their growth and activity fall below normal levels; if food deprivation is prolonged, stunted physical development becomes irreversible and adult size is correspondingly reduced. As a result, their work performance is affected, particularly if they are employed in manual labor (work performance in both agriculture and industry has shown a positive correlation with increased body size and height). Even more ominous than the link between malnutrition and decreased physical development, however, is the finding that severe malnutrition in children, especially very young infants, results in a permanent stunting of brain development, characterized by a decrease in the number of brain cells and an alteration of brain chemistry. Studies have shown that if a nutritional deficiency occurs just before or immediately after birth, the baby will suffer a 15–25% reduction in number of brain cells. If malnutrition afflicts the developing fetus and continues to persist in the post-natal period, the child's complement of brain cells will be lowered by 50–60%. Even milder cases of malnutrition can result in lowered performance on tests designed to measure learning and sensory abilities. Extensive research has been conducted in India, Indonesia, Latin America and elsewhere, comparing intelligence levels of school-age children who had been malnourished during their first years of life but subsequently recovered with other children from similar socioeconomic backgrounds who had not experienced similar nutritional deprivation. The former group, though to all appearances in perfectly good health, exhibited, on average, significantly lower I.Q.s and had much greater difficulty learning to read and write than did the children who had been adequately fed. Malnutrition, by reducing bodily defenses, also greatly increases a child's susceptibility to infectious diseases. Common childhood ailments such as diarrhea and measles are much more likely to prove fatal to an undernourished child than to a well-fed one. The fact that youngsters in poor countries are several hundred times more likely to die of measles than are children in more affluent societies is indicative of malnutrition's impact on infection rates.

Malnutrition takes its toll among older children and adults as well. Undernourished people lose weight and become less able to combat infections or environmental stress. They thereby become less economically productive and less able to care for their families (however, while adults suffering temporarily from severe food deprivation may become listless and apathetic, unable to engage in strenuous physical labor, they seldom experience the permanent damage characteristic of childhood malnutrition). At greatest risk, of course, are pregnant and lactating women. Such women, if malnourished, run a significantly higher risk of miscarriage or premature delivery than do adequately fed mothers. If they manage to carry their babies full-term, the child is likely to suffer from low birth weight (one

BOX 4-1

Nature's Perfect Food

While plant breeders and farmers scramble to find ways of easing the population-food dilemma and nutritionists ponder ways of improving deficient diets, one of nature's finest—and cheapest—foods is being bypassed by a steadily increasing portion of humanity. Human breast milk is the ideal food for babies, an excellent source of high-quality protein providing the perfect balance of nutrients, enzymes, hormones, and growth factors. The immunoglobulins and anti-infective substances in breast milk provide the nursing infant with an important defense against the intestinal pathogens that are a major cause of infant mortality in many developing countries. Unlike cow's milk or special formulas marketed as milk substitutes, human breast milk changes in composition to match the changing needs of the infant, varying during any given feeding as well as during the day (hence recommendations that a baby should be fed "on demand" to the greatest extent possible). Beyond its obvious nutritional advantages, breast-feeding offers an intense "bonding" experience between the nursing mother and her infant, a form of physical communication providing important psychosocial benefits to both mother and child. Although supplemental feeding of solid foods is generally recommended after the age of 5-6 months, groups such as UNICEF advise mothers to continue nursing their babies for at least 11 months after birth.

Unfortunately, in recent decades increasing numbers of mothers have curtailed or totally abandoned breast-feeding in favor of infant formulas, apparently regarding the former as too "old-fashioned" for the sophistication of the modern world. Aside from the increased financial costs which this trend entails (e.g. expenditures for purchased milk or formula, bottles, nipples, sterilizing equipment, fuel for heating the water), for Third World babies, at least, the shift away from nursing to bottle feeding has some serious health implications.

While commercial infant formulas can be a perfectly adequate food for babies when mixed in the proper concentrations, prepared under sanitary conditions with uncontaminated water, and placed in sterile bottles with clean nipples, such ideal conditions are frequently nonexistent in many countries where the transition to bottle-feeding is occurring. As a result, in a number of developing countries the abandonment of breast-feeding has been accompanied by a sharp rise in rates of infant malnutrition and death.

Although causes for the decline in maternal nursing include changing social values, rapid urbanization and modernization among formerly traditional societies (bottle-feeding is largely an urban phenomenon in the developing world—most rural mothers continue to nurse their babies), and simple convenience, the international attention focused on this issue during the 1970s and 1980s laid much of the blame on the aggressive marketing strategies of multinational food companies. In both Africa and Latin America, corporations such as the Swiss food giant Nestlè for years conducted extensive radio advertising campaigns, supplemented by billboard and press advertisements, encouraging mothers to forego breast-feeding in favor of powdered infant formulas marketed under such trade names as *Lactogen* or *Similac*. In some areas, company representatives regularly visited maternity clinics or the homes of new mothers, distributing free samples, while in other places the employment of nurses as sales representatives conveyed the impression that the products had the official endorsement of the health profession. All too often, however, the women who were thus persuaded to give up nursing soon found that purchasing formula consumed a significant portion of the family budget. Often uneducated and unaware of the importance of proper dilution ratios, mothers frequently watered down the formula (often with microbially contaminated water) to make it last longer. In some Latin American countries, mothers added a popular brand of cornstarch to the diluted formula, assuming that because it *looked* like milk it must have the food value of milk. Little wonder, then, that infants fed on such a diet frequently developed malnutrition or gastrointestinal ailments. The phenomenon became so common in some African cities that certain hospitals featured beds labeled "Lactogen Syndrome." At one time in Freetown, Sierra Leone, all but 4 of 717 babies hospitalized for malnutrition were bottle-fed; in parts of Chile, death rates among "bottle babies" were triple those found among breast-fed infants.

In Europe and the United States, outrage prompted by media exposés of such practices led to a consumer boycott of Nestlè products in an effort to pressure the world's largest food manufacturer to cease promoting the use of infant formula in Third World countries. Organized by an international coalition of voluntary, nonprofit organizations, the boycott remained in effect from 1977 to 1984, when Nestlè agreed to sign the World Health Organization's *International Code of Marketing of Breast-Milk Substitutes*.

Adopted in 1981, this agreement prohibits distribution of free samples or supplies to hospitals or to mothers; it also forbids any form of direct promotion of infant formulas to consumers. The truce was a temporary one, however. Adherence to the WHO *Code's* provisions were voluntary, and it soon became apparent that Nestlè, as well as even more aggressive competitors such as American Home Products (the number two marketer of infant formulas in developing nations) were defying WHO guidelines by continuing to dump milk substitutes on Third World hospitals. Extensive television advertising promoting bottle-feeding as chic and modern remained as widespread and as misleading as ever. In the Philippines, Nestlè brochures claimed that their *Nestrogen* formula was "health-giving for baby . . . cost-saving for mommy." Plunging into the fray once again, the Minneapolis-based Action for Corporate Accountability, a successor of the groups that organized the original anti-Nestlè protest, announced a resumption of the boycott in October of 1988. While not attracting the same fervor that attended the earlier campaign, this second boycott achieved its objective when, in the spring of 1991, both Nestlè and American Home Products publicly committed themselves to cease providing free or low-cost infant formula to developing countries—a watershed event in which these giant corporations in essence acknowledged that free samples, while seemingly well-intentioned, adversely affected Third World health by interfering with the initiation of breast-feeding.

The recent termination of infant formula giveaways in the developing world is good news, but reversing the trend toward bottle-feeding requires more than thwarting the Madison Avenue tendencies of multinational corporations. National strategies to halt the decline of breast-feeding must now concentrate on such fundamentals as training hospital staff, providing health and nutritional education, using mass media to project a positive image of breast-feeding as opposed to bottle-feeding, and influencing employers to provide for the needs of nursing mothers in the labor force. Interestingly, in Western countries, where the image of the "liberated female" served as the role model for millions of Asian, African, and Latin American women to adopt infant formulas, there has been a renewed interest in breast-feeding in recent years, particularly among the better-educated and more affluent segments of society (71% of American women in this group are nursing their babies at the time they leave the birth site, as opposed to a 54% national average; by the time their babies are five to six months of age, 31% of better-educated U.S. women are still nursing, compared to just 9% of low-income women). U.S. health officials, like their Third World counterparts, have identified the promotion of breast-feeding as a priority objective. In its 1990 report, *Healthy People 2000*, the U.S. Department of Health and Human Services has set a turn-of-the-century goal calling for 75% of American mothers to be breast-feeding their babies during the first several months after birth, with 21% continuing to do so at five to six months of age. Not content with merely setting ambitious goals, the Canadian province of Quebec for years has encouraged breast-feeding by paying supplements to low-income mothers who nurse their babies, citing the health benefits to children and long-term reductions in national health care expenditures as justification for the nursing allowance. In their efforts to convince modern women that Nature's way is still the best, health officials in developing and industrialized nations alike might reiterate the comments of a French obstetrician who remarked nearly a century ago that ". . . the mother's milk belongs to her child."

Reference
Sasson, Albert. 1990. "Feeding Tomorrow's World," *UNESCO/CTA*.

of the most frequent causes of infant mortality) or to be stillborn (Sasson, 1990). The old myth that nursing mothers draw on their own nutritional reserves to provide top-quality food for their infants is untrue—the milk of undernourished mothers is lower than normal in vitamins, fat, and protein content.

Nutritional Deficiency Diseases

To be well-nourished implies not only an adequate caloric intake, but also a proper balance of carbohydrates, fats, proteins, vitamins and minerals. If amounts of any of these are insufficient, certain deficiency symptoms may become apparent even when all other vital nutrients are in adequate supply. Some of the more common deficiency diseases include the following.

Kwashiorkor.   The single largest contributor to high child mortality rates in Third World countries, kwashiorkor is a protein deficiency disease

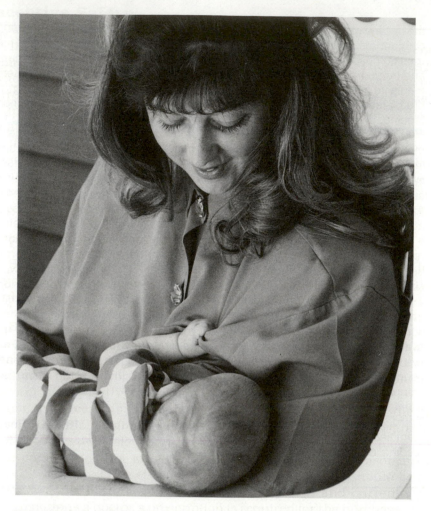

While there has been renewed interest in breast-feeding among American women, reversing the trend toward bottle-feeding in Third World countries is more problematic. [David C. Arendt, photo courtesy of La Leche League International]

that affects millions of children in tropical areas, particularly in Africa. Kwashiorkor most frequently develops in babies who are weaned early and given only starchy, low-protein foods such as rice, cassava, or bananas to eat—common baby foods in many tropical regions. Symptoms of mild kwashiorkor include discoloration of the hair and skin (in dark-haired children, hair may assume a reddish cast), retardation of physical growth, development of a protruding abdomen due to accumulation of fluids, and a loss of appetite. In more severe cases the hair may fall out painlessly in tufts, digestive problems arise, fluid collects in the legs and feet, muscle wastage and enlargement of the liver may occur, and the child becomes listless and apathetic. Once this stage of the disease is reached, death is likely unless the child receives medical attention. In its milder forms,

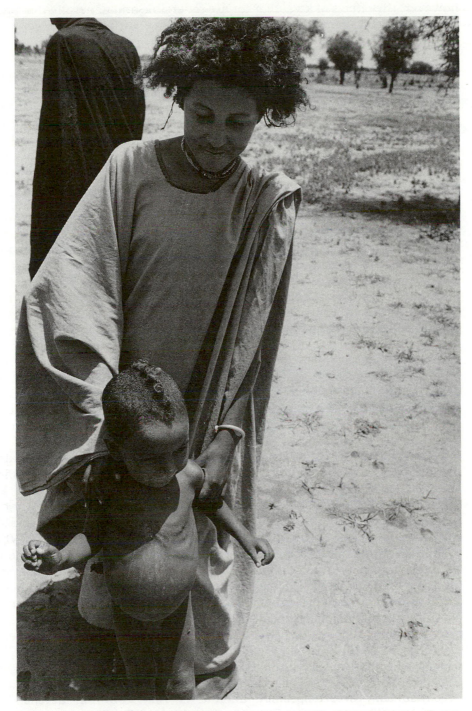

This child exhibits the protruding abdomen characteristic of kwashiorkor sufferers. [Agency for International Development]

however, the effects of kwashiorkor are reversible and generally disappear as the child becomes older and is given a more varied diet.

Marasmus. The second of the two most commonly observed deficiency diseases among children, marasmus is an indication of overall protein-calorie deprivation. Most frequently striking babies under one year of age, especially those no longer being breast-fed, marasmus often occurs after the child has been suffering from diarrhea or some other disease. Victims of marasmus can be distinguished by their thin, wasted appearance, with skin hanging in loose wrinkles around wrists and legs and eyes appearing unusually large and bright because of the shrunken aspect of the rest of the body.

Xerophthalmia (Blindness).   A deficiency in vitamin A, often associated with protein shortages, can result in a drying of the eye membranes or a softening of the cornea, leading to night-blindness and, if not treated, progressing to total blindness in its victims. Lack of sufficient vitamin A is common in Bangladesh, southern India, Sri Lanka, Vietnam, the Philippines, Indonesia, countries of the Middle East, many parts of Africa, Central America, Haiti, and northeastern Brazil. It is estimated that 250,000 children each year become blind due to vitamin A deficiency and that an additional 10 million develop clinical signs and symptoms of xerophthalmia. Recently scientists have confirmed that not only can vitamin A deficiency lead to blindness, but it also is an important determinant of child mortality due to its deleterious effect on the immune system. The micronutrient stimulates maturation of white blood cells which aid the body in fighting disease; its deficiency provokes changes in the mucous membranes lining the respiratory, gastrointestinal, and urinary tracts, rendering them less effective in protecting the body against invading pathogens. Studies conducted among Indonesian preschoolers suffering from night blindness have shown that these children were 4 to 12 times more likely to die than their nonaffected peers, apparently due to their greater susceptibility to respiratory and diarrheal infections. Field trials conducted in both Indonesia and Nepal demonstrated that when vitamin A supplements are administered to young children at 4–6 month intervals, mortality rates can be significantly reduced. Responding to these findings, the U.S. Agency for International Development recently launched a $50 million project to combat xerophthalmia and other diseases caused by micronutrient deficiencies and is now working with governments, research institutions, and private not-for-profit groups in 37 countries to save the sight and lives of children threatened by this deadly but preventable disease (Sommer, 1985; Irving, 1993).

Anemia. Iron deficiency anemia is very common in the less-developed countries where 20–25% of children, 20–40% of women, and 10% of men may suffer from this disorder, caused primarily by strict vegetarian diets and the prevalence of parasitic worm infections. Anemia is characterized by lack of energy and low levels of productive activity. It is especially dangerous—and especially common—in pregnant women, where anemia increases the likelihood of maternal death, premature delivery, or stillbirth. Repeated pregnancies rapidly drain a woman's reserve supplies of iron; in Pakistan and India, where more than 60% of pregnant women are anemic, iron deficiency is held responsible, at least in part, for the high female mortality rates. While women need three times as much iron as men to replace losses during menstruation and pregnancy, their food intake is generally lower than that of their husbands, sons, and brothers. While increasing the consumption of red meat (the best source of easily assimilated iron) among poor women in developing nations may not be a practical option due to religious prohibitions or lack of purchasing power, the frequency of iron deficiency anemia could be significantly reduced by supplying ferrous salt tablets to pregnant and lactating women, as well as to children, living in areas with a high prevalence of this deficiency disease (Sasson, 1990).

Goiter.   Iodine deficiency, affecting about 20 million people world-wide, results in the swollen growth of the thyroid gland on the front or side of the neck known as goiter. Iodine deficiency in pregnant women can result in their babies being born dwarfed and mentally retarded. The World Health Organization estimates that in parts of central Africa, the Andean mountain area of South America, and in the Himalayan foothills, cretinism caused by endemic goiter may affect up to 5% of the population (Pino and Martinez, 1981). Goiter has largely been eliminated in the United States by the simple expedient of adding iodine to table salt.

Other deficiency diseases that are much less common today than they were in the past due to fortification of dietary staples with the missing vitamin or mineral include: scurvy (vitamin C), beri-beri (thiamine-vitamin B1), pellagra (niacin), and rickets (vitamin D).

Prospects for Reducing World Hunger

When confronted with stark pictures of starving babies or cold statistics on the growing prevalence of malnutrition, the typical reaction among most Americans is to say, "let's do something about it!"—send a donation to CARE or OXFAM, eat a vegetarian meal once a week, write a letter to a congressional representative urging a "yes" vote on the next food aid bill. Certainly there has been no shortage on suggestions as to what might be done to ease the population-food crunch. Newspapers and magazines regularly describe the latest "solution" to the problem of world hunger. Some of the approaches being tried have real merit, as well as limitations, while others are merely wishful thinking. It's important that the public have some understanding of the key elements in the ongoing debate as to how best to eradicate hunger, since this issue is certain to assume even greater urgency in the years ahead. Some of the most frequently mentioned ways of increasing the world food supply are discussed in the following sections.

Expanding the Amount of Land Under Cultivation

From the beginning of the Agricultural Revolution right up to the early 1950s, increasing acreage put to the plow was the major, often the only, way of increasing food supply. Expanding the amount of cultivated land was accomplished by clearing forests, terracing mountainsides, or building irrigation systems—all of which permitted hitherto unproductive lands to be farmed. During the 1950s the Soviet Union vastly increased its agricultural acreage by opening up the "virgin lands" of Kazakhstan; at the same time the Chinese completed some major irrigation networks and thus substantially expanded their cultivated acreage. Since that time, significant increases in highly productive farmland have been quite limited. The hard truth is that the world's prime farmland is in finite supply, and after approximately 10,000 years of agricultural expansion most good land is already being cultivated. Since the 1950s most of the additional land cleared for farming has been so-called "marginal land"—land which, because of its poor soil, erodability, or steep slope is incapable of sustaining moderately good yields over any extended period of time. Farmers who today are moving onto marginal lands, desperately trying to eke out a living for their families, do so only because the better lands are already over-crowded. The additional food that such lands will contribute to world harvests is negligible and the long-term ecological damage caused by removing the natural vegetative cover from such lands may eventually have an adverse impact on better lands elsewhere.

Some optimists look hopefully to areas of the world such as the Gangetic Plain of northern India, the Mekong River basin of Southeast Asia, the Niger basin in Africa, or the Amazon region in Brazil, envisioning these lands as future world breadbaskets (or rice bowls, as the case may be) if large irrigation projects could be developed there. Such schemes may be technologically possible (though ecologists worry about large-scale environmental disruption and possible climatic changes if such visions should become reality, especially regarding development of Amazonia), but would require huge amounts of capital investment, far beyond the financial capabilities of the nations involved. Extensive grassy areas in the central African nation of Sudan also look promising for greatly increased livestock and crop production—but only if the tsetse fly can be brought under control. Thus even in parts of the world where potentially productive lands remain uncultivated, the prospects for their future agricultural development are uncertain. The long time period and enormous financial commitment required continue to be major obstacles to turning their potential into a reality (Borlaug, 1981).

When assessing the contribution that additional farm acres could make to the total world harvest, commentators frequently overlook the other side of the coin, i.e. the substantial amounts of good cropland that are currently being lost every year to erosion, desertification, salinization and water-logging of irrigated fields, and urban development. It is now recognized that the increase in world food production witnessed during the 1970s and early 1980s was achieved in part by plowing marginal lands unsuitable for sustained cultivation and by over-irrigating, which has resulted in drastic drawing-down of groundwater reserves in many areas. Today in many of the major grain-producing areas of the world, the cropland base is beginning to shrink as highly erodible lands are abandoned. According to a United Nations-sponsored study, since 1945 nearly 11% of the world's vegetated lands have experienced moderate to extreme degradation, while another 6% have suffered limited damage. Such figures, however, understate the problems in regions such as Central America and Mexico where the percentage of seriously degraded land is as high as 24% (compared to only 5% in North America). On moderately degraded lands restoration is theoretically possible, though the cost of such an undertaking might be prohibitive. Extremely degraded soils—those on which the soil's biotic functions have been destroyed—cannot be reclaimed (Ehrlich, Ehrlich, and Daily, 1993). The following chapter will examine these trends in more detail, but it is important to bear in mind that while most of the lands currently being added to our agricultural base are marginal acres, those being lost are, for the most part, prime croplands that will never be returned to production.

Increasing World Fish Catch

When one considers that 71% of the earth's surface is water, it's understandable that many people, confronted with the prospect of impending food shortages, look to the oceans as the source of apparently limitless high-quality animal protein. Such optimism seemed justified during the years between 1950-1989 when total world fish catch soared from about 22 million tons annually to 100 million tons—a 4.6-fold increase which, even at a time of unprecedented population growth, resulted in a doubling in the per capita availability of seafood. Since fish provide more than 50% of all the animal protein consumed by humans on a worldwide basis, this bounty from the sea raised hopes for substantial progress in combating malnutrition if the 2 million ton/year increase in global fish catch could be sustained. Unfortunately, recent trends indicate that the record 1989 catch, valued at $72 billion, represented an historic watershed, following which heavily-stressed fish stocks began a gradual decline. By 1993 the per capita global fish harvest had fallen 7% below its 1989 peak and marine scientists openly expressed their concerns that the oceans' maximum sustainable yield may have been surpassed (Brown, 1994). The FAO recently declared 9 of the world's 17 major fisheries to be in "serious decline," with 4 more classified as "commercially depleted." The remainder are characterized as "fully exploited" or "overexploited." The FAO concludes that overexploitation of ocean resources has pushed some commercially important fish species to the brink of biological extinction and has unintentionally, though quite predictably, disrupted aquatic food chains to the point that higher trophic level species such as whales, porpoises, and sea turtles have been seriously harmed as well. Such trends have ominous implications for food security and economic well-being in countries heavily dependent on commercial fisheries. On the whole experts agree that the situation is getting worse rather than better (Pitt, 1993).

Figure 4-1

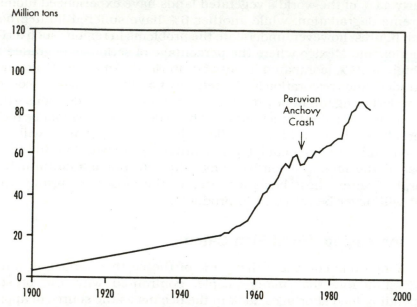

World Marine Fish Catch, 1900–2000

Million tons

Peruvian
Anchovy
Crash

Source: Worldwatch Institute (Worldwatch Paper 116, Nov. 1993), based on data from FAO;
Ray Hilborn, "Marine Biota," in B. L. Turner et al., eds., *The Earth as Transformed
by Human Actions*, 1993; U.N. Department of International, Economic, and Social Affairs.

Contribution of Fish to Diet by Region, 1987–1989

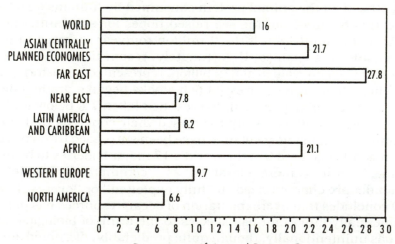

Percentage of Animal Protein Consumption

Source: Worldwatch Institute (Worldwatch Paper 116, Nov. 1993), based on data from "Marine
Fish Supply and Use As a Food Source," *Marine Fisheries and the Law of the Seas:
A Decade of Change,* FAO circular #853, 1993.

Figure 4-2 Declines in Selected Commercial Fisheries since 1970

Atlantic Cod

1970	3.1 million metric tons
1991	916,000 metric tons

Atlantic Redfishes

1976	688,000 metric tons
1989	344,000 metric tons

Western Pacific Yellow Croaker

1970s	300,000 metric tons
1980s	70,000 metric tons

Northwest Atlantic Herring

1970	848,000 metric tons
1989	275,000 metric tons

Atlantic Mackerel

1973	418,000 metric tons
1989	56,000 metric tons

Source: FAO

One ray of hope in an otherwise gloomy outlook is the rapid growth of aquaculture (i.e. fish farming) in recent years. Practiced with both freshwater fish and marine species, aquaculture now provides 12% of the total world fish harvest, up from less than 5% in 1970. Some countries, notably China, Japan, India, Korea, Indonesia, and the Philippines, now obtain a significant portion of their seafood products from aquaculture. Fish farming in the United States, while lagging behind that of the above-mentioned nations, has steadily expanded over the past decade. Already aquaculture accounts for most of U.S. catfish and crayfish production and is the main source of the salmon supplied by American supermarkets. Trout are also successfully raised by means of aquaculture. The recent leveling off of ocean fish harvests suggests that any hopes for maintaining current per capita supplies of fish and seafood in the years ahead depend on an enormous expansion of aquaculture enterprises. Such growth, while theoretically possible, would require vast areas of land, water, and feed—all of which would have to be diverted from other types of agricultural production. Although fish are among the most efficient energy converters, requiring just two pounds of feed to produce one pound of flesh, relying on aquaculture to provide the desired two million ton annual increment in world fish catch would nevertheless consume *four* million tons of feed grains. Obviously, "there's no such thing as a free lunch"—as rising seafood prices amply demonstrate!

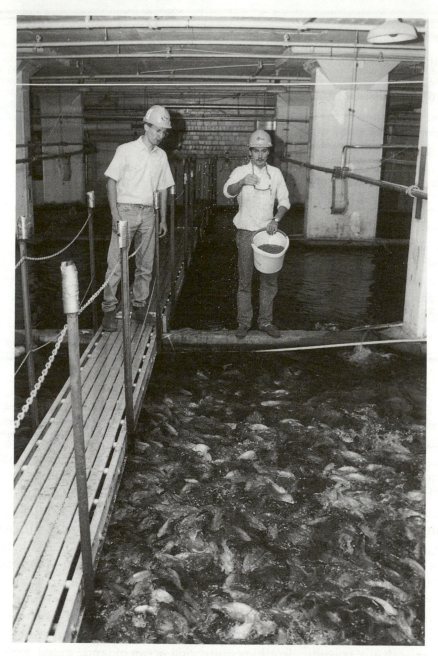

Aquaculture (fish farming) provides 12% of the total world fish harvest. Species that can be successfully raised include catfish, crayfish, salmon, trout, and tilapia (shown above). [Archer Daniels Midland]

Reducing Post-Harvest Food Losses

Implementation of better methods of handling and protecting food between the time it is harvested and the time it appears on the consumer's plate may not sound particularly exciting—rat-proof grain bins are not the

BOX 4-2

Empty Nets

They that go down to the sea in ships,
that do business in great waters.
—Psalms 107:23

Thus sang the ancient psalmist, but if an event that recently transpired in Boston Harbor is any indication of what lies ahead, those who go down to the sea in coming years will do precious little business indeed. In early March of 1994, descendants of ten generations of New England fishermen sailed their boats into the harbor, sounding their horns in a plaintive protest at a human-created disaster which threatens to destroy their way of life. From the legendary cod fisheries of the Grand Banks to the oyster beds of Chesapeake Bay to the salmon runs of the Pacific Northwest, catastrophic declines in marine fish stocks have brought economic ruin to thousands of commercial fishermen. The problem is global in scope and worsening rapidly. The Food and Agriculture Organization (FAO) of the United Nations has identified four major ocean fishing areas (i.e. southeast Pacific, northwest Pacific, eastern portion of the Indian Ocean, and the Mediterranean Sea) where catches already exceed maximum sustainable yields. Ominously, the FAO reports that the vast majority of commercially important fish species are already fully exploited and any intensification of fishing pressure would be unlikely to result in larger catches—and could result in further declines in total harvest.

A number of factors share the blame for the present sad state of affairs. The most obvious explanation for depletion of stocks is **overfishing,** an activity that has resulted in the collapse of several important fisheries during the last few decades. Since the late 1960s herring catches in the northwest Atlantic have dropped by nearly 70%; halibut, whose harvest is down by more than 90%, is now considered commercially extinct (meaning that the species is so rare it is no longer profitable to fish for it). In the early 1970s, overfishing, plus a shift in the Humboldt Current off the coast of South America, reduced the Peruvian anchovy catch from 12 million tons annually to a mere 2 million—a level that has not risen appreciably since then. Increasingly efficient "floating factories"—huge ships using sonar and satellite communications to track schools of fish—have greatly increased the catch of nations like Russia, Poland, and Japan but threaten the long-term viability of the industry, since they harvest young and mature fish indiscriminately and thus prevent the replenishment of fish stocks. Even more damaging has been the use of enormous driftnets, roundly condemned by the United Nations General Assembly because of their efficiency in capturing non-target fish, birds, turtles, and marine mammals (mainly dolphins). Hanging vertically in the water like giant curtains, driftnets may stretch 5–50 kilometers, suspended at or near the surface by floats, snaring by the gills any hapless fish that attempt to swim through the mesh. Utilized primarily by Japanese, Taiwanese, and Korean fishermen, high seas driftnets have been the target of a U.N. worldwide moratorium. In an effort to gain greater control over the predatory activities of foreign fishing fleets which were driving their American counterparts out of business and to protect existing fish stocks, the U.S. Congress in 1976 passed the

Magnuson Fisheries Management and Conservation Act which expanded U.S. territorial waters from the traditional 3 miles offshore to 200 miles. Unfortunately, American fishermen responded to the banishment of their competitors by over-building their own fleets and substituting domestic exploitation for foreign exploitation. As a result, in areas like the Georges Bank east of Cape Cod, once-abundant stocks of haddock, flounder, and cod are all but exhausted and the government has recently approved plans for restricting fishing to a level that will lower catches off the New England coast by 50% over the next five to seven years.

A second factor adversely affecting the sustainability of ocean fisheries is the growing extent of **pollution of the seas**. It has not yet been possible to demonstrate a decline in the abundance of entire species in the open ocean due solely to pollution, but experiments have shown that toxic contaminants such as hydrocarbons, heavy metals, and synthetic organic compounds—all common water pollutants—can kill or injure aquatic organisms. In coastal waters that constitute some of the world's most productive fishing grounds, nutrients—primarily nitrates and phosphates from sewage discharges or farmland runoff—constitute the most extensive and serious pollution problem. The decline of Chesapeake Bay's crab and oyster harvest, once among the world's richest, can be traced largely to contamination from such sources. Shellfish and crustacean populations are particularly susceptible to pollution of near-shore areas; if not directly killed by toxic contaminants, they are often declared unmarketable because of the health threat they pose to human consumers.

Development activities that destroy coastal habitats, particularly coastal marshes, mangroves, and sea grasses, also play a role in reducing populations of ocean fish because 90% by weight of the world's fish catch is comprised of species that depend on coastal or estuarine waters for survival during some phase of their life cycle. Burgeoning urban populations along most of the world's coastlines are rapidly increasing development pressures in these areas, yet few countries are managing such growth in a manner that will protect the ocean's biotic resources.

The sudden decline in world fish harvests, following nearly 40 years of growth, may provide the stimulus policymakers need to change course before it's too late. A follow-up session on threatened fisheries mandated by the 1992 Earth Summit was held in the summer of 1993, attended by diplomats, marine biologists, lawyers, and fisheries officials. In the first international effort at negotiating comprehensive fishing regulations in more than a decade, all agreed that the crisis is real—but no consensus was reached on what to do about it. Some nations are not waiting for coordinated international action. In 1993 Russia angered neighboring nations by demanding a three-year moratorium on fishing in seas off its Pacific coast, following the collapse of pollock stocks there. That same year U.S. Interior Secretary Bruce Babbitt announced a two-year buyout of Greenland's salmon fishing industry, proclaiming the hope that such action would ultimately help restore North American runs of Atlantic salmon. On the West Coast, several conservation groups were threatening lawsuits to force regional fishing councils to protect certain fish species (a salmon-fishing ban considered in 1992 was ultimately rejected, and salmon runs everywhere but in Alaska subsequently fell to their lowest levels ever). In 1994 Congress began a reexamination of the Magnuson Act, considering whether or not to alter current policy whereby eight industry-dominated regional councils essentially regulate commercial fishing in the United States. To date such councils have had minimal success in setting catch limits for themselves. Although skeptics doubt that nations—or individuals—will muster the will to sacrifice current profits for the sake of long-term sustainability of marine resources, the consequences of failing to do so are too dire to cease trying.

References

Egan, Timothy. 1994. "U.S. Fishing Fleet Trawling Coastal Water Without Fish." *New York Times*, March 7.

Safina, Carl. 1994. "Where Have All the Fishes Gone?" *Issues in Science and Technology*, (Spring).

stuff of which poetry is made—but, in the short-run at least, such simple, well-understood measures could do more than anything else to increase the availability of food in the marketplace. Each year enormous amounts of harvested foods are lost to pests and spoilage, particularly in tropical countries. Rats, birds, insects, and molds all consume or render unfit for human use large amounts of stored foods which would otherwise have been available for people. Cultural practices are partially responsible for such losses. In many countries grains are stored in the open or in easily penetrated sacks or bins. Lack of adequate refrigeration promotes spoilage, while poor transport facilities delay rapid movement of food from fields to consumers, thereby increasing chances of loss or spoilage. The FAO estimates that the development of improved storage and transport facilities alone could increase market availability of food by 20% or more in the Third World countries (FAO, 1974).

Eating Lower on the Food Chain

Humanitarians are frequently troubled by the apparent inefficiency of converting a substantial portion of the world grain harvest into meat or poultry to satisfy consumers' carnivorous cravings. The same amount of corn, wheat, or oats, they argue, could satisfy the caloric needs of millions of additional people dining on vegetarian fare (to be consistent, they might also target the 10% of the U.S. corn crop diverted to the manufacture of corn syrup, much of which is used for sweetening soft drinks; that same amount of corn could make a lot of tortillas!)

The impact of diverting feed to food, even if fully implemented, might not be as great as proponents suggest, however. The percentage of the world grain crop used for fodder has already begun declining slightly—37% in 1992, down from a high of 40% in 1986 (Brown, 1994). It has been estimated that abandoning the use of grain for feed entirely would increase market supplies of food by 20%–30% at most (Ehrlich, Ehrlich, and Daily, 1993). If world population continues to grow as projections indicate, the one-time gains achieved by going vegetarian would soon be erased by the continuously mounting food demands generated by more and more people.

Regardless of whether promoting meatless diets would be an advisable or effective approach to increasing food availability, it is not a realistic option. While health concerns are prompting some individuals to reduce their consumption of high-fat animal products, no society in modern times has voluntarily reduced meat-eating by any significant amount. Indeed, as we have seen, the trends in newly affluent areas of the world are in exactly the opposite direction. Contrary to common perceptions, a large portion of feed grain use occurs in the Third World; next to the United States, China is the second-leading nation in terms of amounts of grain fed to livestock, poultry, and fish (USDA, 1992). While consumers might simplify their diets in response to scarcity-induced higher prices, an appeal to altruism—asking diners to forego their steaks and sauerbraten so that strangers far away could enjoy a temporary increase in food supplies—is unlikely to meet with a positive response.

Improving Yields per Acre

Since mid-century the largest gains in world food supply have been obtained not by expanding our cropland base but by dramatically increasing per acre or per hectare (metric unit for land measurement, equivalent to 2.47 acres) yields on existing farmlands. In the United States, corn yields, which had remained stable for almost 70 years, more than quadrupled from 1940 to 1985. Impressive increases in yields were also achieved for wheat, rice, barley, rye, peanuts, and sorghum. In Great Britain, where wheat yields are the world's highest, per hectare wheat production tripled from 1940 to 1984. These enormous gains were accomplished through the application of research and technological improvements gradually developed and perfected since the late 1800s, the major elements of which included new hybrid crop varieties, better farm machinery, tremendous expansion in the use of chemical fertilizers and pesticides, and increased use of irrigation.

The developed nations were not alone in realizing major gains in agricultural productivity during the past several decades. In the late 1960s, twenty years of plant breeding experiments to improve grain yields in tropical and semi-tropical regions resulted in the development of several strains of so-called "miracle wheat" and "miracle rice" which heralded the advent of what commentators have dubbed "The Green Revolution." Within a few years of its introduction, the new hybrid wheat was giving farmers from Mexico to India yields two to three times greater than the best formerly obtained from traditional strains. Since the introduction of the first miracle wheat in India in 1966, that country has more than doubled its wheat production. Pakistan, Turkey, and Mexico were among more than 30 other countries whose farmers eagerly adopted the new technology and witnessed a corresponding surge in their wheat production statistics. Similarly, the miracle rice varieties developed at the International Rice Research Institute in the Philippines have approximately doubled the yields

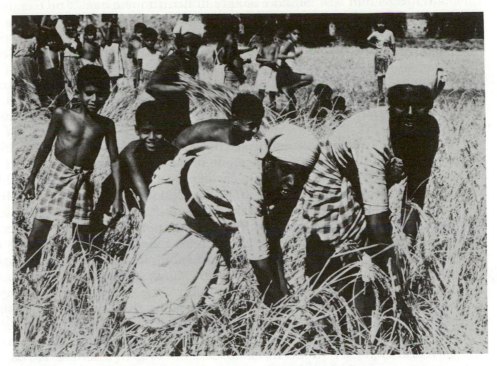

Traditional farming methods, such as those pictured here in southern India, were augmented by the gains of the "Green Revolution," which included hybrid seeds and increased use of agrichemicals and irrigation. Many experts doubt, however, that these same techniques can be relied upon to produce the future harvest gains necessary to keep pace with a growing population. [Author's photo]

of this grain in situations where the hybrid seeds, along with proper fertilization and adequate irrigation, were employed.

The spectacular gains of the Green Revolution led many political leaders during the early 1970s to relax on the population issue, assuming that continued dramatic increases in food production had erased the Malthusian image of starving millions. Agricultural experts, however, were less sanguine regarding the food-population crunch and warned that it would be a fatal mistake to assume that plant scientists would be able to achieve another quantum leap in crop yields in the foreseeable future. Agronomist Norman Borlaug, "Father of the Green Revolution" and recipient of the 1970 Nobel Peace Prize for his key role in developing miracle wheat, cautioned dignitaries assembled for the awards ceremony in Oslo that his contribution would, at best, buy mankind about 30 years of food security—years which he warned they must use to tame the population monster. Unfortunately, Borlaug's gift of time has largely been squandered; in developed and developing nations alike the gains of the Green Revolution are losing momentum even as population figures continue to climb. The fact that many of the world's farmers are already fully exploiting the technologies which enabled them to double, triple, or even quadruple yields in the years prior to 1984 means that future gains will come in ever-smaller increments and will be increasingly difficult to achieve. The trends are starkly evident in U.S. Department of Agriculture graphs (see Figure 4-3) indicating a leveling off of grain harvests in all the major producer nations since the mid-1980s. In Japan, where rice yields had been rising for almost 100 years, they have been falling for the past decade, in spite of the advanced state of Japanese agriculture and strong government support of farmers in that country. Per hectare rice yields in China and India, the world's two largest producers, have also ceased growing since 1990 (Brown, 1994).

Some observers predict that in the not-too-distant future we are likely to encounter an absolute yield ceiling imposed by plants' photosynthetic efficiency, resulting eventually in a widening gap between food production and baby production (Jensen, 1978). Such a ceiling would undoubtedly be reached sooner in the United States and other advanced agricultural countries simply because improved crop varieties and modern farming techniques have been in use longer here than elsewhere, leaving less margin for further improvement. As an example of this, take the case of nitrogen fertilizer use in the American Midwest. Heavy applications of fertilizer accounted for a substantial portion of the increase in corn harvests witnessed since 1950, but in recent decades the Law of Diminishing Returns has become increasingly evident. During the 1950s and 1960s, for every extra pound of nitrogen fertilizer applied a farmer could expect a yield increase of 15–20 extra bushels of corn. By the late 1970s that increment was 5–7 bushels and falling. By the 1990s growth in fertilizer use in the United States halted after a 30-year rise, partly due to more efficient application methods but also in response to farmers' recognition that additional fertilizer inputs were not economically justified by the minimal boost in yields per acre.

Outside the Corn Belt, the trends in fertilizer use are much the same. As high nitrogen-demanding miracle grains rapidly replaced more traditional varieties, fertilizer use worldwide soared, climbing from 14 million tons in 1950 to 126 million tons in 1984. Yield gains from these additional inputs were phenomenal, averaging nine tons for each extra ton of fertilizer applied. After 1984, however, more fertilizer use failed to translate into ever-higher yields; by the early 1990s, the increment was less than two tons of grain per additional ton of fertilizer (Brown, Kane, and Ayres, 1993). Unless plant geneticists can develop new varieties of wheat, rice, and corn that are even more responsive to heavy fertilization than the currently utilized Green Revolution varieties, it is unlikely that the slowdown in annual growth of world harvests witnessed during the past few years will be reversed.

Other components critical to the success of Green Revolution technologies—irrigation and chemical pesticides—also may be approaching practical limits. High-yielding varieties can only achieve their maximum potential when supplied with abundant water. Today approximately one-third of all crops harvested come from the 17% of world cropland under irrigation (Ehrlich, Ehrlich, and Daily, 1993). For a number of reasons, the rapid expansion in irrigated acreage which occurred annually from 1950 to 1978 has tapered off since that time to less than 1% a year (Brown, 1994).

Figure 4-3

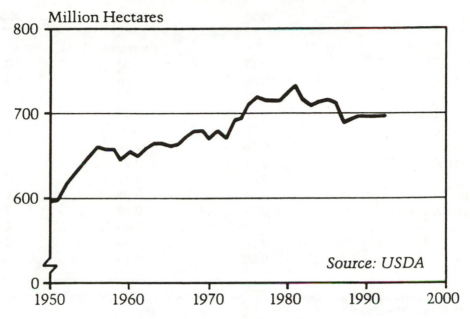

World Grain Harvested Area, 1950–1992

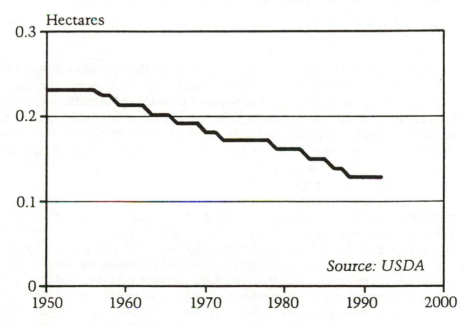

World Grain Harvested Area Per Person, 1950–1992

Source: Worldwatch Institute (*Vital Signs 1993*), based on USDA data.

Figure 4-4 Grain Harvested Area Per Person, by Country, 1950 and 1990, With Projections to 2030

Country	1950	1990	2030*
		(hectares)	
China	0.17	0.08	0.06
United States	0.53	0.26	0.22
India	0.22	0.12	0.07
Former Soviet Union	0.57	0.35	0.27
Bangladesh	0.20	0.10	0.05
Pakistan	0.18	0.10	0.04
Indonesia	0.07	0.07	0.04
Iran	0.21	0.17	0.06
Egypt	0.08	0.04	0.02
Ethiopia & Eritrea	0.24	0.07	0.02
Nigeria	0.23	0.09	0.03
Brazil	0.13	0.14	0.07
Mexico	0.20	0.11	0.06

* Assumes no change in total grain harvested area from 1990 to 2030; reductions in area per person due entirely to population growth.

Source: Lester Brown and Hal Kane, *Full House*, W. W. Norton, 1991 and U.S. Bureau of Census data.

In the absence of irrigation, "miracle grains" perform less well than lower-yielding traditional varieties—another reason why the recent slowdown in grain production is likely to continue. Chemical pesticide use, another factor critical in optimizing yields from new crop strains highly susceptible to insects and fungal pathogens, is also less effective than it was several decades ago. Overuse of these products has promoted development of resistant pest populations that are once again having an adverse impact on agricultural production.

For all these reasons, experts seriously doubt that a doubling or tripling of world harvests can be repeated through a "more of the same" approach. In most of the world's major agricultural areas farmers have already reaped the full potential offered by "miracle crops"; in regions not yet touched by the Green Revolution, natural conditions such as lack of water resources or inadequate technology transfer may preclude them from ever enjoying its fruits. Even within countries where the new technologies have boosted food self-sufficiency, large areas remain mired in poverty and backwardness—northwest China, the Andean Mountain area, the highlands of Mexico, and large areas of central India are all notable examples. The outlook for improvement is perhaps most clouded in the semiarid regions of sub-Saharan Africa where the proportion of high-yielding versus

BOX 4-3

Supercorn and Supercows

With the 1980 Supreme Court ruling (*Diamond vs. Chakrabarty*) confirming patent rights for living organisms, what some commentators have dubbed the "Second Green Revolution" was off and running. During the 1970s significant advances in recombinant DNA techniques had made it possible to "genetically engineer" new forms of life; that is, to insert hereditary material from one organism (most commonly a virus or bacterium) into another species, thereby producing a "designer" microbe. It was the landmark Court decision regarding patent rights that made such painstaking techniques profitable, however, and in the 1980s the new field of biotechnology began to grow by leaps and bounds. Comprising methods of manipulating living organisms for a specific purpose, biotechnology offers the potential for significant advances in crop and livestock production, as well as for controlling human genetic disorders—but at the same time raises fears of scientists' "playing God" by regarding life forms as mere commodities to be altered at will.

While controversy over the ethical aspects of biotechnology is likely to simmer on for years, corporate giants such as Monsanto, Ciba-Geigy, Unilever Royal Dutch-Shell, and dozens of other chemical, pharmaceutical, and energy companies around the world are funding multibillion dollar research and development efforts to commercialize the supercrops and supercows promised by the genetic engineers. It is widely believed that by the turn of the century biotechnology's impact on agriculture will be significant, perhaps leading to more environmentally sound farming practices, free of their current heavy dependence on agrichemical inputs.

The most rapid progress to date has been with genetically engineered plants and plant-bacteria combinations. Field experiments are now being carried out on corn plants within whose vascular tissues lurk genetically altered bacteria, waiting to attack any luckless corn borer larva which decides to nibble on them. In Australia testing is underway on a high-protein strain of alfalfa; Dutch researchers have developed a potato variety that carries a foreign gene enabling the plant to fight off virus infections; and in Louisiana a scientist is striving to produce the "perfect potato"—one which, through gene transfer, could produce all eight essential amino acids, giving it the nutritional value of meat. Many of the world's major food plants are now the subjects of intensive genetic research, with improvement efforts focused on goals such as improving their nutritional value, pest resistance, salt tolerance, or drought resistance. Some laboratories are striving for genetically engineered corn plants with higher photosynthetic efficiency or cereals that could manufacture their own nitrogen, thereby reducing the need for chemical fertilizers.

Gene-tinkering with livestock lags behind that directed at crop plants, but researchers are excited about future possibilities. Since 1981, when a mouse with a rabbit gene attained fame as the first transgenic animal, the pace of genetic research on livestock has accelerated. Work is progressing on pigs that are 30% more efficient at converting feed into meat; mice have been given a sheep gene which allows them to produce higher protein milk (not that mice-breeders are intending to go into the dairy business—the experiment simply showed that transfer of genes into dairy animals represents real potential for producing milk with higher nutritional value). Dreams of creating a race of supercows moved a step closer to reality in November of 1993 when the FDA approved use of rBGH (alternatively referred to as rBST), a genetically engineered growth hormone administered to dairy cattle. Manufactured by Monsanto and marketed under the trade name *Posilac*, the hormone promises to boost milk production 5–20% per cow. For the future, genetic engineers envision custom-designed chickens that are disease-resistant and lay larger eggs; genetically improved salmon; perhaps even caterpillar farms for generating medically useful human proteins!

Exciting as these developments sound, what hope do they provide for increasing world food supply at a time when the number of new mouths to be fed is inexorably escalating? Opinion seems divided among experts who anticipate super-high yielding crops guaranteed to satisfy the food demands of teeming millions and others who welcome a badly needed new weapon in humanity's war against hunger but are convinced the fruits of biotechnology cannot fill the projected food gap. One of the most articulate proponents for the latter viewpoint, Lester Brown of the Worldwatch Institute, points out that developing nitrogen-fixing grains, for example, would help farmers reduce their dependency on chemical fertilizers, but would not enhance yields, since the metabolic energy the plant expends in capturing nitrogen can no longer go into seed production. Public impressions to the contrary, genetic engineering is not magic, but simply represents a faster, more precise way of doing what plant breeders have been doing for thousands of years.

There is no doubt that biotechnology offers immense potential for helping farmers reduce dependence on costly, environmentally damaging agrichemicals; for alleviating nutritional deficiencies; for permitting use of lands too dry or waters too salty for cultivation of existing crop varieties. Whether the dream will become a reality, particularly for poor Third World farmers who most need the new technologies, is an open question. Because the lion's share of research is being conducted by giant multinational firms who have been rapidly acquiring seed companies and livestock genetics firms and claiming exclusive patent rights for the new species they create, there is a very real possibility that Third World countries will be barred access to the "Second Green Revolution." Throughout the industrialized world, gene power is bound to corporate power, and developing countries which lack the scientific and technical infrastructure to carry out their own research programs may find themselves growing ever more dependent on imported agricultural commodities and technologies they can ill afford. It is also possible that corporate goals of genetic research will differ from public goals. Companies, after all, are in business to make a profit, and it might be too much to expect that a chemical company, for example, would deliberately develop a designer plant that no longer needs any agrichemical inputs. For this reason, it shouldn't come as a surprise that the first genetically engineered plant to go commercial was one resistant to herbicides, permitting farmers to continue using chemical weed-killers without fear of damaging their crop. In the spring of 1994, however, societal interests were better served when Calgene Inc., a California-based biotechnology company introduced its

Flavr Savr tomato, the first (though undoubtedly not the last!) genetically engineered food to go commercial. While the *Flavr Savr* still can't compare with the mouth-watering homegrown varieties of summer, it offers a tremendous taste improvement over the "plastic tomatoes" which are standard supermarket fare. By inserting a gene to prevent the rapid softening of ripe tomatoes, Calgene scientists have made it possible for growers to leave the fruits on the vine a few extra days until they begin to flush red and develop more flavor, while still remaining firm enough for shipping to market without damage. A spokesperson for the biotechnology industry has hailed the *Flavr Savr* as "a significant step forward for consumers" in improving the quality of the most frequently complained-about produce item. Although groups such as Jeremy Rifkin's Pure Food Campaign continue to oppose the introduction of genetically altered foods into the marketplace, it is likely that the *Flavr Savr* will soon be followed by other test tube products such as cooking oils and salad dressings with less saturated fat, higher-protein grains, and potatoes that absorb less fat when deep-fried.

Whatever its potential pitfalls, biotechnology promises to revolutionize the future agricultural landscape. Whether it proves to be the panacea for solving world food problems remains to be seen.

References

Doyle, Jack. 1985. *Altered Harvest*. Viking Press.

Leary, Warren E. 1994. "Tomato Altered to Remain Fresh Year Round Is Backed by F.D.A." *New York Times,* May 19.

traditional grains now being cultivated is far lower than elsewhere in the world (e.g. improved rice varieties comprise just 14% of total rice acreage in sub-Saharan Africa as opposed to 95% of all rice varieties grown in Asia). According to FAO, of all the grain varieties grown in Africa as a whole, only 10% are of high-yielding types (Sasson, 1990). Such statistics suggest that food production in these chronically food-deficit areas could improve, despite maximum *genetic* yield barriers, if the use of existing production technology is further expanded. More on-site research to develop improved seed varieties adapted to local growing conditions, more attention to efficient water use and proper planting dates, greater emphasis on educational outreach programs to transfer the latest agricultural developments to cultivators in the field, adoption of government financial and economic policies which make it profitable for farmers to adopt new technologies—all offer potential for boosting currently modest yields in some Third World areas. However, continued rapid rates of population growth in those same areas demand that the governments of those nations give priority attention to modernizing their agricultural sectors in order to realize this potential. In addition, bountiful harvests alone will not eradicate hunger. By the late 1970s the Green Revolution had increased production to such an extent in countries such as India and Pakistan that those nations were declared self-sufficient in food grains; yet millions of their people still suffer the ravages of malnutrition because they are too poor to purchase the food they need. Finally, as population pressures mount, establishment of food reserves as a buffer against bad harvest years and widely fluctuating prices is regarded by many food experts as an urgent necessity. Yet despite much rhetoric, the bulk of world grain carryover stocks (a pivotal indicator of food security, carryover stocks represent the amount of grain remaining in the bin at the time a new harvest begins) consists of surpluses within the United States and in 1993 were equivalent to about 73 days of world consumption—a sharp decline from 1987's record-high 104 days of consumption (Brown, Kane, and Ayres, 1993). This amount is regarded as adequate to maintain relatively stable prices in the world market, but could be depleted rapidly if there were a serious food emergency in any of the major grain-growing regions of the world.

As we approach the end of the 20th century, humanity is confronted by demographic projections indicating that global population will continue to climb by nearly 95 million each year—at a time when growth in per capita food supply has leveled off or even declined in some key areas of the world. While optimists continue to insist that human inventiveness will somehow find the means for feeding future billions of hungry mouths, there are no new technologies on the horizon offering the quantum leaps in food production witnessed during the recent past. With a shrinking cropland base, falling water tables, diminishing impact of chemical fertilizers, and the long-term specter of adverse climatic change in some of the world's most productive agricultural regions (see chapter 11), farmers will be hard-pressed to meet future food demands at prices hungry people can afford. More vigorous efforts at stabilizing population size and reversing land degradation are urgently needed if we are to prove Malthus wrong ■

References

Borlaug, Norman. 1981. "Using Plants to Meet World Food Needs." In *Future Dimensions of World Food and Population*, edited by Richard Woods. Westview Press.

Brown, Lester R. 1994. "Facing Food Insecurity." *State of the World 1994*. Worldwatch Institute, W. W. Norton.

Brown, Lester R, Hal Kane, and Ed Ayres. 1993. *Vital Signs 1993*. Worldwatch Institute, W. W. Norton.

Chen, R., ed. 1990. *The Hunger Report: 1990*. The Alan Shawn Feinstein World Hunger Program, Brown University.

Ehrlich, Paul R., Anne H. Ehrlich, and Gretchen C. Daily. 1993. "Food Security, Population, and Environment." *Population and Development Review* 19, no. 1 (March).

Food and Agriculture Organization (FAO). 1974. "State of Food and Agriculture."

Irving, Ellen C. 1993. "Benefits of Vitamin A Confirmed." *Front Lines* (July).

Jensen, Neal F. 1978. "Limits to Growth in World Food Production." *Science* 201 (July 28).

Kristof, Nicholas D. 1993. "Riddle of China: Repression as Standard of Living Soars." *New York Times*, September 7.

Pitt, David E. 1993. "Despite Gaps, Data Leave Little Doubt that Fish Are in Peril." *New York Times*, August 3.

Pino, John A., and Andres Martinez. 1981. "The Contribution of Livestock to the World Protein Supply." In *Future Dimensions of World Food and Population*, edited by Richard Woods. Westview Press.

Presidential Commission on World Hunger. 1980. *April Report*.

Sasson, Albert. 1990. *Feeding Tomorrow's World*. UNESCO/CTA.

Sommer, Alfred. 1985. "Xerophthalmia, the Deadly Disease." *American Journal of Ophthalmology* 99, no. 2 (Feb. 15).

U.S. Department of Agriculture. 1992. *World Grain Database*.

CHAPTER 5

Fall-Out From the "Population Bomb"

Impacts on Human Resources and Ecosystems

Man has lost the capacity to foresee and to forestall. He will end by destroying the earth.

—Albert Schweitzer

Certainly the issue of how to feed additional billions in the years ahead, when close to half a billion of our present population is malnourished, looms as a monumental task for future world leaders. However, there are many other equally pressing problems inherent in a situation of rapid population growth—problems that are less dramatic and less publicized than famine, yet nearly as devastating in their impact on human well-being.

Some Consequences of Population Growth

Unemployment

The hapless souls discharged into the surf offshore from Queens, New York, on June 6, 1993, epitomized the desperation of millions of able-bodied young people around the world whose overpopulated homelands are incapable of providing enough new jobs to absorb an exponentially growing work force. On that early summer day the *Golden Venture*, a smuggling ship laden with human cargo, ran aground on a sandbar near the dunes of Ft. Tilden, disgorging nearly 300 illegal Chinese immigrants into the choppy waters. In the ensuing panic and confusion, 10 drowned or died of hypothermia; the remainder were picked up by the Coast Guard and incarcerated. Subsequent interrogation of survivors by Immigration and Naturalization Services personnel revealed a harrowing tale of exploitation and victimization involving "snakeheads" (criminal smuggling gangs that charge would-be immigrants tens of thousands of dollars to bring them to America), inhuman living conditions on a freighter where hundreds of poor, frightened passengers were crammed in the dark hold without ventilation or toilet facilities and provided minimal food and water. Their story was depressingly similar to accounts provided by other Chinese brought into the United States by criminal smuggling rings. In addition to the rigors of the journey itself, they described abominable working conditions after arrival, under which workers are compelled to labor 12–14 hours a day, 7 days a week, for wages as low as $2 per hour (Kleinfeld, 1993). Sadly, the story of the *Golden Venture* is unusual only in the fact that those involved were apprehended. While illegal immigration has been a feature of the American scene for many years, the scope of the problem is steadily growing as population pressures mount overseas and aspirations for a higher standard of living permeate even the most remote villages in distant lands. Why do individuals in ever-larger numbers willingly face unknown dangers and submit to conditions which some officials describe as a "modern-day slave trade"? Simply because, if lucky, they can earn more money in a day in the United States (or in Germany, Canada, France,

Sweden, the U.K.—other favorite destinations for illegal immigrants) than they could in a week in China, Mexico, El Salvador, or any of the dozens of other nations of origin from which hopeful job seekers hail. They can find jobs in the sweatshops of New York or the restaurants of San Diego when none are available in their homelands. In spite of a 1986 law aimed at curbing illegal immigration by prohibitions on the hiring of undocumented workers, the inability of government agents to search every approaching ship, to raid every workplace, or to erect an impermeable wall around our borders guarantees a repetition of *Golden Venture*-type episodes as determined migrants continue to pour into the United States, legally or illegally, in search of employment.

News photos of poverty-stricken Haitians and Cubans arriving in Florida in dangerously overloaded boats has in recent years dramatized the fact that providing jobs for ever-growing populations is already a problem of crisis proportions, particularly in the underdeveloped countries. In the past 25 years the working-age population of most such nations has doubled (in comparison with a 45% increase in the United States) and, since the creation of job opportunities has not kept pace, unemployment rates are climbing rapidly. Over the next two decades, the demand for jobs by new workers is projected to take a sharp upturn because of the very large number of children who will be of working age within a few more years. This rapid growth in the labor force also means that a large proportion of all workers are young and inexperienced. Since inexperienced workers are generally less productive, average productivity is lower with a youthful labor force. As a result, both per capita income and resources available for new investment are lower than they would otherwise be. According to Lester Brown of the Worldwatch Institute, for every 1% increase in the labor force, a 3% increase in the rate of economic growth is needed to generate jobs. Thus countries that are experiencing growth rates in the range of 3% annually need a 9% economic growth rate just to maintain the status quo. Large armies of unemployed and underemployed mean an increase in hunger and malnutrition, since people who have no income can't purchase food even when harvests are abundant. More ominous, unemployed youth—especially the educated unemployed—represent a serious and growing threat to the political stability of the global community.

Literacy

It seems paradoxical that after decades of intensive efforts to build schools and train teachers there are more illiterates in the world today than there were 30 years ago. The *percentage* of illiteracy has dropped considerably, from 44% in 1950 to 26% in 1990, but continued high rates of population growth have boosted the total number of adult illiterates from 700 million in 1950 to 1.4 billion today. Some gains have been achieved quite recently, however; between 1985 and 1990, the number of illiterate adults dipped by 2.4 million—the first decline in total numbers ever recorded (Brown, Kane, and Ayers, 1993). Not surprisingly, illiteracy is most prevalent in areas undergoing high rates of population increase.

Although most developing countries spend about the same percentage of their GNP on primary education as do the industrialized nations (approximately 1.7% GNP), the fact that the developing countries have proportionally so many more children of school age (about 39% of the total population) than do the industrialized nations (21%) means that poor countries must distribute their resources much more thinly. Spending on education per child is considerably less in the developing nations than in the developed ones both because their GNP is lower and because the amount they do spend has to be divided among so many more children. As a result, millions of children in the Third World never have a chance to attend school at all, while many others drop out of primary school without ever learning basic reading and writing skills.

Housing

The slums encircling Third World cities and rural shantytowns as well illustrate that the rising demand for building materials and the physical space on which to erect a dwelling have exceeded the financial capabilities of growing numbers to live in a decent home. In many cities it is not uncommon to see families living in packing crates, lean-tos, or other jerry-built structures assembled from whatever materials could be begged, borrowed, or stolen. Along the highway from Bombay's Santa Cruz International Airport into the city the author has observed an entire colony of pipe-dwellers—people who were living in large clay drainage pipes that had been set along the roadside prior to construction work, but were occupied by squatters before they could be put to their intended use. Families moved in, hung rags over the pipe openings for privacy, and doubtlessly considered themselves fortunate to have such a convenient shelter from the monsoon rains in a city where thousands are born, live, and die on the sidewalks. Housing shortages currently plague many industrialized countries as well; the United States can ill-afford to be smug about other nations' shelter problems, since the crisis of the homeless in American cities has become a cause for national shame.

Poverty

High rates of population growth and poverty are mutually reinforcing; rapid population growth within a nation reduces the per capita availability of investment resources, thus slowing the creation of jobs, schools, and public health facilities. At the family level, large numbers of children reduce the amount of time and money parents can devote to each individual child. In many countries, rapid population growth has offset any economic growth and has prevented any gains in per capita income. In general, the higher a country's fertility, the lower are its GNP and average life expectancy (obviously there are some exceptions to this pattern, oil-rich Kuwait being a notable example). At the same time, high infant mortality, high illiteracy rates, lack of women's employment opportunities outside the home, lack of low-cost family planning services—all common among the poorest

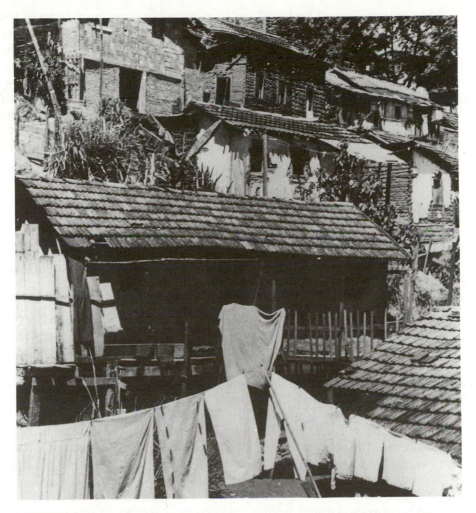

Shantytowns are a common sight along the hillsides of Rio de Janeiro. Millions of Brazilians have migrated to large cities looking for work, only to end up living in slums. [AP/Wide World Photos]

segments of society in developing nations—contribute to the likelihood that poor parents will continue to produce large numbers of children. Sociologists and government planners are still trying to devise a way of breaking this vicious cycle.

Political Unrest

As more and more people exert increasing pressure on the world's finite amount of land, minerals, water, and other resources, conflict both among and within nations will result. As indicated earlier, many current world tensions are intimately related to problems of overpopulation. Record-high birthrates among Palestinians in the West Bank and Gaza undoubtedly contribute to the territorial disputes between Arabs and Jews in Israel; the appalling tribal violence between Hutu and Tutsi in Rwanda and Burundi, the two most densely populated countries in Africa, reflects a desperate competition for limited natural resources; and the upsurge of radical Islamic fundamentalism in countries like Egypt and Algeria is fueled, at least in part, by the inability of secular governments to meet the basic needs of populations doubling every 28–30 years. As human numbers continue to climb, it will be surprising indeed if civil turmoil and international conflict do not grow apace. In an age when both nuclear and chemical weapons are proliferating, nations may not be content to starve peacefully.

Impacts of Growth on the Stability of Ecosystems

> *We abuse land because we regard it as a commodity belonging to us. When we see land as a community to which we belong, we may begin to use it with love and respect.*
> —Aldo Leopold, *A Sand County Almanac*

Commentators who optimistically predict that science and technology will somehow miraculously provide a way of producing ever-increasing amounts of food, fiber, and lumber to sustain the demands of additional billions of people ignore the growing evidence that in many parts of the world large human and livestock populations already have exceeded the carrying capacity of the land itself, resulting in a steady deterioration of the earth's ability to support life. In effect, at a time when we are trying to produce more and more from a given land area to sustain growing human numbers, the activities of those populations are damaging natural ecosystems to the extent that they are becoming incapable of supporting present numbers, much less future additions.

The disruption of natural cycles resulting from human pressures on land resources is undermining the carrying capacity of ecosystems in many parts of the world today. A recent U.N.-sponsored study reveals that since 1945 an area representing nearly 11% of the entire vegetated surface of the earth (i.e. barren deserts, arid mountain regions, and ice-covered land masses were not included in the survey) has been either moderately or severely degraded. Although much of this land is still being cultivated, some of its natural productivity has been lost and could be restored only through implementation of expensive national programs to provide farmers with technical assistance and financial incentives. In the absence of such efforts, the condition of these lands will only deteriorate further. A small portion of this acreage has experienced such an extreme level of degradation that, for all practical purposes, restoration is impossible. The factors largely responsible for the problems identified by the U.N. team include agricultural practices, overgrazing, and deforestation. While the environmental damage provoked by such activities theoretically could occur anywhere, certain natural areas are more vulnerable to long-lasting destruction than others. Tundra, desert, tropical rain forest, and arid grasslands are more easily impaired and take much longer to recover from disruption than does, for example, temperate deciduous forest. Because several of these areas today encompass the homelands of many millions of people whose well-being, and indeed survival, depends on the continued productivity of their land, it is important for us to take a closer look at some specific ways in which humans, consciously or not, are radically undermining the stability of natural ecosystems.

Overgrazing

Of the various activities contributing to soil degradation, none is more significant than overgrazing. Conditions on 35% of all lands classified as degraded can be attributed to excessive pressure generated by too many cattle, goats, or sheep (World Resources Institute, 1992). Under natural conditions, grassland communities are well-adapted to a moderate level of grazing; herds of bison, antelope, wild horses, and so forth, have for millennia been the dominant animals in the grassland biome, evolving and adapting in conjunction with the native plants on which they are dependent. However, when herdsmen increase the number of livestock beyond a certain size or when they introduce types of grazing animals foreign to a particular plant community, the resulting pressure on that community often leads to an unraveling of the ecosystem. The effects of overgrazing are first seen in the declining populations of those plant species least able to tolerate the increased cropping. As these plants disappear, species more tolerant of heavy grazing are then relieved of competition and expand to fill the niche vacated by the more vulnerable types. The loss of the latter, however, results in an overall reduction in the height, biomass, and total coverage of the grassland. If overgrazing persists, even the more resistant native plants will be unable to withstand the pressure and give way to invader weed species that were not members of the original community. Such plants are generally much inferior to the native plants in nutritive qualities and, as a result, the vitality of the herd is adversely affected. Eventually the weeds themselves may be trampled to such an extent that they, too, are reduced in coverage. The soil, thus exposed to the forces of wind and water, may be worn away, leaving a barren mud flat or rocky hillside, devoid of any community (Whittaker, 1975).

While land degradation due to overgrazing is most pronounced in Australia (80%) and in Africa (49%), extensive areas of rangeland in the American West are severely affected as well. For years U.S. environmentalists have complained that nearly 30,000 western ranchers have been grazing their cattle and sheep on public lands at bargain-basement prices ($1.86/month for every cow and calf or for every five sheep) which encourage overexploitation of land resources. In the fall of 1993 Interior Secretary Bruce Babbitt proclaimed a "new land ethic" when he announced plans to increase grazing fees on 260 million federally owned acres in 16 western states and to improve general environmental conditions on those lands. This policy change, expected to be implemented in late 1994 over the bitter opposition of western Senators, represents one of the most far-reaching changes in federal land management since the 1906 introduction of grazing fees—a change which environmental groups like the Sierra Club hail as "a milestone in protecting the last great open stretches of land in the 48 contiguous states" (Schneider, 1993; National Wildlife Federation, 1994).

Soil Erosion

Throughout much of the world, including the rich farmlands of the American Midwest, the fertile topsoil that is the basis of agricultural productivity is thinning at an alarming rate. Around the globe, over 25 billion tons of soil is lost to erosion annually, destroying over a billion acres (430 million hectares) of farmland—about 30% of the land currently under cultivation (Lal and Pierce, 1993; Stutz, 1993). An even larger area (500 million hectares) is losing soil at such a rate that it is likely to lose its productive capacity within the next few decades if effective conservation strategies are not promptly implemented (WCED, 1987). The Food and Agriculture Organization of the United Nations has warned that unless Third World countries give much higher priority to soil erosion control efforts, they could witness a 30% reduction in harvests by the end of the next century—at which time their populations will have increased by as much as sixfold over current levels.

Some degree of soil loss is, of course, a natural process and occurs even in the absence of human intervention. Poor agricultural practices, however, greatly increase the rate of erosion, and when the amount of topsoil lost exceeds that of new soil formed through the gradual decomposition of organic matter (an amount referred to in agricultural circles as **T-value** or, more simply, **"T"**), then the layer of topsoil becomes thinner and thinner until it disappears completely, leaving only the unproductive subsoil or, in extreme cases, bare rock. Topsoil loss has a direct negative impact on cropland productivity, though in recent decades the relationship between soil erosion and diminishing yields has been largely masked by the greatly expanded use of chemical fertilizers. We have, in a sense, been substituting chemical nitrogen and potash for topsoil in order to maintain good harvests. However, while chemicals can replace nutrients lost through erosion, they can't substitute for the lost organic material necessary for maintaining a porous, healthy soil structure. Some studies suggest that heavy fertilizer use can actually damage the soil by disrupting natural nutrient cycles and predict that in the future per acre yields, even on lands receiving chemical inputs, will begin to drop if erosion trends aren't reversed (Smil, 1991; *Yearbook of Agriculture*, 1981).

Serious erosion control efforts in the United States grew out of the disastrous Dust Bowl years of the mid-1930s when millions of tons of rich Great Plains topsoil were literally "gone with the wind" as a result of drought and unwise cultivation practices. In 1935 the Soil Conservation Service (SCS) was created and Congress funded a major research effort to learn more about the processes of erosion and effective methods of control. By the 1940s and 1950s soil loss on U.S. farmlands was declining noticeably as American farmers followed the advice of Cooperative

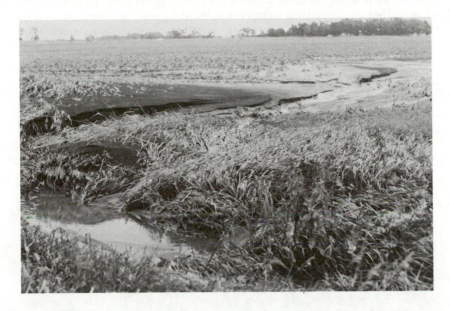

Sheet erosion after heavy rain robs farmland of valuable topsoil and causes water pollution and sedimentation problems in nearby streams and ditches. [Gary Fak, Soil Conservation Service]

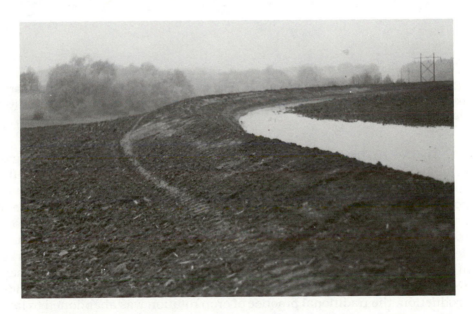

An effective erosion-control method is the construction of grass ridge terraces such as the one pictured here. A terrace reduces soil runoff by shortening the length of the slope and diverting water in a horizontal direction. When planted in perennial grasses, the approximately 10-foot-wide area has the additional benefit of providing valuable wildlife habitat. [Gary Fak, Soil Conservation Service]

Extension advisors ("county agents") or SCS personnel to install terraces, plant windbreaks, contour strip-crop, build grass waterways—whatever method or combination of methods was most suitable to reduce erosion rates on the lands they were cultivating.

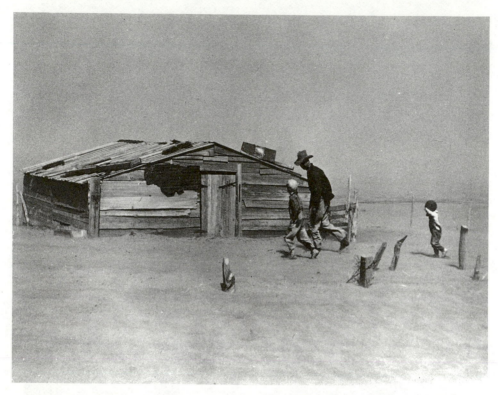

"Dust Bowl" years: an Oklahoma family runs for shelter during one of the numerous sky-blackening storms which afflicted the Great Plains states during the 1930s. [U.S. Department of Agriculture]

By the 1970s, however, soil loss due to farmland erosion once again began to accelerate, reversing the gains of the previous two decades. High commodity prices and the demand for agricultural exports to feed growing populations overseas while simultaneously easing U.S. balance-of-payments problems combined to boost farm production—and promoted record levels of erosion. Citing the link between farm exports and land degradation, an official at the Illinois Department of Agriculture remarked at the time that ". . . for every bushel of corn we ship overseas, we send 1½ bushels of topsoil down the Mississippi River." In the push for expanded production, the traditional practice of crop rotation was abandoned in favor of continuous cropping of corn or soybeans, a practice that greatly increases erosion rates since this leaves the soil surface without any plant cover during a considerable portion of the year. Strong export demand prompted farmers to plow "from fencepost-to-fencepost" to reap the maximum possible profit. By doing so, however, they brought into production much highly erodible land which would have been better left in pasture—and it promptly began to wash away. In the Midwest fall plowing came into vogue and contributed to substantial amounts of erosion by both wind and water during winter and early spring when fields are bare. By the late 1970s it was evident that soil loss was once again becoming a serious national problem. In 1981 the USDA estimated that the inherent productivity of fully one-third of American farmlands was declining because of high rates of erosion. Efforts were launched at both the state and federal level to reduce soil loss to tolerable levels (*i.e.* to T-value). The main strategy for achieving this goal was the promotion of **conservation tillage**, a cultivation practice which involves leaving 30% or more of the soil surface covered with the previous year's crop residue. Variants on conservation tillage include **no-till**, in which crops are planted in the undisturbed residue of an old crop; **ridge-till**, where seeds are planted in ridges developed by cultivation of the field during the previous growing season and left undisturbed after the harvest; and **mulch-till**, a situation where crops are planted in a field where the entire surface has been disturbed, but at least the minimum amount of residue remains after planting. These crop residues perform a number

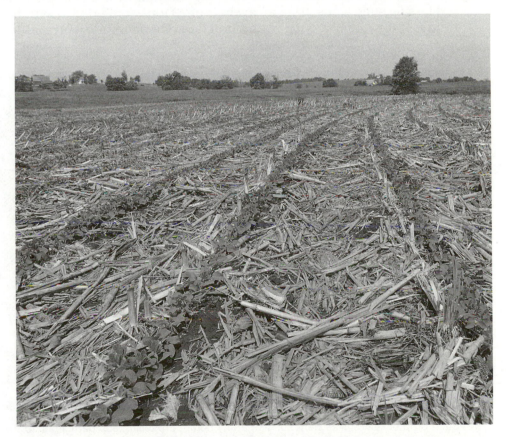

No-till farming: young soybean plants emerge from a field whose surface is protected from erosion by a cushioning layer of corn stubble. [U.S. Department of Agriculture]

of protective functions: cushioning the impact of falling raindrops, decreasing wind access to bare soil, serving as mini-dams to restrict overland runoff from fields, and improving soil characteristics which resist erosive forces. Alone or in combination with such soil conservation measures as terracing or construction of grass waterways, conservation tillage can substantially reduce erosion rates while maintaining or even increasing crop yields. While conservation tillage is not appropriate for all crops, the practice has expanded rapidly during the past decade, particularly in corn- and soybean-producing areas of the Midwest (Illinois leads the nation in acreage devoted to conservation tillage—over 50% by the early 1990s).

Erosion control efforts in the United States were given a major boost when Congress passed the **Food Security Act of 1985**, creating the **Conservation Reserve**. Under this landmark program, excessive production and soil loss are both being curbed by offering farmers financial incentives to take highly erodible lands out of crop production for 10 years, converting them to pastures or woodlands. By 1990, approximately 34 million acres, about 11% of all U.S. cropland, had been enrolled in Conservation Reserve contracts (*Yearbook of Agriculture*, 1991). Surveys carried out on lands idled under the program indicated a sharp decline in soil loss on such lands, from an average of 29 tons/acre prior to withdrawal to just 2 tons after a year in the program. On acres not enrolled in the

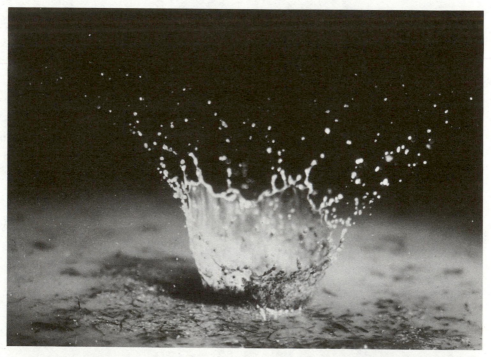

Each drop of rain strikes bare soil like a tiny bomb, propelling soil particles into the air; subsequent overland flow of rainwater across a field carries these loosened particles into waterways, resulting in the annual loss of enormous quantities of topsoil. [U.S. Department of Agriculture]

Reserve but still experiencing unacceptably high erosion rates, the Act required farmers to develop an approved soil conservation plan by 1990—and to complete implementation of that plan by 1995—or risk losing their eligibility for farm program benefits such as crop insurance and price support programs (Berg, 1987; USDA, 1987).

Currently the United States is the only major agricultural nation pursuing systematic efforts to reduce excessive soil erosion, yet outside this country the situation is even more serious. Indian agronomists estimate their country is losing five billion tons of topsoil annually, almost double the soil loss in the United States where the cropland area is about the same (Brown, 1988). In Ethiopia erosion is depriving that nation's hard-pressed farmers of 1.5–2 billion cubic meters of topsoil every year; as a result, 4 million hectares (about 10 million acres) of Ethiopian highlands are now termed "irreversibly degraded." At the foothills of the Himalayas, in eastern Nepal, 38% of the land area consists of barren fields, abandoned because their topsoil has been lost to erosion (Stutz, 1993). In the lush farmlands of central Chile, the current prosperity may be short-lived because excessive rates of soil loss are undermining agricultural productivity even on the best lands; on the marginal lands where over half the country's peasant farmers live, erosion is seriously depressing crop yields and threatening farmers with large financial losses if current trends are not reversed (Faeth, 1994). In China, soil erosion is endangering increases in crop production desperately needed to feed a still-growing population. In China's northwestern Gansu Province, half or more of all arable land has already been lost to erosion and encroaching deserts. Alarmed by the shrinking resource base, a Canadian scientist who recently completed a study on environmental problems in China commented, "You can clean up air pollution, but once you ruin your soil it is very difficult to go back. Land is the irreplaceable foundation of China's food production" (Tyler, 1994).

Deforestation

For the last ten thousand years humans have been cutting and burning woodlands at an ever-increasing pace in their quest for additional farmland, fuel, and building material. Experts estimate that trees now cover approximately three-fourths of the area that was forested prior to *H. sapiens*' arrival on the scene—26% of the earth's surface today versus 34% in pre-human times. Such figures are somewhat misleading, however, for when biologists look closely at the world's remaining woodlands, they find that slightly less than half of these areas consist of intact forest ecosystems—scarcely one-third the total before human activities set in motion the processes of deforestation which have continued over the centuries and which have markedly accelerated within recent decades (Durning, 1993). As the rate of forest loss accelerates, so do pressures on ecosystems as species loss, soil erosion—even climate change—become increasingly apparent.

Deforestation, defined as the permanent decline in crown cover of trees to less than 10% of its original extent, is regarded as particularly worrisome in regard to tropical forests, which have shrunk by as much as 50% in just the last 25 years. Unfortunately, rates of loss continue to accelerate. Results from a recently completed tropical forest inventory conducted by the Food and Agriculture Organization (FAO) show an alarming 40% increase in the pace of tropical forest loss during the 1980s— a 15.4 million hectares/year decline during that 10-year period as compared with an 11.3 million hectare/year loss during the 1970s. While these numbers are disturbing enough, investigations by other researchers suggest that areas adversely impacted by tree loss in the tropics are even more extensive than FAO figures suggest, since *degraded and fragmented forests*, while still providing tree cover, are no longer capable of supporting the rich diversity of plant and animal life they formerly harbored (Skole and Tucker, 1993).

While tropical forests can be divided into a number of different categories depending on precipitation and type of vegetation, the environmental threats posed by deforestation are nowhere more acute than in the rain forest and moist deciduous forests. These lush laboratories of life are

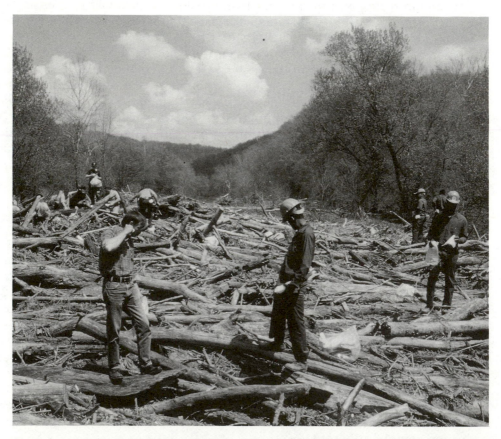

Forest loss can have devastating impacts on terrestrial ecosystems, including soil erosion, species loss, increase in the amount of runoff and flooding, and, perhaps, even climate change. [Thomas A. Schneider]

home to more than half of all plants and animals on earth and their demise would inevitably result in the extinction of millions of species. While most tropical countries have experienced a decline in forest cover over the past decade, deforestation has been most extensive in Brazil and Indonesia where the number of hectares lost each year has averaged 3.7 million and 1.2 million, respectively. *Rates* of tree loss, as opposed to total *area affected*, have been highest on the Southeast Asian mainland (Thailand, Vietnam, Cambodia, and Burma) and in Central America/Mexico. These two regions exhibit current rates of deforestation twice as high as the 0.8% annual average for tropical forests as a whole (World Resources Institute, 1994).

Elsewhere, in the semiarid regions of Asia, Africa, and Latin America where forests have always been scanty, existing trees have almost entirely vanished. Only in Europe and, quite recently, in North America are forests being managed on a sustained-yield basis. In these regions of temperate and boreal forest, tree cover actually increased by about 5% from 1980 to 1990. However, this overall increase in forest biomass obscures the fact that significant areas of temperate old-growth forest have been replaced by commercial woodlands that are much less biologically diverse than the natural forest ecosystems which formerly flourished in those regions.

The largest single cause of deforestation today, as in the past, is the **clearing of land for agriculture**. The population pressures behind this trend and the ecological damage caused by exploitation of marginal lands not suited for sustained cultivation have already been described. A second major contributor to deforestation, also a direct result of human population growth, is the **gathering of wood for fuel**. For approximately 90% of the people in the world's less-developed nations, today's true energy crisis is the scarcity of firewood. In most tropical countries wood is used largely for cooking, but in colder climates and mountainous regions it's used for heating as well. Spiralling population growth rates in such nations have boosted demand for firewood to such an extent that trees are being cut at a pace which far outraces nature's ability to grow new ones. As a result, treeless areas around towns and villages throughout Africa, Asia, and Latin America are expanding rapidly as desperate people gather every twig and sometimes even leaves and bark in their never-ending search for fuel.

The problem is particularly acute in semiarid regions where removal of vegetation leaves land at the mercy of wind and water, subject to rapid rates of soil loss. In once heavily forested lands such as Nepal, whole mountainsides are being stripped by villagers who now spend most of the day searching for a supply of firewood which two decades ago could have been gathered in an hour. The investment in time and physical energy required just to obtain enough fuel to cook the family meal has thus increased tremendously in just one generation. Of greater concern to Nepali officials, however, and to their counterparts in the vast Indian subcontinent to the south is the fact that the progressive denudation of the Himalayan slopes is resulting in a massive increase in soil erosion in this ecologically fragile mountain region. As a result, not only is the productive capacity of the land rapidly decreasing, but also much more frequent and severe flooding, with corresponding heavy loss of life, is occurring downstream

Figure 5-1 Deforestation Hot Spots

Region	Forest remaining as of 1990 (thousands of hectares)	Annual deforestation 1981–1990 (thousands of hectares)	Annual rate of deforestation (percentage)
Africa	527,586	4,100	0.7
East Sahel Africa	65,450	595	0.9
West Africa	55,607	591	1.0
Central Africa	204,112	1,139	0.5
Tropical Southern Africa	145,868	1,345	0.9
Asia	310,597	3,904	1.2
Continental S.E. Asia	75,240	1,314	1.6
Insular S.E. Asia	135,426	1,926	1.3
Latin America	918,115	7,407	0.8
Central America and Mexico	68,096	1,112	1.5
Tropical South America	802,904	6,173	0.7
World Total in Tropics	1,756,297	15,411	0.8

Source: FAO

in the river valleys of northern India, Pakistan, and Bangladesh due to greatly increased amounts of runoff in the headwaters area of the Ganges, Indus, and Brahmaputra rivers. The devastating floods that left 25 million Bengalis homeless and killed 1200 during the 1988 monsoon season in Bangladesh represented an "unnatural disaster" caused by increased runoff from the denuded Himalayan watershed upstream and increased rates of siltation in lowland deltas, diminishing their water-holding capacity. While flooding of such severity used to occur perhaps twice in a century, five "50-year floods" occurred during the 1980s and threaten to become a regular occurrence if deforestation in the Himalayas is not reversed. In 1993, after monsoon floods once again inundated one-third of Bangladesh, that nation demanded action on the part of India and Nepal to devise long-term solutions to what has in recent years become almost an annual problem. Pointing out that river beds in Bangladesh are steadily rising due to the two billion tons of silt washing down from the Himalayas each year, Bangladeshi officials reiterated their insistence that Nepal control downstream flow by building dams and reservoirs on its major rivers. In spite of the fact that flood damage and death tolls have been high in Nepal and India also, neither country has indicated any inclination to heed their neighbor's request, and diplomatic relations among the three countries continue to deteriorate over this issue (Hazarika, 1993).

As the supply of fuelwood continues to diminish, prices rise accordingly, imposing additional burdens on already impoverished populations.

In the West African nation of Niger, for example, an average laborer's family must spend close to 25% of its income for firewood; in neighboring Burkina Faso the figure may approach 30% (exploitation of forest resources for fuel is more acute in African nations than anywhere else in the world; fully 90% of all the wood harvested in Africa is burned directly or used for making charcoal). Where people can't afford the high cost of wood, women and children spend much of their time scrounging the countryside for anything burnable—dry grass, fallen leaves, animal dung, garbage. In the industrialized nations, which until about 100 years ago had been just as dependent on wood for fuel as the developing countries are today, the substitution of coal, petroleum products, and natural gas for wood forestalled a growing pressure on their forests for fuel. Until recently it was widely hoped that increasing use of kerosene or bottled gas stoves in Third World countries would ease the burden on those nations' timber resources. The virtual overnight quadrupling of world oil prices which OPEC imposed on the world economy in 1973 and further escalation in the price of petroleum products since then have placed wood substitutes such as kerosene out of reach of millions of the world's poorest people and guaranteed continued overexploitation of forest products. Thus can economic decisions in Riyadh or Tripoli upset the ecological stability of a mountain hamlet in Peru or a dusty village in Ethiopia.

BOX 5-1
Drugs and Deforestation: The Coca Connection

The montane forests of South America's Andean highlands, extending along the "backbone" of the continent from Venezuela to Argentina, constitute a veritable treasure-trove of biodiversity. Although Brazil's Amazon rain forest has been the focal point for world concerns about species loss in recent years, the once-vast expanse of trees, ferns, mosses, and herbaceous flowering plants covering the foothills of the Andes are today even more seriously threatened by human activities than are the forests of Amazonia. In the northern Andes, particularly in Peru and Colombia, 90% of the original forest cover has already been destroyed, with more disappearing daily. Since montane forests provide critical habitat to 40,000 species of flowering plants alone (compared with 30,000 identified in the Amazon), deforestation of this immensely rich and varied bioregion is an ecological tragedy.

While some of the pressures responsible for dwindling forest cover in the Andes are the same as those confronting woodlands throughout the tropics—subsistence farming, fuelwood gathering, cattle ranching—a more sinister influence is more directly responsible for the accelerating pace of destruction: the international trade in illicit drugs.

For centuries the native American populations inhabiting the Andean highlands have cultivated the coca shrub, utilizing its dried gray-green leaves for a wide variety of ceremonial purposes and for treating such ailments as headaches, upset stomach, altitude sickness, and hunger pangs. Over time, selective breeding by native cultivators produced coca varieties which could thrive in poor soil and could be harvested as many as six times a year. Nevertheless, production remained at a low level, sufficing only to meet limited local demands, until the late 1960s when cocaine use in North America began to soar. To supply the burgeoning market, drug dealers turned to the highlands of the Andes, particularly to the Huallaga Valley of Peru where an especially potent variety of coca is grown. Although the fertile soil supports a wide range of crops— bananas, beans, corn, rice, citrus, etc.—none are half so profitable as coca; as a consequence, production increased exponentially on the steep slopes. Over the past 25 years, more than 700,000 hectares (1.7 million acres) of mountain forests have been cleared in Peru alone to grow and process coca. Researchers estimate that a minimum of three acres of forest around the Huallaga Valley are cleared daily to provide space for fields, processing labs, and secret airstrips servicing the illicit trade. Such estimates are no more than educated guesses, however, since fear of retribution from narco-traffickers deters scientists from entering the so-called "red zone" dominated by *Sendero Luminoso* ("Shining Path"), a Maoist guerilla group which forces peasants to grow coca in order to use drug trade profits to finance its revolutionary aims.

Aside from the obvious ecological damage caused by removing tree cover from erosion-prone slopes, coca cultivation has imposed numerous environmental insults on the northern Andes. As in the Brazilian rain forest, fire is often employed as the quickest, easiest way of clearing forests; pilots who fly over the area during the dry burning season (June–August) report that the air is so thick with smoke they're forced to switch to radar to navigate. Growers attempting to maximize leaf yield commonly employ five times the recommended amounts of chemical fertilizers; they similarly misuse pesticides, poisoning everything that isn't coca. With absolutely no vegetative cover left between the rows of coca shrubs, heavy rainfall on the thin mountain soil washes tons of pesticide-laden mud into waterways. Erosion isn't the only source of toxic chemical pollutants in the region's rivers, however. Crude cocaine processing labs set up in the jungle feature plastic-lined holes where piles of dried coca leaves are soaked in a series of chemical baths, then in kerosene, to yield an oily sludge that is filtered through toilet paper into shallow drainage trenches. The filtrate, a grayish powder which comprises a crude cocaine base, is generally flown out to Colombia for final processing into cocaine powder; the waste liquid—a witches' brew of acids, ammonia, acetone, and kerosene—is simply discharged into the nearest waterway. Little wonder that Peruvian biologists report the disappearance of many species of fish, amphibians, and other aquatic organisms throughout the region. Since the mid-1980s, cooperative efforts by the Peruvian police and the U.S. Drug Enforcement Agency to apprehend growers and destroy their crops has only exacerbated problems of deforestation. Because drug trade profits are so high, growers targeted by police have simply moved deeper into the jungle where the cycle of destruction is perpetuated. If current trends persist, experts estimate that Peruvian coca production in the year 2000 will be double that of 1990.

An observed decline in U.S. cocaine consumption in the early 1990s prompted initial hopes that market forces might act as a brake on continued exploitation of Andean forest resources. Recent reports, unfortunately, give little hope for optimism. While cocaine use has indeed been on the decline, heroin use is rising in both the United States and in Europe. The South American drug cartel, taking note of this change in consumer preference, has begun diversifying its product line, planting opium poppies across vast areas of Colombia's central cordillera. Between 1991 and 1993, poppy cultivation expanded from 1000 hectares to 20,000 hectares, with an additional 30,000 cleared and ready to plant. Since protection of national forest resources is a low priority in most financially strapped Andean nations, preservation of the region's remaining biodiversity would seem to hinge on winning "the war against drugs" here at home. Unless the demand for such products declines, reducing the enormous profits they currently generate, the future of Andean forests is bleak indeed.

References

Goodman, Billy. 1993. "Drugs and People Threaten Diversity in Andean Forests." *Science* (July 16).

Joyce, Stephanie. 1990. "Snorting Peru's Rain Forest." *International Wildlife* 20, no. 3 (May/June).

While the clearing of land for subsistence farming and the increasing demand for fuelwood are two of the most prominent factors resulting in destruction of forests on a worldwide basis, in some areas, most notably in Southeast Asia but recently in South America as well, **commercial lumbering** is decimating valuable tropical hardwood reserves in order to supply the increased demands of industrial nations for furniture, plywood, and paper pulp. Until relatively recently, tropical forests largely escaped the logging pressures which earlier had decimated the virgin forests of Europe and North America, primarily because they were sparsely populated and not easily accessible. In addition, in tropical forests commercially valuable tree species are widely dispersed over a broad geographic area, interspersed with many less-desired species, a fact which made their large-scale exploitation economically unfeasible. This situation changed dramatically in the 1960s when mechanization of the timber industry and the arrival of giant multinational lumber companies made possible the ever-more-rapid felling of tropical forests. The methods employed by these companies have been particularly destructive and wasteful; in a typical operation only 10–20% of the trees are cut and removed (*i.e.* those species with commercial value), but 30–50% of non-target trees are destroyed in the process. On many tracts, trees are felled by utilizing giant tractors, working in tandem, to drag huge link chains across the forest floor, pulling down everything in their path. This process causes such extensive soil damage that the land may never fully recover. In other cases, less desirable tree species are burned or left to decay in wide expanses of clear-cut forest land. Although experience on a few demonstration plots shows that it is possible to harvest tropical hardwoods selectively, leaving the forest to regenerate, in practice this is seldom done—it is estimated that only 0.1% of all tropical wood is cut on a sustained-yield basis (Durning, 1993).

While commercial lumbering in the tropics has taken its greatest toll thus far in Southeast Asia, the near-exhaustion of primary forests in that region has prompted timber barons to shift their attention to South America, particularly to Bolivia, where logging concessions have been granted for more than half that nation's forest lands; to Guyana, where more than 80% of government-owned forests have been leased to wealthy Korean and Malayasian timber companies on terms extremely generous to the Asian firms; and to Chile, where the world's largest remaining expanse of still-pristine temperate rain forest is being felled at an alarming rate to meet the insatiable demands of Japanese paper producers for wood chips. Environmentalists fully expect to see the same well-documented pattern of land degradation and abuse which have accompanied logging operations in Africa, Malaysia, Indonesia, and Papua New Guinea repeated in South America. In political systems where politicians control the distribution of timber concessions, bribery and corruption ensure the over-exploitation of forest resources with minimal regulation of environmental damage. Careless logging practices frequently result in permanent ecological degradation and those charged with enforcing sound forest management practices are either bought off or become totally frustrated by their inability to prosecute loggers whose political connections insulate them from any enforcement actions. Land rights of indigenous forest peoples, 50 million of whom still make their home within the tropical rain forest, are another casualty of commercial logging operations in the tropics. Preexisting tribal claims are seldom considered when timber concessions are granted and native peoples frequently suffer total impoverishment after logging destroys the forest resources which sustained these groups for millennia (Colchester, 1994; Nash, 1993, 1994).

International efforts to promote sustainable timber harvesting in the tropics have been hampered by a North-South divergence of economic interests. At the 1992 Earth Summit in Brazil, attempts to produce a world forestry agreement calling on developing nations to adopt tougher conservation policies to protect tropical forests were defeated by Third World insistence that the industrialized North similarly pledge its members to observe environmentally friendly logging practices in temperate forests. A compromise agreement hammered out early in 1994 just prior to expiration of the 1983 International Tropical Timber Agreement pledged all signatories to place forest preservation on a level of equal importance with commercial demands of the global timber industry. Although the agreement requires regular reports on progress toward the goal of sustainable use of forests, environmental groups are skeptical that the treaty will have any meaningful impact, regarding it as merely a public-relations ploy to conceal an unwillingness by both sides to deal seriously with problems of tropical deforestation (Pitt, 1994).

In Latin America, **cattle-ranching** has imposed additional pressures on threatened forests. In such Central American nations as Costa Rica and Panama, cattle ranching has destroyed more hectares of tropical forest than any other activity—70% of the land formerly covered by trees in both countries is now utilized as pastureland (Coffin, 1993). During the 1980s much of this destruction was driven by the demand for cheap beef to supply fast-food chains in the United States—the infamous "hamburger connection," now largely curtailed. In Brazil, cattle ranching is by far the leading cause of deforestation in the Amazon basin, the largest continuous tract of tropical forest in the world. Since the 1970s, ranchers have cleared more than 10 million hectares of rain forest for pastureland, a practice originally encouraged by generous tax breaks and subsidies from a Brazilian government eager to develop the vast interior of that nation while providing an abundant supply of inexpensive meat for working-class consumers in the country's large coastal cities. In recent years subsidy programs have been terminated, but ranchers continue to clear new pasture as a form of land speculation—a means of obtaining legal title to such lands at a time of rapidly rising property values. Unfortunately, as in the case of agricultural exploitation in Amazonia, grazing pressures on these deforested tracts can be sustained profitably for only a few years. When the fragile tropical soils wear out, their content of phosphorus and other nutrients depleted, ranchers simply move on, burn or cut down more trees, and thus perpetuate the destructive cycle. Although the abandoned pasturelands are subsequently revegetated by invader plant species, the new biotic community bears little resemblance to the original forest either in biomass or in biodiversity. Observations of ecological succession in areas of rain forest denuded by ranching operations suggest that regeneration of such areas to mature forest conditions may require several centuries (World Resources Institute, 1990).

That destruction of the earth's forest cover will have a serious and adverse impact on terrestrial ecosystems—and on their human inhabitants as well—is undisputed. Past history should have taught us that heedless deforestation can lead to excessive erosion rates, decrease the soil's water-absorbing capacity, increase the amount of runoff and flooding, and lead to the transformation of once-productive environments into desert-like conditions. Today we have growing evidence to indicate that loss of forest cover can also lead to local climatic changes, with an increase in temperature and drop in annual rainfall when large expanses of woodland are cleared. More ominous is the possibility that heedless deforestation will hasten the onset of global warming, due to the pivotal role forests play as a "carbon sink," absorbing CO_2 and thereby counteracting the so-called "Greenhouse Effect."

One might suppose that since the consequences of deforestation are well understood, a serious attempt to reverse current trends would be well underway. Unfortunately, in many of the countries most seriously affected reforestation efforts are negligible. Even where the political will exists and funds are available, large-scale tree-planting programs encounter serious difficulties which are inextricably related to the cultural, political, and economic facts of life in rural societies. In many areas saplings planted with high hopes are promptly devoured by overabundant and freely-roaming goats, sheep, and cattle. In some places nomads passing through an area may decimate a village's efforts at reforestation, while in still other areas villagers themselves may uproot young trees because they simply have no other source of fuel. Successful reforestation efforts require extensive administrative efforts to protect the plants for years—efforts which may be politically unrewarding to officials trying to win voters' approval for next year's election rather than a "job well done" 20 years in the future. There have been some reforestation success stories, most notably in India where approximately four hectares of trees are being planted for every one that is deforested. Although these tree plantations, which consist primarily of fast-growing eucalyptus or pine, lack the diversity of species which characterized the native forest cover, they nevertheless provide soil and watershed protection while serving as windbreaks and a renewable source of fuel for local residents.

Ultimately the most serious obstacle to curbing forest loss is the continued rapid growth of human populations in the countries most affected. As a Costa Rican squatter on a partially forested ranch poignantly stated, "By subsisting today I know I can destroy the future of the forest and the people. But I have to eat today" (Hamilton, 1989).

Desertification

That humans can create desert-like conditions on once-productive land has been known, though largely ignored, since the time 2300 years ago when Plato bewailed the ecological fate of his native Attica, writing that "our land, compared with what it was, is like the skeleton of a body wasted by disease. The soft, plump parts have vanished and all that remains is the bare carcass." This sorry situation was brought about by the cutting of forests and overgrazing of livestock which in that semiarid climate inevitably resulted in erosion of topsoil and the drying up of springs which were no longer being recharged, since rainwater quickly ran off the bare ground rather than percolating through the soil. The formation of cultural wastelands which occurred over two millennia ago in Greece and the lands around the eastern Mediterranean is a process which has so increased in extent during the 20th century that it has been graced with the somewhat unwieldy, though descriptive term **"desertification."** Defined by delegates at the 1992 United Nations Conference on Environment and Development (UNCED) as "land degradation in arid, semiarid, and dry sub-humid areas resulting from various factors including climatic variations and human activities," desertification today is adversely affecting the lives and economic well-being of an estimated 900 million people in over 100 countries.

Contrary to the prevailing image of sand dunes relentlessly sweeping down over green fields and pastures, desertification seldom involves the steady influx of sands along a uniform front. Most often the process is set in motion when climatic fluctuations and abusive land use practices interact to extend desert-like conditions irregularly over susceptible land. Spots of extreme degradation are especially likely to grow around water holes when nearby pastures are heavily grazed and trampled and around towns when people denude adjacent lands in their search for fuelwood. Since desertification first captured world attention in the 1960s and 1970s, it has generally been assumed that pressures generated by growing human populations have been the primary cause of the adverse environmental trends evident in many arid and semiarid regions. Recently, however, data obtained from a decade's worth of satellite photos indicate that climatic variations exert a much more pronounced influence on the expansion of desert-like conditions than do human pressures. In the world's arid grasslands and semi-desert regions, year-to-year fluctuations of rainfall can be moderately destructive to biotic communities even under natural conditions, but in the long run natural processes can correct the imbalance and quickly reestablish pre-drought vegetational patterns. However, when environmental stresses due to normal climatic variation are coupled with pressures created by human activities (e.g. overgrazing, fuelwood gathering, poor cultivation practices), problems of land degradation are seriously aggravated. If such human pressures persist and intensify, they can sharply limit the regenerative capabilities of the land, hindering its recovery even after climatic conditions improve (Hulme and Kelly, 1993; Stevens, 1994).

Whatever its cause, desertification is a process occurring today on an unprecedented scale. The human tragedy embodied in the great dust storms that blackened the skies in the American prairie states during the 1930s is being repeated today in sub-Saharan Africa where the nomadic herdsmen and their oversized flocks seem to have pushed the carrying capacity of the land beyond the point of no return; in northwest India, the world's most densely populated arid zone and, thanks to the large herds of cattle, camels, goats, etc., also perhaps the world's dustiest area; in North Africa, where excessive rates of soil erosion are accelerating the pace of desertification on lands that were once the granary of the Roman Empire; in China, where sand-break forests are being planted in a desperate effort to combat sandstorms which are threatening almost 9 million hectares of agricultural lands and causing direct economic losses valued at approximately $800 million annually; and in the American Southwest where overgrazing during the past several hundred years may be largely responsible for the formation of Arizona's Sonoran Desert. Many of these areas still have the potential to reestablish their former grassland ecosystems if the constant pressure of overgrazing and overplowing could be lifted, but some have been irreversibly degraded by complete loss of topsoil. If human pressures continue to mount, degradation of arid lands will result in the permanent destabilization of existing ecosystems and a continuing impoverishment of both ecological and cultural conditions. Ecosystems, like civilizations, can decline and fall if pushed too far.

Wetlands Loss

Swamps, bogs, fens, tidal marshlands, pocosins, estuaries, ponds, river bottoms, flood plains, and prairie potholes all fall under the designation of **wetlands**, ecosystems characterized by soils which are inundated or water-saturated for at least a portion of the year and by the presence of certain water-loving plants ("hydrophytes"). In the not-too-distant past, most people viewed wetlands as a nuisance, useful only to frogs and mosquitoes, and thus prime candidates for draining or filling to convert them into more "profitable" areas for farming, mining, or urban development. As a result, over half the wetlands which existed in the contiguous 48 states at the time European settlers first arrived (estimated at more than 200 million acres in A.D. 1600) have now disappeared; although the rate of wetlands loss has declined somewhat over the last quarter-century, an additional 290,000 acres continue to be lost each year. Today, wetlands cover just 5% (104 million acres) of the land surface in the lower 48 states. Alaska has another 200 million acres, with wetlands extending across half the North Star State. Outside Alaska, Florida and Louisiana have the largest remaining expanses of wetlands, though they are also among the states with the highest rates of wetlands loss in recent years. California has lost a greater percentage of its original wetlands than any other state (91%), but Florida has lost the largest number of acres (*America's Wetlands*, 1988; World Resources Institute, 1992). In recent years the significance of this loss has finally begun to be realized, and belated efforts to control wetlands conversion are now underway at both the federal and state level.

Figure 5-2 Relative Abundance of Wetlands in the U.S.

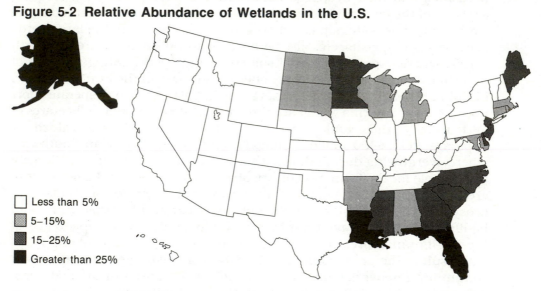

☐ Less than 5%
▨ 5–15%
▤ 15–25%
■ Greater than 25%

Source: U.S. Fish and Wildlife Service, *Wetlands of the United States: Current Status and Recent Trends*

Today the importance of wetlands in both ecological and economic terms is unquestioned. Their ability to retain large amounts of water makes them extremely valuable as nature's own method of preventing devastating floods. Not surprisingly, as wetlands along the Mississippi River Valley have been destroyed, the severity and frequency of floods in that region has escalated—a fact made tragically clear during the disastrous flooding along the upper Mississippi River Valley in the summer of 1993. Wetlands provide the major recharge areas for groundwater reserves and also serve as "living filters" for purifying contaminated surface waters as these percolate into the ground. Indeed, taking advantage of wetlands' capacity to act as "nature's kidneys," some communities are now utilizing constructed marshes to treat stormwater or secondary wastewater effluent by directing the flow through **engineered wetlands** where living organisms remove pollutants efficiently and inexpensively. The sustained productivity of commercial fisheries is also heavily dependent on the existence of wetlands. Between 60–90% of fish caught along the Atlantic and Gulf coasts spend at least some portion of their life cycle, usually the vulnerable early stages, in coastal marshes or estuaries. Further inland in the Midwest, the system of lakes, marshes, and prairie potholes extending from the Gulf of Mexico north into Canada provides the major life-support system for millions of migratory waterfowl (half of all ducklings in North America are hatched in the prairie potholes of the Dakotas and Canada). A $1 billion recreational hunting industry, attracting 2.5 million duck hunters each year, is thus totally dependent on preservation of these vital wetlands breeding areas. Wetlands also provide a habitat not only for ducks and geese but for many other bird and mammal species—whooping cranes, river otters, black bears, and so on.

BOX 5-2

New Hope for the Everglades

The Everglades, Florida's legendary "River of Grass" and the world's largest freshwater marsh, is today one of the most threatened ecosystems in the United States. Under incremental attack for more than a century by humans who have dredged, drained, and diked this once-vast swampland, the Everglades has shrunk to little more than half of its original 4 million acres, stretching from Lake Okeechobee in central Florida more than 100 miles south to Florida Bay. The insatiable water demands of irrigated agriculture and of thirsty cities lining the Sunshine State's "Gold Coast," along with flood control projects and natural droughts, have disrupted the natural sheet flow of water which for millennia sustained the natural rhythms of life throughout the Everglades. The ecological damage caused by disruption of the region's hydrologic cycle has been further compounded by serious degradation of water quality due to fertilizer-laden drainage from adjacent sugarcane fields. Phosphate pollution in particular has precipitated massive fish kills and algal blooms, as well as the explosive growth of cattails which now cover 34,000 acres, replacing native vegetation and depriving wading birds of feeding areas. Another major threat to ecosystem stability in the Everglades has been the melaleuca tree, an exotic Australian species introduced in 1906 to help drain the swamp; it did its job only too well and, in the absence of natural enemies, is now displacing many of South Florida's native plant and animal species. As a result of this triple onslaught (i.e. drainage projects, water pollution, and melaleuca), wildlife populations in the Everglades have plummeted in recent decades— breeding pairs of waterbirds are down 90% from former levels and 33 species of indigenous animals are listed as either threatened or endangered. In the long run, degradation of the Everglades threatens not only flamingoes and alligators but Floridians as well, since the groundwater supplies on which the southern part of the state depends, naturally replenished through hydrologic contact with the Everglades, are not being recharged as rapidly as in the past. Soil resources are threatened as well, thanks to drainage projects and intensive agricultural production which have exposed the rich topsoil to oxidation and erosion. Soil loss in these areas has averaged an inch per year since the late 1970s and in some places topsoil now is completely gone.

The slow ecological decline of this invaluable wetland resource has not gone unnoticed; from the early years of this century, activists have loudly protested the activities which, they warned, would destroy the very features that attracted people to South Florida in the first place. By 1947 proponents of preservation were successful in persuading Congress to set aside the southern portion of the giant marshland as Everglades National Park. More recently, the Everglades Coalition, an assemblage of 28 national and local environmental groups, began pressing toward a far more ambitious goal—reengineering, and in some places undoing, the elaborate plumbing system that makes the Everglades the most intensively managed region on earth. The ultimate objective of this effort to "Save Our Everglades," as proclaimed in 1983 by then-Governor Bob Graham, was nothing less than to make ". . . the Everglades look and function by the year 2000 more as it did at the turn of the century."

Restoration of the Everglades moved a giant step closer to reality in the fall of 1992 when Congress authorized the Corps of Engineers to commence a 15-year, $558 million project to restore 29,000 acres of wetlands and oxbow lakes along the central stretch of the Kissimmee River, a once-meandering 103-mile waterway converted during the post-World War II years into a 56-mile canal unaffectionately known as the "Big Ditch." The Kissimmee restoration project represents an historic turning point—the first time ever that a major U.S. public works project (*i.e.* the Central and Southern Florida Project) has been "un-done" for ecological reasons.

Engineering projects alone, however, won't be enough to restore the Everglades to good health. The water quality problems caused by nutrient runoff from 440,000 acres of cane fields and 60,000 acres of vegetable farms present a more politically charged dilemma than putting meanders back into the Kissimmee. "Big Sugar" is a powerful force in South Florida, and growers didn't take kindly to demands that they control polluted runoff from fields. Court battles pitting agricultural interests against state officials and environmentalists stymied a solution to the Everglades' woes for years. The logjam was finally broken in May 1994, when Florida Governor Lawton Chiles signed the Everglades Forever Act, legislation mandating the construction of 40,000 acres of filtration marshes around Lake Okeechobee to reduce phosphate concentrations in farmland runoff. The cost of the project, estimated at $700 million, will be shared by growers (one-third) and Florida taxpayers (two-thirds)—a compromise which angered local environmentalists who felt that agribusiness should have been forced to pick up the whole tab. Nevertheless, U.S. Interior Secretary Bruce Babbitt hailed the new law as "a historic step toward systematic restoration of the Everglades." Responding to environmentalists' worries that Florida's initiative would result in a slackening of federal resolve to implement a more encompassing Everglades recovery program, Babbitt pledged that a comprehensive master plan, demonstrating how the region's original pattern of water flow could be restored, would be presented by year's end. Viewing the success of this effort as a crucial test of his ecosystem approach to resource management, Babbitt acknowledged that Florida's new law was but the latest step, albeit an important one, in a widening program of Everglades restoration which he hopes will one day encompass the entire southern portion of the state. While progress toward that ultimate goal will be slow, arduous, and expensive, the task is now underway, offering Floridians and all who love wetlands a realistic hope of one day experiencing "Paradise Regained."

References

Cushman, John H. 1994. "Florida Adopts Bill on Everglades Pollution." *New York Times*, May 4.

Derr, Mark. 1993. "Redeeming the Everglades." *Audubon* (Sept./Oct.).

Stevens, William K. 1994. "Everglades: Paradise Not Quite Yet Lost." *New York Times*, March 22.

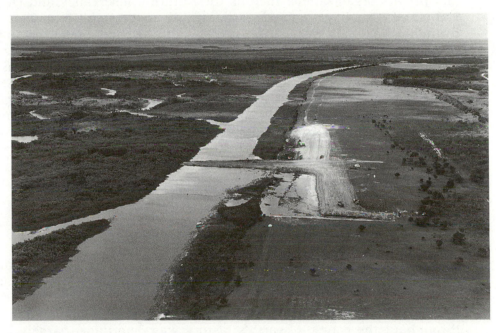

Plans are underway to restore 22 miles of the channelized Kissimmee River to its original form, which will restore 26,500 acres of wetlands. This 1000-foot linear "test-fill" crossing the river will provide valuable information for the larger restoration project. [South Florida Water Management District]

Although some wetlands are lost due to natural causes such as erosion, land subsidence, storms, or salt water intrusion, human activities account for by far the greatest amount of loss. Draining swamps or bottomlands for agricultural purposes is the leading cause of wetlands destruction (historically, about 85% of all wetlands have been lost to farmland conversion, though since the 1970s this percentage has been declining), but urban development, dredging for canals and port construction, flood control projects, and road building have also taken a significant toll. In the southeastern states, one of the leading causes of wetlands loss in recent years has been the clearing and draining of deep-soil swamps by timber companies who subsequently used the land for pine plantations. In 1994, responding to a lawsuit filed by a coalition of environmental groups protesting the practice, EPA banned further conversion of wetlands for this purpose (Hilts, 1994). While there are no federal laws expressly prohibiting the draining, filling or converting of most wetlands, Congress took a small step toward protecting our remaining wetlands when it included a section in the 1985 farm bill referred to as the "Swampbuster Provision," aimed at discouraging draining of wetlands for agriculture by stating that farmers who do so will lose their farm program benefits. The Conservation Reserve Program, enacted under that same legislation, provided farmers with financial incentives to protect lands taken out of cultivation and thereby fostered the restoration of critical wetlands habitat. Government agencies and private organizations such as the Nature Conservancy and Ducks Unlimited also have worked cooperatively to reestablish habitat for dwindling wetlands species. The success of these efforts, resulting in the restoration of hundreds of thousands of acres of prairie potholes, was dramatically evident by the mid-1990s when breeding populations of waterfowl rebounded to their highest levels since the 1970s (Stevens, 1994).

Since almost three-fourths of all wetlands acreage in the United States is privately owned, the ultimate success of wetlands preservation attempts hinge on efforts by both government and environmental organizations to educate landowners on the intrinsic value of wetlands, to encourage wetlands conservation and restoration, and to provide the technical assistance and financial incentives which will persuade property owners to protect our nation's precious wetland resources.

Loss of Biodiversity

Extinction of a species, like the death of an individual, is a natural process. As fossil evidence clearly indicates, many groups of plants and animals which dominated life on earth in past millennia have died out, only to be replaced by newly evolving organisms. The rise and fall of species throughout the course of earth's history was determined largely by a population's ability to adapt to changing environmental conditions or to become increasingly specialized for life in a particular ecological niche. As evolution proceeded the number of plant and animal species proliferated as populations dispersed into far-flung geographic regions and adapted to life in a seemingly endless variety of ecological niches. Today biologists have classified approximately 1.8 million species of living things, but estimate that the actual number currently in existence, many yet undiscovered, ranges from 3 to 30 million, the largest number being small creatures living in tropical forests and in the deep oceans. Unfortunately, it is widely feared that many of these species will vanish before their existence is ever noted or recorded.

The sad truth of the present situation is that human actions have greatly accelerated the rate at which species are becoming extinct; indeed, for the first time since the last great die-off at the end of the Cretaceous Period 65 million years ago, species are vanishing more rapidly than new ones are evolving, resulting in a diminishing diversity of life forms. The first recorded animal extinction—that of the European lion—was documented in A.D. 80; more than half of the animal species which have disappeared since that time have become extinct since 1900. Just as human populations have been increasing at an ever-faster pace in recent centuries, so has the rate of species loss. While estimates indicate that over the vast span of geologic time one mammalian species suffers extinction every 400 years and one bird species every 200, the record for the past 400 years shows a dramatic acceleration in the rate of extinction: 58 mammalian species and 115 bird species (World Conservation Monitoring Centre, 1992). Even these numbers don't accurately represent the true toll, especially for recent decades, since, by international agreement, a species isn't classified as extinct until 50 years after its last sighting. In addition, with millions of species still undiscovered and unnamed, it is quite likely that large numbers are quietly disappearing, unnoticed and unmourned, with their names never appearing on the obituary list (Wilcove, McMillan, and Winston, 1993). By 1990 approximately 12% of mammalian species and 11% of bird species worldwide were regarded as threatened. When *all* types of organisms are considered—not just the feathered or furry creatures which appeal to human emotions, but the myriads of insects, mollusks, fish, fungi, plants, and other organisms which greatly enrich the diversity of life—then current rates of extinction are even more alarming. Harvard biologist E.O. Wilson estimates that in tropical forest areas alone, home to a conservatively estimated 10 million species, the world is currently losing 3 species every hour, 74 per day, 27,000 each year—and the rate of loss continues to accelerate. If present trends of rain forest destruction are not reversed, 10–20% of all rain forest species will be extinct within 30 years—a number equivalent to at least 5–10% of all species on earth (Wilson, 1992).

The magnitude of such a loss is staggering. Species diversity is generally considered a prime determinant of ecological stability; extinction of key species, particularly plant species, may lead to the collapse of whole ecosystems. Less spectacular but equally distressing from a human viewpoint is the prospect of many potentially useful plant species being lost before their food or medicinal value is discovered. Even today, one-fourth of all pharmaceutical products bought by Americans contain active ingredients derived from plant products. The discovery of taxol, a potent anticancer drug derived from the bark of the Pacific yew (formerly regarded as a weed tree in old-growth forests of the Pacific Northwest) is but one of the more recent additions to a long list of valuable medicinal products extracted from forest plants. From a philosophical viewpoint also, the implications of the wholesale destruction of nonhuman life is profoundly disturbing. Over a century ago Thoreau proclaimed that "In wildness is the preservation of the world." Much ethical discussion in recent years has centered around the question of whether humans have the moral right to exterminate another form of life, to abruptly terminate the product of millions of years of evolution. Undeniably, "extinction is forever."

Although the causes of accelerating species loss are by now fairly well understood, reversing the trends which have brought about the current situation will be extremely difficult, particularly in regions where rapidly growing human populations are in direct competition with wildlife. Human pressures on other species can assume a variety of forms:

Direct Killing or Collecting of Wildlife for Food, Pleasure, or Profit. From the Paleolithic hunters who decimated the wooly mammoths and mastodons with primitive weapons to the modern Russian and Japanese fishing fleets which have brought several species of whale to the brink of extinction, predatory humans have totally eliminated a number of bird and mammalian species. Of all the animal extinctions known to have occurred within the past 400 years, the World Conservation Union estimates that nearly one-fourth (23%) were caused by overhunting. Collectors who dynamite reefs to obtain chunks of coral or capture rare tropical fish for sale to aquarium hobbyists; cactus "rustlers" who steal plants from nature preserves to satisfy the growing demand for rare houseplants; African poachers who shoot the endangered rhinoceros for the high profits its horn will bring in the markets of the Orient (powdered rhinoceros horn has long been considered an aphrodisiac in China and the Far East)—all contribute to the demise of species, as do the consumers who provide the incentive for such actions.

In an effort to remove the financial incentives for exploitation of wildlife, conservation groups mustered enough support to secure passage of the 1973 **Convention on International Trade in Endangered Species of Flora and Fauna (CITES)**. Meeting twice a year, CITES' governing body regulates international trade in and shipments of specified animal and plant products and flatly prohibits trade in products from endangered species. CITES has received much credit for stemming the slaughter of African elephants after issuing a ban in 1989 on ivory trading. CITES has been less effective in curbing the illicit trade in tiger parts which just in the last few years has resulted in such a precipitous decline in populations of the big cats that many wildlife biologists hold out little hope for the survival of tigers outside of zoos. In countries such as China and Taiwan, virtually every part of the animal's body brings premium prices due to their supposed medicinal benefits: tiger bones for potions to cure rheumatism, tiger whiskers to provide strength, tiger eyes to calm convulsions, and tiger penis, simmered in a soup, to rekindle male sexual prowess among senior citizens (only *wealthy* senior citizens need apply, however—a bowl of tiger penis soup may cost over $300!). The apparent lack of effort on the part of government officials to stem illegal commerce in tiger and rhino products has brought strong CITES criticism of both Taiwan and China and led the Clinton Administration in April of 1994 to impose trade sanctions on Taiwan, the first time the U.S. government (or *any* government, for that matter) has ever employed such measures for the protection of endangered wildlife. However, inasmuch as the body has no enforcement powers of its own, effective punishment of transgressor nations can only come about through trade sanctions imposed by individual member countries (Linden, 1994). The willingness of treaty signatories, such as the United States, to stand up for beleaguered wildlife may determine whether such magnificent creatures as tigers, elephants, and whales remain our coinhabitants on this planet or whether they are relegated, like the dodo and the passenger pigeon, to the status of nostalgic images in a picture book.

Introduction of Exotic Species.   Until relatively recently, the single most important factor accounting for the demise of many plant and animal species has been the accidental or deliberate introduction by humans of nonnative species into environments where such organisms had no natural enemies to curb explosive rates of growth. These alien invaders frequently decimated indigenous species by preying upon them or by outcompeting them for food or living space. The examples are legion: the melaleuca, an Australian tree that is taking over the Everglades; European starlings which have driven many less-aggressive songbirds from their original range; zebra mussels which are outproducing and overwhelming native mussel species throughout inland waterways in much of the United States. The fish-stocking programs that have introduced exotic species such as carp, blue tilapia, Chinook salmon, or large-mouth bass into waterways where they previously didn't exist have put native species under extreme pressure and have driven some to extinction. Experts estimate that over two-thirds of the fish extinctions which already have occurred in the United States were caused, at least in part, by the introduction of alien species, while half the fish now on the "endangered" list are thus imperilled because of introduced exotics (Luoma, 1992). The impact of nonnative species can be seen most dramatically in island ecosystems such as that of Hawaii, site of fully three-fourths of all known bird and plant extinctions in the United States. The goats, pigs, sheep, rats, and mongooses that came ashore with European settlers in the years after Captain Cook's voyage to the islands in 1778 are the most notorious of approximately 3900 plant and animal species arriving in Hawaii over the past two centuries. Today, of the remaining native Hawaiian plants, one-fifth are endangered; for native bird species, the proportion at risk rises to nearly half, primarily due to the impact of exotic newcomers. On the Pacific island of Guam, the brown tree snake, a recent arrival from New Guinea, has virtually wiped out native bird populations since it was first introduced 30 years ago. Nowhere, however, has the impact of alien species been more devastating than in Africa's Lake Victoria, a waterway once renowned for its amazing diversity of cichlid fishes—more than 300 species found nowhere else in the world. In 1959 Nile perch, a type of carnivorous fish growing up to six feet in length, were introduced into the lake by British settlers who thought they would enhance sports fishing opportunities. Within 25 years the invaders had gobbled up so many of the native cichlids that several species disappeared completely; it is expected that eventually over half the native species will become extinct. The demise of the plant-eating cichlids has had far-reaching effects on the Lake Victoria ecosystem, leading to algal blooms, oxygen depletion, and the decline of many other lake species. While the decision to introduce the perch had no malicious intent, the catastrophic results of this act led a team of biologists to observe: "Never before has man in a single ill-advised step placed so many vertebrate species simultaneously at risk of extinction and also, in doing so, threatened a food resource and traditional way of life of riparian dwellers" (Wilson, 1992).

Pollution of Air and Water with Toxic Chemicals.   The death of entire aquatic ecosystems due to acid rainfall is but one of the more recent examples of the effect toxic pollutants are having on other forms of life. Particularly since the introduction of the synthetic organic pesticides after World War II, numerous wildlife species, especially carnivorous birds, have suffered sharp population declines and contamination of rivers, lakes, and estuaries with poisonous industrial effluents threaten the sustained productivity of those ecosystems. The impact of pollution on wildlife was a major topic of international discussion in the summer of 1988 when beaches along Europe's North Sea and the U.S. East Coast were littered with the bodies of dead and dying seals and porpoises. Though the cause of the marine mammals' demise was ultimately determined to be a type of pneumonia, it was theorized that swimming in highly polluted coastal waters weakened the animals' resistance to disease and thereby contributed to their death. More recent casualties have been the beluga whales inhabiting the St. Lawrence River. Once numbering in the thousands, the belugas have dwindled to an estimated population of 500 animals, large numbers of which are afflicted with various types of tumors, ulcers, lesions, cysts, pneumonia, and reproductive problems. Scientists attribute the whales' plight to chemical contamination of the river with mercury, lead, PCBs, and various organochlorine pesticides. Analyses of tissue samples from dead belugas show concentrations of all these chemicals at levels far above those in whales from Arctic waters. One researcher commented that beluga carcasses contain such high concentrations of PCBs that they ought to be regulated as hazardous wastes! (Dold, 1992). While marine mammals and fish are particularly hard-hit because of the toxic soup that constantly surrounds them in many waterways, polluted air also is taking its toll on sensitive species. In western Europe fungi appear to be dying off *en masse*, with a 40–50% loss of species in certain areas of Germany, Austria, and the Netherlands. Among those adversely affected are the mycorrhizal fungi which live in symbiotic association with plant roots, promoting the uptake of dissolved nutrients. The fact that these inconspicuous organisms play an important role in the normal functioning of many plant species gives their demise far-reaching significance (Wilson, 1992). Efforts to safeguard human health by curbing pollutant emissions will have a beneficial impact on the health of ecosystems as well.

Habitat Destruction.   By far the greatest threat to biodiversity today—and the most difficult to control— is the destruction of those natural areas which wildlife require for breeding, feeding, or migrating. As the pressures of expanding populations and economies increase, forests are chopped down, swamps are drained, prairies are put to the plow, rivers are dammed. Some wildlife species can thrive in close proximity to humans—most cannot and perish when their natural habitat is destroyed or reduced in size below a critical minimum.

While there is little disagreement that preservation of biodiversity is a lost cause without a significantly greater commitment to conserving natural habitats, the question of how to maintain the integrity of dwindling expanses of forest, savannah, and grasslands at a time of exponentially increasing human needs is a vexing one for policymakers everywhere. Since 1872 when Yellowstone was established as the world's first national park, the conventional approach to preserving wild areas of great beauty or biological richness has been to set aside **protected areas** as wildlife refuges, national parks, or wilderness areas. Today 4% of the earth's total land surface has been thus preserved in approximately 8000 protected areas worldwide, their natural wealth safeguarded by limiting human access to such areas. Although in the past this approach has been somewhat successful, particularly in regions such as North America where population pressures are modest, trends suggest that in the years ahead preservation of critical habitat through reliance on government-established exclusion zones cannot adequately protect biodiversity and is ultimately doomed to failure. This is true for a number of reasons: 1) in most cases, the protected areas are too scattered, small, and fragmented to sustain the long-term stability of their biotic communities; ecologists have amply documented the adverse impact of crowding species into isolated "islands" of woodland or tropical forest, surrounded by a "sea" of farmlands or urban development. The "edge effect" experienced around the periphery of these fragmented habitats (i.e. increased exposure to wind, sunlight, decreased humidity, vulnerability to new predators) may result in the loss of many species highly adapted to life within a narrow range of environmental conditions; 2) many so-called protected areas, particularly those in developing countries, are protected in name only, since governments frequently lack the financial resources, the technical expertise, or the will to enforce their borders. The widescale poaching of endangered rhinos in East Africa or of tigers in India—both legally protected animals—is indicative of the difficulty many poor countries face in trying to safeguard their natural heritage through a reliance on protected reserves; 3) finally, and perhaps most importantly, the protected area strategy doesn't take into account the fact that humans are an integral part of ecosystems also. Most of the areas set aside for wildlife once sustained the needs of local people who are now forbidden to hunt, fish, or grow crops on lands they once considered theirs to use. As growing human populations press against park boundaries, it will be impossible and, indeed, unjust, to forbid them the use of their own surroundings without providing viable alternatives for survival.

Accordingly, within the past two decades a radically different approach to conservation of habitat has slowly gained adherents, an approach which attempts to make local communities both the *beneficiaries* and the *custodians* of efforts to safeguard biodiversity. Referred to as **community-based conservation**, this new concept recognizes that the exclusionary policies of the past, as embodied in the wildlife reserves, cannot be sustained in the face of mounting human poverty and hostility to programs which seem to place greater value on elephants or pandas than on people. Community-based conservation relies on positive grassroots participation, relinquishing the traditional top-down planning by central government officials in favor of involving local people in the planning, design, and implementation of conservation efforts which will benefit them directly and give them a personal stake in the successful outcome of such ventures. Community-based conservation efforts are quietly underway in a number of areas around the world and involve situations as diverse as the "extractive reserves" in Brazilian Amazonia, subsistence farming combined with ecotourism in Papua New Guinea, forest management by community councils in India, or incentive payments to private landowners for fostering biodiversity in England (Wright, 1993). The shift in focus from preserving wildlife to acknowledging the need to factor human needs into the equation may be the only practical approach to saving as much biodiversity as possible at a time when human-modified landscapes are relentlessly expanding. Convincing local people that their own well-being can best be ensured by conserving and sustainably using the biological wealth of their surroundings may ultimately be the key to species preservation. Whether motivated by poverty or greed, those who today are engaged in mindless destruction of habitat, thereby driving untold numbers of species to extinction, might well consider the words spoken over 30 years ago by Julius Nyerere, a leader in the African independence movement and first President of Tanzania:

> The survival of our wildlife is a matter of grave concern to all of us in Africa. These wild creatures amid the wild places they inhabit are not only important as a source of wonder and inspiration but are an integral part of our natural resources and of our future livelihood and well-being.

Protecting Biodiversity: The Endangered Species Act

Since its enactment in 1973, the **Endangered Species Act (ESA)** has constituted the nation's most effective weapon for ensuring the survival of native plants and animals. Probably the toughest wildlife protection law anywhere in the world, the ESA prohibits the killing, collecting, harassment, or capture of any species listed by the U.S. Fish and Wildlife Service (FWS) as "endangered" or "threatened." It also provides strict protection for the critical habitat of endangered species and requires FWS to develop recovery programs for each species listed. By 1994, 760 U.S. species had been officially declared endangered or threatened, 532 foreign species had been similarly listed, and an additional 382 new U.S. species (90% of them plants) are scheduled for addition to the list by 1996.

While environmentalists hail the ESA for noticeably slowing the pace of wildlife extinction in the United States, citing as evidence the fact that 60 endangered species have increased their numbers or expanded their range over the past 20 years, opponents are working hard to weaken the law when it comes up for reauthorization. Charging that the Act has excessive power to supersede individual property rights, hinder economic progress, and threaten jobs, such disparate constituencies as land

BOX 5-3
Making Preservation Profitable

Conservationists acknowledge the futility of initiatives to preserve bio-diversity unless local people, convinced that their economic security will be enhanced by such efforts, lend their active support. Everywhere in the world biological resources are undervalued, a fact which contributes to thoughtless and wasteful destruction of Nature's bounty. This situation may be changing, thanks to an innovative project now underway in the small but ecologically rich Central American republic of Costa Rica—a project which may provide a model to emulate for countries struggling to safeguard their biological heritage while simultaneous-ly promoting sustainable development policies.

In 1989 the Instituto Nacional de Biodiversidad (National Institute of Biodiversity), commonly referred to as **INBIO**, was founded as a private non-profit organization, working in close cooperation with the Costa Rican government, to serve as an information clearinghouse on that country's plant and animal wealth. Now in the process of compiling a comprehensive inven-tory of the estimated half million to one million species indigenous to Costa Rica, INBIO hires and trains local people as designated "parataxono-mists," sending them into the field to collect specimens and perform preliminary identifications. These para-taxonomists come from every walk of life—students, farmers, housewives, park rangers—and their efforts have already greatly expanded the nation's existing body of scientific knowledge. In just the first six months after the program was initiated, parataxonomists collected four times as many insect specimens as Costa Rica's national

collection had received in a century—and the number continues to grow by approximately 100,000 specimens each month. Field identifications are subsequently confirmed by experts and information pertaining to the name, collection site, conservation status, and potential commercial value of each species is entered into a computerized data base at INBIO headquarters on the outskirts of San Jose. This infor-mation constitutes a veritable treasure-trove for researchers looking for previously unknown organisms of potential medicinal, pesticidal, or agricultural value, and INBIO has agreed to make its data available, for a fee, to commercial interests search-ing for new products.

Recognizing a golden opportunity, Merck & Co., Inc., the world's largest pharmaceutical corporation, in 1991 entered into a contract agreement with INBIO, paying the Costa Rican organization $1 million to send the company a steady supply of plant, animal, and microbial specimens to be analyzed for possible medicinal properties. Sometimes referred to as **chemical prospecting**, such wide-scale screening of wild species for new pharmaceuticals or other useful biochemical products is now economically feasible, thanks to the perfection of automated analytical techniques which allow up to 50,000 samples per year to be processed using mere bits of fresh tissue or extracts sent to drug company labs from anywhere in the world. As part of the contract agreement, Merck will pay royalties to INBIO for any commercial products developed from Costa Rican specimens (it is assumed that once the biochemically active ingredient of a newly discovered species is identified, it will be possible to mass-produce an identical synthetic compound, thereby avoiding further exploitation of the species in its native habitat). Since even now 40% of U.S. prescription drugs, worth billions of dollars in annual sales, derive their active ingredients from wild species, it is highly probable that the collaborative effort between Merck and INBIO will be mutually beneficial. Costa Rican conservation programs will get a boost from the arrangement as well, since INBIO has earmarked 10% of Merck's initial payment, as well as half of any royalties earned, to be spent on Costa Rica's national parks.

By intimately involving local people in cataloguing their country's biodiversity, INBIO gives Costa Ricans an in-depth understanding of their natural heritage and a personal stake in protecting it. By demonstrating that it can be more profitable to conserve than to extract the nation's biological resources, the Institute and Costa Rica are in the vanguard of a promising new approach to ensuring that future generations will continue to enjoy—and to utilize—the myriad species, large and small, which so greatly enrich the quality of life on this planet.

References

Wilson, E. O. 1992. *The Diversity of Life*. Harvard University Press.

World Resources Institute. 1992. *World Resources 1992–93*. Oxford University Press.

developers, Gulf Coast shrimpers, and loggers in the Pacific Northwest would like to see the Act significantly weakened. These groups raise the question of how much biological diversity can or should be preserved, especially when the species in question isn't particularly cute or fuzzy. Some people find it hard to get emotional about the Colorado squawfish or the scrub plum!

ESA defenders counter-charge the assertion that the Act is blocking the inexorable march of progress (and profits) by pointing out that, for the vast majority of protected species, recovery plans seldom provoke conflict. Indeed, out of almost 2000 projects or activities evaluated by the Fish and Wildlife Service for potential adverse impacts on endangered species between 1987 and 1991, only 23 were denied or dropped from consideration. Perhaps one explanation for increasing antagonism toward ESA is the fact that in recent years the Act has begun to affect entire regions rather than just isolated projects, as was generally the case in the past. The acrimony in Northwest logging regions over attempts to save the northern spotted owl by declaring large areas of old-growth forest off-limits for timber harvesting has prompted vociferous complaints that current policy favors wildlife over people.

In fact, contrary to detractors' claims, the Act *does* make an effort to accommodate societal concerns. Economic considerations are taken into account to some degree when designations of critical habitat are made; in situations where proposed projects threaten endangered species, the Act requires that an effort be made to find alternative means of carrying out the activity without endangering survival of the species in question. In those rare cases where the conflict is irreconcilable, an official panel (the "God Squad") can give the green light to projects deemed of sufficient importance, even if this action constitutes a death sentence for an endangered species.

Even supporters admit, however, that implementation of ESA is in need of improvement. To some extent, problems center around insufficient money and personnel to carry out the intent of the Act. The responsibility for enforcing the prohibitions against hunting, harassing, capturing, or collecting listed species rests on the shoulders of just 210 federal agents nationwide. Little wonder, then, that from 1988 to 1992 only 53 cases were filed against violators, with just 39 convictions obtained. Even more problematic is the cumbersome process of officially listing rare species as threatened or endangered. Frequently the official designation comes so late that populations of the species in question may already be too low to halt the slide into oblivion. In other cases, only costly rescue missions such as captive breeding programs can guarantee long-term survival, when earlier action could have achieved success through less extreme measures. Although studies suggest that a minimum population in the low thousands is a prerequisite for viable vertebrate populations, the average number of individuals remaining in vertebrate groups listed as endangered was just 1075; for invertebrates it was even lower—999. For plants, the average number of remaining specimens in at-risk populations at the time of official listing is a mere 120, making recovery of such species extremely difficult. Biologists suggest that the minuscule number of species which have rebounded and been removed from the endangered list can be explained by the fact that official designation often comes too late to implement effective recovery plans. FWS staffers concur with this assessment, but are laboring under such an immense backlog of candidates for consideration that a 1990 report from the General Accounting Office estimated that, at existing levels of staff and funding, it would take 50 years to determine the status of the 3000 species then under consideration, not to mention the additional species whose names would be submitted for review during that time! Subsequent to this report, FWS approximately doubled the rate at which it was adding species to the list; nevertheless, as federal officials deliberate, species continue to slide toward extinction.

In spite of such problems, the Endangered Species Act can claim its share of notable success stories. While only six species to date have been delisted entirely after attaining the goals for complete recovery (gray whale, Atlantic population of the brown pelican, Rydberg milkvetch, and three Pacific island birds), a number of others have made a remarkable comeback from near-extinction: the bald eagle, which in 1994 was reclassified as "threatened" rather than "endangered" after its population in the lower 48 states climbed from just 791 nesting pairs in 1974 to approximately 4000 at present; the American alligator, which remains on the "threatened" list despite full recovery only because it is easily mistaken for the American crocodile which *is* still endangered; whooping cranes, peregrine falcons, California sea otters, grizzly bears, black-footed ferrets, the red wolf—all now have a new lease on life, thanks to the Endangered Species Act (World Resources Institute, 1994).

While ESA historically has focused on protecting individual species on a case-by-case basis, a 1982 amendment to the Act established an alternative approach to preserving biodiversity in the form of **habitat conservation planning (HCP)**. Devised as a way of striking a balance between pressures for economic growth and habitat preservation, HCP allows landowners to develop property occupied by endangered species if they agree to minimize the loss of critical habitat or offset that loss by providing additional land nearby. While this approach implicitly permits the loss of *some* members of the endangered species in question, it guarantees that enough critical habitat will be preserved to sustain the remainder of that population indefinitely. Drawing up an acceptable plan may involve years of negotiations among developers, environmentalists, local governments, and Fish and Wildlife Service personnel who supervise the process and must ultimately approve the plan. Nevertheless, both environmentalists and property rights advocates are supportive of the concept, the former seeing it as a way of winning concessions from land-owners who might otherwise ignore the law, the latter preferring negotiated plans to restrictions on land use.

Although to date habitat conservation planning has been used only sparingly (just 17 plans had been approved by 1994, most of them in California; work on 75 more is now in progress), the concept has won the ringing endorsement of Interior Secretary Bruce Babbitt. Deploring the long legal process set in motion when the Endangered Species Act is invoked, Babbitt hopes to make that law unnecessary by protecting entire ecosystems. A major test of whether HCP is capable of saving species was initiated in southern California in 1993 when Secretary Babbitt worked out an agreement (the Natural Communities Conservation Program) between developers and environmentalists who had been at loggerheads for years over the fate of a diminutive songbird, the California gnatcatcher. Since fewer than 3000 nesting pairs of the birds remain in the 250,000 acres of sage scrub stretching along the Pacific coast from Los Angeles to San Diego, environmentalists had been demanding that FWS list the gnatcatcher as endangered; developers were adamant that such action, automatically triggering prohibitions on use of valuable real estate, would impose serious economic hardships. Under the HCP brokered by Babbitt, the gnatcatcher would be listed as merely "threatened," permitting a more flexible recovery plan than would be allowed under "endangered" status; in return, development interests agreed to protect critical habitat by setting aside up to 12 reserves, an act which would benefit not only the gnatcatcher, but as many as 40 other species as well (Hulse, 1993; National Wildlife Federation, 1994).

While experience with habitat conservation planning is not yet extensive enough to render a verdict on its ability to save species, hopes are high that it provides a means for avoiding bitter confrontations and halting the decline of species long before their situation deteriorates beyond redemption ■

References

Berg, Norman A. 1987. "Making the Most of the New Soil Conservation Initiatives." *Journal of Soil and Water Conservation* (Jan./Feb.).

Brown, Lester. 1988. "The Changing World Food Prospect: The Nineties and Beyond." *Worldwatch Paper 85* (Oct.).

Brown, Lester, Hal Kane, and Ed Ayres. 1993. *Vital Signs 1993*. Worldwatch Institute, W. W. Norton.

Coffin, Tristam, ed. 1993. "The Damage Done by Cattle-Raising." *The Washington Spectator* 19, no. 2 (Jan. 15).

Colchester, Marcus. 1994. "The New Sultans." *The Ecologist* 24, no. 2 (March/April).

Dold, Catherine. 1992. "Toxic Agents Found to Be Killing Off Whales." *New York Times*, June 16.

Durning, Alan Thein. 1993. "Saving the Forests: What Will It Take?" *Worldwatch Paper 117* (Dec.).

Environmental Protection Agency. 1988. *America's Wetlands: Our Vital Link Between Land and Water*. OPA-87-016 (Feb.).

Faeth, Paul. 1994. "Building the Case for Sustainable Agriculture: Policy Lessons from India, Chile, and the Philippines." *Environment* 36, no. 1 (Jan./Feb.).

Hamilton, John Maxwell. 1989. "Rescuing the Bounty of Rain Forests." *The Christian Science Monitor*, Jan. 26.

Hazarika, Sanjay. 1993. "Bangladesh Faces Dispute on Floods." *New York Times*, Aug. 1.

Hilts, Philip J. 1994. "Government Halts Wetland Practice." *New York Times*, Feb. 8.

Hulme, Mike, and Mick Kelly. 1993. "Exploring the Links Between Desertification and Climate Change." *Environment* 35, no. 6 (July/Aug.).

Hulse, Carl. 1993. "Building Near Endangered Species." *New York Times*, Dec. 28.

Kleinfeld, N. R. 1993. "Immigrant Dream of Heaven Chokes in a Journey of Misery." *New York Times*, June 8.

Lal, R., and F. J. Pierce. 1991. "The Vanishing Resource." In *Soil Management for Sustainability*, edited by R. Lal and F. J. Pierce. Soil and Water Conservation Society.

Linden, Eugene. 1994. "Tigers on the Brink." *Time*, March 28.

Luoma, Jon R. 1992. "Boon to Anglers Turns into a Disaster for Lakes and Streams." *New York Times*, Nov. 17.

Nash, Nathaniel C. 1994. "Vast Areas of Rain Forest Are Being Destroyed in Chile." *New York Times*, May 31.

_____. 1993. "Bolivia's Rain Forest Falls to Relentless Exploiters." *New York Times*, June 21.

National Wildlife Federation. 1994. "26th Environmental Quality Index." *National Wildlife* 32, no. 2 (Feb./March).

Pitt, David E. 1994. "Rich and Poor Countries Negotiate Accord on Preservation of Forests." *New York Times*, Jan. 23.

Schneider, Keith. 1993. "Pact Would Raise U. S. Grazing Fees." *New York Times*, Oct. 8.

Skole, David, and Compton Tucker. 1993. "Tropical Deforestation and Habitat Fragmentation in the Amazon: Satellite Data from 1978 to 1988." *Science* 260 (June 25).

Smil, V. 1991. "Population Growth and Nitrogen: An Exploration of a Critical Existential Link." *Population and Development Review* 17, no. 4.

Stevens, William K. 1994a. "Threat of Encroaching Deserts May Be More Myth Than Fact." *New York Times*, Jan. 18.

_____. 1994b. "Praire Ducks Return in Record Numbers." *New York Times*, Oct. 11.

Stutz, Bruce. 1993. "The Landscape of Hunger." *Audubon* 95, no. 2 (March/April).

Tyler, Patrick E. 1994. "Nature and Economic Boom Devouring China's Farmland." *New York Times*, March 27.

USDA. 1991. *Yearbook of Agriculture: Agriculture and the Environment.*

_____. 1987. *Agricultural Resources: Cropland, Water, and Conservation Situation and Outlook Report.* Economic Research Service, Washington, DC.

_____. 1981. *Yearbook of Agriculture: Will There Be Enough Food?*

Whittaker, Robert H. 1975. *Communities and Ecosystems.* Macmillan.

Wilcove, David S., Margaret McMillan, and Keith C. Winston. 1993. "What Exactly Is an Endangered Species? An Analysis of the U. S. Endangered Species List, 1985–91." *Conservation Biology* 7, no. 1.

Wilson, Edward O. 1992. *The Diversity of Life.* Harvard University Press.

World Commission on Environment and Development. 1987. *Our Common Future.* Oxford University Press.

World Conservation Monitoring Centre. 1992. *Global Biodiversity: Status of the Earth's Living Resources.* Chapman and Hall.

World Resources Institute. 1990. *World Resources 1990–1991.* Oxford University Press.

_____. 1992. *World Resources 1992–1993.* Oxford University Press.

_____. 1992. *The 1993 Information Please Environmental Almanac.* Houghton Miflin Co.

_____. 1994. *The 1994 Information Please Environmental Almanac.* Houghton Miflin Co.

_____. 1994. *World Resources 1994–1995: People and the Environment.* Oxford University Press.

Wright, Michal, ed. 1993. *The View from Airlie: Community-Based Conservation in Perspective.* Liz Claiborne and Art Ortenberg Foundation, narrative sampling of discussions during workshop held at Airlie, Virginia, week of Oct. 17.

PART II

Our Toxic Environment
Does Everything Cause Cancer?

It can be said that each civilization has a pattern of disease peculiar to it. The pattern of disease is an expression of the response of man to his total environment (physical, biological, and social); this response is, therefore, determined by anything that affects man himself or his environment.

—René J. Dubos

Newspaper headlines screaming "Ozone Alert!"; a $1 million damage settlement to an asbestos worker's widow; public protests over a leaking hazardous waste dump; migrant workers hospitalized for pesticide poisoning; accidental sewage discharge forcing closure of public beaches— such situations represent but a handful of the issues daily facing modern society in which some aspect of environmental quality has a direct impact on human health.

From primitive times up until the mid-19th century the idea that health and disease were determined, at least in part, by environmental factors was widely accepted (witness the belief that night air precipitated fever and chills). The middle 1800s, however, marked a period of rapid progress in research relating to disease causation. The discovery of the anthrax bacterium by the German microbiologist Robert Koch and his demonstration in 1877 that this organism was responsible for an important human disease revolutionized society's view of health. For the next 70 years virtually all human ailments were blamed on pathogenic organisms such as bacteria, viruses, and protozoans. It was widely assumed that the development of preventative vaccines or curative antibiotics should be our main focus in protecting public health.

More recently, however, recognition of the role that deprivation or stress can play in initiating serious health problems and the sharp increase, particularly in more affluent societies, of the so-called "degenerative diseases" (cardiovascular disease, cancer, hypertension) have led to the realization that good health depends on more than just the absence of disease-causing microorganisms. Some of today's most prevalent ills are increasingly blamed on toxic environmental contaminants—synthetic chemical wastes carelessly dumped in waterways or landfills, products of combustion spewed into the air, pesticide residues and chemical additives in the food we eat. Other illnesses are associated with personal habits that in the broad sense can be considered aspects of environmental quality— smoking, drinking, high-fat diets, lack of regular exercise. Perception of the threat that such factors pose to human well-being provided the main thrust behind the environmental movement of the last 25 years. Preservation—or restoration—of environmental quality means far more than protecting bald eagles or ensuring that the last coastal redwood isn't converted into a picnic table; the prime emphasis among environmental advocates has always been the protection of human health, with the implicit recognition that human well-being is inextricably intertwined with the health and stability of the natural ecosystems of which we form an integral part.

While not a perfect standard, the health status of societies is often measured in terms of life expectancy—the number of years an average individual in that society can expect to live. In terms of longevity, health conditions in the Western world have improved markedly in recent centuries. Whereas in the days of Roman emperors the average lifespan was about 30 years, today in most industrialized countries it has reached 75 years, up from 50 years at the turn of the century (Japanese are currently the world's longest-lived people, with an average life expectancy of 79, compared to 76 in the United States). Among the developing nations average longevity is more variable, ranging from the lower to mid-40s in Afghanistan and some African countries to the mid-70s in parts of Latin America and the Caribbean. Many people, looking at such statistics, assume that the major factor accounting for increased longevity worldwide was the introduction of modern medicines and pesticides that provided the first really effective weapons against many of the infectious epidemic diseases. While medical science undoubtedly played a part in reducing mortality rates, many observers feel that a more fundamental factor was a general improvement in living conditions: better nutritional levels made possible by increased agricultural productivity; improved sanitary conditions as a result of sewer system construction; the provision of safe drinking water supplies; refuse collection; sewage treatment; the enforcement of housing codes, and so forth. Rising incomes, increasing levels of education, mass communications, and improved standards of personal hygiene have also been extremely important determinants in furthering the health advances observed in most parts of the world.

However, we seem to have now reached a longevity plateau and are no longer observing a continued rapid drop in death rates such as characterized the years between 1950–1960. Indeed, longevity is actually declining in Russia, where high levels of pollution, added to the ravages of alcoholism and substandard health care, have caused male life expectancy to fall to just 60 years, the lowest for any industrialized country (female life expectancy has remained stable at 72 years). There appears to be general agreement that future gains will come, not so much through new medical discoveries, but when—and only when—currently unmet essential preconditions of better health are everywhere available. These essential preconditions relate largely to environmental considerations: sufficient quantities of uncontaminated water, elimination of malnutrition, proper handling and disposal of human wastes, control of toxic pollutants, adoption of healthier personal life-styles. The environmentally induced diseases currently plaguing much of humanity can best be controlled through a strategy of prevention, rather than cure, requiring not only application of technology but also social, political, and behavioral changes. Adopting such a strategy and enlisting the public support necessary to attain the goal of a healthful society require a thorough understanding of the issues and dilemmas involved. The following chapters will delineate the major concerns regarding our increasingly toxic environment and the health implications inherent in our present life-style; they also attempt to show that improving human health and enhancing environmental quality are but two sides of the same coin ∎

CHAPTER 6

Environmental Disease

> *The most important pathological effects of pollution are extremely delayed and indirect.*
>
> —René J. Dubos

Polluted air and water, excessive levels of noise, sunshine, nuclear weapons fall-out, overcrowded slums, toxic waste dumps, inadequate or overly adequate diet, stress, food contaminants, medical X-rays, drugs, cigarettes, unsafe working conditions—these comprise but a partial listing of the many environmental factors which, through their adverse impact on human health, can be regarded as causative agents of environmental disease. In recent years public concern about rising levels of pollution and environmental degradation has increasingly focused on the question of whether such trends may be influencing disease rates, particularly ailments such as heart disease, cancer, stroke and other ills that have assumed major importance following the conquest of the microbial killers of yesteryear. If such a connection exists, as virtually all authorities agree it does, then society's response should be clear: most environmentally induced diseases, unlike those caused by bacteria or other pathogens, are difficult to cure but theoretically simple to prevent—remove the adverse environmental influence and the ailment will disappear. In other words, by preventing the discharge of poisons into our air, water, and food, by avoiding exposure to radiation, by refusing to fill our lungs with cigarette smoke or our stomachs with synthetic food colorings we can protect our health far more effectively and cheaply than we can by desperately searching for an often nonexistent cure after our bodies succumb to a malignancy or degeneration of vital organs or when our children are born deformed. The old adage, "Prevention is the best cure," has never been more true than when applied to environmentally induced disease.

Historically the environmental health profession has concentrated primarily on reducing the incidence of epidemic diseases spread through contaminated food and water. Their success, through implementation of such now taken-for-granted procedures as drinking water purification, sewage treatment, and vector control can be seen in a comparison of present and past statistics of mortality rates for diseases such as cholera and typhoid fever. These filth-related killers are now extremely rare in the United States, though the causative organisms are still present and would undoubtedly return with a vengeance if we were to relax the environmental controls that hold them at bay. The threat posed by these water- and food-borne diseases, as well as the hazards related to air contaminants, radiation, pesticides, and noise—all features of the modern environment—will be discussed in greater detail in the chapters dealing with those topics.

In spite of the fact that environmental factors can affect human health in many ways, the focus of most environmental health concern today in this age of toxic pollutants is on those substances that, in ways not yet completely understood, act at the cellular level to initiate often irreversible changes that can kill or damage the cell in question. Although health

BOX 6-1
General Disease Classification

Human disease conditions can be categorized in various ways: infectious or noninfectious; endemic or epidemic; acute or chronic. It is important to have an understanding of the basic nature of any particular disease state in order to know how to respond to the problem in an appropriate manner.

Infectious vs. Noninfectious

Infectious diseases are those caused by pathogenic organisms such as bacteria, viruses, protozoans, parasitic worms, and so on. Infectious diseases can be spread from one person to another by inhalation of airborne pathogens released when an infected person coughs, sneezes, or talks; by direct contact with food, water, soil or clothing that has been contaminated with fecal matter or saliva from an infected person; through sexual intercourse or other close physical contact with a diseased individual; or as a result of activities of a nonpathogenic disease-carrier, or vector, such as mosquitoes or body lice which transfer the disease agent from an infected person to a healthy one. Many of the leading killers of the past included such infectious diseases as malaria, smallpox, cholera, typhoid, measles, and tuberculosis.

Noninfectious diseases, currently the major cause of mortality in industrialized societies, are those that are not caused by pathogenic organisms and are not transmitted from one person to another (except in the case of hereditary conditions). Noninfectious diseases frequently have multiple causes, often related to adverse environmental conditions, and may develop slowly over a number of years.

Unlike many infectious diseases which, if survived, are of short duration, most noninfectious diseases are irreversible. Although many can be kept under control with proper medical treatment, few such conditions can be permanently cured. Examples of some of the leading noninfectious diseases include cardiovascular disease, cancer, diabetes, emphysema, sickle-cell anemia, asthma, and cerebral palsy.

Endemic vs. Epidemic

When the causative agent of an infectious disease such as typhoid is carried by many individuals within a population without leading to a rapid and widespread outbreak of illness and a high death rate, the disease is said to be endemic within that population. An epidemic disease, by contrast, involves a sudden severe outbreak of an infectious disease affecting a large number of people. The term "pandemic" refers to an epidemic that is worldwide in extent.

Acute vs. Chronic

Generally used in reference to certain infectious diseases such as smallpox, plague, or cholera which can be quite severe but are of short duration, an acute illness can also be caused by a short-term, high-dose exposure to a toxic substance. In most cases, if the victim survives the initial attack, the effects of the illness are reversible. With chronic conditions (e.g. malaria, tuberculosis, heart disease, cancer, emphysema) the illness is of long duration, often lasting a lifetime, occasionally flaring up, sometimes going into remission, or, in some cases, growing progressively worse as the years pass.

damage due to environmental pollutants may be manifested by outward symptoms, research has shown that the action of such contaminants in fact occurs at the level of an individual cell or cells. In spite of its small size, the cell is an exceptionally complex structure—the end product of billions of years of evolution and natural selection in response to existing environmental conditions. Thus it should not be surprising to find that a sudden change in the environment (e.g. exposure to X-rays, synthetic organic chemicals, heavy metals, etc.) to which a cell has become so finely adapted can kill or injure the cell. Cell death, in many respects, is a lesser concern than cell injury because it has no further implications—the cell is dead. Cell damage, on the other hand, has more ominous implications. The subject of extensive scientific and medical research for the past half century, cell damage can be manifested as mutations, birth defects, or cancer.

Mutation

Mutation, defined as any change in the genetic material, is perhaps the most worrisome type of cell damage because of its potential for harming not only the person or organism harboring the mutant cell but, if the mutation occurs in an egg or sperm, unborn generations as well. To understand the significance of mutation, it is necessary to examine the nature of the hereditary material itself.

The most conspicuous organelle in most cells is the nucleus, readily visible under an ordinary light microscope. The nucleus contains thread-like structures called **chromosomes**; each species of plant or animal has its own characteristic number of chromosomes per cell—in humans the normal chromosome number is 46. When cells undergo **mitosis** (cell division), each chromosome splits longitudinally into two daughter **chromatids**, one of which goes into each of the two newly forming cells. Thus the number of chromosomes per nucleus remains constant and the hereditary material contained within the chromosomes is equally shared.

Chemically, chromosomes consist of a single giant molecule of DNA (deoxyribonucleic acid) and associated histone and non-histone proteins. The DNA molecule itself is composed of two parallel strands of alternating units of a five-carbon sugar and phosphate molecules, cross-linked by one of four different nitrogenous bases (adenine, guanine, thymine, and cytosine), and twisted into a helical configuration. The pairing of the nitrogenous bases is quite specific: adenine can pair only with thymine and guanine with cytosine. Along any one strand bases can occur in any sequence, but once the order on one side is given, the sequence on the parallel strand is automatically determined. The adenine-thymine (A-T) or guanine-cytosine (G-C) combination making up each cross-connection is referred to as a **base pair**.

DNA is vitally important to cellular function and is often referred to as the "Master Molecule" because 1) it passes genetic information from one generation to the next and 2) it controls cellular metabolism by giving the instructions for protein synthesis.

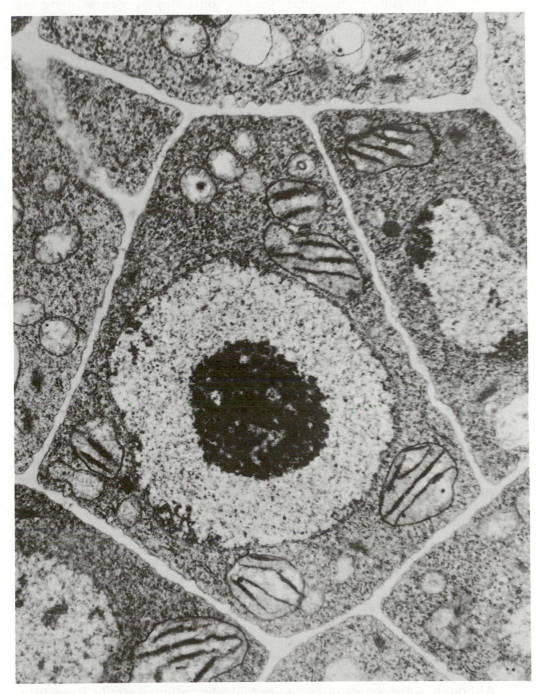

The complexity of cell structure can be seen in this electron micrograph of a plant cell showing such organelles as nucleus, chloroplasts, ribosomes, endoplasmic reticulum, mitochondria, and vacuoles. Environmental toxins act here at the cellular level within organisms. [Mathew Nadakavukaren]

The hereditary characteristics are controlled by **genes** along the length of the chromosome. In essence, a gene is a section of chromosome consisting of approximately 1500 base pairs. Genes are responsible for the production of proteins necessary for proper cell function. It is absolutely essential that the integrity of the DNA molecule be maintained if the correct information for protein synthesis is to be passed from one generation to the next. Any change within the gene, resulting in production of the wrong protein, constitutes a mutation.

Types of Mutations

There are three basic types of mutations recognized.

"Point" Mutation (gene mutation).   By far the most common type of mutation, point mutations involve a change at the molecular level within a gene. Such a change usually consists of the deletion or substitution of a base pair, resulting in the "misreading" of the genetic code (the sequence of bases along a DNA strand is all-important; any change can result in the wrong protein being formed). The severity of a point mutation depends on precisely where within a gene the change occurs; it can range from being lethal to causing an almost imperceptible loss of vigor. Point mutations are now known to be responsible for several serious human ailments. These include sickle-cell anemia, hemophilia, diabetes, and achondroplastic dwarfism. Though such ailments are tragic for the victim (prior to modern forms of treatment, which are only partially effective, these diseases invariably resulted in death at a fairly early age), many geneticists are more concerned about the accumulation of sub-lethal mutations in populations. Such sub-lethal mutations don't kill their victims outright, but render them less fit than they would otherwise be. Examples of the types of impairment that could result from a sub-lethal mutation include reduced physical or mental vigor, shortened life span, increased susceptibility to disease, or varying degrees of malformation of some organ. Such changes, though possibly debilitating, nevertheless permit afflicted individuals to survive, reproduce, and pass defective genes on to succeeding generations, resulting in what some researchers refer to as the "contamination of the human gene pool."

Chromosomal Aberrations.   These represent gross structural changes in the chromosome, usually caused by the loss or addition of sizeable pieces of a chromosome or the reversing of chromosome parts which frequently occurs during a stage of meiosis (reduction division) when the homologous chromosomes are in synapsis and crossing-over occurs. Although some types of chromosomal aberration seem to have little outward effect, the loss of part of a chromosome usually is fatal to the cell— that is, it represents a lethal mutation.

Change in Chromosome Number.   Caused by the nondisjunction (failure to separate) of paired homologous chromosomes during meiosis,

Figure 6-1 DNA Double Helix

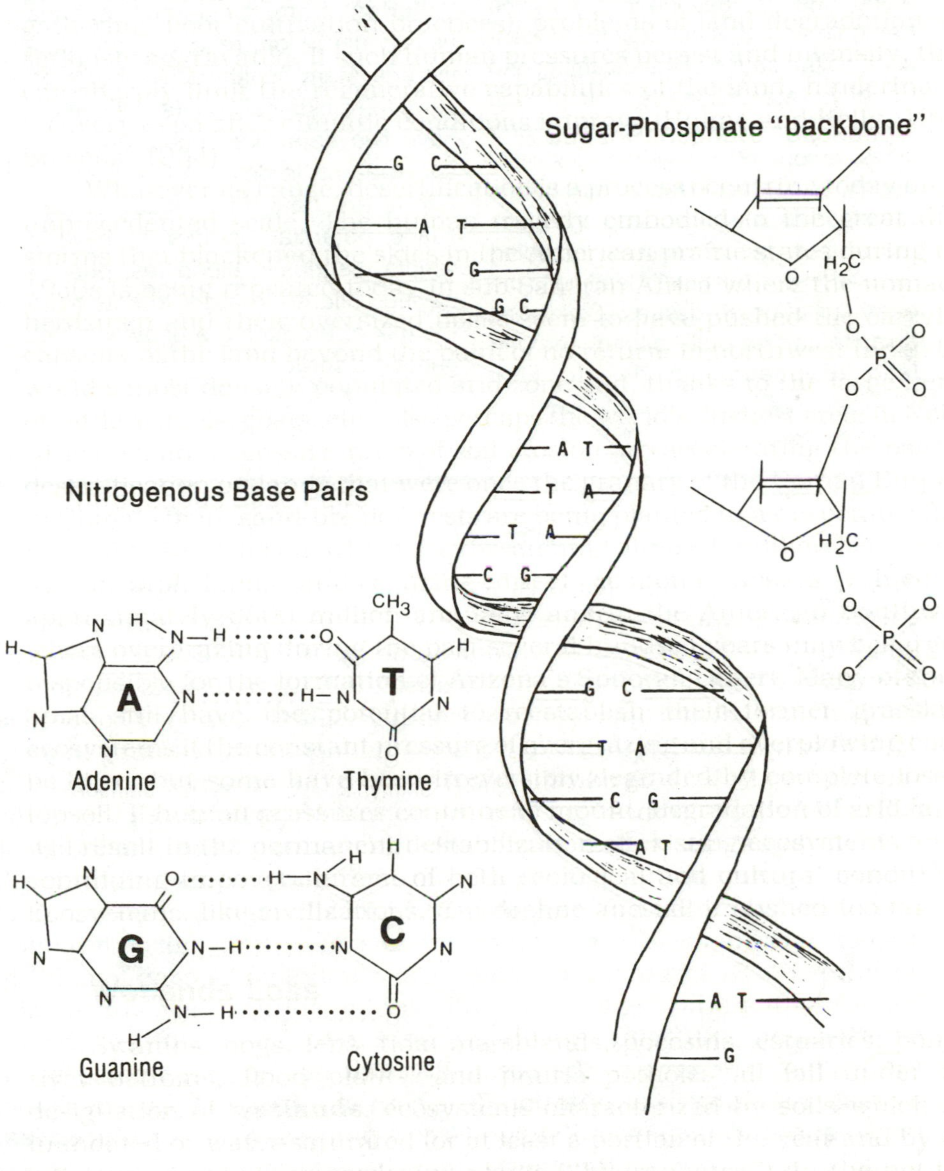
Sugar-Phosphate "backbone"
Nitrogenous Base Pairs
Adenine
Thymine
Guanine
Cytosine
A
T
G
C

BOX 6-2

Sickle-Cell Anemia

A single base pair substitution, resulting in the selection of the amino acid valine instead of glutamic acid along one polypeptide chain of the hemoglobin molecule, has been identified as the cause of the disabling and usually fatal disease, sickle-cell anemia. The most common long-term illness among black children, sickle-cell anemia is characterized by misshapen red blood cells which clump and block the smaller blood vessels, impeding circulation and eventually leading to the death of affected tissues. Sickle-cell disease can be quite painful and can lead to pneumonia due to lung damage, rheumatism as a result of muscle and joint deterioration, and damage to heart and kidneys. Victims suffering from sickle-cell anemia usually die before reaching reproductive age. Many healthy adults, however, carry the sickle-cell trait (a victim must have two defective genes, one from each parent, to develop the disease). Efforts are now being made to persuade potential carriers to have a simple diagnostic blood test prior to having children in order to determine the risk of producing a baby with this genetic disorder.

this type of mutation features some cells with more than the normal chromosome number, others with less. The best known human ailment resulting from a change in chromosome number is Down's Syndrome (sometimes called "mongolism" because the flattened facial features give a superficial Oriental appearance to victims). Afflicting about 14 out of every 10,000 babies born in the United States and inevitably resulting in mental retardation, Down's Syndrome occurs due to the presence in the victim's cells of 47 chromosomes instead of the normal 46 (to be more precise, three #21 chromosomes rather than two). Interestingly, the likelihood of a woman's giving birth to a Down's Syndrome child increases as the mother gets older. Whereas on average only 13.5% of all pregnancies occur among women over 35, these older mothers produce more than half of the children with Down's Syndrome. Prevailing theory is that since each female child is born with all the egg cells she will ever have, these eggs are subject to deterioration with aging or with exposure to toxic substances. The older the woman, the greater the possibility that her egg cells could sustain damage resulting in a mutation. It is common medical procedure today for pregnant women over 35 to undergo a process called **amniocentesis**. Usually performed in the fourth month of pregnancy, amniocentesis involves inserting a needle through the woman's abdomen into the uterus and withdrawing about 20 ml of amniotic fluid. An analysis of the fetal cells that have sloughed off into this fluid can reveal the presence of Down's Syndrome as well as approximately 100 other genetic diseases. If tests for such disorders are positive, the parents then have the option of terminating the pregnancy (Norwood, 1980).

Two other human abnormalities resulting from a change in chromosome number are Klinefelter's Syndrome, found only in males, and Turner's Syndrome, restricted to females. Whereas a normal man has an X and a Y sex chromosome, victims of Klinefelter's Syndrome have an extra X, or 47 chromosomes altogether. This condition, one of the most common of all genetic abnormalities, can cause a variety of problems, ranging from learning disabilities, language difficulties, behavioral problems, infertility, and, in about one-third of cases, enlargement of the breasts following puberty. Many of these symptoms respond to therapy, enabling Klinefelter males to lead normal, productive lives even though they will never be able to father children (nevertheless, many marry and are sexually active). The frequency of Klinefelter's births is relatively high—about 1 in 800—and is only slightly more prevalent among children of older mothers. Turner's Syndrome, by contrast, occurs when one X chromosome is missing; i.e., the victim has only one sex chromosome, for a total of 45 instead of the normal 46. This malady is outwardly expressed by retarded sexual development (no breast development, failure to menstruate or ovulate), unusually short stature, and lower-than-average intelligence in some Turner's females. Treatment methods developed within recent years have made it possible for an increasing number of Turner's Syndrome women to live near-normal lives. Interestingly, the incidence of Turner's Syndrome is far lower than that of Klinefelter's—only 1 in 3500. This discrepancy appears to be due to a very high rate of intrauterine deaths among fetuses with only one sex chromosome. Indeed, examinations of spontaneously aborted fetuses reveal that fully 10% were afflicted with this chromosomal condition (Volpe, 1975).

Cause of Mutations

That mutations occur is not in question; their underlying cause is less well understood. A great many mutations occur spontaneously due to natural causes. Some of these spontaneous mutations have been attributed to radiation exposure from cosmic rays and radioactive minerals in the earth's crust. However, it is thought that such relatively low levels of background radiation are insufficient to account for the majority of spontaneous mutations, the cause of which remains a mystery.

During the 20th century a number of artificial substances identified as capable of inducing mutations have been introduced into the human environment and have raised serious concerns within the scientific community regarding their potential for increasing mutation rates. Such substances capable of inducing a mutation are known as **mutagens**. X-rays were the first mutagens to be recognized, their mutagenic effect on fruit flies being described in 1927 by the great geneticist H. J. Muller at Indiana University. Subsequently a number of chemical compounds have been found to possess mutagenic properties, among them formaldehyde, mustard gas, nitrous acid, colchicine, and vinyl chloride. Many other candidates are now under suspicion as being possible mutagens.

Mutation Rates

Although the probability of any given human gene in an egg or sperm cell undergoing a spontaneous mutation is difficult to estimate accurately, it is generally regarded as low. However, one must keep in mind that each person has millions of genes. The chances of a mutation occurring in at least one of those genes is thus quite large. In fact, the English geneticist Harry Harris asserts that, on the average, every newborn child may be "expected, as the result of a new mutation in either of its parents, to synthesize at least one structurally variant enzyme or protein." Since only those mutations which occur in an egg or sperm have the potential to be passed on to subsequent generations, studies of mutation frequency have focused on these so-called "genetic mutations." Typically mutations occurring in a person's sex cells have no effect upon him or her but present a risk to succeeding generations of offspring. On the other hand, a mutation occurring in any cell other than an egg or sperm (somatic mutation) can adversely affect the person who sustained the mutation, but such injury will not be inherited by his or her children and thus represents no threat to the human gene pool.

In this context it is of interest to note that 10–15% of all human conceptions spontaneously abort within the first month of pregnancy; 12–15% more are miscarried before the 27th week; and 2% terminate as stillbirths. Thus approximately 30% of all human conceptions fail to survive until birth (Volpe, 1975). Much of this reproductive failure is thought to be due to mutations. Chromosomal studies of miscarried fetuses reveal that fully half have gross chromosomal abnormalities, while lethal point mutations are suspected in many of the others.

The great concern among geneticists today is that exposure of populations to the artificial mutagens so common in the modern environment could further increase mutation rates. Since most mutations are harmful to some degree, it is in humanity's long-term interest to keep mutation rates as low as possible.

Birth Defects

As we have seen in the previous section, mutations in parents' sex cells can result in their children being born with structural or functional abnormalities, but by no means are all birth defects due to mutations. Of the roughly 110,000–150,000 infants in the United States whom the Centers for Disease Control and Prevention (CDC) estimates are born with birth defects each year, mutations are believed to account for approximately 25% of the total. Since birth defects constitute the leading cause of infant mortality in the United States, efforts to understand why fetal malformation occurs and how to prevent such a tragic course of events assume added urgency.

Living things are far more sensitive to adverse environmental influences during their early stages of development than they are at any other time. Embryos that are perfectly normal genetically can be seriously or fatally damaged if exposed to extraneous hazards. Investigations over the past several decades have revealed the sad truth that the womb is not the safe haven it was once assumed to be.

The likelihood that all abnormal development is triggered by some aspect of the environment (even hereditary disorders were at some point initiated by a mutation caused by some mutagenic influence) has given rise to the science of **teratology**—the study of abnormal formations in animals or plants (originally, "the study of monstrosities")—and to the search for **teratogens**, substances that cause birth defects.

Figure 6-2 Some Known Human Teratogens

TERATOGEN	EFFECT
Ionizing Radiation	
X-rays	central nervous system disorders, micro-cephaly, eye problems, mental retardation
nuclear fall-out	
Pathogenic Infections	
German measles	congenital heart defect, deafness, cataracts
syphilis and herpes simplex type 2	mental retardation, microcephaly
cytomegalovirus	kidney and liver disorders, pneumonia, brain damage
toxoplasmosis	fatal lesions in the central nervous system
Drugs and Chemicals	
thalidomide	phocomelia
methyl mercury	mental retardation, sensory and motor problems
DES	vaginal cancer in girls, genital abnormalities in boys
dioxin	structural deformities, miscarriages
anesthesia	miscarriages, structural deformities
alcohol	mental retardation, growth deficiencies, microcephaly, facial irregularities
cigarette smoke	low birth weight, miscarriage, stillbirth
dilantin	heart malformations, cleft palate, harelip, mental retardation, microcephaly
valproic acid	spina bifida
Accutane	cardiovascular abnormalities, deformation of the ear, hydrocephaly, microcephaly
Tegison	same effect as for Accutane

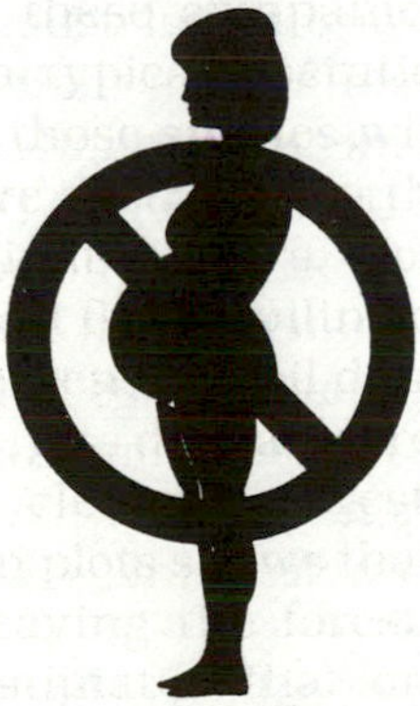

Interest in birth abnormalities is undoubtedly as old as humanity itself, although prior to the present century most ideas regarding birth defects involved considerably more fantasy than fact. From ancient times until fairly recently, some societies believed that the emotional state and visual impressions of an expectant mother could influence the physical development of her child. For this reason women in ancient Greece were encouraged to gaze at statuary representing the ideal human form, while Norwegian mothers-to-be were cautioned against looking at rabbits, for fear their babies would be born with harelip! The Babylonians and Sumerians regarded certain types of malformations as portents of coming events; medieval Europeans regarded them as evidence that the mother had indulged in intercourse with Satan or other demons and occasionally used this event as an excuse to execute the unfortunate mother and child. The so-called "Theory of Divine Retribution," also prevalent in Europe during the Middle Ages, viewed the birth of a defective child as God's punishment on the parents for past sins. With the rebirth of scientific inquiry in the Western world following the Renaissance, less mythical interpretations of teratogenesis were sought. In the 17th century birth defects were attributed to such factors as the narrowness of the mother's uterus, poor posture of the pregnant woman, or to a fall or blow on the abdomen during pregnancy. Though inaccurate, these explanations at least were an attempt to find a rational explanation for what remained a mysterious phenomenon. Gregor Mendel's discovery of the laws of genetics, followed by an explosion of research into the mechanism of heredity, led in the early 20th century to acceptance of the idea that all developmental errors could be attributed to faulty genes. This view prevailed for the first 40 years of this century, but a series of significant discoveries and observations since that time has once again altered our perception regarding teratogenesis and has given new impetus and urgency to the field of teratology.

The first key discovery to change the prevailing view that heredity is all-important emerged from animal studies investigating the influence of maternal diet on the outcome of pregnancy. In 1940 a report was published showing that specific types of nutritional deficiencies in pregnant rats caused predictable types and percentages of malformations in their offspring (Warkany, 1972). This finding effectively shattered old ideas about the overriding importance of genes and the conviction that the fetus could parasitize the mother if necessary to ensure normal development. Continued research into the influence of maternal diet on fetal development has confirmed and broadened these original findings. It is now known that a wide range of nutrients, from proteins to trace minerals to specific amino acids, are essential for normal development. Conversely, an excess of some of these necessary substances (e.g. phenylalanine, vitamin A) can exert teratogenic effects.

In 1941 an unusually large number of babies in both the United States and Australia were born suffering from congenital cataracts, heart defects, or deafness. Epidemiological studies launched to try to determine the cause for such an outbreak found that the only common thread linking all the victims was the fact that during the first trimester of pregnancy, their mothers had contracted German measles (*Rubella*) which had reached

BOX 6-3
Folic Acid to the Rescue in China

Neural tube defects such as spina bifida ("open spine"—a condition in which a portion of the spinal cord protrudes from the spinal column, frequently causing paralysis of the lower extremities) and anencephaly (a severe malformation in which most of the brain is missing) are among the most common—and most serious—types of birth abnormalities. In the United States approximately 2500 babies are born with neural tube defects each year, but that figure pales by comparison with the 80,000–100,000 Chinese infants born with the affliction annually. China leads all other nations in the world in the incidence of neural tube defects, a fact totally unrecognized even by the Chinese until the early 1980s when a limited surveillance program was established in the Beijing area to study birth abnormalities. Chinese physicians at Beijing Medical University's National Center for Maternal and Infant Health, working in cooperation with an American researcher from the Centers for Disease Control and Prevention (CDC), discovered that neural tube defects were the leading cause of stillbirths among the sample population studied—ten times more prevalent among Chinese babies than among their counterparts elsewhere in the world. And while Western infants born with spina bifida generally receive the medical care that permits them to survive into adulthood, those in China, if born alive, typically die before they reach their first birthday.

Coincident with growing realization of the scope of China's problem, researchers in both Hungary and Great Britain announced the results of some major nutritional studies that had been underway in those countries for a number of years: neural tube defects could be reduced by as much as 75% by increasing a pregnant woman's intake of **folic acid**, one of the B vitamins. The news reverberated worldwide, and nowhere was it received more enthusiastically than among the medical team in Beijing. For the first time ever, a major birth defect could be prevented simply by taking a vitamin pill!

As researchers scrutinized the situation more closely, the reasons for China's excess incidence of neural tube defects became more clear. Folic acid deficiencies seldom occur among women who eat a plentiful amount of green vegetables such as spinach or broccoli, as well as fresh fruits. In northern China, however, the winter diet consists primarily of steamed cabbage, a food quite low in folic acid. Because Chinese New Year (generally falling in late January or early February) is regarded as an auspicious time for weddings, many babies are conceived at a time of year when maternal nutritional levels are deficient in folic acid. The solution to this problem appeared obvious: provide prospective Chinese mothers with Vitamin B supplements. With $1 million per year in financing from the CDC, in the fall of 1993 (a few months prior to the peak marriage season!) China's Health Ministry launched a pilot project in 12,000 villages, dispensing millions of low-cost folic acid pills while simultaneously displaying color photographs of dead, deformed babies as an inducement for women to enroll in the program.

Chinese leaders are not alone in recognizing the enormous public health benefits offered by folic acid. In the United States, the Public Health

Service now recommends that all women of childbearing age take 0.4 milligrams of the vitamin daily—about double the amount consumed in the typical American diet. Since the types of birth defects caused by folic acid deficiency occur during the first weeks of fetal development, before many women realize they have conceived, the advice to begin taking folic acid at the time pregnancy is confirmed comes too late to be of real benefit. For this reason, many nutritionists have urged that foods be fortified with folic acid, just as they are with iodine, niacin, Vitamin D, and other important micronutrients. Accordingly, in the fall of 1993 the Food and Drug Administration (FDA) proposed that 140 micrograms of folic acid be added to every 100 grams (3.5 ounces) of bread and grain products—not enough to meet a woman's entire daily requirement of the vitamin, but enough to fill the gap between the amount normally consumed in a well-balanced diet and the amount considered optimal for preventing neural tube defects. (Because too much folate can have adverse health implications for the elderly, FDA was reluctant to recommend a larger dose of the supplement.) If the regulation is finalized before the end of 1994 as expected, folic acid-fortified flour, cornmeal, grits, rice, and noodles will be on the plates of over 90% of American women by early 1995—the first time in U.S. history that a food additive has been used to prevent birth defects.

References

Tyler, Patrick E. 1994. "Chinese Start a Vitamin Program to Eliminate a Birth Defect." *New York Times,* Jan. 11.

Williams, Rebecca D. 1994. "FDA Proposes Folic Acid Fortification." *FDA Consumer,* (May).

epidemic proportions that year. The fact that a virus could cross the placental barrier and damage the fetus was thus established.

While these two developments demonstrated that mammalian embryos are vulnerable to such commonplace environmental influences as inadequate diet and infections, the most dramatic confirmation that certain environmental factors (in this case an artificially synthesized drug) must be regarded as a potential risk to the unborn came only in the early 1960s with revelation of what has since come to be referred to as the "Thalidomide Tragedy."

Thalidomide was a drug first synthesized by a pharmaceutical company in Germany in 1953 and subsequently developed and widely marketed in Western Europe as a mild sedative. Preliminary testing on laboratory animals indicated that thalidomide had little injurious effect even when taken in quantity (in fact, humans who attempted to commit suicide using the drug survived extremely large doses). With evidence of its safety regarding overdosing, but with virtually no testing for other side effects, the German manufacturer put thalidomide on the market as a nonprescription sleeping pill and, thanks to an aggressive advertising campaign stressing its safety, thalidomide (sold under the trade name *Cantergan*) became the most widely used sedative in Germany and was extensively sold in Great Britain and several other European countries as well. Two American drug companies initially showed interest in acquiring thalidomide but concluded from their own tests that the drug was less effective than the brands they were already marketing. Somewhat later another American firm, impressed by the growing popularity of thalidomide in Europe, began another series of tests and released the drug for prescription use in Canada. In the United States, however, a doctor with the Food and Drug Administration had nagging doubts about some unexplained neurological results among long-term thalidomide users and restricted use of the drug in this country to a small clinical human trial. At about this time (1960) the European medical community was becoming increasingly puzzled by the sudden increase in what had formerly been an extremely rare type of birth abnormality. In near-epidemic proportions children were being born with a condition known as **phocomelia** ("seal-limb"), in which there is typically a hand or foot attached directly to the torso without an arm or leg. In some cases, however, even the hands and feet were absent, the babies being born with only a head and torso. The presence of large numbers of babies with such an obvious deformity couldn't be overlooked, but intense questioning of the parents regarding their hereditary background, blood type, radiation exposure, or chromosomal aberrations in other children failed to reveal a common link. Finally two alert physicians made the connection between thalidomide use early in pregnancy to the birth of limbless babies. Subsequent studies revealed that 40% of the women who had taken thalidomide during their first trimester of pregnancy delivered babies afflicted with phocomelia. As proof of thalidomide's teratogenic properties gained acceptance, use of the drug was gradually discontinued in country after country, but not before nearly 10,000 children had been permanently disabled (Glasser, 1976). Ironically, thalidomide's unsavory reputation may yet be redeemed by recent animal research which suggests that by inhibiting blood vessel growth in the cornea of the eye, the drug offers hope for treating diabetic retinopathy and macular degeneration, the two leading causes of blindness in the United States (it is hypothesized that thalidomide's teratogenic effects were a result of the drug's stunting blood vessel growth in the arm and leg buds of developing fetuses).

The thalidomide saga not only emphasized the importance of testing new drugs for their teratogenic effects, but also raised the profoundly disturbing question of what other drugs and medicines widely used by pregnant women might be doing to their unborn babies. That harmful effects could indeed result from medications used by pregnant women was confirmed again in the early 1980s when a French physician linked numerous cases of spina bifida to maternal use of valproic acid to control epileptic seizures (Harris and Wynne, 1994). A very beneficial medication for the mother's health problems, valproic acid proved devastating for unborn children exposed to the medication *in utero*. Valproic acid and thalidomide produced such distinctive types of abnormalities that they could scarcely go unnoticed. Conceivably, however, other teratogens that result in slight impairment of mental abilities, slight physical abnormalities, or diminished vigor might never be suspected as harmful. These episodes, tragic though they were, stimulated research, still ongoing, into what other substances present a threat to the unborn. Though much

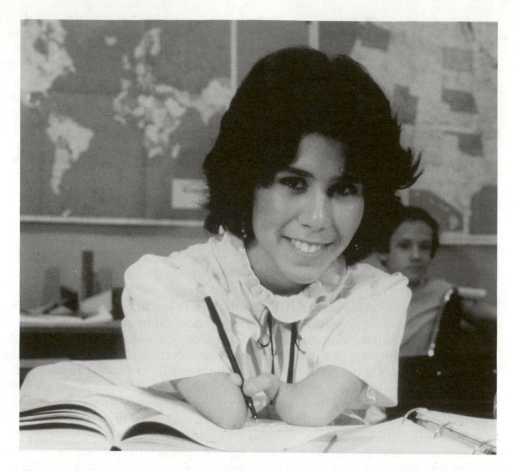

This young girl is but one of the more than 10,000 children born with missing arms or legs as a result of fetal exposure to thalidomide—a nonprescription sedative widely used in Europe during the early 1960s. [March of Dimes Birth Defects Foundation]

remains to be learned, investigations over the past three decades have implicated an increasing number of drugs and chemicals as proven or suspected teratogens. Among them, in addition to thalidomide: dioxin, organic mercury, diethylstilbestrol (DES), lead, cadmium, anesthetic gases, alcohol, and—responsible for by far the largest number of birth abnormalities and miscarriages—cigarette smoke. In spite of the gruesome lessons of past tragedies, pregnant women continue using various drugs (e.g. aspirin, antacids, barbiturates, tranquilizers, cough medicines), drinking, and smoking, even though it is generally accepted that excess use of any of the above substances carries some risk of fetal damage.

Self-administered drugs or medications are not the only source of teratogenic exposure, of course. Hundreds of thousands of American workers currently are employed in occupations that expose them to reproductive hazards—lead, anesthetic gases, ethylene oxide (used as a sterilant for many hospital supplies), and certain pesticides. While few well-documented associations between specific workplace chemicals and

Maternal consumption of alcohol during pregnancy is now recognized as a serious problem worldwide, its most dramatic consequences manifested here in the birth defect known as Fetal Alcohol Syndrome (FAS). FAS children generally suffer from low IQ, attention deficits, memory problems, and hyperactivity. The majority exhibit abnormalities of the upper lip, teeth problems, and an unusual shape of the head, face, ears, palms, and back/neck/spine. [From "Fetal Alcohol Syndrome in Adolescents and Adults" by Ann Pytkowicz Streissguth, PhD., et al., JAMA, April 17, 1991, Vol. 265. Courtesy of FAS Research Fund]

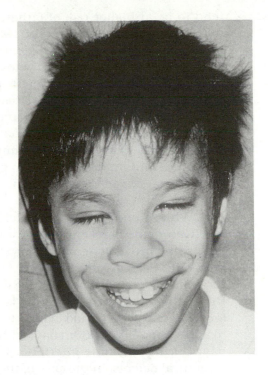

reproductive problems (i.e. miscarriage, reduced fertility, neonatal death, birth defects) exist at present, this doesn't mean such a linkage is nonexistent. Very few well-designed clinical or epidemiologic studies on the issue have been conducted, making it impossible to draw definitive conclusions. Nevertheless, a 1985 review of 2800 chemicals evaluated for their ability to induce birth defects in animals indicated that more than a third exhibited some teratogenic potential (Chivian et al., 1993). Unfortunately, most workplace teratogens are identified only after significant numbers of employees experience personal tragedies. Among the more recent reproductive hazards to make headlines are two glycol ethers, widely used as solvents in the manufacture of computer chips. Studies conducted on female workers exposed to the chemicals during the chip-making process found that the women suffered miscarriages 40% more frequently than did nonexposed women in the industry and experienced 30% fewer pregnancies. As a result of these findings, several of the corporate giants in the semiconductor industry are allowing pregnant female employees to work outside the chip fabrication area of the plant and have announced their intention to phase the hazardous chemicals out of the production process altogether (Markoff, 1992; "Solvents Used," 1992). The widespread assumption that workplace precautions against exposure to known teratogens need apply only to female workers is now being challenged by provocative, though inconclusive, evidence that a *father's* exposure to environmental hazards may also lead to defective offspring. It has long been observed that men working as painters, farmers, or mechanics—jobs involving exposure to certain solvents and pesticides—

tend to be at higher risk of fathering children with birth defects than do men in other occupations. In 1990 a British epidemiologist published research results purporting to demonstrate elevated incidence of childhood leukemia among youngsters whose fathers worked at Britain's Sellafield nuclear fuel reprocessing plant, suggesting occupational exposure to radiation as the culprit. These results have been strongly challenged by other scientists who claim to have found no such association in studies at other nuclear facilities. Whatever the case, the controversy has stimulated a new look at the impact which mutagenic or teratogenic substances might have on sperm production or on the chemical composition of semen, and thereby on the development of a fertilized egg (Stone, 1992).

While some progress in elucidating the mechanism of teratogenesis has been made in recent years, much more research is needed. Nevertheless, some broad generalizations about the causation of birth defects can be made. Perhaps most critical is the finding that fetal vulnerability to teratogens depends on the stage of development at the time of exposure. By far the most sensitive period is the time of tissue and organ formation (organogenesis), a period lasting from about the 18th day after conception to approximately the 60th day, with the peak of sensitivity around the 30th day. During this time interference with development can result in gross structural defects. In the case of the thalidomide episode, it was found that virtually all of the thalidomide mothers had taken the drug precisely during those few days when the limb buds were forming. Those women who used thalidomide before or after this critical time gave birth to normal babies. During the first week after conception, when the embryo is a relatively undifferentiated mass of cells, any damage caused by teratogenic exposure will be lethal to the developing embryo. After the 8th week, though the fetus is barely an inch long, its organs are already basically formed. Exposure to teratogens after this time can cause such harm as mental retardation, blindness, or damage to the external sex organs, but the time for major structural deformation has passed. It must be recognized, however, that individual genetic differences in both mother and child will determine the extent of damage caused by teratogenic exposure. No teratogen causes birth defects in 100% of those exposed; if a group of women, all at the same stage of pregnancy, were exposed to equal concentrations of the same teratogen, some would give birth to babies with serious abnormalities, others with only moderate damage, and some would deliver infants who were perfectly normal (Harris and Wynne, 1994).

A second widely accepted generalization about teratogenesis is that as the dosage of a teratogen increases, the degree of damage increases. Basing their assumptions on the results of animal studies, teratologists thus presume the existence of a threshold below which no injury of any kind can be demonstrated. Determining exactly where that threshold is for any particular substance is, however, uncertain at best, and expectant mothers are well advised to limit their exposure to potential teratogens to the greatest extent possible.

BOX 6-4

Accutane—Boon or Bane?

Severe, recalcitrant cystic acne is neither infectious, fatal, nor even debilitating, but for those young men and women suffering its ravages it can leave both physical and psychological scars. The scourge of adolescents since time immemorial, cystic acne has been treated with an untold number of home remedies or bona fide pharmaceutical formulations, but until recently nothing provided any significant, long-term relief. Thus when a highly effective new drug, Accutane (isotretinoin), received FDA approval in 1983, it encountered an enthusiastic reception.

Accutane is the first—indeed, the only—medication that can totally cure this particularly severe type of acne. While other forms of treatment are lengthy and only effective in holding the condition at bay as long as medication continues, after a few months of taking Accutane, drug use can be stopped and, in most cases, the skin remains clear. For males, who comprise by far the largest number of cystic acne sufferers, this is unmitigated good news—they now have access to a cure for their problem. For females, however, (and 40% of all Accutane prescriptions are for young women), deciding whether or not to use Accutane may entail choosing between a beautiful face or a healthy baby. For Accutane is a known teratogen; of women using the drug during pregnancy, one out of four has given birth to a defective child. Since Accutane is a Vitamin A derivative and large doses of Vitamin A also are known to be teratogenic, Accutane received FDA approval with the stipulation that its use during pregnancy be forbidden. Nevertheless, it is now apparent that such use contrary to label requirements has occurred, with predictable results— malformed infants, miscarriages, and induced abortions by women wishing to avoid the birth of a defective child.

Alarmed by what was happening, representatives of such prestigious groups as the Centers for Disease Control and Prevention and the American Academy of Pediatrics urged the FDA to pull the drug from the market. Equally concerned dermatologists and pharmaceutical company representatives pleaded for the rights of acne sufferers, the majority of whom are not pregnant, to have continued access to the only medication that can help them. After lengthy consultations among the various concerned parties, a compromise agreement was reached whereby the FDA will continue to allow marketing of Accutane under very stringent conditions. Henceforth labeling information for the patient will provide explicit descriptions and warnings of Accutane's teratogenic potential. The patient will be told not to use the drug unless she is protected by an effective form of contraception; to safeguard against the possibility that she may already be pregnant but not yet realize it, the patient is told not to begin using the drug until the second or third day of her normal menstrual cycle.

Instructions to physicians have also been drastically revised under the new agreements. Doctors are being told not to prescribe Accutane to any woman of child-bearing age unless she 1) has severe, disfiguring cystic acne which won't respond to any other type of treatment, 2) can be relied upon to follow instructions, 3) is using an effective method of contraception, 4) has had a negative pregnancy test within 2 weeks of the beginning of Accutane use, and 5) has received verbal and written warnings of Accutane's teratogenic potential, as well as the risks of contraceptive failure, and has signed a statement saying she understands these. Hoffmann-LaRoche, the manufacturer of Accutane, has agreed to undertake extensive professional education efforts and to conduct follow-up studies on drug use.

Officials are hopeful that with these increased efforts to inform women about the inherent danger of Accutane use and to prohibit access by pregnant or potentially pregnant women, an otherwise valuable drug can continue to be available to those for whom nothing else is effective.

Reference

Willis, Judith. 1988. "New Warnings About Accutane and Birth Defects." *FDA Consumer* 22, no. 8 (Oct.)

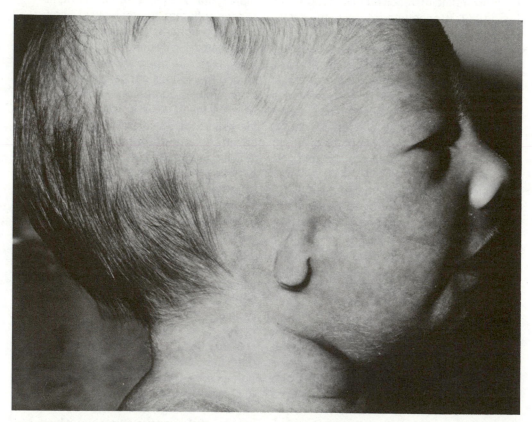

This infant has obvious defects which were caused by the mother taking Accutane during pregnancy. [Dr. Reba Michels Hill, St. Luke's Episcopal Hospital]

Cancer

Few words arouse such emotions of sheer terror and hopelessness today as does the term "cancer." As the second leading cause of death in the United States at the present time (heart disease ranks first), cancer appears to have assumed epidemic proportions. Cancer now accounts for approximately 20% of all deaths each year, both in the United States and in the industrialized world as a whole—and although improved treatment methods are reducing cancer death rates among victims under age 45, overall age-adjusted rates of cancer mortality continue to rise. While 143 out of every 100,000 people in the United States died of cancer in 1930, by 1950 that figure had risen to 157; by 1970 the cancer death rate had climbed to 163, and by 1990 it reached 174. The American Cancer Society estimates that U.S. cancer deaths now total 1400 daily, with an annual toll well exceeding half a million. Cancer is not age-specific; although incidence rates increase with age (the majority of cases occur among middle-aged or elderly adults), cancer causes more deaths among children aged 1–14 than any other disease (American Cancer Society, 1994). In general, cancer death rates are considerably higher in developed countries than in the developing world, but the *types* of cancer which are most prevalent in various parts of the world differ sharply. Malignancies associated with cigarette smoking, asbestos exposure, or high-fat diets are far more common among populations in industrialized countries, while cancers linked to certain food preservatives, viral infections, or fungal toxins in food are more prevalent in the developing world.

Contrary to popular belief, death rates are not increasing for all types of cancer. In the United States, mortality rates for cancer of the uterus, the cervix, and of the stomach have all fallen by approximately 70% over the last 50 years. In the case of uterine and cervical cancers, credit for the decline in death rates is attributed to widespread use of the Pap smear test which provides early diagnosis when the disease is still treatable. Experts estimate that a further 90% reduction in the current annual number of U.S. cervical cancer deaths (est. 4600) could be achieved if all American women would take advantage of this simple procedure. Regarding stomach cancer mortality, which is lower today in the United States than anywhere else in the world (at present the East Asian and eastern European countries have the highest incidence of stomach cancer mortality), favorable trends are probably due to improved methods of transport and to refrigeration which have made fresh produce available year-round. These advantages of modern life are significant in terms of cancer prevention because they have led to increased consumption of fresh fruits and vegetables (known to contain anticarcinogenic compounds), thereby lessening dependence on the salted, pickled, or smoke-preserved foods that are thought to pose a cancer risk. Colorectal cancers, currently the second leading cause of cancer mortality in the United States, have also begun to decline in both North America and Western Europe; liver cancer, bladder cancer, and leukemia death rates exhibit similar downward trends. Unfortunately, however, these gains in reducing cancer's toll have been offset by still-rising

Figure 6-3

Cancer Death Rates by Site, Males, United States, 1930–90

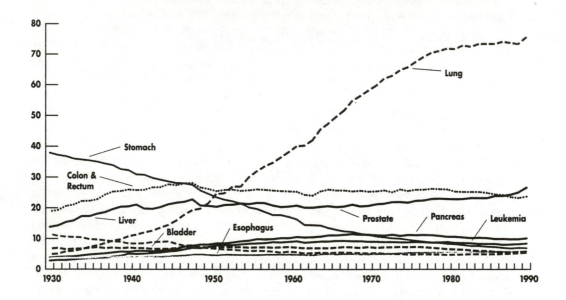

Cancer Death Rates by Site, Females, United States, 1930–90

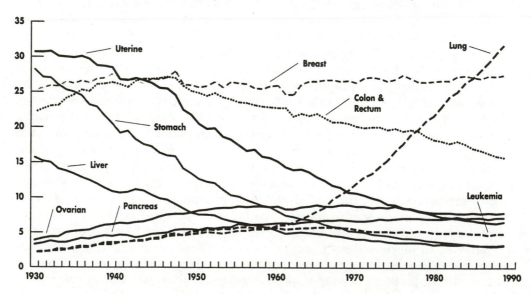

Rates are per 100,000 and are age-adjusted to the 1970 U.S. census population.

Source: American Cancer Society, *Cancer Facts & Figures—1994*. Used with permission. © 1994 American Cancer Society, Inc.

mortality from several other forms of cancer: prostate, breast, brain, kidney, and pancreatic malignancies, melanoma, non-Hodgkins lymphoma, and multiple myeloma—all are on the upswing (Davis and Hoel, 1992; Squires, 1990). By far the major factor to which the rise in cancer death rates can be attributed, however, is the explosive increase in lung cancer. Lung cancer alone accounts for close to one-third of all U.S. cancer deaths each year.

Cancer, of course, is not a new disease; ancient societies, like their modern counterparts, were familiar with the ravages of cancer. Indeed, all multicellular organisms, plant and animal, are subject to the occasional development of malignancies. However, cancer's rapid rise to prominence as a leading cause of illness and death during the present century has embued the malady with an aura of dread and fatalism. Until recently, progress achieved in the so-called "War Against Cancer" remained disappointingly limited after decades of intensive medical research and the expenditure of billions of dollars. Although some successes had been scored in reducing deaths from childhood leukemia and Hodgkins lymphoma, the "magic bullet" that would provide a cure for cancer was nowhere in sight. Research and observation strongly suggested that a majority of cancers were associated with environmental causes (using the term "environment" in its broadest sense to include diet, smoking, sun exposure, chemical pollutants, and so forth), yet the mechanism for such interaction remained unknown. Within the past few years, however, several major breakthroughs in cancer research have revolutionized our understanding of carcinogenesis. While a great deal more remains to be learned, these findings have provided important information on how once-healthy cells become malignant and offer new hope for both prevention and treatment of this formidable killer.

What Causes Cancer?

"Cancer" is a collective term used to describe a number of diseases that differ in origin, prognosis, and treatment. It is essentially a condition in which the regulating forces that govern normal cell processes no longer function correctly, leading to uncontrolled cell proliferation. Cancerous cells, unlike normal ones, continue to divide and spread, invading other tissues where they interfere with vital bodily functions and eventually lead to death of the organism. The search for agents responsible for initiating this chain of events has been ongoing for years and has focused on a number of possibilities including pathogens, hereditary factors, oxidation damage within cells due to normal metabolic processes, and exposure to a wide range of environmental **carcinogens** (substances that can cause cancer) such as toxic chemicals and radiation.

Viruses are definitely known to cause some forms of cancer in animals (e.g. viral leukemia in cats, Rous sarcoma in chickens) and are suspected of being involved in the type of human cancer known as Burkitt's lymphoma. Similarly, there appears to be an association between hepatitis-B infection and the development of liver cancer, as well as between a herpes-type virus and some cases of cervical cancer, the latter suspicion based on the fact that cervical cancer is most common among women who have had intercourse with various partners. For decades it had been assumed that **bacteria** had no part to play in the cancer drama, but in 1994 researchers at Stanford University reported that the risk for non-Hodgkins lymphoma of the stomach is markedly higher among people infected with the bacterium *Helicobacter pylori*, the common microbe that was recently recognized as the leading cause of stomach ulcers (three years earlier another research team demonstrated an association between this same bacterium and a different form of stomach cancer, gastric carcinoma). Interestingly, while non-Hodgkins lymphoma of the stomach is extremely rare in the United States, it is relatively common in the Veneto region of Italy where 90% of the population is infected with *H. pylori* (Parsonnet et al., 1994; Isaacson, 1994).

Since the rediscovery of Mendelian principles of genetics at the turn of the century, **heredity** has been a prime suspect for cancer causation, particularly because certain kinds of malignancies are more common in some families than in others. It is well-established that a few types of cancer *are* hereditary; one of the best known hereditary cancers is retinoblastoma, a cancer of the eye. For the most part, however, studies carried out earlier in this century discounted heredity as a significant factor in cancer causation. These studies compared the incidence of specific types of cancer among descendants of immigrants to the United States and members of the same ethnic group remaining in the homeland. For example, a 1944 study of the incidence of liver cancer showed that African-Americans have much lower rates of this disease than do native African populations; similarly, Japanese-Americans exhibit low rates of stomach cancer—comparable to those of the general American population—while stomach cancer remains very common in Japan. By contrast, these Japanese-Americans, like other U.S. residents, experience typically high rates of colon cancer, a disease quite rare in Japan. Such results appear to indicate that environmental factors (e.g. diet), rather than genetic predisposition, account for the development of these types of malignancies.

However, within the past few years, a tidal wave of new discoveries demonstrating the existence of an inherited *predisposition* to cancer has been flowing out of research laboratories throughout the United States and Canada. By the late spring of 1994, at least three dozen genes which mediate malignant tumor formation in humans had been identified. Such findings not only help to explain for the first time why some people exposed to known carcinogens remain hale and hearty while others sicken and die, but also offer promising therapeutic approaches for reducing cancer mortality among those likely to develop the disease.

An important breakthrough, announced in late 1993, involved discovery of a **mutator gene** associated with a common type of colon cancer (hereditary nonpolyposis colorectal cancer) which afflicts as many as 22,000 Americans each year—10 to 15% of all colon cancers. In its normal form, this gene (dubbed "hMSH2") produces a protein that acts as a cellular "spell checker," correcting errors in the order of nucleotide base pairs during DNA replication. In mutated form, the gene is no longer able to produce its key protein and mistakes occurring after replication accumulate throughout the genetic material, creating a situation that may eventually result in cancer. Researchers estimate that over a million Americans—1 out of every 200 people in this country—carry this mutator gene (Leach et al., 1993; Fishel et al., 1993). In March 1994, the discovery of a second mutator gene linked to colorectal cancer was announced (this one called "*hMLH1*"). Cumulatively, these two genes, when defective, are believed to account for nearly 20% of diagnosed colon cancer cases. For those who carry one of these mutator genes, the chances of eventually developing colon cancer ranges between 70–90%, with many victims developing tumors before the age of 50. The practical significance of these recent findings is therefore immense: if carriers could be identified through genetic screening programs, they could begin having regular colonoscopic examinations at an early age in order to detect precancerous polyps when they can be easily removed. Similarly, identified bearers of the defective gene could be strongly advised to adopt the low-fat, high-fiber diet which is known to reduce the risk of colorectal cancer (Papadopoulos et al., 1994; Bronner et al., 1994).

A great many **environmental agents** such as cigarette smoke, radon gas, sunlight, heavy metals, X-rays, chemical pesticides, some air pollutants, and high-fat diets are known to be carcinogenic and are believed responsible for many human cancers. The exact mechanism by which such agents induce cancer is still not completely understood, but recent progress in unravelling cancer's mysteries has brought us tantalizingly closer to that goal.

Carcinogenesis, in most cases, is thought to involve a multi-step process, often with a time gap of many years between the initial mutational event and the development of malignant growth. The first step, termed **initiation**, involves a change in the genetic material (i.e. an induced mutation), caused by a brief interaction between the target organ or tissue and a carcinogenic substance. It has been demonstrated that many environmental carcinogens bond tightly with DNA nucleotides to form DNA-carcinogen **adducts**, causing genetic damage that can eventually lead to cancerous growth. Cells which have undergone initiation do not inevitably give rise to malignancies unless this first step is followed by a second event called **promotion**, a process by which initiated cells are exposed to another group of agents called **promoters**. In general, promoters by themselves are neither mutagenic nor carcinogenic but can stimulate cells to divide. If an initiated cell is present, it may thus be stimulated by a promoter to multiply and form a clone of initiated cells, thereby greatly enhancing the likelihood that additional mutations of "primed cells" (i.e. cells containing oncogenes, tumor-suppressor genes, etc.) will occur, leading eventually to cancer. A number of environmental agents have now been identified as initiators, others as promoters, while many act as both. In some cases, **demotion** of cancer can occur when certain anticarcinogenic compounds reverse the spread of a malignant growth or switch off initiated cells. The characteristic **latency period** between the initial exposure to a carcinogenic substance and the development of a malignancy after a period typically ranging from 10–20 years is more understandable in light of the findings regarding initiation and promotion of cancer and the realization that it usually takes considerable time for a cell to accumulate the five to six mutations generally required to cause cancerous growth. A number of researchers now hypothesize that the most effective way of reducing cancer incidence would be to reduce exposure to promoting agents or increase exposure to antipromoters. Since long-term exposure to a promoting agent is necessary to trigger malignant growth, eliminating or reducing such exposure will result in initiated cells remaining permanently in the latent phase.

A number of highly significant findings emerging from cancer research centers recently have further clarified the nature of the molecular changes within genes that lead to the development of cancer and suggest radical new approaches for combatting the disease *after* an adverse environmental exposure has provoked cellular damage. Molecular biologists working with a number of different species have now identified more than one hundred so-called **oncogenes** which tell the cell when to commence dividing. In their normal form, oncogenes play a beneficial— indeed, essential—role in regulating the cell cycle. When functioning properly, oncogenes orchestrate orderly fetal development, the routine replacement of worn-out cells, healing of wounds, and so forth. However, in mutant form an oncogene may cause the complex system by which normal cell replication is controlled to go awry, resulting in runaway cell proliferation. By contrast, **tumor-suppressor genes** typically act to *halt* uncontrolled multiplication of cells. In their normal form, oncogenes and tumor-suppressor genes act in concert with cellular replication processes to regulate cell growth, but if a mutation should occur in either type of gene, the finely-tuned mechanism of the cell can be thrown into a fatal malfunction, leading to cancerous growth.

In recent years mutant forms of several important oncogenes and tumor-suppressor genes have been identified as key contributors to the development of many cancers. The *Hras* oncogene, one of the first oncogenes described, is now known to be present in 50% of colon cancers and 90% of pancreatic cancers. Another significant development in cancer research recently was the discovery of the tumor-suppressor gene *p53*, important because it controls the synthesis of a protein that inhibits the formation of malignant tumors. It has been shown that the protein resulting from the activity of the *p53* gene can stimulate production of a second protein which, in turn, inhibits key enzymes needed for completion of the cell cycle. In addition, *p53* gives instructions for a cell to self-destruct when it detects unrepairable damage to DNA during cell division. Because of its role in thus preventing the dangerous proliferation of mutant cells, *p53* is sometimes referred to as "the guardian of the genome." Mutations to the *p53* gene which result in a dysfunctional protein product can thus have devastating consequences to the organism. Mutations along the *p53* gene have now been detected in more than 50% of all human cancers studied. Some of those mutations have been linked to specific environmental chemicals which leave their unique "biomarkers" at a characteristic location along the gene. Thus researchers can now examine an individual's *p53* gene, note the position of the mutated segment and the nature of the change, and thereby identify which agent—various components of cigarette smoke, aflatoxin, UV light, etc.—caused the damage (a development with obvious implications for environmental lawyers representing clients claiming harm from toxic pollutants!). Ongoing research using animal models, combined with data from human cancers, indicate that there may be specific molecular patterns of mutant *p53* genes associated with particular forms of cancer. Thus there is exciting potential for the *p53* gene as a diagnostic tool in the detection of cancers. Other data suggest a role for *p53* in the treatment of cancers (Culotta and Koshland, 1993; Harris, 1993; Blakeslee,1994).

Undoubtedly, the next few years will witness unprecedented expansion of our knowledge regarding cancer causation—knowledge that will provide an increasing number of weapons for fighting and eventually controlling this dreaded disease. In the meantime, however, society must continue ongoing efforts to prevent exposure to the myriad of environmental agents which are believed responsible for the majority of cancers. While new evidence of inherited predisposition to specific cancers explains why some people are more likely to develop cancer than others, it holds true nevertheless that with most cancers (retinoblastoma being a notable exception) even susceptible individuals are unlikely to develop a malignancy in the absence of adverse environmental exposure. Conversely, even individuals who are not genetically predisposed can experience the DNA damage leading to carcinogenesis if exposure to cancer-causing agents is excessive. By eliminating contact with known carcinogens, one can drastically reduce the incidence of a malignancy—as in so many other realms of life, prevention is the best cure for cancer.

Environmental Carcinogens

The fact that an environmental agent can cause cancer was first reported more than two hundred years ago when, in 1775, an English physician, Sir Percival Pott, recognized an association between cancer of the scrotum and exposure to soot. Every patient he examined with this relatively rare ailment had, as a child, worked as a chimney sweep, being lowered naked into chimneys to clean out the soot that accumulated there. In the process, the boys were covered with soot and grime themselves and with the low standards of personal hygiene which characterized those times, some of this soot remained in the folds of the scrotum for long periods, eventually resulting in the development of scrotal cancer years later (more recently the active ingredient in this soot was identified as benzopyrene, known as a very potent carcinogen). Not until the present century, however, was much research directed toward detecting environmental carcinogens. Work during the early 1900s revealed the cancer-causing properties of a number of coal tar products and of X-rays, but not until mid-century as age-adjusted cancer rates began to soar did the search for cancer causation acquire new urgency. Since that time the public has been bombarded with so many dire warnings that the average

BOX 6-5

Lab Tests for Carcinogenicity—Are They Valid?

In 1977 a Canadian study documenting an excess incidence of bladder cancer among male rats fed a 5% diet of saccharin created a furor among an American public unconvinced that the food additive posed a real health threat and dismayed at the possible banning of the only non-caloric sweetener on the market at that time. Intelligent assessment of the implications of the saccharin research was not helped by the statement by a top FDA official that humans would have to drink 800 cans of diet soda daily to consume an amount of saccharin equivalent to that fed the experimental rats. The issue was widely aired in outraged letters to Congress and newspaper opinion pages, laughed about on late-night talk shows, and used as the butt of many a cartoonist's jokes. The public was given the impression that the tests were meaningless as far as human health was concerned, an attitude most aptly expressed by Congressman Andrew Jacobs of Indiana who proposed that his colleagues pass a bill requiring that products containing saccharin bear the label: "Warning: the Canadians have determined that saccharin is dangerous to your rat's health."

Unfortunately, the Congressman's remarks, echoed by millions of his fellow Americans, reveal a profound lack of understanding regarding the methods routinely used for determining the safety of new chemicals. The objections raised to the Canadian saccharin tests—and to animal testing procedures in general—focus primarily on the following two points:

1) *The question of dosage*—does *everything* cause cancer when present in excess? Contrary to popular belief, only carcinogens cause cancer. A test animal might be fed a mountain of sugar or salt and die of toxemia, but it will not develop a malignancy because neither substance is a carcinogen (some would qualify this statement by pointing out that because hyper-obesity is a risk factor for certain types of cancer, excessive consumption of chocolate fudge sundaes could lead to cancer; nevertheless, it would be difficult to argue that ice cream is an environmental carcinogen in the same sense that aflatoxins or nitrosamines are known to be). Feeding or exposing test animals to extremely high doses of a suspected chemical is a widely accepted procedure necessary for obtaining meaningful results within a reasonable period of time, given the constraints of such experiments. In a typical study, for reasons of expense and space considerations, only 50 to 100 experimental animals are used in each test group. Such animals have a relatively short life span in comparison with humans, so in order to compensate for the long latency period involved in cancer initiation and to increase the chances for a weak carcinogen to be revealed in the small study population, massive doses are used. This method simply facilitates the collection of data within a reasonable time and at considerably less expense than would be possible using larger test populations and lower dosages. That such tests are valid and that administration of large doses, *per se*, does not lead to carcinogenesis are supported by the results of past experimentation. A researcher at the National Cancer Institute some years ago reported that of 3,500 suspected carcinogens tested in the routine manner, only 750 proved, in fact, to be carcinogenic—hardly

support for the thesis that large doses in themselves are cancer-causing.

2) *Animals aren't humans*—do the substances that cause cancer in mice, monkeys, or rats (Canadian or otherwise!) predict cancer causation in humans? The prevailing assumption among researchers is that the basic biological processes in all mammals are fundamentally the same. For ethical reasons it is impossible to prove the thesis that any chemical which causes cancer in animals also causes the disease in humans—to do so would require deliberately exposing humans to a known animal carcinogen and waiting to see if cancer develops! However, numerous tests have been successfully carried out to prove the reverse: every substance known to induce human cancer causes cancer in animals as well (with the sole exception of arsenic, a heavy metal that is a human carcinogen, is mutagenic to bacteria and to cells grown in tissue culture, yet has never been shown to have carcinogenic potential in animals). Thus it seems logical to assume that the opposite is true also and that animal testing is a valid method for determining which chemicals are carcinogenic. What animal testing cannot tell us, however, is how strong or weak a given carcinogen will be in humans. This is because different species show varying degrees of sensitivity to the same substance, some developing cancer only at high levels of exposure while others are vulnerable to relatively low doses. Unfortunately it is not possible to calculate the level of human risk to a carcinogen based on the risk level in animals. We may be more vulnerable or less vulnerable; the tests indicate only which substances are a potential threat, not how much of the substance can be expected to result in a given number of human cancer cases.

Animal models, of course, provide but one of several methods for studying the mechanism of carcinogenesis. Other approaches for advancing our understanding of cancer include: **mutagenesis studies using bacteria** which, due to their very large population size and short generation time, allow rapid screening of numerous potential carcinogens; **tissue culture research** which permits examination of DNA damage and mutagenesis in eukaryotic cells (as opposed to prokaryotic bacterial cells); and **epidemiologic studies** of cancer incidence among human populations. Each of these lines of investigation has inherent limitations, and results yielded by one type of study may not always correspond with conclusions drawn from an alternative mode of inquiry. For example, nickel compounds are potent carcinogens in both humans and animals but are not mutagenic to bacteria. Conversely, organic mercury compounds damage DNA in bacterial cells and are mutagenic to cells in tissue culture, but have not been shown to induce cancer either in humans or animals. Cadmium and chromium, on the other hand, show carcinogenic potential in all four systems.

The disturbing lack of consistency in results among these various test models has led some observers to question the validity of current testing procedures and to challenge government regulations based on the results of carcinogenicity studies on animals. Most investigators would argue, however, that in an admittedly imperfect world, we must continue to use the only tools currently available, always bearing in mind their limitations and exercising due caution when interpreting data or extrapolating results from such experiments. As one cancer researcher remarked in defense of animal tests, "... half a loaf is better than no loaf at all!"

citizen may be excused for thinking that indeed everything causes cancer. This of course is untrue, but the very large number of new chemicals and products that have been coming into widespread use each year, many without adequate testing for harmful side effects, justifies concern. Surveys carried out on the "geography of cancer" indicate that the incidence of certain types of cancer are elevated in heavily industrialized areas. Results from an epidemiologic study recently conducted by the New York State Health Department confirmed the suspicions of Long Island residents worried about their region's unenviable status as a hot spot for breast cancer incidence. In a report that scientists describe as "the first credible study outside a laboratory to suggest a possible link between breast cancer and industrial pollution," Health Department researchers found that women living within 1 kilometer (0.6 miles) of chemical factories on Long Island had a 60% higher risk of developing post-menopausal breast cancer than did women living farther away. While the study didn't prove that chemical emissions from the factories were a direct cause of the observed cancers, it raised concerns among state officials and spurred demands for additional research (Schemo, 1994; "Studies Yield," 1994).

Debate currently rages over the extent to which present cancer rates reflect exposure to chemical pollutants as opposed to personal habits such as smoking or diet. The outcome of this controversy is obviously of political and economic importance, since extensive regulation would be required to control the former, while education and persuasion represent the practical limits to modifying the latter. Several of the most prominent public concerns in relation to cancer causation include the following.

Smoking.　Tobacco use, particularly cigarette smoking, is now recognized as far and away the leading contributor to cancer mortality in the United States. Rates of lung cancer are most reflective of the impact of smoking on health, and the drastic rise in this disease neatly parallels the increase in the smoking habit in American society. Today about one-third of all cancer deaths are due to lung cancer and of the 170,000 new lung cancer victims diagnosed annually in recent years, 87% are cigarette smokers (most of the others are individuals industrially exposed to carcinogens such as asbestos fibers or those exposed to radon gas inside their homes). Death rates among lung cancer victims, as opposed to victims of some other types of cancer, are quite high largely because lung malignancies are seldom diagnosed before the mass has reached a size of about 1 cm in diameter. By that time it has been growing for about 10 years and has usually spread to other parts of the body. Lung cancer rates began their steady rise in the mid-1930s, approximately 20 years or so after cigarette smoking became popular. Interestingly, until the mid-1950s it was widely assumed that women were resistant to the disease because the incidence of lung cancer among females was negligible compared to that among men. Since the mid-1950s, however, lung cancer mortality among women has been rising rapidly in a fashion parallel to that of males several decades earlier, reflecting social pressures which inhibited women's smoking prior to the "female emancipation" of the 1920s and 1930s. By the late 1980s, lung cancer had surpassed breast cancer as the leading

BOX 6-6

Synergism 1 + 1 = 5

Virtually all laboratory tests to determine carcinogenicity of suspected substances are based on responses to single-source exposures. Results of such testing methods may significantly underestimate risks in the real world because it is now well known that certain substances in combination are far more hazardous than either one would be if acting independently. For example, people who smoke cigarettes are 10 times more likely to develop lung cancer than are nonsmokers; asbestos workers incur significantly higher risk of lung cancer than do people not exposed to asbestos. However, a person who both smokes cigarettes and works with asbestos is 90 times more likely to get lung cancer than is a person exposed neither to cigarette smoke nor to asbestos—far higher than the risk factor for either type of exposure separately. This phenomenon, where the interaction of two or more substances produces an impact greater than the sum of their independent effects, is known as synergism and can perhaps be most easily thought of as a situation where $1 + 1 = 5$.

Synergistic effects are well documented in relation to interactions between various air pollutants, water pollutants, and so forth and will be mentioned again in the chapters dealing with those topics. Synergism has been most studied, however, in the context of cancer and smoking in an effort to demonstrate the degree of risk inherent in various types of smokers' lifestyles. In addition to the smoking-asbestos connection, other synergistic associations with smoking include:

1. Smoking and alcohol consumption—much higher rates of cancer of the mouth, larynx, and esophagus

2. Smoking and living in areas of high air pollution—elevated risk of lung cancer

3. Smoking and working with chemicals or in uranium mines—high lung cancer risk

cause of cancer mortality among women, making it for the first time the number one cancer killer among both sexes. As the advertisement for Virginia Slims puts it, "you've come a long way, Baby"—all the way from virtually no lung cancer to approximately 72,000 new cases among American women in 1994 (American Cancer Society, 1994). Thanks to increasing public awareness of the many adverse health impacts of tobacco use following the 1964 Surgeon General's report, the incidence of cigarette smoking among American adults steadily declined from 42% in 1965 to 25% in 1991. In the early 1990s, the consistent downward trend of the past 25 years was reversed by a slight upswing in smoking prevalence, almost entirely due to increased tobacco use by African-Americans and by young women. The growing popularity of smoking among teenage girls is particularly disturbing in view of the now well-documented adverse impact of smoking in relation to problem pregnancies and birth defects.

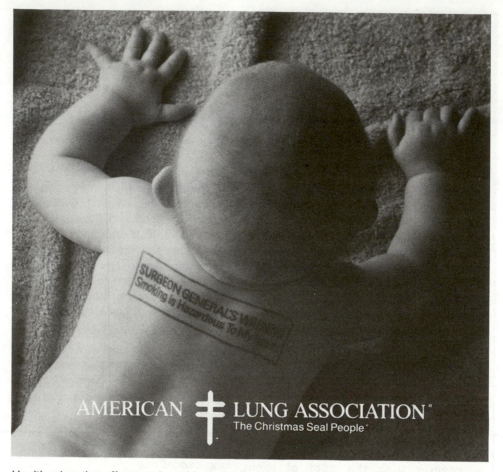

AMERICAN ✚ LUNG ASSOCIATION®
The Christmas Seal People®

Health education efforts such as this poster from the American Lung Association emphasize the danger of cigarette smoke on developing fetuses.

Another unfortunate trend in recent years, ironically motivated at least in part by concerns about the health hazards of *inhaling* cigarette smoke, has been the upsurge in use of smokeless tobacco, particularly by teenage males. A CDC Youth Risk Behavior Survey in 1991 revealed that 19% of male high school students were using snuff or chewing tobacco (keeping company with five million adults), a practice that exposes the user to amounts of nicotine equivalent to that in cigarettes. While use of smokeless tobacco products circumvents concerns about *lung* cancer, it certainly is not risk-free—the incidence of oral cancer is several times higher among snuff-dippers than among nonusers, while risk of cancer of the cheek and gums is nearly 50 times higher.

Elsewhere in the world, the number of smokers and the number of cigarettes smoked per person continue to climb. With a few notable exceptions, effective anti-smoking campaigns are rarely encountered outside the United States and Canada. Newly affluent developing countries

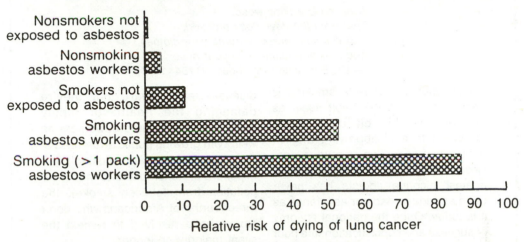

Figure 6-4 Relative Risk of Dying of Lung Cancer Due to Smoking and Occupational Asbestos Exposure*

*Includes asbestos workers, but not other workers exposed to asbestos.

Source: Surgeon General of the United States.

in particular are witnessing an explosive increase in cigarette sales—South Korea, China, and Brazil have experienced significant increases in per capita cigarette consumption. In a number of countries where smoking by females has long been socially unacceptable, increasing numbers of women are now taking up the habit. In Spain, for example, half of all 20-year-old women now smoke, compared with just 3% in their grandmothers' generation. Russia and the eastern European nations constitute several of the most rapidly expanding markets for tobacco sales. In those formerly Communist countries, so voracious is the craving for cigarettes that demand far exceeds supply, and Western companies are rushing in to fill the void. R. J. Reynolds, for one, has recently entered into a joint venture with the Russians to build several new plants in their country, capable of producing 22 billion cigarettes a year; watch for the Russian cancer statistics of 2020! (Brown, Kane, and Ayres, 1993).

Such trends cause dismay to those who realize that cigarette smoke contains more than 4,000 chemical compounds, of which at least 43 are known carcinogens, including benzo(a)pyrene, arsenic, cadmium, benzene, and radioactive polonium. Since these substances are inhaled, it is not surprising that the lungs are the tissue most directly affected. However, smoking has also been documented as a major cause of cancer of the mouth, esophagus, larynx and pharynx—and contributes to the development of bladder, kidney, and pancreatic cancer. In addition, research results published recently by the National Cancer Institute indicate that cigarette smoking can also lead to colon cancer, an enhanced risk that persists for a lifetime, even if the smoker subsequently kicks the

---

BOX 6-7

Public Outcast #1

Tobacco is a filthy weed,
That from the devil does proceed;
It drains your purse, it burns your clothes,
And makes a chimney of your nose.
  —Dr. Benjamin Waterhouse (1754–1846)

Vilification of cigarette smoking is nearly as old as the habit itself, as attested by this bit of doggerel attributed to a disapproving English physician nearly two centuries ago. However, the opprobrium directed against nicotine addicts has never been as widespread nor as intense as it is today. Once the national epitomy of success and sophistication, the poor smoker is rapidly becoming a social outcast, banished to the hallways at professional meetings, passed over for promotions, excluded from some restaurants and many public places, and nagged unmercifully by spouse and children. "Nonsmokers' Rights" has become a battle cry across the nation, relegating the once-admired Marlboro Man to the status of second class citizen. Why this sudden evaporation of public tolerance for a habit still prevalent among one out of every four American adults? Why do most states now restrict smoking in public places? Why has the U.S. government banned smoking on all commercial domestic flights? Nonsmokers have always suffered physical discomfort when forced to breathe air polluted with tobacco smoke, yet as long as the belief persisted that smokers were only endangering their own health, nonsmokers felt they had no right to complain. Personal grumbling turned to open militancy only with medical evidence proving that not only are cigarette smokers killing themselves in record numbers (approximately 419,000 Americans die from tobacco-related diseases each year), but they're damaging the health of family members, friends, and coworkers as well. With growing public awareness of the impact of "passive smoking" (i.e. exposure of nonsmokers to indoor air pollution from tobacco smoke), the three-fourths of Americans who don't smoke have resolved to remain the silent majority no longer.

Tobacco smoke inhaled by a nonsmoker can originate either from the "mainstream" smoke exhaled by a smoker or from the "sidestream" smoke emanating from the burning end of the cigarette. The latter accounts for approximately 85% of the pollution in the proverbial "smoke-filled room" and contains higher concentrations of carcinogens per unit weight than does mainstream smoke. While the sidestream smoke is significantly diluted by the volume of air in the room, two of its major components—carbon monoxide and nicotine—nevertheless have been measured at concentrations exceeding the ambient air quality standards in public places and meeting rooms. For nonsmokers who frequent these smoky environments, blood levels of carboxyhemoglobin are as high as if they had just smoked five cigarettes; their nicotine levels also are equivalent to those of a light smoker.

Much of the health research on passive smoking has focused on a possible association with enhanced lung cancer rates among nonsmokers. Numerous studies have been conducted in several different countries, and while the evidence is not yet universally accepted, EPA researchers estimate an average of 3000 nonsmoking Americans die annually due to working or living in an atmosphere contaminated with tobacco smoke. Studies in Japan and Greece likewise support a link between passive smoking and lung cancer mortality. EPA's recent designation of **environmental tobacco smoke (ETS)** as a Class A carcinogen added further weight to nonsmokers' demands for pollution-free indoor air.

Far more prevalent than nagging worries about lung cancer are the more mundane health complaints by nonsmokers forced to inhale someone else's smoke. While the following problems may not be life-threatening, they seriously diminish the nonsmoker's sense of well-being: 1) eye irritations—experienced by 69% of those reporting problems; 2) headaches—33%; 3) nasal symptoms—33%; 4) cough—33%. While these represent the most common problems reported, a sizable number also mention allergic reactions, wheezing, or sore throats. Angina patients report more frequent attacks when exposed to passive smoke and bronchial asthma sufferers show sharp declines in pulmonary function when in a smoky environment.

The most tragic victims of passive smoking, however, are those members of society least able to speak out in their own defense—infants, children, and the unborn. That parental smoking could be considered another form of child abuse has been amply documented in numerous studies. The EPA estimates that a minimum of 150,000 serious respiratory ailments among young children are caused each year by exposure to environmental tobacco smoke, with those under the age of 18 months facing the greatest risks. Bronchitis, pneumonia, asthma, and wheezing all occur more frequently among children whose parents smoke.

Researchers estimate that ETS causes 8,000–26,000 additional cases of asthma each year and aggravates symptoms in many more. Medical researchers have demonstrated that asthmatic children exposed to significant levels of secondhand smoke suffer 70–80% more attacks than children subjected to little or no such exposure. A significantly greater number of children whose mothers smoke are hospitalized for respiratory conditions than are children of nonsmoking mothers. Children suffering from asthma have been shown to experience marked improvement when their parents quit smoking.

Even more vulnerable to tobacco's insidious effects are children in the womb. When a pregnant woman smokes (and 20% of pregnant Americans *do* smoke), she is exposing her fetus to nicotine, carbon monoxide, radioactive polonium, and numerous other toxic chemicals. Carbon monoxide appears to be the most fetotoxic of these, causing a rise in carboxyhemoglobin in the blood of both mother and child and resulting in retarded fetal growth rates. Medical experts estimate that 20–40% of all low-weight births can be directly attributed to maternal smoking during pregnancy. Infants born to smoking mothers weigh on the average about 10% less at birth than do babies of nonsmokers. Since low birth weight is a major risk factor for infant mortality, it is not surprising that approximately 10% of all U.S. neonatal deaths each year are blamed on maternal smoking. Smoking during pregnancy is also blamed for an estimated 50,000 miscarriages annually and for 11–14% of all premature births, the risk of which rises the more heavily the mother smokes. Nor does the harm done by fetal exposure to secondhand smoke end with childbirth. Recent studies conducted on 3- and 4-year-olds have shown that preschoolers whose mothers smoked heavily during pregnancy score lower on IQ tests, and many experience subtle difficulties with speech and attention span compared to children who were not exposed to ETS in the womb.

Considering the extent to which a smoker's habit can adversely affect those around him or her, it's no wonder that smoking is increasingly viewed as antisocial behavior. With the proliferation of clean indoor air regulations in cities and states across the country sharply curtailing smokers' freedom to light up in public, the possibility of the Surgeon General's dream of a "smoke-free America" becoming a reality by the turn of the century seems ever more likely.

References

"EPA Says Smokers' Children at Risk." 1992. *New York Times,* June 19.

Fackelmann, K. A. 1994. "Mother's Smoking Linked to Child's IQ Drop." *Science News,* Feb. 12.

Pear, Robert. 1992. "U.S. Reports Rise in Low-Weight Births." *New York Times,* April 22.

habit. Altogether, it is estimated that smoking is responsible for fully 30% of all cancer-related deaths. In light of these realities, those who look forward to a long and healthy life would do well to consider the categorical advice offered by a former U.S. Surgeon General:

> There is no single action an individual can take to reduce the risk of cancer more effectively than to stop smoking—particularly smoking cigarettes.

Dietary Factors.   Recent scares about everything from coffee to charcoal broiled meat to peanut butter having the potential to cause cancer have prompted consumers to fear that many food additives and contaminants are potential carcinogens—a concern that is reflected in the growing popularity of so-called "natural" or "organic" foods. This topic will be discussed at greater length in the chapter on Food Quality. Suffice it to say here that although some food additives—particularly the coal tar dyes used for artificial coloring and sodium nitrite in hot dogs—are known to be carcinogenic in tests on laboratory animals, no solid evidence yet exists to indicate that human cancer rates are rising because of these substances in food. However, bearing in mind the long latency period of many forms of cancer and the fact that many additives have been widely used for only a few decades, it may yet be too early to state categorically that such chemicals won't cause future problems.

Ironically, while many people worry, perhaps unjustifiably, about synthetic food additives, they pay little attention to findings regarding naturally occurring carcinogens in food. Substances called **aflatoxins**, potent carcinogens produced by the fungus *Aspergillus flavus*, are known to cause liver cancer in animals and are suspected of being responsible for the high rates of human liver cancer observed in parts of Africa and Southeast Asia (although lung cancer accounts for the majority of cancer deaths in the United States, liver cancer is the leading cancer killer in the world as a whole). The toxin-producing mold grows on peanuts, pistachios,

BOX 6-8

The Benefits of Broccoli

Broccoli—along with its cruciferous cousins cauliflower, cabbage, kale, and brussels sprouts—may prove to be a potent weapon in the ongoing war against cancer. Lurking in the cells of these humble, though tasty, vegetables is **sulforaphane**, a chemical compound recently isolated by scientists who call it the most powerful anticarcinogen yet discovered. Though still imperfectly understood, sulforaphane, which belongs to a group of chemicals known as isothiocyanates, appears to stimulate the body's production of certain enzymes (i.e. "phase 2 enzymes") which detoxify cancer-causing agents and help flush them out of the system. Rats that were injected with sulforaphane and subsequently given a shot of dimethyl benzanthracene (DMBA), a known carcinogen, developed strikingly fewer malignant tumors than did rats exposed solely to DMBA, demonstrating the ability of sulforaphane to block carcinogenesis.

Such results buttress observations that people whose diets include generous amounts of broccoli and other cruciferous vegetables experience significantly lower rates of cancer incidence than people who avoid such foods. Fortunately, sulforaphane is not degraded by cooking, so diners who don't particularly care for crudites can pop their broccoli or cauliflower into the microwave, steam it, or bake it in a casserole—its anticancer attributes remain unaltered. While broccoli, the consumption of which has risen by 800% in the United States over the past two decades, constitutes perhaps the most notable example of a "must eat" food for those serious about avoiding cancer, it is by no means the only dietary anti-carcinogen. Numerous fruits and vegetables contain a treasure-trove of chemicals which fight cancer in a variety of different ways (for confirmed carnivores, the news is not so cheerful—a meat-heavy diet is associated with increased incidence of several different types of malignancies). Among plant constituents which have been shown to inhibit cancerous growth are the following:

- *Antioxidants* such as beta carotene and Vitamins C and E have been acclaimed for years due to their ability to disable "free radicals"—unstable oxidizing chemicals which form within the body during normal metabolic processes or enter the body from outside. Because they are highly reactive, free radicals can damage protective cell membranes, providing environmental toxins access to sensitive tissue; conversely, free radicals may cause mutations in DNA, leading to cancerous growth. Foods rich in the antioxidants beta carotene and Vitamin C include a wide variety of yellow and green vegetables, as well as citrus fruits, apricots, and cantaloupe. Vitamin E, another powerful antioxidant, is found in oatmeal, brown rice, wheat germ, peanuts, and nuts.

- *Genistein*, associated primarily with diets rich in soybean products (e.g. *miso* soup) or, to a lesser extent, cabbage-family vegetables (another benefit of broccoli!), this plant chemical inhibits cancerous growth by blocking the growth of new blood vessels into tumors, a process called **angiogenesis**. Since malignant tumors must receive a blood-borne supply of oxygen and nutrients to continue growing and to metastasize, the capillary growth inhibitor genistein keeps tumors too small to pose any real danger.

• *Allylic sulfides* are believed to protect against carcinogens by boosting production of a detoxification enzyme. Allium compounds are readily obtained by eating a generous amount of onions and garlic (also considered good preventatives for cardiovascular disease and a host of other ills).

• *Ellagic acid*, found in grapes, nuts, and a number of other fruits and vegetables, inhibits the initiation of carcinogenesis by aflatoxin by binding itself with DNA, thereby preventing aflatoxin from forming a DNA-carcinogen adduct.

• *Curcumin*, a constituent of turmeric, the spice which gives Indian curries their distinctive color, has antimutagenic properties.

These natural anticarcinogenic compounds represent but a small fraction of the disease-fighting chemicals present in fruits and vegetables; scientists admit that they know less than 10% of the substances existing in plant tissues. While it would be consoling for veggie-haters to believe that identification of certain active agents such as sulforaphane could lead to development of dietary supplements in tablet form (an "anticancer pill"), most nutritionists caution against such an approach. Current evidence suggests that interactions among the multitude of chemicals present in plant cells confer benefits that a single nutrient is incapable of matching. As evidence, researchers point to a study of lifelong smokers conducted in Finland, where daily supplements of Vitamin E, beta carotene, or a combination of the two taken over a six-year period conferred no apparent protection against lung cancer—a disease against which antioxidants are thought to be a deterrent (earlier epidemiologic studies in both the United States and Switzerland demonstrated that men who ate few foods containing beta carotene and Vitamin C were more likely to die of lung cancer than those whose diets included generous amounts of such foods). While the design of the study could be criticized on several grounds, researchers conclude that one of the most important lessons it offers is that a nutritious, vegetable-rich diet is a far better defense than pills against chronic disease.

So, meat-eaters of the world, shed your aversion to green and heap your plates with broccoli! Pass by the barbecue pit in favor of the salad bar— a dietary transformation could have a profound impact on the cancer rates of tomorrow.

References

Angier, Natalie. 1994. "Benefits of Broccoli Confirmed as Chemical Blocks Tumor Growth." *New York Times,* April 12.

Davis, Devra Lee. 1990. "Natural Anticarcinogens: Can Diet Protect Against Cancer?" *Health & Environment Digest* 4, no. 1, (Feb.).

corn, rice, and certain other grains and nuts when temperatures and humidity are high. If large quantities of aflatoxin are present in the food, liver damage and death may occur very quickly; in small amounts, consumed over a period of time, aflatoxins are among the strongest carcinogens known. Other natural carcinogens in food include safrole, an extract of sassafras long used to flavor root-beer until banned by the FDA in 1960, and oil of calamus, used until 1968 to flavor vermouth.

Perhaps most important of all in reference to food and cancer is the conviction among many researchers that there is a direct correlation between high fat intake and rates of colon and prostate cancer, as well as a relationship between stomach cancer and consumption of smoked, salt-pickled, and salt-cured foods. In addition, being excessively overweight seems to favor development of cancer of the endometrium in women (Willett, 1994; National Research Council, 1982). Consumption of high-fiber foods rather than the refined flours and heavily processed foods so common in the American diet has also been suggested as a way of reducing the risk of colon and rectal cancer, presumably because a high fiber content hastens passage of waste materials through the intestines, allowing less time for carcinogens to form and act on the intestinal surfaces (Oppenheimer, 1982). These findings reinforce the recommendations given by many doctors to heart patients concerning the unhealthfulness of high-fat, low fiber diets and suggest that a dietary regimen aimed at preventing coronary disease should be beneficial in reducing cancer risk as well.

Air Pollution.   It is well known that urban air contains a number of carcinogenic substances, benzo(a)pyrene included. It has not been possible, however, to prove conclusively that breathing polluted air, by itself, induces cancer. The fact that many cancer victims living in polluted areas are also smokers makes it difficult to say which factor was the decisive one, and the fact that even nonsmokers are simultaneously exposed to a variety of potentially carcinogenic substances further clouds the picture. Although the "gut feeling" of many researchers is that air pollution is probably, at the least, a contributing factor to the development of some cancers, the impossibility of carrying out a controlled scientifically valid experiment on humans makes obtaining conclusive evidence unlikely. Nevertheless, it is an observed fact that people living in cities larger than 50,000 in population run a 33% higher risk of developing lung cancer than do people living in small towns or rural areas. The reasons behind this phenomenon, referred to as the "Urban Factor," have never been conclusively determined.

Occupational Exposure.   Since the days of Sir Percival Potts' observations on scrotal cancer among chimney sweeps, it has been recognized that certain occupations entail heightened risk of specific diseases. In recent decades the proliferation of new synthetic chemicals in industry, as well as the continued use of older substances only recently recognized as hazardous, has been reflected in cancer rates far higher among certain segments of the work force than among the general public. Estimates of the number of American workers potentially exposed to chemicals considered by the National Institute of Occupational Safety and Health (NIOSH) to be proven or likely carcinogens range from three to nine million; many others work with materials suspected to be carcinogens but on which the necessary testing has not yet been done. Although there has been considerable difference of opinion between industry and labor regarding the health impact of exposure to carcinogens in the workplace, researchers estimate that occupational exposure accounts for 4–38% of U.S. cancer incidence (Chivian et al., 1993). Until passage of the Toxic Substances Control Act in 1976, giving the federal government the power to require testing of potentially hazardous substances before they go on the market, hundreds of new chemicals with unknown side effects came into industrial use each year. Unfortunately, the carcinogenicity of many substances was recognized only after exposed workers, like human "guinea pigs," fell sick or died. Some of the most significant industrial carcinogens thus discovered include:

- **asbestos**, one of the best known occupational hazards which is expected to cause the death of 30–40% of all asbestos workers
- **vinyl chloride**, a basic ingredient in the manufacture of plastics, found in 1974 to induce a rare form of liver cancer among exposed workers
- **anesthetic gases** used in operating rooms have been identified as the reason nurse anesthetists develop leukemia and lymphoma at three times the normal rate—and also experience higher rates of miscarriage and birth defects among their children
- **benzene**, long known to be a powerful bone marrow poison, capable of causing aplastic anemia, has now been shown to cause leukemia as well
- **coke oven emissions** have been linked with cancers of the lung, trachea, bronchus, and kidneys and are now regulated as hazardous air pollutants when vented to the outdoor air
- **benzidine**, **naphythylamine**, and several other chemicals associated with rubber and dye manufacturing pose an excess risk of bladder cancer to exposed workers in those industries
- **hardwood dust** inhaled by cabinet and furniture makers can lead to malignant nasal tumors
- **radioactive mine dusts** have been a particular problem in uranium mines, resulting in lung cancer rates among miners four times higher than the national average

Although pressure from labor unions and adoption of protective government legislation have resulted in some improvements in reducing occupational hazards, standards set for protecting workers are far less stringent than those set for protecting society at large. In addition, until a few years ago workers often lacked basic information about the nature of the materials with which they worked and were thus unable to take precautionary action even if they desired to do so. A major step forward in this regard was promulgation by the Occupational Safety and Health Administration (OSHA) in 1983 of its Hazard Communication Standard, intended to provide employees in manufacturing industries access to information concerning the hazards of chemicals which they encounter in the workplace. Essentially a federal "Employee Right-to-Know" law, this ruling requires that manufacturers inform their employees of any workplace hazards and how they can minimize risk of harm. Manufacturers must also ensure that all chemicals are properly labeled and that Material

Safety Data Sheets for each chemical are available for any employee who requests them.

Reproductive/Sexual Behavior. The National Cancer Institute estimates that 7% of all cancer deaths can be linked with reproductive factors or sexual practices. For reasons thought to relate to hormone levels, breast cancer incidence is significantly higher among women who experienced early onset of menstruation, childless women or women who first gave birth at a late age, and women who were older than average at the time of menopause. Conversely, research suggests that mothers who breast-feed, especially *teenage mothers* who nurse their babies for at least six months, cut their risk of developing breast cancer before menopause nearly in half. For women in their 20s and 30s, prolonged breast-feeding reduces cancer risk by approximately 22%. Although such risk factors are largely beyond the control of the women involved, those who fall into one or more of these categories should be especially conscientious about having regular mammograms once they reach age 40.

Risk factors for cervical cancer are more subject to self-control: early age at the time of first intercourse and multiple sex partners predispose a woman to subsequent development of this type of cancer. Chances of contracting uterine cancer are enhanced by early onset of menstruation, late menopause, a failure to ovulate, a history of infertility, or by excessive obesity. Estrogen replacement therapy, sometimes given to women to control symptoms experienced during menopause, may also increase the risk of uterine cancer (American Cancer Society, 1994).

Preventing Cancer

The preceding discussion should make it apparent that while we still have much to learn about the nature of carcinogenesis, we have already discovered enough to suggest a variety of personal actions which individuals can take to reduce substantially their own risk of developing cancer. Cancer biologist S. B. Oppenheimer (1983) lists the following guidelines, based on current medical research, which if generally followed could result in a significant reduction in cancer rates through prevention of this dreaded, but certainly not inevitable, disease:

1. stop smoking
2. avoid excessive exposure to sun
3. avoid exposure to known carcinogens
4. avoid heavy alcohol consumption
5. reduce consumption of fats and increase consumption of high-fiber foods
6. reduce consumption of salt-cured, salt-pickled, smoked, and charred foods
7. maintain life-style that prevents obesity
8. avoid unnecessary exposure to radiation
9. eat foods rich in vitamins A, C, and E
10. avoid or try to limit psychosocial stress ■

References

American Cancer Society. *Cancer Facts and Figures—1994.*

Blakeslee, Sandra. 1994. "Genes Tell Story of Why Some Get Cancer While Others Don't." *New York Times*, May 17.

Bronner, Eric C., et al. 1994. "Mutation in the DNA Mismatch Repair Gene Homologue hMLH1 Is Associated with Hereditary Non-polyposis Colon Cancer." *Nature* 368 (March 17).

Brown, Lester R., Hal Kane, and Ed Ayres. 1993. *Vital Signs 1993*, Worldwatch Institute, W. W. Norton.

Chivian, Eric, M.D., et al., eds. 1993. *Critical Condition: Human Health and the Environment*. Physicians for Social Responsibility. The M.I.T. Press.

Culotta, E., and D. E. Koshland, Jr. 1993. "p53 Sweeps through Cancer Research." *Science* 262 (Dec. 24).

Davis, Devra Lee, and David G. Hoel. 1992. "International Trends in Cancer Mortality." *Health & Environment Digest* 6, no. 2 (May).

Fishel, Richard, et al. 1993. "The Human Mutator Gene Homolog MSH2 and Its Association with Hereditary Nonpolyposis Colon Cancer." *Cell* 75 (Dec. 3).

Glasser, Ronald J. 1976. *The Greatest Battle*. Random House.

Harris, C. C. 1993. "At the Crossroads of Molecular Carcinogenesis and Risk Assessment." *Science* 262 (Dec. 24).

Harris, John A., M.D., and Jackie W. Wynne. 1994. "Birth Defects Clusters: Evaluating Community Reports." *Health & Environment Digest* 7 (Feb.).

Isaacson, Peter G., D.M. 1994. "Gastric Lymphoma and Helicobacter Pylori." *New England Journal of Medicine* 330, no. 18 (May 5).

Leach, F. S., et al. 1993. "Mutations of a mutS Homolog in Hereditary Nonpolyposis Colorectal Cancer." *Cell* 75, no. 6 (Dec. 17).

Markoff, John. 1992. "Danger of Miscarriage Found for Chip Workers." *New York Times*, Dec. 4

National Research Council, National Academy of Sciences. 1982. *Report on Diet, Nutrition, and Cancer.*

Norwood, Christopher. 1980. *At Highest Risk*. Penguin Books.

Oppenheimer, S. B. 1983. "Prevention of Cancer." *American Laboratory* (Feb.).

Oppenheimer, S. B. 1982. *Cancer: A Biological and Clinical Introduction*. Allyn Bacon.

Papadopoulos, Nickolas, Nicholas C. Nicolaides, et al. 1994. "Mutation of a mutL Homolog in Hereditary Colon Cancer." *Science* 263 (March 18).

Parsonnet, Julie, M.D., et al. 1994. "Helicobacter Pylori Infection and Gastric Lymphoma." *New England Journal of Medicine* 330, no. 18 (May 5).

Schemo, Diana Jean. 1994. "Chemical Plants Seen as a Factor in Breast Cancer." *New York Times*, April 13.

"Solvents Used in Making Computer Chips Linked to Workers' Miscarriages at IBM." 1992. *Environmental Health Letter*, Sept. 16.

Squires, Sally. 1990. "The Importance of Pap Tests." *Washington Post*, July 24.

Stone, Richard. 1992. "Can a Father's Exposure Lead to Illness in his Children?," *Science* 258 (Oct. 2).

"Studies Yield Conflicting Findings on Environment's Link to Cancer." 1994. *Environmental Health Letter*, April 27.

Volpe, E. Peter. 1975. *Man, Nature, and Society*. Wm. C. Brown.

Warkany, J. 1972. "Trends in Teratologic Research." *Pathobiology of Development*, edited by E. Perrin and M. Finegold. Williams and Wilkins.

Willett, Walter C. 1994. "Diet and Health: What Should We Eat." *Science* 264 (April 22).

CHAPTER 7

Toxic Substances

Being born a human being, but not being able to live as a human being, is the most painful thing to me.
—Tsuginori Hamamoto, Minamata Disease victim

Human illness or death due to contact with toxic materials in the environment is certainly not unique to the modern age. Hippocrates described the symptoms of lead poisoning as early as 370 B.C.; mercury fumes in Roman mines in Spain made work there the equivalent of a death sentence to the unfortunate slaves receiving such an assignment; for centuries Turkish peasants living in homes built of asbestos-containing volcanic rock have been dying of lung disease. Yet for the most part, such examples of illness caused by direct contact with toxic substances have been confined to certain occupational groups or to people who, by chance, happened to be living in an area where there was an unnaturally high concentration of some toxic material. By and large, in the past large populations seldom, if ever, were exposed to significant amounts of poisonous substances on a sustained basis. Today, however, that situation is changing, thanks in part to the tremendous increase in industrial production during the present century, as well as to the "chemical revolution" that has witnessed the introduction of thousands of new synthetic compounds into widespread use in recent decades. Some of these substances, several of which were briefly mentioned in the preceding chapter, are largely confined to an occupational setting and pose little threat to the general public, although of course they are a major concern to workers and their families. Others, however, are now virtually omnipresent throughout the human environment and are generating considerable controversy as to the degree of public health threat they present. In this chapter we will take a closer look at several of these substances—some naturally occurring, others artificially produced—to which human exposure is nearly universal and which are known to cause serious health damage.

Polychlorinated Biphenyls (PCBs)

In 1964 Dr. Soren Jensen, a Swedish chemist at the University of Stockholm began a project to determine DDT levels in human fat and wildlife samples; instead he discovered that the tissues he was examining contained large amounts of synthetic organic chemicals called PCBs. His findings, published in 1966, were greeted with widespread surprise and disbelief because PCBs, unlike DDT and other chlorinated hydrocarbon pesticides, were not being deliberately released into the environment but were restricted to use in an industrial setting. Despite the initial skepticism, subsequent studies by researchers in many countries confirmed Dr. Jensen's findings. Virtually every tissue sample tested, from fish to birds to polar bears to animals living in deep sea trenches, contained detectable levels of PCBs. Humans also were shown to have accumulated large amounts of the chemical. The U.S. Environmental Protection Agency calculated that 91% of all Americans have detectable levels of PCBs in their fatty tissues, and human breast milk contains significant amounts—the average level being seven times higher than the amount legally permissible in cow's milk! (Environmental Defense Fund, 1979). As the evidence continued to mount, it became generally accepted that PCBs, whose toxic properties were already well documented, are the most widespread chemical contaminant known.

How Could This Situation Come About?

Polychlorinated biphenyls were first synthesized in 1929, their production being taken over in 1930 by Monsanto, which sold the chemical under the trade name Arochlor. PCBs, which range in consistency from oily liquids to waxy solids, are extremely stable substances with a high boiling point, high solubility in fat but low solubility in water, low electrical conductivity, and high resistance to heat—all qualities which made them valuable for a wide variety of industrial uses. Primarily employed as cooling liquids in electrical transformers and capacitors, PCBs have also been used in hydraulic fluids, in carbonless carbon paper, insulating tapes, adhesives, paints, caulking compounds, sealants, and as road coverings to control dust.

The chemical stability that made PCBs so attractive to industry, however, is the very characteristic that has made them such an environmental and health hazard. Although designed for industrial use, there are many ways in which PCBs can inadvertently escape and contaminate the environment: 1) discharge of PCB-laden wastes from factories into waterways have resulted in mammoth pollution problems, the most notorious episodes being Outboard Marine Corporation's dumping of PCBs into Waukegan Harbor (on Lake Michigan), which currently holds the dubious distinction of containing the highest PCB concentrations documented in the United States, and a similar situation in the Hudson River, traced to two General Electric plants; 2) vaporization from paints or landfills or burning of PCB-containing material can result in the chemical becoming airborne and then reentering the ecosystem with precipitation. It's estimated that 11,000 pounds of PCBs enter Lake Michigan with rain and snow each year (Great Lakes Basin Commission, 1980). A classic example of fire causing extensive PCB contamination occurred early in 1981 in Binghamton, New York, where PCB-containing electrical equipment in the basement of the newly built 17-floor State Office Building caught fire. Although the blaze was quickly extinguished, inspectors subsequently discovered that contaminated soot had been carried through the air conditioning system and deposited throughout the entire building. Air sampling indicated that this soot contained 10–20% PCBs, as well as lesser amounts of dioxin and dibenzofurans formed during the combustion process. The ensuing cleanup operation took seven years to complete and cost New York taxpayers $37 million (Fawcett, 1988); 3) leaks in industrial equipment have resulted in numerous instances of PCB contamination, such as the case during the summer of 1979 when 200 gallons of PCBs

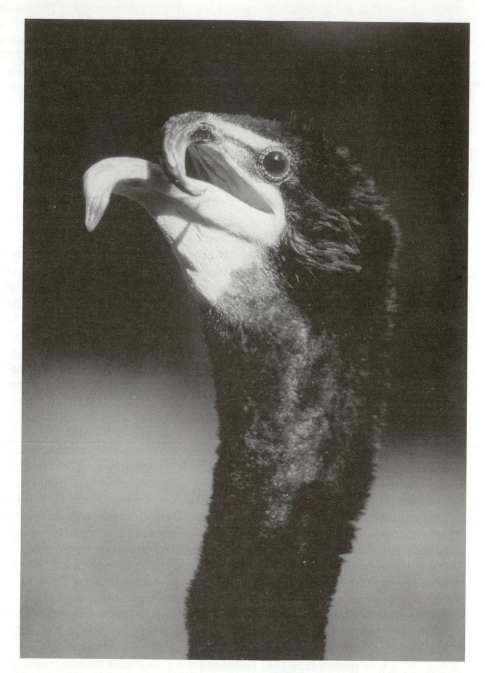

This double-crested cormorant, with its twisted and deformed beak, is a glaring example of the toxic effects of PCBs. [Thomas A. Schneider]

leaked from an electrical transformer at a feed processing plant in Billings, Montana, contaminating about a million pounds of meal used in chicken feed. Subsequently, $2.7 million worth of chickens and eggs had to be destroyed because the birds had eaten the contaminated meal before the leak was discovered (Regenstein, 1982); 4) accidental spills or illegal dumping are a source of increasing concern because the high cost of legally disposing of PCB wastes has tempted some haulers to dump such materials along roadsides, in ditches, or other out-of-the-way places. In August of 1978 such "midnight dumpers" opened the discharge pipe of their truck while driving along 210 miles of back roads in North Carolina, releasing 31,000 gallons of PCB-laden waste oil along the roadside where most of it remains to this day.

Whatever the route, once PCBs enter the environment they persist there for decades, resisting breakdown. Contamination of living organisms with PCBs generally occurs via the food chain, the concentration of the chemical increasing as it moves from lower to higher trophic levels ("bio-magnification"—see chapter 8). Within an individual organism, especially among higher-level consumers such as carnivorous birds, fish, and humans, PCBs accumulate in fatty tissues such as liver, kidneys, heart, lungs, brain, and breast milk, and increase over a period of time, a process known as **bioaccumulation**. Though ingestion of PCBs with food is the primary route of human exposure to these chemicals, PCBs can also be inhaled or absorbed through the skin.

PCB Threat to Health

Widespread human exposure to PCBs has concerned health and regulatory officials because laboratory testing has shown the chemicals to be toxic to several animal species even at very low concentrations. In experiments with rodents, minks, and Rhesus monkeys, PCB exposure has resulted in the development of a number of adverse health effects: liver disorders, miscarriage, low birthweight, abnormal multiplication of cells, and (in rats only) liver cancer. Researchers presumed that chemicals which could produce such effects in some mammalian species were likely to have similar effects on humans, and the knowledge that virtually everyone on the planet has been exposed to at least trace amounts of PCBs was considered cause for alarm. Evidence that many foods, especially freshwater fish, were contaminated with PCBs prompted the U.S. government to take regulatory action. In 1973 the FDA established tolerance levels for PCBs in food; passage of the Toxic Substances Control Act in 1976 specifically banned the production, sale, distribution, and use of PCBs in open systems; and in 1977, Monsanto, the sole U.S. manufacturer of the chemicals, terminated PCB production.

In the meantime, research on the human health impact of PCBs continued. Evidence documenting adverse health effects among workers occupationally exposed to the chemicals began accumulating in the early 1930s, soon after production of PCBs began. The most frequent complaint among these individuals was the appearance of an acne-like skin disorder now referred to as "chloracne" and regarded as the most characteristic symptom of PCB poisoning (or poisoning with any of the related group of chemicals known as chlorinated hydrocarbons). Some workers complained of a burning sensation in their eyes, nose, and throat; others experienced

Box 7-1
Good News for Lake Michigan Fisheries

The presence of PCBs in Lake Michigan would have generated little public attention were it not for the fact that these toxins bioaccumulate in fish and can be passed along the food chain to humans, becoming increasingly concentrated as they move from one trophic level to the next. High PCB readings in Great Lakes fish have dealt a serious blow to the commercial fisheries of the area, particularly to the Green Bay region of Lake Michigan, where the alewife fishery has been virtually wiped out. The FDA has set 2 ppm as the maximum allowable level of PCBs in fish sold for human consumption. While the catch of sports fishermen cannot be regulated, they too are warned by state and federal agencies to avoid frequent consumption of fish species known to exhibit high PCB concentrations. Since PCBs are stored in fatty tissues and increase in concentration as the fish ages, fish with the highest PCB levels tend to be the larger individuals among such fatty species as lake trout, brown and steelhead trout, Chinook and coho salmon, chubs, and carp. By contrast, lean fish species such as perch, sunfish, pike, bluegills, bass, and brook trout seldom contain dangerous levels of toxins.

Health advisories issued by Illinois and Michigan regarding fish from Lake Michigan recommend that pregnant and nursing mothers, as well as small children, avoid eating lake trout and other fatty fish such as those mentioned above. They also advise everyone to restrict consumption of such species to less than 1/2 pound per week.

Certain methods of preparing Great Lakes fish can help limit PCB consumption for those who can't resist a tempting lake trout or salmon. As much fat as possible should be removed during the cleaning and filleting process; significant amounts of PCB are eliminated by cutting off the fatty belly flap and the dorsal back flap. Rather than frying the fish, cooks are encouraged to bake, broil, or grill the fish to allow additional fat to drip off during cooking.

Fortunately, after more than a decade and a half of declining PCB use, studies show that PCB levels in Great Lakes fish have been steadily falling. A recent health assessment performed on people who reported frequent consumption of Lake Michigan fish (following the preparation recommendations mentioned above), indicated no significant health problems when compared with a control group of non-fisheaters. Assuming PCB levels continue to decline, certain Great Lakes fisheries may become economically viable once again—good news for fishermen and consumers alike!

Reference

Hovinga, Mary. 1993. "Environmental Exposure to Lead, Cadmium, PCBs, and DDt—Blood Levels, Lifestyle Predictors, and Health," *Health and Environment Electronic Seminars*, presented by the Association of State and Territorial Health Officials and the Association of State and Territorial Health Risk Assessors, Oct. 7.

liver ailments. Additional problems reported during the early years of PCB use included a range of vague symptoms such as general tiredness, loss of appetite, diminished sex drive—all now recognized as classic signs of PCB intoxication.

All of these cases, however, involved acute health effects resulting from relatively high levels of workplace exposure and left unanswered the question of whether the public at large need fear chronic health damage (liver cancer being a major worry) due to long-term, low-level PCB exposure in food, air, and water. A large outbreak of what was thought at the time to be PCB poisoning occurred in Japan in 1968 when 1300 Japanese developed chloracne, swelling and pain in the joints, eye discharges, weakness, headaches, and a host of other acute symptoms after consuming rice oil that had been contaminated when a PCB-containing heat exchanger fluid leaked from a pipe into the vat of oil during processing. Referred to as "Yusho (rice oil) disease," this incident provoked alarm around the world as an example of how easily food supplies can inadvertently be contaminated with toxic chemicals. In 1978–79 a similar accident occurred in Taiwan, where it was dubbed "Yu-cheng disease." While most of the adverse health effects reported by victims of these two episodes were short-term (i.e. acute effects), consumption of the contaminated cooking oil by pregnant women resulted in some babies being born with dark skin discoloration and low birthweight; in other cases, infants were born with erupted teeth and follow-up studies in later years showed that among these children, dentition of the permanent teeth was affected. For years following the Yusho incident, close medical monitoring of the affected population was carried out in hopes of gaining information on chronic health effects of PCB exposure. Eventually, however, it was concluded that the troubles experienced by both Japanese and Taiwanese victims of contaminated rice oil were not due to PCBs at all, but rather to a related, more toxic group of chemicals called dibenzofurans which were also present in the heat exchanger fluid. As a result, investigators are left without a single convincing case of chronic human health damage caused by low-level environmental PCB exposure. In fact, even among those occupationally exposed to the chemical, there is no convincing evidence that PCBs cause cancer—or any other chronic health problems—in humans.

Although PCB production in the United States halted in 1977, the chemicals remain very much a part of the American scene. During the years 1929–1977, 1.4 billion pounds of PCBs were produced in the United States. Hundreds of millions of pounds are still in use in closed systems, especially by the utility industry as coolants in high voltage capacitors (common on ordinary utility poles) and in electrical transformers. In addition, approximately 500 million pounds of PCBs have been dumped into landfills and waterways where they continue to pose an environmental threat. As existing PCB-containing equipment becomes obsolete and is replaced, safe methods for disposing of this material must be found. While several promising new technologies for treating PCB-contaminated soils have been developed recently and are undergoing feasibility testing, high-temperature (2200°F or above) incineration is the EPA-approved method at present for destroying wastes containing high concentrations of PCBs.

Dioxin (TCDD)

In the wet spring of 1983 public apprehension about the dangers of dioxin soared when the U.S. Environmental Protection Agency announced that inhabitants of the tiny riverside community of Times Beach, Missouri, should abandon their homes and evacuate the town. Soil analyses had revealed high levels of dioxin contamination due to oiling of roads for dust control in the early 1970s; the oil had been scavenged from a trichlorophenol factory by a waste hauler and was heavily laced with the toxic chemical.

Times Beach is but one of numerous places around the world where industrial accidents, deliberate dumping, or inadvertent use of dioxin-tainted pesticides have resulted in environmental contamination which has provoked alarm, sometimes panic, among local residents. Public concerns, in turn, have been generated by debatable statements by some researchers that "dioxin is the most toxic substance ever created by humans," and by allegations of a wide range of health problems and genetic disorders among American servicemen exposed to dioxin during their tour of duty in Vietnam. Widespread fears that serious human health damage can be caused by infinitesimally small amounts of the chemical have led to such controversial regulatory actions as the evacuation of Times Beach and the suspension of the selective herbicides 2, 4, 5-T and silvex, yet the results of numerous follow-up studies on exposed populations fail to show a single case where human death has resulted from dioxin exposure. What are the facts about this chemical whose very name seems to generate hysteria?

Chemically related to PCBs and other chlorinated hydrocarbons, dioxins form a large group of chemicals of widely varying levels of toxicity. The most dangerous dioxin is 2, 3, 7, 8-tetrachlorodibenzo-p-dioxin, generally referred to as TCDD or, simply, "dioxin." TCDD, unlike its chemical cousin PCB, has no industrial usefulness and has never been intentionally manufactured; it is formed as an unwanted by-product in the production of certain herbicides and the germ-killer hexachlorophene. Dioxin can escape into the atmosphere when it evaporates from TCDD-contaminated soil and water or when dioxin- or PCB-containing materials are burned (EPA researchers say that hospital incinerators currently constitute the leading source of dioxin emissions in the United States, thanks to the large amounts of plastics being burned at temperatures between 1400° and 1600°F—hot enough to kill pathogens but not sufficiently high to destroy dioxins). Airborne dioxins can be carried long distances before they eventually are rained out or settle as dry deposits on soil, plant surfaces, or bodies of water. There they bind tightly to soil particles or sediment at the bottom of lakes and streams. Although TCDD undergoes rapid photolysis, if protected from light exposure dioxin breaks down very slowly—experimental evidence suggests that its half-life in soil may exceed 10 years. TCDD in minute quantities is now very widespread throughout the environment, present in soil, dust, chimneys of wood-burning stoves and furnaces, eggs, fish tissues, and animal fat. Most humans have accumulated small amounts of dioxin in their fatty tissues largely through consumption of meat, fish, and dairy products, with only 1% or less of the total body burden coming from such sources of exposure as contaminated air or water.

Statements asserting that dioxin is the "most toxic of all synthetic chemicals" are somewhat misleading because they are based on the observation that extremely low doses of TCDD are fatal to guinea pigs, by far the most sensitive species to the chemical's lethal effects. Hamsters, by contrast, can tolerate doses of dioxin up to 1900 times the amount that would kill a guinea pig. For other test species, dioxin's lethality ranges somewhere between the extremes represented by guinea pigs and hamsters. However, dioxin is capable of producing many adverse effects other than death, and while any given species may exhibit a biological response at the far end of the range for a particular TCDD-induced problem, most species, humans included, respond similarly for most effects. For example, dioxin produces chloracne in rabbits, monkeys, mice, and humans at roughly equivalent levels of exposure. Interference with immune system function, fetal toxicity, and cancer are other adverse effects of dioxin exposure to which humans, rats, guinea pigs, and hamsters exhibit similar sensitivity. On the other hand, some of TCDD's effects are strikingly species-specific. Teratogenic effects of dioxin are apparent only in mice, which develop cleft palates at doses below the lethal level. Similarly, while dioxin acts as a liver toxin in a number of species, no signs of liver damage have yet been observed in highly exposed humans. By contrast, TCDD is carcinogenic in most species, producing malignant tumors at multiple sites—but only at high levels of exposure. Perhaps most significant among dioxin's long-term effects revealed by animal tests (presumed valid for humans as well) is the chemical's ability to disrupt the hormonal systems that control reproduction. Evidence from both wildlife and laboratory studies shows that exposure to dioxin (and to chlorinated organic chemicals in general) may result in reduced fertility, fetal loss, changes in sexual behavior, thyroid dysfunction, and suppression of the immune system. Indeed, some scientists conclude that these effects are far more significant than the carcinogenicity concerns that have been the focus of most toxicological research in relation to dioxin (Birnbaum, 1994; Dickson and Buzik, 1993; Schneider, 1992; Luoma, 1992).

The implications of all this so far as human exposure is concerned remains somewhat problematic. Over the years thousands of people, particularly chemical industry workers, have had extensive exposure to the chemical at relatively high levels (e.g. a 1949 incident in a Monsanto plant in Nitro, WV, exposed more than 200 workers to dioxin; more spectacularly, a 1976 explosion at a trichlorophenol factory near Milan, Italy, released a toxic cloud that settled on the nearby suburb of Seveso, exposing 37,000 people of all ages to considerable amounts of dioxin). It is estimated that additional millions have been exposed to low concentrations (e.g. the farmers and ranchers using dioxin-contaminated herbicides, military personnel exposed to Agent Orange, residents of Times Beach and other communities where dioxin-laced waste oils were sprayed on dirt roads, consumers of TCDD-tainted fish, etc.). With the exception of the chemical industry workers whose dioxin exposure was 500 times greater than that experienced by the general public, the only confirmed human health problems associated with TCDD have been acute symptoms such as chloracne, muscle aches and pains, nervous system disorders, digestive upsets, and some psychiatric effects. However, a statistically significant increase in deaths due to soft tissue sarcoma (a type of cancer) and respiratory cancer has been confirmed among a group of men who were highly exposed while working for more than 20 years in chemical manufacturing plants. Among this group, workers who had been exposed to dioxin for the longest period of time had TCDD blood levels of 3600 ppt. By comparison, for adults living in the industrialized world, the average blood level of dioxin is 6 ppt, while members of the U.S. military who handled dioxin-contaminated Agent Orange exhibited peak levels around 400 ppt. In 1993, publication of a study carried out by a team of Italian researchers reviewing the medical records of thousands of Seveso residents documented an increase in soft tissue sarcomas, cancer of the gall bladder, and multiple myelomas among citizens exposed to the highest levels of dioxin ever recorded among civilian populations. However, the overall cancer rate for the region was lower than expected. Another study of U.S. chemical industry workers whose exposure to TCDD averaged less than one year revealed average blood concentrations of 640 ppt—a level 90 times higher that the national norm—yet the cancer death rate among these men 20 years after exposure was scarcely distinguishable from that of the general public. Such findings have led most researchers to the conclusion that while dioxin *does* cause cancer in humans at very high levels of exposure, it poses a minimal threat of malignancies at the low concentrations commonly encountered.

For those charged with protecting the public health and setting regulatory requirements regarding TCDD exposure, the dioxin issue presents some difficult decisions. Without question the chemical is acutely toxic to laboratory animals and produces serious chronic health problems in many animal species as well. However, in spite of extensive human exposure to TCDD, only a handful of transitory acute effects have been confirmed in people. It must be noted that one of the problems in determining the health effects of dioxin is the fact that TCDD virtually never occurs alone; rather, it is but one of many chemicals in a mixture which may include PCBs, dibenzofurans, chlorophenols, and other dioxins. Since the identity of these other chemicals is frequently not known or not reported, it could be risky to attribute a given observed health effect to TCDD alone. While some investigators argue that dioxin presents less of a health threat to humans than to other animal species, others are convinced that the subtle effects observed in laboratory animals are having an impact on people as well. Citing animal data regarding TCDD's adverse impact on reproduction and on immune system function as justification for continued regulatory controls, such authorities are convinced of the necessity to limit human exposure to dioxin as much as possible (Fingerhut et al., 1991; Dickson and Buzik, 1993; Tschirley, 1986).

Asbestos

Probably no other hazardous substance has resulted in so many deaths and cases of disabling disease as has asbestos, the collective term for a group of six fibrous silicate minerals (amosite, chrysotile, tremolite, actinolite, anthophyllite, and crocidolite) found almost worldwide. Utilized by humans ever since Stone Age potters employed the substance to reinforce their clay, asbestos was woven into cloth during Greek and Roman times and was regarded as having magical properties because of its invulnerability to fire.

In modern times asbestos has acquired great economic value as an essential component in thousands of commercial products and processes. By the late 1970s, over six million tons of asbestos were being produced worldwide. About two-thirds of the asbestos used in the United States is employed in building materials, brake linings, textiles, and insulation, while the remaining one-third is consumed in such diverse products as paints, plastics, caulking compounds, floor tiles, cement, roofing paper, radiator covers, filters in gas masks, conveyor belts, potholders, ironing board covers, theater curtains, fake fireplace ash, and so on.

Unfortunately, in addition to being very useful, asbestos also represents an occupational hazard of major proportions. It is now estimated that of the 8–11 million current and retired workers exposed to large amounts of asbestos on the job, 30–40% can be expected to die of cancer. Exposure

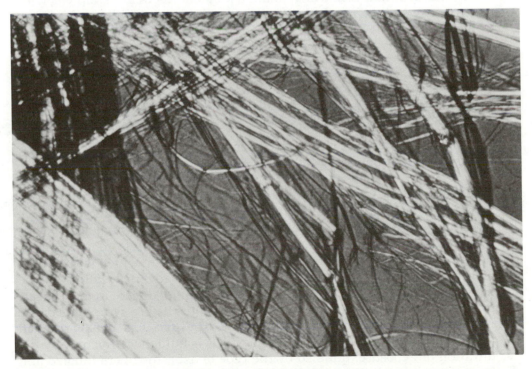

Asbestos fibers magnified to show the needle-like configuration of these hydrated silicate minerals. [Illinois Department of Public Health]

to asbestos is primarily through inhalation of tiny fibers suspended in the air. While airborne fibers may occur naturally in regions characterized by outcroppings of the mineral, they are more commonly associated with the deterioration of manufactured asbestos-containing materials or with the demolition or renovation of buildings containing asbestos. Fiber levels tend to be highest near asbestos mines or factories and are higher in cities than in rural areas, but virtually any air sample, regardless of where it is taken, will contain some asbestos fibers. Once inhaled, asbestos fibers are deposited in the air passages and cells within the lungs. Most of these are quickly carried away by the mucus that lines the respiratory tract, being transported up to the throat where they are swallowed, carried to the stomach, and eventually excreted with the feces. Some, however, remain trapped deep in the lungs and may never be removed.

Although inhalation represents the primary route by which asbestos enters the human body, people may also be exposed to the mineral in drinking water. Asbestos fibers can be released into water supplies when cement asbestos pipes corrode or when asbestos-containing wastes piled near mine sites are washed into lakes or rivers. While most municipal drinking water supplies experiencing asbestos contamination have relatively low concentrations, under one million fibers per liter, residents of cities such as San Francisco, Philadelphia, Seattle, New York, Atlanta, and Boston may be consuming water with fiber levels 10 to 100 times this amount. Asbestos that is swallowed, fortunately, presents much less of a health hazard than that which is inhaled. Most fibers are simply carried through the stomach and intestines and are excreted within a few days. A small portion, however, may lodge in the cells lining the gastrointestinal tract, while a few may move through the intestinal lining and enter the blood stream. These may either become trapped in other tissues or be excreted in the urine.

Asbestos-Related Diseases

Several different types of asbestos-related diseases are known, the most significant being the following.

Asbestosis.   A chronic disease characterized by a scarring of the lung tissue, asbestosis most commonly occurs among workers who have been exposed to very high levels of asbestos dust (once inhaled, asbestos fibers remain in lifelong contact with the lung tissue). It is an irreversible, progressively worsening disease, the first symptom of which is shortness of breath following exertion. Lung function is adversely affected, the maximum volume of air a victim can inhale being reduced. In most cases, it takes 20 years or more of exposure to asbestos before symptoms of the disease appear; unfortunately, by this time asbestosis has usually reached an advanced state. The severity of asbestosis is influenced not only by the duration of exposure, but also by the type of asbestos fibers inhaled and by the synergistic effects of cigarette smoking. Until about 40 years ago when concerns about workers' health led to regulations regarding dust

Figure 7-1 Summary of Asbestos-Containing Products

Product	Average percent asbestos	Binder	Dates used
Friction products	50	Various polymers	1910–present
Plastic products			
Floor tile and sheet	20	PVC, asphalt	1950–present
Coatings and sealants	10	Asphalt	1900–present
Rigid plastics	<50	Phenolic resin	?–present
Cement pipe and sheet	20	Portland cement	1930–present
Paper products			
Roofing felt	15	Asphalt	1910–present
Gaskets	80	Various polymers	?–present
Corrugated paper pipe wrap	80	Starches, sodium silicate	1910–present
Other paper	80	Polymers, starches, silicates	1910–present
Textile products	90	Cotton, wool	1910–present
Insulating and decorative products			
Sprayed coating	50	Portland cement, silicates, organic binders	1935–1978
Trowelled coating	70	Portland cement, silicates	1935–1978
Preformed pipe wrap	50	Magnesium carbonate, calcium silicate	1926–1975
Insulation board	30	Silcates	Unknown
Boiler insulation	10	Magnesium carbonate, calcium silcate	1890–1978
Other uses	<50	Many types	1900–present

Source: U.S. Environmental Protection Agency

levels in asbestos factories, asbestosis was the leading cause of death among asbestos workers. Since the 1940s, however, rates of severe asbestosis have been substantially lowered. Nevertheless, even today standards for permissible levels of asbestos exposure are based on those amounts deemed low enough to protect workers from asbestosis, in spite of the fact that this disease is no longer the most significant asbestos-related health threat.

Lung Cancer. With the gradual reduction in dust levels in asbestos factories, deaths due to asbestosis have been decreasing, allowing workers to live long enough to develop today's leading cause of asbestos-related mortality, lung cancer. Compared to the 4–5% of the general population who die of lung cancer, as many as 20–25% of asbestos workers now succumb to this disease. The risk is especially great when exposure to asbestos fibers is accompanied by exposure to cigarette smoke. Studies have shown that while asbestos exposure alone increases an individual's risk of lung cancer death by a factor of seven, exposure to both asbestos and cigarette smoke entails a 60 times greater risk of lung cancer than that experienced by persons who are not exposed to asbestos and don't smoke.

Mesothelioma.   This previously rare cancer of the lung or stomach lining today kills more than 5% of all asbestos workers. Like many other forms of cancer, mesothelioma is characterized by a long latency period, onset of disease symptoms occurring 25–40 years after initial exposure. Mesothelioma is of special interest to researchers because, unlike other forms of cancer, the only known causative agent for this disease is asbestos. Thus mesothelioma is considered a "marker disease" indicating asbestos exposure. Since no effective treatment exists, mesothelioma is an invariably fatal ailment, with death generally occurring within two years of diagnosis. Even very low levels of asbestos exposure can result in mesothelioma, and since asbestos is now so widespread throughout the environment, it is expected that the incidence of this disease will continue to rise for the next 20 years.

Gastrointestinal Cancer.   Cancer of the GI tract, which includes cancer of the colon, rectum, esophagus, and stomach, strikes asbestos workers with greater frequency than it does the general public, although a direct causative link is still not conclusively established. It is known that inhaled asbestos fibers can pass from the lungs to the stomach, colon, or intestines, and cell culture studies have demonstrated that the epithelial cells of the human intestine are particularly sensitive to damage by asbestos. There is also some evidence to suggest that people whose drinking water contains high concentrations of asbestos fibers may be at slightly elevated risk of gastrointestinal cancer. With the exception of esophageal cancer, the risk of gastrointestinal cancer is not enhanced by smoking.

Although research has not yet been able to establish conclusively the degree of asbestos exposure necessary to initiate cancer, evidence suggests that some individuals who were exposed to high levels of asbestos for only one day developed cancer years later as a result. For this reason the current presumption is that there is *no safe level for asbestos exposure*. In recent years some scientists have argued that the development of asbestos-related disease is dependent on the mineral type of asbestos to which an individual is exposed. Several studies have suggested that chrysotile (the asbestos mineral most widely used in the United States) is considerably less dangerous than other forms of asbestos, particularly crocidolite. However, most researchers believe that fiber *size* is a more important determinant of asbestos' cancer-causing potential than are its chemical or physical properties. Experimental data suggest that long fibers (those exceeding 1/5000 of an inch in length) are more injurious than short fibers (less than 1/10,000 of an inch).

While *any* amount of asbestos exposure entails some degree of hazard, the extent of that risk is determined by a combination of several factors, among the most important of which are:

- level and duration of exposure
- time since exposure occurred
- age at which exposure occurred
- personal history of cigarette smoking
- type and size of asbestos fibers

While asbestos workers constitute by far the largest percentage of victims, others may be affected through indirect exposure. Mesothelioma has claimed casualties among people living in the vicinity of asbestos factories and among children of asbestos workers, whose only exposure to the fibers was from their fathers' work clothes when they returned from the factory. When asbestos is brought into the home, it becomes a permanent part of the domestic environment, embedded in carpets and draperies and suspended in the air where it constitutes a 24-hour/day source of exposure not only to the less vulnerable healthy adults of the household but also to the very young, the sick, and the elderly who are the groups most susceptible to any type of environmental irritant. For this reason, asbestos workers today are cautioned to shower and change clothes at the workplace in order to avoid inadvertent contamination of their homes with asbestos fibers.

Asbestos Problems in Public Buildings

Until fairly recently, most asbestos-related health concerns were focused on the millions of American workers who had experienced significant levels of occupational exposure to the hazardous fibers. It thus came as an unwelcome surprise when the EPA warned that the general public has been receiving asbestos exposure for years simply by working or living in any of the estimated 700,000 commercial, governmental, or residential buildings which contain friable asbestos ("friable" refers to asbestos material which, when dry, can be crumbled to a powder by hand pressure). Of greatest concern was the revelation that as many as two to six million school children and 300,000 teachers in 31,000 primary and secondary schools across the nation might be inhaling asbestos fibers on a daily basis. During the years 1946–1973, asbestos-containing fireproofing materials were extensively used in constructing or renovating schools throughout the country. By 1973 increasing documentation of the health threats posed by asbestos had caused the EPA to ban all spray applications of asbestos in insulating and fireproofing materials and in 1977 new restrictions totally halted the spray application of asbestos. Such regulation had no effect, however, on existing asbestos-containing materials which, by this time, were beginning to deteriorate in many schools, releasing potentially dangerous asbestos fibers into the classroom environment. When asbestos-containing dust is swept up by janitors or disturbed by students' coming and going, it becomes resuspended and can remain in the air—at breathing level—for as long as 80 hours. The high levels of asbestos fibers measured in the indoor air of many schools have prompted concerns for elevated rates of lung cancer and mesothelioma among today's schoolchildren 20–40 years hence. The initial EPA response to this perceived threat was to issue an advisory to school districts throughout the country, informing them of the situation and requiring that they inspect their buildings for the presence of asbestos-containing materials (ACM). If friable asbestos was found, the districts were to notify parents or the PTA of that fact. The federal authorities apparently assumed that if an asbestos hazard was identified, parental concerns about their children's safety would be sufficient to ensure prompt remediation of the problem. Such did not prove to be the case, however, as financially strapped school districts, in the absence of a firm federal mandate, postponed expensive remediation projects. By 1983, 66% of the nation's school districts had not yet even inspected for asbestos or had failed to report doing so to the EPA.

Consequently, in the fall of 1986, President Reagan signed into law the far-reaching Asbestos Hazard Emergency Response Act (AHERA), requiring that all primary and secondary schools be inspected for the presence of asbestos; if such materials are found, the school district must file and carry out an asbestos abatement plan. EPA was charged with promulgating rules detailing correct inspection procedures, establishing asbestos abatement standards, certification programs for contractors, and standards for the transportation and disposal of asbestos. Although AHERA created a $50 million revolving fund to be used for grants and no-interest loans to needy school districts, the amount available represents a tiny fraction of the total cost. In spite of the maximum $5000 fine that can be imposed on school districts which violate AHERA's mandate, it is expected that many school districts simply do not have the financial resources to comply with the law. In 1989 additional legislation (the Asbestos School Hazard Abatement Reauthorization Act) was enacted to require that contractors involved in asbestos abatement projects in public or commercial buildings meet the same training and accreditation standards required for those doing asbestos work in public schools. It also directed EPA to provide information to local school districts on the advantages and disadvantages of various asbestos abatement alternatives and to promote the selection of options which would impose the least financial burden while still protecting human health and the environment.

Asbestos Abatement

When an asbestos hazard is identified, those charged with remedying the situation have several options from which to choose:

1. **encapsulation**—a technique in which exposed asbestos is heavily coated with a polymer sealant to prevent further release of fibers.
2. **enclosure**—feasible when the area affected is relatively small, this process involves building a nonpermeable barrier between the source of exposure and surrounding open areas.
3. **removal**—a labor-intensive process whereby all asbestos-containing materials are physically removed from the structure.

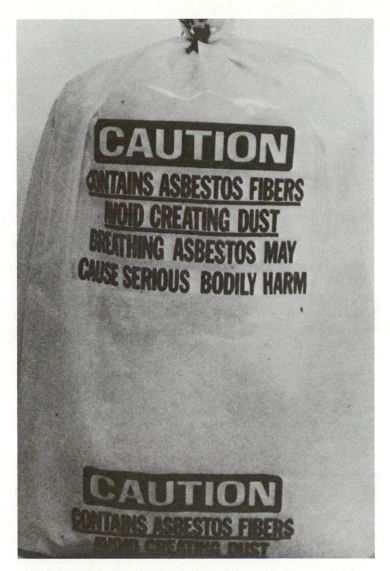

Damp asbestos-containing materials must be placed in thick plastic bags or plastic-lined containers, tagged with a warning label, and disposed of in a sanitary landfill. [U.S. Environmental Protection Agency]

Of the various abatement alternatives, complete removal is the most expensive and time consuming. It also entails the risk of worker exposure to asbestos fibers and, if carelessly done, could endanger the public as well. However, since removal absolves a building's owner of future liability and because encapsulated asbestos requires periodic reinspection, removal may, in the long run, be cheaper than encapsulation. In addition, federal laws require that any buildings that are going to be demolished or renovated, other than private homes or apartments with four or less dwelling units, must have all asbestos-containing materials removed before work can commence. Essentially this means that if a school district chose encapsulation as its asbestos abatement option and subsequently decided to tear down or substantially renovate that building, it would first have to hire a contractor to remove all encapsulated asbestos materials, thereby paying twice to have the job done. For these reasons, even though encapsulation is an acceptable method of reducing asbestos exposure, most asbestos abatement projects today involve complete removal.

Asbestos removal projects must adhere to strict federal and state regulations to protect both workers and the general public. Under the Clean Air Act provisions for hazardous air pollutants, EPA has set a standard of "no visible emissions" for any asbestos removal activities. Asbestos-containing materials must be wet down before work commences and must be kept damp throughout the course of the project, right up to final disposal. Damp asbestos wastes must be containerized in thick plastic bags or plastic lined containers, tagged with a warning label, and transported in a covered vehicle to a sanitary landfill. Since asbestos is not classified as a hazardous waste, the EPA-approved method of asbestos disposal is to bury the material in an area of the landfill separate from other household wastes, covering the containers with at least six inches of soil or other nonasbestos materials before compacting. Final cover of an additional 30 inches of non-asbestos material is required.

Legal Status of Asbestos

The mass of evidence documenting asbestos' adverse health impact has led to passage of legislation in several countries restricting the use of this otherwise valuable material. The United Kingdom, Germany, and Sweden have all banned some uses of asbestos and are searching for acceptable substitutes. Japan is similarly discouraging imports of the material. In the United States, action against asbestos is proceeding on several fronts. Occupational exposure, which in the 1970s was lowered first to 5 and subsequently to 2 fibers/cm^3 of air, has now been reduced to 0.2 fibers/cm^3 over an eight-hour time-weighted average. Employers are required to sample at factory sites every six months and daily at construction sites unless employees are wearing respirators. In situations where fiber levels exceed 0.1/cm^3, employers must install exhaust ventilation and dust control systems and air vacuuming methods to reduce worker exposure to asbestos dust. Medical surveillance of workers, provision and laundering of protective clothing, maintenance of respirators, provision of showering and changing facilities—all are employer responsibilities to enhance the health and safety of asbestos workers (ATSDR, 1990; Brodeur, 1980).

Lead

Lead poisoning is entirely preventable, yet it is the most common and societally devastating environmental disease of young children.
—Dr. Louis Sullivan, former Secretary of Health and Human Services

Dr. Sullivan's remarks regarding the impact of lead on childhood health were prompted by recent estimates that three to four million American youngsters, representing 17% of all preschoolers in the United States, have blood lead levels high enough to impair their intellectual abilities. Future medical historians may regard it as ironic that in the last decade of the 20th century a substance whose toxicity has been well established for millennia is regarded as the single most important environmental health problem affecting American children.

Human contact with lead, a mineral element naturally occurring throughout the environment, dates back to at least 4000 B.C. when it was first smelted as a by-product of silver processing. Because it is malleable and easy to work, doesn't rust, corrode, or dissolve in water, and binds readily with other metals, lead has been widely used since ancient times as an alloy; as an ingredient in paints, glazes, and cosmetics; and for gutters and piping. Indeed, the word "plumbing" is derived from the Latin word for lead, *plumbum*—hence lead's chemical symbol, Pb.

Among those who worked with the metal, it early became apparent that in addition to being commercially valuable, lead is a potent human poison. Over the centuries, evidence of the multifaceted aspects of lead's toxicity has continued to mount. More than two thousand years ago, Roman doctors were describing patients suffering with symptoms of gout, an ailment associated with chronic lead poisoning; modern commentators theorize such problems may have been caused by the Roman practice of lining wine casks, cooking pots, and aqueducts with lead. Lead poisoning may also have contributed to the low birth rate and high incidence of mental retardation among the Roman aristocracy. A major source of exposure to the metal among wealthy Romans is thought to have been a grape juice syrup, *frumentum*, which was brewed in lead pots and subsequently used to sweeten foods and wine; even one teaspoonful of this syrup would have been more than enough to cause chronic lead poisoning. Unfortunately, later generations learned little from the Roman experience, since even in the 16th century widespread outbreaks of lead poisoning were occurring in France as a result of storing wine in lead-lined vessels.

Sources of Lead

Today, as in centuries past, lead is used in a wide range of industrial products. The single largest use of lead, over 70% of total U.S. consumption of the metal, is for lead storage batteries (virtually every car on the road contains 20 pounds of lead in its battery); other lead-containing products include ammunition, brass, coverings for power and communication cables, glass TV tubes, solder, and pigments. With world production estimated at more than three million tons annually, lead is produced in larger amounts than any other toxic heavy metal. Not surprisingly, lead is now found throughout the environment—in soils, water, air, and food. Until the mid-1980s, automobile emissions constituted the major source of environmental lead. With the phaseout of leaded gasoline in the United States and a number of other countries, amounts of lead entering the atmosphere have declined sharply in recent years. Airborne lead today originates primarily from the burning of lead-contaminated used oil, from the smelting of ores and other industrial processes, and from the incineration of municipal refuse. Currently more lead is released into soil than into the air, primarily as the result of lead-containing solid wastes being dumped in landfills (aware of this hazard, a number of states have passed laws banning landfill disposal of lead batteries). Weathering of lead-based paints, particularly around the foundations of older structures, and fallout of airborne lead further contribute to the buildup of lead in soils.

Route of Entry into Body

Until recently, ingestion of lead-tainted food and water constituted the main source of lead intake for most Americans. Canned foods and beverages represented a significant hazard because over 90% of such cans had lead-soldered seams. Leaching of the toxic metal from the solder into the cans' contents was commonplace, especially when the food items were acidic (e.g. tomato products, citrus, or carbonated drinks). One study of lead contamination in canned tuna showed that while the fresh fish contained a mere 0.3 ppm lead, tuna from the supermarket shelf in a lead-soldered can measured 1400 ppm lead! (Settle, 1980). Airborne fallout of lead from automobile emissions onto vegetables or fruits growing near busy highways was responsible for lead concentrations as high as 3000 ppm on such crops. Drinking water, too, has been identified as a source of exposure for as many as 40 million Americans whom EPA estimates live in homes where tap water contains elevated levels of lead due to the presence of lead pipes or lead solder in household plumbing (see chapter 15). Fortunately, human exposure to lead from all these sources has been declining sharply in recent years, thanks to the phaseout of leaded gasoline, the substitution of plastic (PVC) for metal piping in new and replacement home plumbing systems, and to a precipitous reduction in the use of lead-soldered cans by U.S. food processing companies. Today less than 1% of all domestically produced cans contain lead solder; imported foods continue to pose a hazard, however, since few other countries restrict the use of lead solder.

Ironically, housepaint remains the most important source of lead poisoning problems, even though the use of lead in paints was halted years ago. Until 1953 the use of paint containing as much as 50% lead by weight was common in the United States. In that year a consensus was reached within the industry to reduce paint lead levels, resulting in a steady decline in the manufacture and use of interior lead-base paint (most European countries had recognized the problem decades earlier, signing a treaty in 1921 to prohibit the use of *interior* paints containing lead). Exterior lead-base paint continued to be widely available until the mid-1970s, although its lead content by then was considerably less than that of paint produced prior to the 1950s. In 1977 the Consumer Product Safety Commission banned all house paints, interior or exterior, as well as paints on toys or furniture, which contained more than 0.06% lead by weight. Lead-base

BOX 7-2

Poison on Your Plate?

What do such apparently disparate items as ceramic coffee mugs, crystal decanters, pewter goblets, earthenware dishes, foil capsules on wine bottles, and bone china dinnerware have in common? All are food containers that may contain varying amounts of leachable lead, thus posing a risk of lead poisoning to unwary consumers.

The hazards of ingesting lead with food or beverages has been recognized for centuries and both manufacturers and government regulators have made commendable efforts in recent years to reduce such contamination to the greatest extent possible. Thanks primarily to the drastic reduction of airborne lead fallout onto food crops (due to the phaseout of leaded gasoline) and to the voluntary elimination of lead solder by the canning industry, levels in U.S. food products are lower today than at any time in history and are down fully 90% over the levels prevailing in 1980. Nevertheless, some previously unsuspected items have recently been identified as constituting potential sources of toxic exposure. Concerns focus primarily on types of china, porcelain, and earthenware coated with a lead-containing glaze. When such glazes are poorly fired, copious amounts of lead can migrate into foods. In one notable episode, five members of an affluent Idaho family developed acute lead poisoning as a result of using an improperly glazed earthenware pitcher to pour their breakfast orange juice each morning. Even when manufactured according to the strict regulations that prevail in such countries as the United States, Japan, and the United Kingdom, glazes can gradually break down and begin leaching lead after repeated scouring or when in prolonged contact with acidic liquids such as tomato or citrus juices, wine, tea, or coffee. Because they are generally used several times daily to hold a hot, acidic beverage, ceramic coffee mugs have been identified by the FDA as the type of hollowware contributing the largest amount of adult lead exposure from this source. Accordingly, for a separate category consisting solely of mugs, cups, and pitchers, the agency recently set a new lead leaching action level (guideline informing manufacturers the point at which FDA may take regulatory action) of 0.5 ppm—the lowest for any type of ceramic ware.

In further efforts to protect the public from lead exposure in food, especially in relation to china and pottery, the FDA performs spot checks for lead leaching on both domestically manufactured and imported dinnerware. Nevertheless, with its limited resources, FDA is incapable of testing all but a small percentage of such articles sold in the United States, nor does it monitor items brought into the country by returning travelers or those made by hobbyists or handicrafters. Thus wary consumers would be well advised to take precautionary actions to limit their exposure to lead in food by observing the following FDA recommendations:

- If you are pregnant, avoid daily use of ceramic mugs for drinking hot beverages such as coffee or tea.
- Don't store wine or other alcoholic beverages in lead crystal containers.
- Limit the use of antique or collectible dinnerware to special occasions (items manufactured years ago are more likely to contain lead than those made more recently).

- Discontinue using items that show a dusty or chalky gray residue on the glaze after they are washed.
- If a wine bottle is sealed with a foil capsule, wipe the rim of the bottle with a damp cloth before removing the cork.

Consumers desiring further information may telephone the National Lead Information Center toll-free at 1-800-532-3394 to request an English or Spanish language information package. Questions regarding home test kits for lead leaching from ceramic ware or other lead-related matters can be directed to FDA headquarters at 1-301-443-4667.

Bon appetit!

Reference

Foulke, Judith E. 1993. "Lead Threat Lessens, But Mugs Pose Problem." *FDA Consumer* (April).

paint can still be used, even today, for painting bridges, ships, and other steel structures and for a variety of industrial and military applications—and sometimes this paint ends up being applied in homes by workers who have access to the material and fail to realize its hazardous nature ("Preventing Lead Poisoning," 1991).

Although the use of leaded paint has been illegal for almost 20 years, it is estimated that three million tons of lead from paint remains in the 57 million U.S. homes and apartment complexes built before 1980. In such structures, deterioration or renovation activities may expose older layers of paint, providing access to toddlers who may inadvertently consume the poison chips or paint dust. While at one time it was believed that chewing on window sills or eating flakes of the sweet-tasting paint was the major lead-poisoning hazard to children, researchers are now convinced that the prime culprit is ordinary household dust, contaminated by tiny particles of lead from the gradually deteriorating paint. Simply by playing in their own homes and doing what children normally do—putting dirty fingers in their mouths—youngsters can swallow enough lead to cause serious health problems. Growing recognition of the extent of lead contamination in the nation's housing supply has prompted action by the federal government, requiring that, as of October 1995, lead hazards in pre-1978 housing be disclosed in any real estate transaction.

Lead presents a hazard outside as well as inside homes. Soil or dust adjacent to housing once painted with lead-base paints may contain lead levels high enough to pose a risk to small children playing in such locations; soil near busy streets or highways frequently features high lead levels also, thanks to airborne fallout of lead emissions from motor vehicles. Once deposited, lead may remain in soils as long as two thousand years; a number of studies have shown that children living in areas where soil lead levels are particularly high (e.g. in the vicinity of a smelter) often exhibit elevated blood lead levels.

Interestingly, *ingested* lead poses a much greater hazard for young children than it does for adults. Whereas only 10% of lead swallowed by adults passes from the intestine into the bloodstream, 40% of the lead

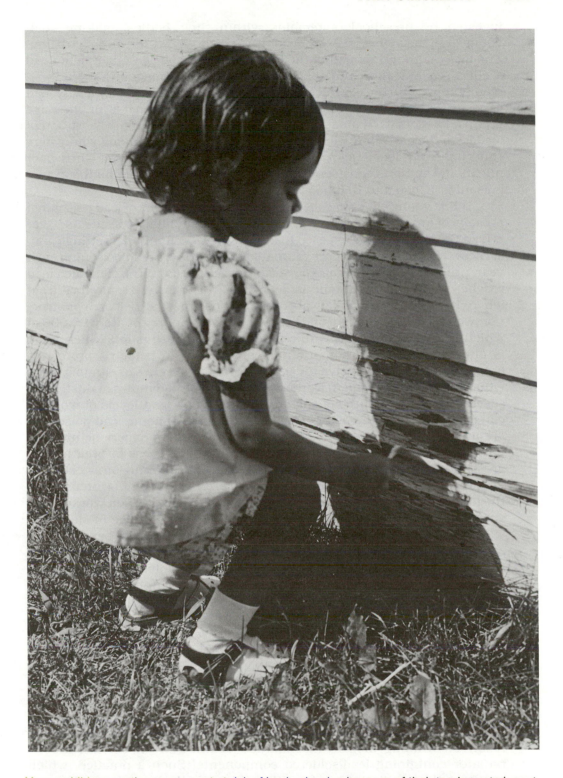

Young children are the group most at risk of lead poisoning because of their tendency to ingest lead-containing materials, such as paint chips. [Illinois Department of Public Health]

ingested by preschoolers remains within their bodies, making such youngsters the highest risk group for lead poisoning within our population. The fact that development of the blood-brain barrier isn't complete until a child reaches approximately three years of age means that lead can readily move into the central nervous system, further explaining why lead exposure is more hazardous for infants and toddlers than it is for other age groups. Particularly vulnerable are malnourished children; absorption of lead from the gastrointestinal tract occurs more readily among youngsters suffering from deficiencies of protein, calcium, zinc, or iron. Thus poor nutritional status is considered an additional risk factor for childhood lead poisoning (Chao and Kikano, 1993).

While young children constitute the primary victims of lead poisoning, persons of any age group are susceptible to the metal's toxic effects. Over 800,000 Americans are exposed to lead in their occupational settings and, of these, tens of thousands are estimated to suffer from lead poisoning each year, primarily through inhalation of airborne lead (30–50% of inhaled lead reaches the bloodstream and is deposited in the lower respiratory tract where it is almost completely absorbed). Those most at risk are construction workers who renovate or demolish bridges, approximately 90,000 of which in the United States are coated with lead-base paints. Such work is often performed without training or the use of personal protective equipment and may involve the use of acetylene torches or sandblasting, either of which can result in workers' inhalation of lead fumes or dust. After several weeks or months of such exposure, blood lead levels of workers can rise well above the point at which symptoms of acute lead poisoning are apparent. Case reports describe affected workers experiencing such poisoning symptoms as light-headedness and shortness of breath, progressing to dizziness, headache, fatigue, vomiting, confusion, weakness, forgetfulness, and abdominal pain—the severity of symptoms intensifying the longer exposure continued. One 23-year-old construction worker who spent three months sandblasting a lead paint-coated bridge in Maryland experienced blood lead levels as high as 175 μg/dL, requiring several years of chelation therapy to flush the toxin out of his system. In addition to bridge maintenance, other occupations that may involve excessive worker exposure to lead include battery manufacturing, shipbuilding, radiator repair, smelter and foundry operations, and certain crafts. Police or military personnel working at firing ranges have also reported symptoms of lead toxicity, a result of inhaling fumes released when lead-containing ammunition is fired (CDC, 1993; Franklin, 1991). Occasionally, some rather bizarre instances of lead poisoning illustrate the challenges facing those in the environmental health profession: over a period of seven months during 1991, eight individuals in Alabama were diagnosed with various symptoms of lead poisoning (e.g. anemia, abdominal pains, weakness in the arms, seizures, and nervous system damage) which developed as a result of drinking illegal "moonshine" distilled in an old automobile radiator containing lead-soldered components! Such a practice, which results in the leaching of lead from the solder into the home-brewed liquor, is a frequent source of lead poisoning in some rural Alabama counties and

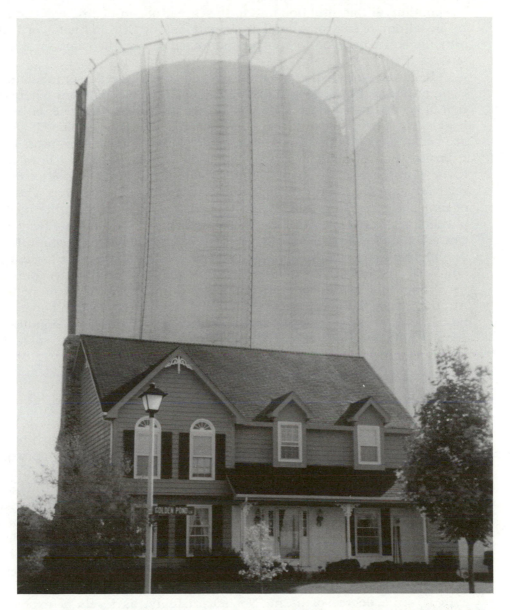

The water tower in Wheaton, Illinois was draped with fabric in order to contain lead dust after the exterior was sandblasted to remove lead-based primer. [Ray Schnurstein, City of Wheaton]

accounts for the fact that moonshine may contain up to 74 μg/L of lead (CDC, 1992).

Although lead concerns understandably focus on human health problems, it shouldn't be overlooked that environmental lead constitutes a hazard to other species as well. Especially vulnerable are waterfowl, large numbers of which have died after eating lead fishing sinkers lost by anglers.

Responding to this situation and to the threat of compelling legal action by a coalition of environmental organizations, the EPA in the fall of 1993 announced its decision to ban the manufacture and distribution of lead sinkers (EDF, 1993).

Regardless of whether the route of exposure is ingestion or inhalation, upon entering the body, lead first moves into the bloodstream where its half-life is estimated at 36 days. For this reason, measurements of blood lead levels, calculated as micrograms of lead per deciliter of blood (μg/dL), are considered to give the most accurate indication of short-term lead exposure. Some lead makes its way into soft tissues such as the brain and kidneys; approximately 50–60% of the lead that enters the body is excreted relatively quickly, mainly through the feces but also in urine. Over a period of time the remaining lead is slowly deposited and stored in the bones, particularly in the long arm and leg bones where it can remain for years (the estimated half-life of lead in bones is 27 years). Lead also accumulates in children's baby teeth, which have been used in research to indicate a child's lead burden. Lead in bones can act as a cumulative poison, becoming increasingly concentrated over an extended time period. Although once thought to be inert, it is now known that lead in bones can be suddenly released back into the bloodstream by a number of conditions such as high fever, osteoporosis, or pregnancy, resulting in cases of acute lead poisoning.

Biological Effects

A potent toxin that can adversely affect people in any age group, lead can damage human health in a number of ways. It interferes with blood cell formation, often resulting in anemia; lead can cause kidney damage, sterility, miscarriage, and birth defects. Because lead has a strong affinity for nerve tissue, injury to the central nervous system is perhaps the most serious manifestation of lead poisoning. Depending on the degree of exposure, lead poisoning can be reflected by hyperirritability, poor memory, or sluggishness at lower levels all the way to mental retardation, epileptic convulsions, coma, and death at high levels.

Lead is a poison that exhibits what health experts refer to as a **continuum of toxicity**; any amount of exposure, however small, carries with it some degree of harm. Not surprisingly, as levels of exposure increase, risk of adverse health effects rise correspondingly (as is the case with exposure to any hazardous substance, identical levels of lead may provoke a varying range of responses in different people). Until about 30 years ago, it was widely believed that a diagnosis of "lead poisoning" was appropriate only when blood lead levels were high enough to cause such overt symptoms of lead poisoning as anemia, kidney disease, brain damage, or death. Such conditions can be manifested when blood lead levels exceed 70 μg/dL (typically, brain damage only occurs at blood lead levels above 100 μg/dL). At that time, levels of blood lead below 60 μg/dL weren't regarded as dangerous enough to warrant monitoring or treatment. By the early 1970s, however, new evidence regarding lead's deleterious effects on biological systems prompted a reevaluation of the U.S. Public Health Service's level of "undue lead absorption"—the blood lead level at which medical intervention is recommended. In 1971 that level was lowered to 40 μg/dL, further lowered to 30 μg/dL in 1975, to 25 μg/dL in 1985, and, most recently, in 1991 was again reduced to an action range of 10–15 μg/dL. Current analytical devices are incapable of measuring blood lead levels below 10 μg/dL (Florini, 1990).

Figure 7-2 U.S. Public Health Service's Changing Perception of "Undue Lead Absorption" Levels Over Past 3 Decades

Year	"Undue Lead Absorption" Level (μg/dL)
1970	60
1971	40
1975	30
1985	25
1991	10 –15

The justification for the steadily declining levels of blood lead that define a case of lead poisoning can be found in the results of numerous studies carried out over the last several decades, which have conclusively shown that even at levels previously considered safe, chronic low-level exposure to lead can inhibit the normal development of children's intellectual abilities. A landmark study launched in 1979 in the Boston suburbs of Somerville and Chelsea among second grade students revealed that those whose baby teeth (which they had willingly withheld from the Tooth Fairy to contribute to science!) had a relatively higher lead level also exhibited a greater incidence of unruly classroom behavior, a lesser ability to follow instructions, and lower scores on I.Q. tests than did classmates with low lead levels in their teeth (Needleman et al., 1979). Yet none of the children would have been categorized as lead-poisoning victims based on the prevailing view at that time regarding "safe" levels of lead. Eleven years later, in 1990, a follow-up study was carried out to see whether the effects of low-level childhood lead poisoning persist into young adulthood. In light of the millions of children who have experienced some lead exposure, the results of this investigation were depressing: in comparison with classmates whose baby teeth had minimal levels of lead, the higher-lead students, now 18-year-olds, exhibited a significantly greater school drop-out rate, higher incidence of reading disabilities, lower class rank, and higher absenteeism—all a legacy of childhood lead exposure (Needleman, 1990).

Lead Poisoning: Treatment and Prevention

Children with blood lead levels of 45 μg/dL or higher typically are treated through the use of **chelation**, a process which employs a drug that binds to lead, sequestering the metal and facilitating its excretion from the body. Most commonly, chelating agents are administered in a hospital setting where the patient must remain for a five-day period of treatment and testing (a relatively new type of chelating agent that can be given orally at home has recently been approved for use in less serious cases). Some forms of chelation therapy can be quite painful and the process, while essential in forestalling further impairment to the nervous system, cannot reverse damage that has already occurred. Nor is chelation a one-time solution to lead poisoning problems. Since the chelating agent is generally unable to reach all of the lead stored in bones and teeth, blood lead levels frequently rebound following chelation therapy, the result of additional lead moving from bony tissues into the bloodstream. Many lead poisoning victims are forced to suffer repeated bouts of hospitalization for years after the initial treatment. Children whose lead poisoning symptoms are relieved by chelation therapy frequently require special education and therapy long after cessation of treatment and, in the all-too-common situation where they return to the same lead-contaminated environment responsible for the initial poisoning, their symptoms will promptly recur. For this reason, removal of the child from the source of exposure or, conversely, removal of lead from the child's environment, is one of the most important aspects in restoring that child to good health.

Figure 7-3 Lead Poisoning: Assessing the Risk

Medicaid guidelines say that doctors should ask these questions to assess the risk of lead poisoning in children 6 months to 6 years old:

1. Does your child live in or regularly visit a house, a day-care center, or a nursery school that was built before 1960 and has peeling or chipping paint?

2. Does your child live in a home built before 1960 that is being remodeled or renovated?

3. Does your child live near a heavily traveled major highway where soil and dust may be contaminated with lead?

4. Have any of your children or their playmates had lead poisoning?

5. Does your child often come in contact with an adult who works with lead—in construction, welding, plumbing, pottery or other trades?

6. Does your child live near a lead smelter, a battery-recycling plant or other industrial sites likely to release lead?

7. Does your home plumbing have lead pipes or copper with lead solder joints?

If the answer to any of these questions is yes, the government says, a child has a substantial risk of exposure to lead and should be given a blood lead test as soon as one can be arranged. If the answers to all questions are negative, the child is said to have a low risk, but should nevertheless be tested for lead poisoning at 12 months of age and again, if possible, at 24 months, federal officials say.

Source: The *New York Times,* Sept. 13, 1992.

Since the health impact of lead, even at very low levels, has been shown to be so devastating and because damage, once it occurs, may never be completely reversed, *prevention* of lead poisoning should be a high-priority societal goal. As mentioned previously, the near-total phaseout of the use of lead in gasoline, paint, food containers, and home plumbing has drastically reduced human exposure to this toxic metal in recent years. Nevertheless, four million U.S. preschoolers continue to exhibit elevated lead levels due to lead-contaminated paint and dust still present in millions of homes. Others are inadvertently exposed when a family member engages in such hobbies as making pottery (lead glaze), stained glass, oil painting (some artists' paints contain lead), or furniture refinishing. Parents who work in occupational settings involving lead exposure may unintentionally carry lead dust home on work clothes, thereby exposing children to the toxic metal. Identifying those children at risk—most of whom exhibit no overt symptoms of lead poisoning and hence are likely to go undiagnosed and untreated—has become the focus of a national effort in the United States following a federal government directive in 1992 that all children from six months to three years of age (the group most vulnerable to lead poisoning) whose families are eligible for Medicaid must be screened for lead toxicity. Some states have carried this mandate further, requiring that all young children, regardless of income level, be evaluated for lead exposure and that those entering day care or elementary school present evidence of a blood lead test.

Since blood lead levels as low as 10 μg/dL are now regarded as cause for concern, it is recognized that identifying and eliminating the source of lead exposure for every child with blood lead at or slightly above this threshold will yield important health benefits. Accordingly, the government currently is recommending the following multi-tier approach to dealing with low-level lead poisoning:

Blood lead level	Recommended action
• < 10μg/dL	no lead poisoning; continue regular screening
• 10–14 μg/dL	community prevention activities; more frequent screening may be necessary
• 15–19 μg/dL	family counseling about symptoms and sources of lead exposure; nutritional intervention; more frequent screening
• 20–24 μg/dL	environmental investigation and remediation; medical evaluation
• 25 μg/dL	prompt medical and environmental evaluation and intervention, including chelation therapy

For the most part, environmental intervention entails removal of lead paint and lead dust from those structures where lead-poisoned children are living; prevention of future lead poisoning cases would require removing lead paint from all homes, with special emphasis on the nearly two million U.S. dwellings where such paint is in a deteriorating condition and presents

BOX 7-3
Dream Turned Nightmare

The old Victorian farmhouse in upstate New York was a homeowner's dream. Built in the mid-19th century, the two-story wood-and-stone structure featured 10 rooms arranged around a central hallway whose focal point was an elegant center staircase. The solid wood floors, moldings, and doorframes had been painted many times and looked a bit dingy, but the young New York City executive and his wife who moved into the house in late June of 1987 knew the basic woodwork was sound and were convinced that with some energetic stripping and varnishing the place would be as good as new—the ideal location to raise their 5-year-old daughter and 20-month-old son, far from the stress and pollution of big-city life.

In early August, after hiring two workmen to perform the renovations, the family left for vacation, hoping that during their absence the job of sanding layers of old paint off floors, walls, and woodwork would be completed. Upon returning in mid-September, however, they found the work only partially finished and signs of work in progress were all too evident. The workmen had neglected to seal off the area undergoing repairs and a thick layer of dust had spread throughout the house, settling in every nook and cranny. Over the next several weeks, renovation activities shifted into high gear as the workmen used torches, heat guns, and chemical woodstrippers to remove over a century's accumulation of paint from door frames and moldings in the central hallway.

In an effort to keep the children out of the work area, a young woman was hired as a babysitter to come to the house five days a week, accompanied by her own toddlers, aged two and three. Whenever possible, she tried to keep all the children occupied outdoors, while the mistress of the house pursued her career from an office in the home. The two family dogs were less easily persuaded to avoid the work area; one of them, a 10-year-old mongrel, took a special liking for one of the carpenters and spent most of her time sitting at his feet, conscientiously licking the fresh paint dust off her coat as he sanded.

By mid-October, renovations were nearly complete, but some unsettling developments indicated all was not well. The dog, previously healthy, was rushed to a veterinarian with symptoms the owners described as "shaking and twisting." Suspecting poisoning, the veterinarian asked the wife about possible lead exposure; upon hearing that the dog lived in a home where extensive renovations were underway, the vet took a blood sample that immediately confirmed his hunch. Chelation therapy was promptly begun on the animal, but in spite of a brief period of initial improvement, the dog died of kidney failure a few days after returning home.

By this time, the paint removal process was taking its toll on the human members of the household as well. In early November the mother reported feeling tired and weak; her daughter frequently complained of stomach aches in the morning prior to catching the bus for kindergarten. The father experienced severe nausea after spending a weekend at home while workmen used acetylene torches for paint removal. After blood tests revealed that all family members, including the baby, were suffering from lead poisoning, the mother and children were admitted to the hospital for a five-day course of chelation therapy. Shortly after returning home, the mother discovered she was two months pregnant; realizing the devastating teratogenic effects of lead, she decided to undergo a therapeutic abortion. Over the next several weeks, the little girl had to endure chelation therapy five times; her brother was treated twice, and both children continued to receive close medical evaluation. Nor were family members the only victims; the babysitter and her two youngsters were subsequently tested and they, too, had elevated blood lead levels requiring chelation. The workmen, however, who might be expected to have the highest lead levels of all, were never tested and no information on their health status has been reported.

While the menace posed by lead-base paints in deteriorating inner-city structures has been recognized for decades, increasing numbers of "yuppie lead poisoning" incidents such as that just described have only recently begun to attract public attention. Suburban or rural homeowners are generally far less aware of the lead hazards of housing renovation than are their urban counterparts who for years have been deluged with such information by public health activists. Anyone intending to engage in structural restorations involving the potential for lead exposure needs to be aware of the hazard and to take appropriate precautions. Small children and pregnant women in particular should not remain in a dwelling while such activities are underway and should not return until a thorough cleanup has been performed. The example described here also demonstrates how health problems experienced by nonhuman species (in this case, the family dog) can be early warning signs of more widespread environmental exposure and illustrates the importance of good communication between family doctors and veterinarians. Awareness that lead poisoning recognizes no ethnic or socioeconomic boundaries, coupled with greater parental vigilance and caution, is essential if we are to eliminate this devastating, yet entirely preventable, childhood disease.

Reference

Marino, Phyllis E., MD, et al. 1990. "A Case Report of Lead Paint Poisoning During Renovation of a Victorian Farmhouse." *American Journal of Public Health*, 80, no. 10 (Oct.).

an imminent and constant hazard. Since soils around homes with exterior lead-base paints commonly exhibit elevated concentrations of lead (in some cases as high as 11,000 ppm), a number of health authorities also recommend soil abatement programs for neighborhoods where childhood lead poisoning is prevalent. Such efforts would involve removing the top 6–7 inches of soil, replacing this with clean dirt, and then revegetating the area. However, recent epidemiologic studies have shown that in urban areas where children were experiencing low-level lead exposure, blood lead levels declined only slightly when soil abatement activities were carried out. Thus although lead in soils *does* contribute to children's body burden of the metal (studies have shown that blood lead levels rise by 3–7 μg/dL for every 1000 ppm increase in soil or dust concentrations), the considerable expense of contaminated soil removal may not be cost-effective; significantly greater health benefits can be achieved by targeting available funds to interior paint abatement. In many situations where potential exposure to lead in soil is a concern, simply covering bare soil with sod or planting foundation shrubs along the base of the structure can eliminate or greatly reduce the opportunity for children to come into contact with contaminated soil—and at a much lower cost than removal activities would entail. However, in situations where soil lead levels are extremely high or where a child suffering from lead poisoning has a condition called **pica**—a tendency to eat nonfood items, including soil—then soil abatement could effect beneficial results (Weitzman et al., 1993; Xintaras, 1992). A national initiative to prevent childhood lead poisoning by a massive lead-base paint removal effort, while providing major long-term public health benefits, would be very expensive. The Environmental Defense Fund, an environmental organization that advocates such a program, estimates the likely cost of de-leading a house at $3000–$10,000 (Florini, 1990). In the absence of a strong federal commitment to such a costly undertaking, universal lead screening of children offers the best hope for identifying youngsters at risk and providing prompt treatment to lower blood lead levels before damage becomes irreversible.

Mercury

This liquid metal, the "quicksilver" of ancient times, has been used for a wide variety of purposes for at least 2500 years—and has been contributing to illness and death among those exposed to it for an equal period of time. Although at very low levels of exposure mercury does not appear to be damaging, the margin of safety is small. Mercury is a valuable constituent of many industrial products and processes. It has been used as a catalyst in the manufacture of plastics, as a slime retardant in paper making, as a fungicide in paints, as an alloy in dental fillings, as an ingredient in many medicinal products (mercury's first medicinal use was for the treatment of syphilis when that disease reached epidemic proportions in 16th-century Europe), in the manufacture of scientific instruments, and for many other purposes.

While mercury has always been present in the environment in trace amounts, concentrations have been increasing during the modern era thanks to such human activities as coal burning, the single largest source of mercury emissions to the atmosphere. Industrial processes such as electroplating, paper milling, mining and ore processing, chlorine and caustic soda production, textile manufacturing, and pharmaceutical production produce a mercury-laden effluent that is sometimes discharged into waterways. Evaporation of mercury from paints during the drying process can add significant quantities of this substance to the air; studies have shown that mercury concentrations in indoor air may be one thousand times higher immediately after a room is painted than they were before painting. Several well publicized cases of children developing symptoms of mercury poisoning after mercury-containing latex paints were applied to their homes led to an agreement among U.S. paint manufacturers to stop adding mercury to their products. Nevertheless, although the production of interior paints containing mercury halted in 1990, followed by similar action regarding exterior paint in 1991, the fact that many people keep partly used containers of paint for future use means that paint will remain a potential source of mercury exposure for years to come. Incineration of mercury-containing wastes contributes to atmospheric levels of mercury, as does vaporization of mercury compounds naturally occurring in the earth's crust (ATSDR, 1992). While U.S. mercury emissions to the air totalled approximately 346 tons in 1990, that amount is now gradually declining due to a decrease in demand for the metal, especially in the paint and chlor-alkali industries and for battery and wire manufacturing. As mercury is used in smaller amounts and in fewer products, emissions of the toxic metal from municipal and medical waste incinerators will correspondingly fall ("Paper Quantifies," 1993).

Health Effects of Mercury Exposure

The action of mercury on the human system depends primarily on the form of mercury to which the victim is exposed, either inorganic metallic mercury or the far more toxic organic mercury.

Inorganic Metallic Mercury. This form of mercury frequently attacks the liver and kidneys; it also can diffuse through the alveolar membranes of the lungs and travel to the brain where it can cause such neurological problems as lack of coordination. Inorganic mercury can enter the system either by inhalation of mercury vapors or by absorption of mercury compounds through the skin after prolonged contact. Examples of human poisoning with inorganic mercury include the malady prevalent among hatmakers in 17th-century France called the "Mad Hatters' Disease" (immortalized by a character of the same name in Lewis Carroll's *Alice in Wonderland*). This neurological disorder, manifested as tremors and mental aberrations, resulted from the practice at that time of soaking animal hides in a solution of mercuric nitrate for purposes of softening the hairs. Since the hatmakers' bare arms and hands were in frequent contact with the solution as they manipulated the hides, skin absorption of mercury led to development of the disease symptoms.

Poisoning by inhalation is more common than skin absorption, however, and represents the most common form of occupational exposure to mercury. A survey conducted by the National Institute for Occupational Safety and Health (NIOSH) estimated that 70,000 American workers may be exposed to mercury vapors on the job. These include nurses, lab technicians, machine operators, miners, plumbers, dentists and dental hygienists, and many others. Even the families of potentially exposed workers may be at risk if mercury is carried home from the occupational setting on contaminated work clothing.

Many people have become ill and some deaths have been reported among persons exposed to mercury fumes when large quantities of mercury were accidentally spilled within confined, inadequately ventilated

BOX 7-4

Mercury in Your Mouth:
Are Amalgam Fillings a Health Hazard?

George Decker may have been street-smart, but he displayed a fatal ignorance about mercury when he began collecting old fillings from dentists' offices several years ago. "Cooking" the amalgam on his kitchen stove, Decker extracted the silver from teeth by boiling off the mercury that constitutes approximately 50% by weight of standard dental fillings. In his quest for easy money to finance drug-trafficking jaunts to Colombia, Decker inadvertently inhaled enough mercury vapors to poison his lungs, initiating tissue damage leading to irreversible pneumonia which eventually killed him. A post-mortem investigation of his home revealed accumulations of mercury one thousand times higher than permissible levels under the floor boards around his stove!

Mr. Decker's demise constitutes an unusual, though not unique, example of mercury poisoning caused by dental fillings. Of far greater public health relevance than the undoing of a greedy drug dealer, however, is the question of whether the millions of people whose teeth contain amalgam fillings are at risk of chronic mercury poisoning. Similarly, occupational safety issues regarding the potential for mercury poisoning among dentists and dental hygienists has been a source of heated debate within the profession ever since mercury-containing amalgams were introduced as a cheaper alternative to gold fillings more than 150 years ago.

The possibility that mercury leaking from fillings can be absorbed via the intestinal tract or inhaled as chewing or tooth brushing release mercury vapor into intra-oral air has been investigated by a number of studies. One such investigation cited autopsy reports showing that mercury levels were significantly higher in the brains and kidneys of individuals who had received amalgam fillings than in those who had not; persons with fillings similarly had elevated levels of mercury in their blood and urine. Nevertheless, despite suggestions that exposure to mercury in fillings may cause such health problems as rheumatoid arthritis, multiple sclerosis, leukemia, or reduced ability to fight infection, no convincing evidence to support such claims has yet been verified and most authorities feel that the amount of mercury that dental fillings contribute to the average person's daily body burden of the toxic metal is too small to pose any credible health risk. (The small group of individuals who experience a pronounced allergic reaction to mercury within a few hours or days after placement of mercury-containing fillings constitute an obvious exception to this generalization.)

If evidence for mass mercury poisoning among dental patients is weak, what about adverse health effects among the professionals who work with substantial amounts of the metal on a daily basis? Dentists and their technicians constantly handle mercury-containing compounds and inhale mercury vapors while preparing, placing, polishing, or removing amalgam fillings. Contamination of dental offices with mercury can easily occur due to accidental spills, vapors leaking from storage containers, vaporization while the amalgam is being heated, or high-temperature sterilization of mercury-contaminated instruments. Poor office ventilation exacerbates the problem—approximately 10% of dental offices have mercury vapor concentrations double the maximum allowable level set by OSHA. Dental professionals experience mercury exposure both through inhalation and direct skin contact. The extent of occupational exposure is evident in the fact that dentists have blood mercury levels almost twice as high as the general public. Nevertheless, in spite of what appear to be worrisome levels of exposure and elevated body burdens of mercury, few dentists report clinical symptoms of mercury toxicity. Statistical analyses of a questionnaire survey of 20,000 dental professionals gave no evidence of an increase in miscarriages or birth defects among offspring of those who were exposed to high levels of mercury in dental offices.

While the weight of current evidence favors the position taken by the American Dental Association that mercury in dental fillings does not present a significant health hazard to patients or to dentists when proper precautions are followed, the debate is unlikely to end any time soon. Data continues to accumulate suggesting that mercury from a variety of sources—consumption of seafood as well as amalgam fillings—can have a subtle adverse impact on various bodily organs, from brain to kidneys. One researcher recently presented controversial evidence that occupational mercury exposure is hindering fertility among dental hygienists who prepare numerous fillings each week. Other studies performed with laboratory animals exposed to mercury vapors documented such adverse reproductive consequences as spontaneous abortions, premature births, low birthweight and learning disabilities among surviving offspring.

Unfortunately, the current debate is being waged with limited experimental evidence. Contenders on both sides agree that much more research is needed to settle the dispute over the safety of mercury amalgam fillings, but the abysmally low level of federal funding for such studies suggests that a definitive answer is unlikely any time soon.

References

Fung, Yiu K. and Michael P. Molvar. 1992. "Toxicity of Mercury from Dental Environment and from Amalgam Restorations." *Clinical Toxicology,* 30 (1:49–61).

Stone, Richard. 1992. "Name Your Poison: Toxicologists Meet." *Science,* 255 (March 13).

Weaver, Daniel C. 1993. "Heavy Metal." *Discover,* (April).

areas. Such a situation occurred during the summer and fall of 1989 in Michigan after a small container of liquid mercury was spilled in a boy's bedroom. The mercury made its way into the pile of carpeting and cracks in the floor and slowly volatilized over a period of months. Vacuuming the contaminated area simply facilitated the spread of mercury throughout the house. By late summer, two young sisters living in the home began experiencing numbness in fingers and toes; their gait became progressively impaired and eventually they were unable to walk at all. At this point the girls were hospitalized and a diagnosis of chronic mercury poisoning was established (a brother had elevated mercury levels but remained asymptomatic). Although chelation therapy resulted in substantial improvement in both girls, the younger sister continued to experience weakness in her arms and legs, blurred vision, and emotional instability— lingering legacies of residual neurologic damage induced by mercury

(Taueg et al., 1992). In contrast to the dangers posed by *inhalation* of mercury fumes, *swallowing* inorganic mercury, such as could occur if an oral thermometer were to break while in the mouth, poses virtually no health threat. Such mercury simply passes through the gastrointestinal tract and is excreted through the kidneys within a few days.

Organic Mercury.   Far more toxic than elemental mercury are the organic mercury compounds such as methyl mercury which, being extremely soluble, can readily penetrate living membranes. Organic mercury circulates in the bloodstream bound to red blood cells and gradually diffuses into the brain, destroying the cells that control coordination. Symptoms of organic mercury poisoning generally don't appear until a month or two after exposure, showing up initially as numbness in the lips, tongue, and fingertips. Gradually speech becomes slurred and difficulty in swallowing and walking becomes apparent. As mercury levels rise, deafness and vision problems may develop and the victim tends to lose contact with his or her surroundings. Before the nature of mercury poisoning was understood, such people were often thought to be neurotic or mentally ill and were occasionally placed in insane asylums.

Several tragic episodes involving methyl mercury poisoning have been documented in past decades. In 1972 more than 6500 Iraqi villagers became seriously ill and 459 died after eating bread that had been made from seed wheat coated with an organic mercury fungicide. A similar situation, fortunately on a much smaller scale, occurred in the United States three years earlier when several members of a family in Alamagordo, New Mexico, suffered permanent neurological impairment after they butchered and ate a hog that had been fed fungicide-treated seed corn. Undoubtedly the most infamous episode of mass poisoning with methyl mercury occurred during the years 1953–1961 in the coastal town of Minamata on the Japanese island of Kyushu. A plastics factory, Chisso Corporation, had for a number of years been discharging inorganic mercury wastes into the waters of Minamata Bay where many of the local residents earned their livelihood by fishing. In the anaerobic conditions among the sediments at the bottom of the bay, the inorganic mercury was converted into highly toxic methyl mercury by the bacterium *Methanobacterium amelanskis*. Readily soluble, the methyl mercury thus began moving through the aquatic food chain, being passively absorbed by microscopic algae which were subsequently eaten by zooplankton, which were eaten by small fish, etc., the methyl mercury becoming increasingly concentrated at each higher trophic level (mercury concentrations in predator fish at the top of aquatic food chains commonly reach levels 100,000 times higher than those present in the surrounding water).

Trouble first became apparent in Minamata when the town cats developed what residents first thought must be a strange viral disease, yowling continuously and sometimes leaping into the sea to drown. When the townspeople themselves started to complain of vague maladies such as extreme fatigue, headaches, numbness in their extremities, and difficulty in swallowing, it was first suspected that they were contracting some sort of illness from the sick cats. Eventually the true nature of their

BOX 7-5

A Brazilian Minamata?

Across the vast expanse of Brazil's Amazon River Basin, the lessons of Minamata are today being relearned the hard way. Amazonia is in the throes of a modern-day gold rush, with an estimated half-million prospectors roaming the region, searching along riverbeds for traces of the precious metal. Watching gold production steadily climbing, Brazilian geologists affirm that "the future of Amazonia is mineral exploration" and are convinced the region's potential yield is two to three times greater than the 100 tons now being extracted each year. While the bonanza promises to make Brazil one of the world's leading gold producers, it is also wreaking havoc on the natural environment and on the health of local populations in the areas beset with gold fever. If present trends are any indication, entire ecosystems may be irrevocably poisoned before the eventual depletion of reserves brings a halt to mining operations.

Amazonia's toxic troubles can be traced to the technique used for extracting the region's treasures. Brazil's gold rush is dominated by hundreds of thousands of individual entrepreneurs employing methods that would have looked entirely familiar to California's "Forty-niners" over a century ago. Digging or pumping mud from riverbeds, the miners scrutinize the muck for a glimpse of telltale glitter. If gold is present, the prospector pours liquid mercury into the mixture, causing the formation of a gold/mercury alloy which is easily separated from the mud. This amalgam is then subjected to treatment with a blowtorch to burn off the mercury, leaving purified gold behind. Unfortunately, this procedure pollutes the surrounding air with mercury vapors, presenting a distinct health hazard to anyone within breathing distance. To make matters worse, prospectors frequently pour mercury into the water where—just as happened at Minamata—it enters the aquatic food chain, poisoning fish and, ultimately, people who have no way of knowing if the fish on their dinner plate contains mercury or not. It is estimated that miners are dumping anywhere from 200 to 1000 tons of mercury into the Amazon every year. An American biologist currently working in Brazil has reported finding fish with mercury concentrations five times higher than the safety limits recommended by the World Health Organization. Bewailing the extent of the problem, the biologist observed that, "Wherever there's gold mining the fish are contaminated, and there's gold mining now across an area half as big as the United States."

The lethal legacy of this situation has become tragically evident. Although no official figures are available, local doctors as well as university research teams report a dramatic increase in the tally of victims claimed by "mercury madness." One physician based in Santarem, one of the region's largest cities, saw his number of mercury-intoxicated patients soar from 20 per month in mid-1989 to more than 130 per month two years later. Medical authorities are convinced that many cases go undiagnosed, since doctors in the region are largely unfamiliar with the symptoms of mercury poisoning and often confuse the ailment with malaria, a widespread condition in Amazonia.

The Brazilian government has finally begun to respond to the situation; in 1988 an edict was issued, banning the use of mercury by miners. Observers doubt that the prohibition will have much, if any, impact however, because there aren't enough inspectors to enforce the law. The area is simply too vast for effective policing, and the miners themselves remain unconvinced that they are a part of the problem. Unfortunately, it appears that until a major health disaster becomes too obvious to ignore, the poisoning of the Amazon will continue—but by that time the damage may well be irreversible.

mutual problem was discovered—methyl mercury poisoning derived from a diet composed primarily of mercury-contaminated fish. By this time more than 100 people had been stricken with such symptoms as mental derangement, inability to walk or use chopsticks, visual disturbances, and convulsions. Forty-four of the Minamata victims died during this period and many others were permanently disabled. As this sad episode unfolded, the teratogenic properties of methyl mercury became apparent. Twenty-two brain-damaged babies were born during this period to mothers who themselves exhibited no outward signs of mercury poisoning, though several mentioned experiencing a slight numbness of the fingers during pregnancy and analysis showed a high level of mercury in their hair. Subsequent studies have revealed that methyl mercury has a special affinity for fetal tissue, easily crossing the placental barrier where it severely damages the developing child while leaving the mother unharmed. The ultimate human toll of Chisso's poisoning of Minamata Bay included 700 deaths and 9000 individuals left with varying degrees of paralysis and brain damage. Estimates are that as many as 50,000 persons living within 35 miles of the bay who consumed its fish have suffered at least mild symptoms of mercury poisoning (Weisskopf, 1987). Follow-up studies on the people of Minamata have indicated that in some areas of the town as many as 25% of the children are regarded as "mentally deficient," though outwardly they appear normal, suggesting that even low levels of methyl mercury in the maternal diet have left their subtle imprint (Smith, 1977).

Cadmium

This soft, silver-white toxic metal plays no beneficial role in the metabolism of living things. Used primarily in the electroplating industry, cadmium is also an important constituent of nickel-cadmium batteries, in the production of pigments and plastics, and as a neutron absorbent in nuclear reactors. Particles of the metal can become airborne during smelting or soldering, or when cadmium-containing wastes are incinerated. Similarly, cadmium can contaminate waterways when industrial wastewaters containing the heavy metal are discharged into rivers and streams. The most common route of exposure to cadmium among the general population is ingestion of cadmium-tainted foods; like organic mercury, cadmium readily bioaccumulates as it moves up the food chain. Cadmium may also be inhaled in cigarette smoke, since tobacco, like most plants, contains some cadmium in its leaves. A single cigarette contains two micrograms of the toxic metal, 50% of which is absorbed through the lungs during active smoking. Those who smoke one pack per day exhibit body burdens of cadmium double those of nonsmokers. The amount of cadmium absorbed by the body is dependent, in part, on an individual's nutritional status. Those suffering from iron, calcium, or protein deficiency appear to be especially vulnerable to cadmium's toxic effects (Grum, 1990).

The largest outbreak of cadmium poisoning documented thus far involved a number of people living near the Jintsu River basin in Japan who, during the 1950s and 1960s, experienced severe bone pains and kidney malfunctions. As their condition worsened, victims developed a condition known as osteomalacia, suffering multiple bone fractures and excruciating pain (hence the villagers' name for the condition: *itai-itai*, or "ouch-ouch" disease). The whole skeleton became abnormally soft and death generally followed, usually due to kidney failure. Most frequently the victims were people who were malnourished or middle-aged women under physiological stress due to numerous pregnancies or menopause. Eventually it was discovered that the mysterious itai-itai disease resulted from cadmium discharges from a lead and zinc mine upstream from the affected farming community. Cadmium fumes and particles from the mining operation, as well as cadmium-laden wastewaters, had contaminated farmland and irrigation water with the toxic metal. Plants readily absorb cadmium from soil and water, and it was found that both rice and soybeans grown in the area contained high levels of the metal; consumption of cadmium-contaminated foods thus proved to be the cause of the disease outbreak (Waldbott, 1978).

Although most Americans exhibit some body accumulation of cadmium, most of it in the kidneys, instances of acute poisoning in recent times are rare. Occasionally outbreaks of food poisoning due to cadmium intoxication are traced to the consumption of acidic drinks (e.g. lemonade) or foods served in galvanized metal containers that contained a cadmium alloy. Nevertheless, while the low concentrations of cadmium most commonly encountered are not acutely toxic, chronic exposure to the metal is a justifiable concern because of cadmium's ability to accumulate in the body over a period of time. Those most at risk are people whose jobs entail the potential for inhaling cadmium particles, since levels of the airborne metal are usually thousands of times higher in the occupational setting than in the general environment.

In addition to the toxic materials discussed in this chapter, there are many other substances capable of causing health damage in humans when present in more than trace amounts or when exposure to even very low levels persists over an extended time period. Fluorides, selenium, copper, nickel, chromium, and arsenic are but a few of the naturally occurring toxins that are known, under certain conditions, to affect human health adversely. Unfortunately, because the symptoms of exposure to toxic substances are often so vague or so similar to those of other more common ailments, they are frequently either ignored or misdiagnosed. Thus it would not be surprising to find that health damage due to such toxins is more prevalent than commonly assumed at present ■

References

Agency for Toxic Substances and Disease Registry (ATSDR). 1992. "Mercury Toxicity." *American Family Physician* 46, no. 6 (Dec.).

Agency for Toxic Substances and Disease Registry (ATSDR). 1990. *Toxicological Profile for Asbestos, TP–90–04.* U.S. Dept. of Health and Human Services (Dec.).

Birnbaum, Linda S. 1994. "The Mechanism of Dioxin Toxicity: Relationship to Risk Assessment." *Environmental Health Perspectives.*

Brodeur, Paul. 1980. *The Asbestos Hazard.* New York Academy of Sciences.

Centers for Disease Control and Prevention (CDC). 1993. "Lead Poisoning in Bridge Demolition Workers—Georgia, 1992." *Morbidity & Mortality Weekly Report* 42, no. 20 (May 28).

Centers for Disease Control and Prevention (CDC). 1992. "Elevated Blood Lead Levels Associated with Illicitly Distilled Alcohol—Alabama, 1990–1991." *Morbidity & Mortality Weekly Report* 41, no. 17 (May 1).

Chao, Jason, M.D., and George D. Kikano, M.D. 1993. "Lead Poisoning in Children." *American Family Physician* (Jan.).

Dickson, L. C., and S. C. Buzik. 1993. "Health Risks of Dioxins: A Review of Environmental and Toxicological Considerations." *Veterinary and Human Toxicology* 35, no. 1 (Feb.).

Environmental Defense Fund (EDF). 1993. "EPA to Ban Lead Fishing Sinkers." *EDF Letter* 24, no. 5 (Sept.).

Environmental Defense Fund and Robert H. Boyle. 1979. *Malignant Neglect.* Random House.

Fawcett, Howard H. 1988. *Hazardous and Toxic Materials: Safe Handling and Disposal.* John Wiley & Sons.

Fingerhut, Marilyn A. et al. 1991. "Cancer Mortality in Workers Exposed to 2,3,7,8-Tetrachlorodibenzo-p-Dioxin." *The New England Journal of Medicine* 324, no. 4 (Jan. 24).

Florini, Karen L. 1990. *Legacy of Lead: America's Continuing Epidemic of Childhood Lead Poisoning.* Environmental Defense Fund.

Franklin, Deborah. 1991. "Lead: Still Poison After All These Years." In *Health* 5, no. 5 (Sept.-Oct.).

Great Lakes Basin Commission. 1980. "PCBs: You Can Store Them Up, But Can You Throw Them Out?" *Great Lakes Communicator* 11, no. 3 (Dec.).

Grum, Emily E., M.D. 1990. *Case Studies in Environmental Medicine: Cadmium Toxicity.* Agency for Toxic Substances and Disease Registry, U.S. Dept. of Health and Human Services (June).

Luoma, Jon R. 1992. "New Effect of Pollutants: Hormone Mayhem." *New York Times,* March 24.

Needleman, H. L. et al. 1990. "The Long-Term Effects of Exposure to Low Doses of Lead in Childhood." *The New England Journal of Medicine* 322:83–88.

Needleman, H. L. et al. 1979. "Deficits in Psychologic and Classroom Performance of Children with Elevated Dentine Lead Levels." *The New England Journal of Medicine* 300:689–95.

"Paper Quantifies Airborne Mercury: Forecasts Decline in Future Levels." 1993. *Environmental Health Letter* (July 7).

Preventing Lead Poisoning in Young Children. 1991. U.S. Dept. of Health and Human Services, Centers for Disease Control.

Regenstein, Lewis. 1982. *The Poisoning of America.* Acropolis Books.

Schneider, Keith. 1992. "Panel Finds No Wide Threat of Cancer Caused by Dioxin." *New York Times,* Sept. 26.

Settle, D. M., and C. C. Patterson. 1980. "Lead in Albacore: Guide to Lead Pollution in Americans." *Science* 207.

Smith, A. 1977. "Congenital Minamata Disease." Proceedings of a Conference on Women and the Workplace, Washington, D.C.: The Society for Occupational and Environmental Health.

Taueg, C. et al. 1992. "Acute and Chronic Poisoning from Residential Exposures to Elemental Mercury—Michigan, 1989–1990." *Clinical Toxicology* 30, no. 1.

Tschirley, Fred H. 1986. "Dioxin." *Scientific American* 254, no. 2 (Feb.).

Waldbott, G. L. 1978. *Health Effects of Environmental Pollutants.* C. V. Mosby.

Weisskopf, Michael. 1987. "Japanese Town Still Staggered by Legacy of Ecological Disaster." *The Washington Post,* April 18.

Weitzman, Michael et al. 1993. "Lead-Contaminated Soil Abatement and Urban Children's Blood Lead Levels." *Journal of the American Medical Association* 269, no. 13 (April 7).

Xintaras, Charles. 1992. "Impact of Lead-Contaminated Soil on Public Health." Agency for Toxic Substances and Disease Registry, U.S. Dept. of Health and Human Services (May).

CHAPTER 8

Pests and Pesticides

And the locusts came up over all the land of Egypt, and settled on the whole country of Egypt . . . they covered the face of the whole land, so that the land was darkened, and they ate all the plants in the land and all the fruit of the trees . . . not a green thing remained, neither tree nor plant of the field, through all the land of Egypt.

—Exodus 10:14–15 RSV

The infestation of locusts which caused Pharaoh and his people such distress was but one of countless incidents recorded throughout history of the harmful, sometimes disastrous, impact which certain insects, fungi, rodents, and so on, can have on human health and well-being. Such organisms are typically referred to as "pests," a term derived from the Latin word *pestis* ("plague"), which was applied to a number of deadly epidemic diseases which periodically swept through the ancient world.

What Is a Pest?

Biologically speaking, there is, of course, no such thing as a "pest"; no classification system divides living things into categories labelled "good species" and "bad species." The term "pest," then, is a purely human concept and refers broadly to any organism—animal, plant, or microbe—which adversely affects human interests. Pest species comprise only a small percentage of the total number of organisms on earth, the vast majority being either beneficial or, more commonly, neutral so far as their impact on humans is concerned. Pests are not restricted to any one taxonomic group; representative species can be found among such invertebrates as insects, mites, ticks, and nematodes. Several bird species such as starlings, pigeons, and English sparrows can be considered pests, as can some mammals—rats, mice, moles, rabbits, and, in some situations, deer, coyotes, or even elephants! Many types of microorganisms, such as disease-causing bacteria, viruses, rickettsia, and fungi, are pests, as are weeds—plants which happen to be growing where they're not wanted (the proverbial petunia in the onion patch could justifiably be considered a pest, for example).

Problems Caused by Pests

Conflict between people and pests has existed since time immemorial and is generated primarily when such organisms compete with humans for the same resources, cause us discomfort, or are vectors of disease. The need to protect human interests by limiting pest damage has created a demand for better methods of combatting such problems and constitutes the chief justification for the development and use of chemical pesticides. Although the use of such toxic compounds has, for a variety of reasons, come under increasing scrutiny and criticism in recent years, it is important to review the types of problems caused by pests in order to understand why suggestions to limit or abolish the use of chemical pesticides generates such controversy.

Resource Competition

Insects, weeds, and plant pathogens (fungi, nematodes, bacteria and viruses) are responsible for the loss of an estimated 30–35% of the global harvest each year, despite 50 years of escalating chemical warfare against agricultural pests. Insect problems are particularly severe on corn and cotton (over 10% of all pesticide use worldwide is directed to cotton production; in the United States, corn, citrus, cotton, and apples account for the largest percentage of insecticide applications). Fungal diseases cause significant losses primarily to fruits and some vegetables, while yield reductions due to weed infestations are most pronounced on acreage devoted to corn and soybean production. In addition to such losses in the field, about 6% of the annual harvest in the United States (and a substantially larger share in developing nations) is lost to pests while in storage or transit.

A reduction in current pesticide use would undoubtedly result in a further increase in crop loss due to pest depredation—a cause for concern both to farmers and to humanitarians worried about feeding a hungry world. The extent of such loss is hotly disputed, however. The U.S. Department of Agriculture estimates that without pesticides, American agricultural production would drop by at least 25% and food prices would rise by 50%. Some agriculturalists, such as Norman Borlaug ("Father of the Green Revolution") and former Agriculture Secretary Earl Butz predict crop losses as great as 50% if all pesticide use were banned. Others, however, calculate that preharvest losses of all crops resulting from a significant reduction in pesticide use would be minimal. A noted entomologist at Cornell University estimates that if American farmers were to adopt a variety of nonchemical control techniques they could cut current levels of agricultural pesticide use by 50% without experiencing any decline in yields. Under this scenario, substituting nonchemical for chemical controls would result in food price increases of less than 1% (Pimental, 1991).

Although loss in farm production is the major example of resource competition between humans and pests, many other instances of conflict can be cited: termites cause millions of dollars worth of property damage annually; clothes moths have destroyed many a fine winter coat or woolen blanket; prairie dogs and fire ants construct burrows and mounds, respectively, on pasture lands, significantly reducing their value; rats and mice cause enormous economic loss, both by consuming vast amounts of food and by damaging property—between 5–25% of the fires of unknown origin on farms are suspected of being caused by rats gnawing the insulation from electric wires (Pratt, Gjornson, and Littig, 1977).

Sources of Discomfort

Itching, buzzing, creeping, and crawling may not seem like serious concerns, but the creatures responsible have been driving people to distraction for millennia and have been the targets of a great deal of pesticide use in recent decades. Some of the major villains involved in producing acute human discomfort, if not illness, include the following.

Lice.   Head lice, body lice, and crab lice are all human parasites which can cause severe itching, secondary infections, and scarred or hardened skin. Lice are typically associated with people living in crowded conditions where opportunities for bathing and laundering clothes are limited. With the introduction of DDT following World War II, the incidence of lice infestations dropped to low levels. As the use of this insecticide became restricted, however, cases of head lice among school children have been increasing.

Fleas.   Aside from the flea species which transmit the deadly plague bacterium (see next section), fleas commonly found on domestic animals can cause severe irritation, loss of blood, and discomfort. Although most fleas prefer to feed on their animal host, they frequently bite humans if the normal host is absent. Such bites can be extremely painful and may cause swelling and a reddening of the skin.

Mites.   These tiny insect relatives are responsible for the serious skin condition known as scabies, as well as a number of other forms of dermatitis such as "grocers' itch," acquired by handling mite-infested grain products, cheese, dried fruits, and so on. Mites that normally live as ectoparasites on birds may become very serious pests of humans when they migrate in large numbers into homes after starlings or sparrows leave their nests. For this reason, householders should discourage birds from nesting on eaves or windowsills or other locations in close proximity to homes. **Chiggers**, a type of mite inhabiting many parts of the southern or midwestern United States, can cause extreme skin irritation lasting for a week or more when they attach themselves to a human host, usually around the waist or armpits.

Bedbugs.   Hiding during the day in mattresses, bedsprings, cracks in the wall, and so on, bedbugs cause many a sleepless night and produce large, intensely itchy welts on sensitive victims. Fortunately they are not known to transmit any disease.

Spiders.   Although many people harbor an irrational antipathy toward spiders, the vast majority of these eight-legged creatures are quite harmless to humans. Even the fearsome-looking tarantula—the loathsome villain in many a B-grade Hollywood thriller—is actually rather docile. Now widely sold as pets, tarantulas can be handled with ease and rarely bite; even when they do, their venom is of little harm to most people. Only three U.S. species present any real danger: the **black widow** (female only), the **brown recluse** (both sexes), and the **aggressive house spider** (males more venomous and more likely to bite than females). The black widow, though more abundant in warmer regions of the country, can be found throughout the United States; primarily an outdoor spider, the black widow is typically found around piles of wood or other debris where the female spins a nondescript-looking web. Black widow venom acts as a nerve poison, but while bites may be quite painful they are very seldom fatal, even in the absence of medical attention. Contrary to popular myth, the diminutive male black widow is *not* devoured after mating by his much larger bride—unless she is unusually hungry!—but generally spends a parasitic post-nuptial existence in the vicinity of her web, waiting for any leftovers that may come his way. The brown recluse spider, whose range covers much of the south-central and southeastern United States as far north as Missouri, Illinois, and Indiana, is most often encountered within dwellings where it hides in attics, closets, and other dark, seldom-disturbed places. It is a shy, retiring species that bites only when provoked—usually when rolled on at night or when clothes are taken out of storage. The poison injected by the bite of a brown recluse differs from that of a black widow in that it is *cytotoxic,* causing tissue death in the vicinity of the wound. Scarcely noticeable at first, the bite gradually becomes very painful and frequently develops into an open ulceration that persists for weeks and eventually leaves a large ugly scar. The aggressive house spider, a European immigrant whose range is currently limited to British Columbia and the states of the Pacific Northwest, has only recently been identified as the source of spider bites long attributed to the brown recluse (which doesn't live in that part of the country). Like brown recluse venom, that of the aggressive house spider is a cytotoxin, causing tissue necrosis very similar to that of a brown recluse bite. *Unlike* the brown recluse, however, aggressive house spiders are true to their name and tend to bite without provocation. Large (40 mm in length) and fast-running, these spiders tend to live in or near houses, often in rock walls, along foundations, or in woodpiles (many bites occur when firewood is being carried inside). Large numbers of males enter basements and ground floor rooms of homes in the autumn and dogs and cats are frequently bitten on the face as they attempt to investigate, occasionally dying as a result. These are *not* nice spiders! (Akre and Myhre, 1994)

In addition to the above, the buzzing of flies, mosquitoes, gnats, cicadas, June bugs, or wasps—even when these insects are not carrying disease organisms—can provoke extreme annoyance. Ants marching across the floor, crickets chirping in a corner, or spiders spinning their webs on the chandelier often sufficiently arouse the householder into reaching for a can of pesticide spray. Certain plant species also, particularly poison ivy and its relatives, have been prime targets of chemical herbicides because of the intensely irritating rash which contact with these plants can produce.

Vectors of Disease

Public health practitioners, along with farmers, were among the first to greet the introduction of synthetic chemical pesticides with great enthusiasm. Compounds such as DDT were viewed as perhaps the ultimate weapon in freeing humanity from the threat of a number of insect- or rodent-borne diseases responsible for millions of deaths and illnesses each year. Quite appropriately, the first use to which DDT was put involved the wartime dusting of refugees in Italy to curb an outbreak of typhus fever. The success of this effort led to extensive spraying campaigns in many parts of the world against the vectors of such dreaded killers as malaria, yellow fever, river blindness, bubonic plague, and encephalitis. Although the medical community's high hopes for complete eradication of the carriers of these diseases have proven overly optimistic, pesticide use has played a significant role in lowering death rates and improving public health in many parts of the world. Some pests of particular public health importance include mosquitoes, flies, body lice, rat fleas, and ticks.

Mosquitoes.   Mosquitoes have probably been responsible for more human deaths than any other insect, though their role as disease-carriers was not recognized until late in the 19th century. Worldwide, even today millions of people become ill each year due to such mosquito-borne ailments as malaria, yellow fever, dengue, filariasis, and encephalitis. In the past, there have been major outbreaks of all these diseases, particularly malaria and yellow fever, in parts of the United States. In recent years, entry of large numbers of infected immigrants from tropical regions where malaria is still endemic has been primarily responsible for the several hundred new cases of malaria being reported in the United States each year. In addition, some cases of so-called "airport malaria" have been diagnosed among Americans returning from trips abroad as a result of visiting countries where malaria is still a problem. One traveler, en route home after a business trip to Australia, was bitten by an infected mosquito during a one-hour refueling stop in Liberia and several weeks later died of malaria when his personal physician in Connecticut misdiagnosed his fever and chills as a bad case of influenza. As malaria rates continue to rise in Africa and southern Asia, such cases prompt warnings to travelers not to neglect taking prophylactics for this very serious disease before visiting affected areas. Of mosquito-borne disease outbreaks within the United States today, only encephalitis continues to occur with some frequency. During times when mosquito populations are high and when the viral pathogen of the disease has been detected in birds or small mammals (the virus is generally carried to humans by a mosquito which has previously bitten an infected bird), chemical spraying may be carried out by local authorities to prevent the possibility of encephalitis, a disease which in severe cases can permanently damage the central nervous system or even kill its victim. Although the last major U.S. outbreak of a mosquito-borne disease occurred in 1975 (a St. Louis encephalitis epidemic which killed 142 and sickened more than 2000 throughout the Midwest), vector-control officials had a new cause for worry in the late 1980s when some unwelcome stowaways arrived with a shipment of used tires in the port of Houston. *Aedes albopictus*, the **Asian tiger mosquito**, quickly spread from Texas throughout much of the eastern United States, presumably hitch-hiking on the truckloads of used tires which ply the interstate highway system (the insect lays its eggs just above the waterline in treeholes or artificial containers—like tires). Because tiger mosquito eggs can overwinter, *A. albopictus* is already

Figure 8-1 Some Serious Pest-Borne Diseases of Humans

Disease	Causative Agent	Vector	Method of Infection
African sleeping sickness	trypanosome	tsetse fly	bite
Cholera	bacterium, *Vibrio cholerae*	house fly	contamination of foods
Dengue fever	virus	*Aedes* mosquito	bite
Dysentery, amoebic	protozoan	housefly	contamination of foods
Dysentery, bacillary	bacterium, *Shigella sp.*	house fly	contamination of foods
Encephalitis	virus	*Culex* mosquito	bite
Lyme Disease	spirochete bacterium *Borrelia burgdorferi*	deer tick	bite
Malaria	protozoan, *Plasmodium vivax*	*Anopheles* mosquito	bite
Onchocerciasis (River blindness)	parasitic worm, *Onchocerca volvulus*	black flies	bite
Plague	bacterium, *Pasteurella pestis*	Oriental rat flea and other fleas	bite or contact with infected rodents
Rocky Mountain spotted fever	rickettsia *Rickettsia rickettsi*	American dog tick	bite
Typhoid fever	bacterium, *Salmonella typhi*	house fly	contamination of food and water
Typhus	rickettsia, *Rickettsia prowazeki*	human body louse	contamination of bite and abrasions
Yellow fever	virus	*Aedes* mosquito	bite

becoming established as far north as Illinois and Ohio. Unlike many other mosquitoes, it can also live inside houses year-round, breeding in pet water dishes and in the saucers under flowerpots. The tiger mosquito is a vicious biter and, in its Asian homeland, is an important disease vector. Although as yet no outbreaks have been attributed to the newcomer, researchers have determined that *A. albopictus* has the ability to pick up and transmit the viral pathogens for dengue fever and encephalitis and fear that it has the potential to become the most important carrier of mosquito-borne diseases in the United States. These fears were given added urgency in 1992 when a tiger mosquito captured in Florida, just 12 miles from DisneyWorld, was found to be harboring the virus for Eastern equine encephalitis, the most deadly form of the disease which, until now, has been carried primarily by salt marsh mosquitoes whose preferred habitat is remote from

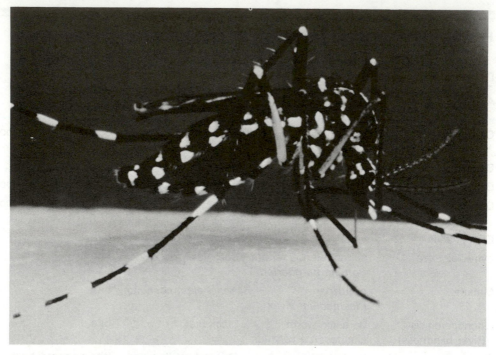

Asian Tiger Mosquito: a vicious biter and potential disease vector, *Aedes albopictus* has spread rapidly through the southern and midwestern states since its accidental introduction to the U.S. in 1985. [American Mosquito Control Association/L. Munstermann]

human settlements. The tiger mosquito, by contrast, lives in close proximity to people and thus represents a more serious public health concern.

Flies.   Many species of flies, particularly the common housefly, are important carriers of serious gastrointestinal diseases such as typhoid fever, cholera, dysentery, and parasitic worm infections due to their habit of feeding on human and animal wastes. If such wastes contain pathogenic organisms, the fly can pick these up either on the sticky pads of its feet or on its body hairs or mouthparts and mechanically transmit them to humans when it alights on food materials. Fly vomitus and feces also frequently contain pathogenic bacteria which can inoculate human food, multiply rapidly in the food medium, and subsequently result in outbreaks of intestinal diseases when the food is consumed by people.

Body Lice.   As mentioned in the previous section, body lice can be a source of intense discomfort, but they are of special public health concern because they are vectors of several serious epidemic diseases. Typhus fever, characterized by elevated temperature, severe headache, and a rash, has been a major killer in past centuries, particularly during wartime when perhaps as many soldiers died from typhus as from swords or bullets. The rickettsial pathogen responsible for the disease is passed from louse to human by the feces of the insect, not its bite. When a person infested with

BOX 8-1
Hantavirus: A New Disguise for an Old Disease

"Navajo flu" the media called it—the mysterious, often lethal ailment that first attracted national attention in the early summer of 1993. Initially reported from the Four Corner region of the American Southwest, the malady's early victims were predominantly Native Americans on the vast Navajo reservation. As the months passed and new cases were reported from as far afield as California, Kansas, Florida, and Rhode Island, it became apparent that the ailment was anything but restrictive in its choice of victims.

Initial manifestations of the infection don't cause particular alarm among those stricken—the fever, chills, headache, cough, muscular aches and pains are similar to symptoms associated with many mundane illnesses. "I thought I was coming down with the flu . . . so I took a couple of Tylenol and went to bed," remarked one survivor. Very quickly, however, the disease takes a nasty turn as the lungs fill with fluids leaking from surrounding capillaries, leading to acute respiratory distress. Within days after the onset of symptoms, two-thirds of patients die of respiratory failure; currently there is no specific treatment for the disease other than supportive intensive care given to severe cases (work is underway to develop a vaccine, but none is yet commercially available).

The Four Corners outbreak of what at the time appeared to be a previously unknown disease precipitated a crash effort by public health officials to determine what was causing the deadly illness. Investigators quickly eliminated such possibilities as plague or environmental toxins and soon obtained laboratory evidence confirming that a pathogenic agent known as **hantavirus** was the culprit behind the outbreak. This discovery caused considerable

surprise among the medical detectives because hantavirus infections, although not unusual in other parts of the world, had never before caused acute human illness in the United States—nor had they ever before been manifested primarily as a respiratory disease. In the U.S. outbreak, hantavirus had assumed a new disguise which initially deceived those who were trying to track it down.

Previous outbreaks of hantavirus-associated illnesses in Asia and elsewhere (usually referred to as "hemorrhagic fever") have always involved kidney failure as a distinctive feature and the absence of renal complications among U.S. victims accounted for much of the initial delay in identifying what is now referred to as **Hantavirus Pulmonary Syndrome** (HPS). In retrospect, it is now known that two cases of HPS had occurred in the Southwest the year prior to the major outbreak but were not reported, the cause attributed at the time to "unknown respiratory illness."

A group of rodent-borne pathogens, hantaviruses can be carried by more than 16 different rodent species (rats, mice, voles, and so forth) and have recently been found to infect cats and chickens as well; most strains of the virus are associated with a specific rodent host—in the Four Corners outbreak the common deer mouse (*Peromyscus maniculatus*) was identified as the carrier, while the rodent vector responsible for the Florida case is assumed to be the cotton rat (*Sigmodon hispidus*). Generally present in its animal host as a non-symptomatic, chronic infection, the virus is shed in urine, feces, and saliva and can be transmitted to other rodents or to humans either by direct contact or by inhalation of aerosolized rodent excreta containing viral particles (person-to-person spread has never been documented). Outbreaks of what was probably hemorrhagic fever have occurred sporadically over the centuries, the first having been described in a 1000-year-old Chinese medical text. Several 20th century episodes, both involving military forces, have occurred in East Asia, the first during the 1930s in Manchuria, followed by an outbreak among U.N. troops during the Korean War ("Korean hemorrhagic fever"). The latter occurrence focused world attention on the disease, prompting intensified research efforts which ultimately led to identification of hantaviruses as the causative agent.

The recent emergence of hantavirus as a dangerous human pathogen in the United States dramatizes several troubling realities: not only do different strains of the virus exhibit extreme variability in their clinical manifestations, but the geographic areas to which hantaviruses have long been endemic now appear to be expanding. As a result, although the disease is still considered quite rare, it is important for the public to be aware of its existence and to take precautionary measures to avoid exposure. Since the primary risk factor for acquiring hantavirus is **exposure to rodents or rodent excretions**, the main strategy for preventing infection is to avoid contact with these animals and their burrows. There is reason to believe that the 1993 outbreak in the Southwest may have resulted, at least in part, from piñon nut-gathering activities by the victims. A bumper crop had been produced that year, supporting a surge in populations of the deer mice, which stored large numbers of the nuts in their burrows. Raids on those burrows by human foragers may well have enhanced the opportunity for viral transmission from infected deer mice to people. Similarly, a Kansas housewife who died of Hantavirus Pulmonary Syndrome in the fall of 1993 was reported by her husband to have routinely trapped and disposed of mice in the old farmhouse they were refurbishing. Since investigators suspect that hantavirus is now well established among deer mice populations and other rodent species throughout the country, a number of public health officials are urging restoration of community rodent control programs, many of which were allowed to lapse due to fiscal belt-tightening by government agencies. Simultaneously, state health departments are issuing advisories to households, warning about new hazards of mice infestations, advising that gloves be worn whenever removing dead mice from traps and recommending that a household disinfectant (e.g. 1-1/2 cups of chlorine bleach in a gallon of water) be used to mop areas frequented by mice. Extra efforts should be made to exclude rodents from buildings and from areas adjacent to structures where people live or work. Those who work in occupations which might expose them to rodent excretions—farm laborers, electricians, construction workers who demolish or renovate old buildings—should wear respirators or face masks to avoid inhaling virus-bearing dust; campers are advised not to sleep directly on the ground in areas where rodent populations are present, since rodent urine and feces are omnipresent in such environments.

For those who not so long ago blithely assumed that vector-borne diseases were no longer a cause for concern among industrialized societies, hantavirus has provided a wake-up call—a reminder that microbial pathogens are still out there, ready and waiting to strike whenever humanity becomes careless or complacent.

References

Larson, Erik, and Eric Morgenthaler. 1994. "Killer Disease, Borne by Rodents, Is Found in Wider Areas of U.S." *Wall Street Journal*, Jan. 14.

Sinnott, John T., MD, et al. 1993. "Hantavirus: An Old Bug Learns New Tricks." *Infection Control and Hospital Epidemiology* 14, no. 11 (Nov.).

Figure 8-2 Distribution of *Peromyscus maniculatus* and Number of Recognized Cases of Hantavirus Pulmonary Syndrome*

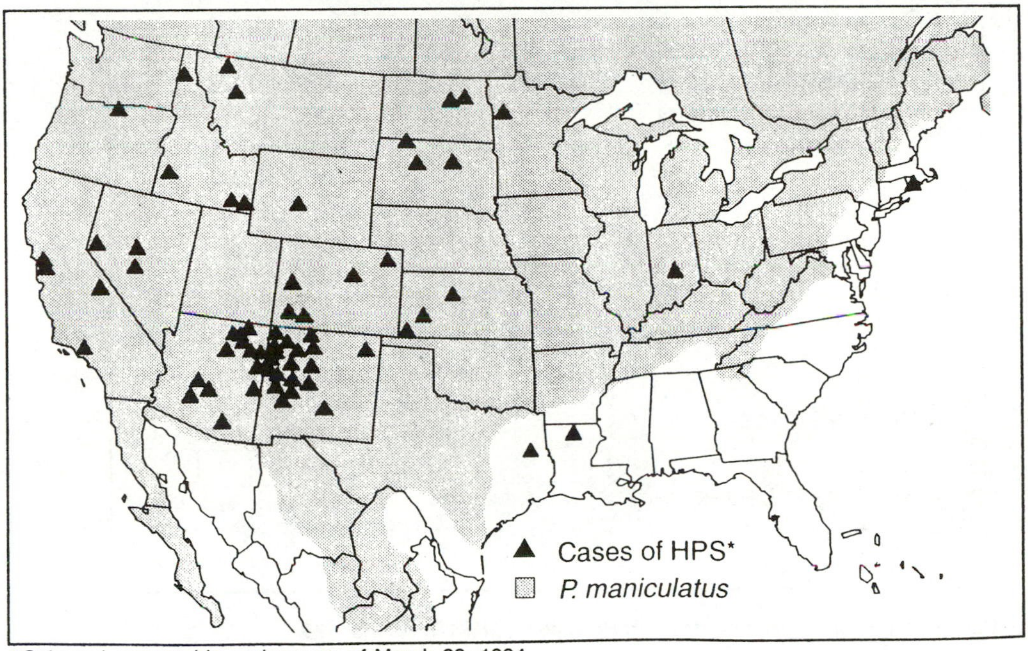

▲ Cases of HPS*
▢ *P. maniculatus*

*Selected geographic regions, as of March 23, 1994
Source: Centers for Disease Control and Prevention.

lice scratches the affected area, minor abrasions on the skin permit entry to the rickettsia. Other lice subsequently feeding on a person infected with typhus ingest the pathogen and spread it as they move from person to person. This method of transmission explains why typhus outbreaks are most prevalent when people are living together in crowded, unsanitary conditions. Insecticidal dusting of louse-infested persons has proven to be an effective method for controlling the spread of typhus fever. Two other louse-borne diseases, also most common during wartime but with much lower fatality rates than typhus, are trench fever and relapsing fever.

Rat Fleas.   Aside from the enormous economic damage caused by rats, these pests are of great public health concern because they are vectors of a number of diseases, the most deadly of which is plague (the "Black Death" of medieval times). In September 1994 the first major plague outbreak in half a century terrorized residents of the Indian city of Surat, killing more than 50 people and reminding the world that the infectious killers of the past remain a threat even as we approach the 21st century. The plague bacterium actually is carried by fleas on rats, not by the rats themselves. When infected fleas feed on their rat hosts, the rats too sicken and die. If rats are living in close proximity to humans, a flea whose host

Figure 8-3 Number of Human Plague Cases Reported, by State and Decade, U.S., 1944–1993

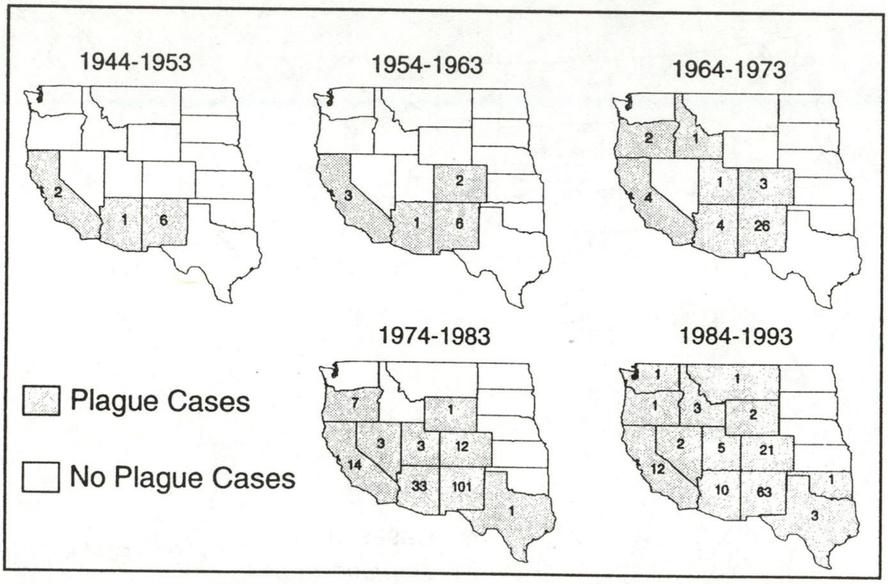

Source: Centers for Disease Control and Prevention, *MMWR*, April 8, 1994.

has died may then hop onto a person for a blood meal and thus spread the plague organism to human populations. Because of the tendency of fleas to substitute hosts when necessary, rat poisoning campaigns should always be preceded by insecticidal spraying of rat-infested areas to kill the fleas first. If this is not done, one runs the risk of transferring rodent diseases to humans.

While most Americans tend to think of plague as a "long-ago and far-away" type of disease, rat fleas infected with the plague bacterium were introduced into California early in this century and quickly became endemic among wild rodent populations in the region. Since that time the focus of plague infection has expanded steadily eastward; today plague-infected rodent populations have been identified in 13 western states and during the past 50 years 363 cases of human plague have been reported from this region. The incidence of plague outbreaks in the United States seem to be increasing, as rapid suburbanization results in growing numbers of people living in close proximity to wild rodent habitat. A worrisome trend noted in recent years is a rise in the number of human cases in which domestic cats were the source of infection—15 such instances between 1977–1993. Because cats typically are allowed to roam freely, those living in areas where plague-infected rodents are common have ample opportunity to contract the disease and subsequently transmit the ailment to their human companions (CDC, 1994). People living, camping, hiking, or hunting in areas where plague is endemic should take precautions to avoid contact with wild rodents and rodent burrows (where infected fleas may be present) and should never approach or handle obviously sick or dying wild animals. Even recently-dead rodents can present a disease hazard: one plague death in the Southwest involved a housewife who picked up a dead ground squirrel which her cat had proudly deposited on the doorstep. She presumably was bitten by a hungry flea who found her an acceptable alternative host and subsequently contracted a fatal case of bubonic plague.

Ticks.   Among our most common parasites, ticks are a source of profound annoyance to campers, hunters, dog owners, and livestock raisers who frequently discover themselves or their pets providing a blood meal to these tiny pests. Ticks are far more than a nuisance, however. They are vectors of several serious human diseases such as Rocky Mountain spotted fever, a condition that frequently results in death within two weeks and which, contrary to its name, is not restricted to mountainous areas but is found throughout the continental United States, with the largest number of cases being reported from North and South Carolina. Lyme disease, an

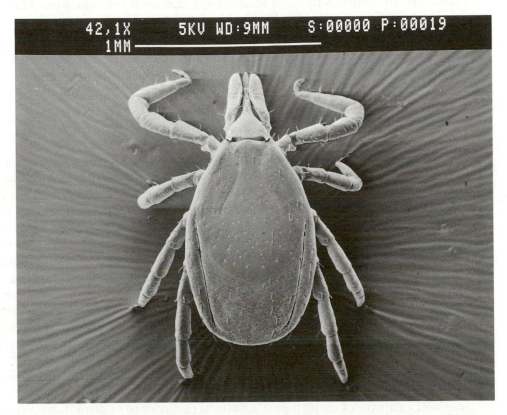

The diminutive deer tick (*Ixodes scapularis*) carries the bacterium that causes Lyme Disease. [Mathew Nadakavukaren]

ailment scarcely heard of by most Americans until a few years ago, has now been reported from 47 states (it also occurs throughout Europe and in parts of Africa, Asia, and Australia) and is currently by far the most commonly diagnosed vector-borne disease in the nation (see Box 8–2). Q-fever, relapsing fever, tularemia, and tick paralysis are just a few of many ailments which can be transmitted by ticks. Species which most commonly feed on humans generally are found in areas of wild vegetation such as woods, high grass, parks, and along paths frequented by wild animals. Here they lie in wait for a potential human or animal host, clinging to bushes or tall weeds, ready to latch onto an unwary passer-by (contrary to popular belief, they don't drop onto victims from trees). People planning outdoor activities in tick-infested areas should take such precautions as applying tick repellent to exposed areas of skin, wearing socks and long trousers, and avoiding sitting on the ground or on logs. They should also be diligent about checking their bodies for the presence of ticks at least twice a day and immediately removing them, since most tick-borne diseases are transmitted only after the creature has been feeding for several hours.

Although the above is by no means a complete listing of the human health problems caused by various pest species, it should convey some realization of the need for pest control and an understanding of why many public health officials feel that abandoning chemical pesticides would entail the risk of increased mortality and morbidity rates due to vector-borne disease.

Pest Control

Early Attempts at Pest Control

Human efforts to control pest outbreaks date back to the development of agriculture approximately 10,000 years ago, when relatively large expanses of a single crop and sizeable numbers of people living close together in none-too-sanitary conditions favored an increase in pest populations which wouldn't have been possible among small, scattered societies living a nomadic, hunter-gatherer type of life-style. Early attempts to reduce pest damage included purely physical efforts—stomping, flailing, burning—as well as the offering of prayers, sacrifices, and ritual dances to the local gods. A few effective measures were discovered even at such early dates, however. The Sumerians, in what now is Iraq, successfully employed sulfur compounds against insects and mites more than 5000 years ago; over 3000 years ago the Chinese were treating seeds with insecticides derived from plant extracts, using wood ashes and chalk to ward off insect pests in the home, and applying mercury and arsenic compounds to their bodies to control lice. Among the Chinese is found the earliest example of using a pest's natural enemies to control it: by A.D. 300 the Chinese were introducing colonies of predatory ants into their citrus groves to control caterpillars and certain beetles.

BOX 8-2
"The Woods are Lovely, Dark, and Deep . . ." but Beware of Lyme Disease!

It was late in the fall of 1975 when the small town of Lyme in southeastern Connecticut became the unlikely setting for the opening chapter of a modern-day medical mystery and ultimately bestowed its name on the vector-borne scourge of the late 20th century, **Lyme Disease**. In November of that year, the Connecticut State Health Department was notified of an abnormally high incidence of juvenile rheumatoid arthritis, normally a very rare ailment, in Lyme and several neighboring communities. Suspecting that something was amiss, Department officials summoned a team of epidemiologists from Yale to investigate the situation. The geographic distribution and timing of disease outbreaks (most of the victims lived in wooded areas and developed disease symptoms between June and late September) suggested that some sort of vector-borne pathogen was involved, but it took several years of extensive investigation by researchers at a number of institutions to solve the baffling puzzles posed by this new ailment.

It is now known that the villain responsible for the wide array of unpleasant symptoms which make life miserable for Lyme Disease victims is a spirochete bacterium, *Borrelia burgdorferi*, transmitted to humans (as well as to dogs and horses which are also susceptible) by the bite of an infected deer tick, *Ixodes scapularis* (on the West Coast the main vector is the closely related species, *I. pacificus*).

That the tiny arthropod should first surface as a troublemaker in the well-to-do residential developments spreading into New England woodlands is, in retrospect, not surprising; deer ticks are most abundant in the transitional vegetation characteristic of woody suburban areas where clearings have been cut in the forest or lawns established amidst woods—the type of habitat attractive to deer and a variety of small mammals and birds which provide the main source of sustenance for *I. scapularis*. Similarly, conservation efforts which have resulted in a population explosion among deer herds have also contributed to a corresponding increase in the prevalence of deer ticks.

The tick's life cycle extends over a two-year period; after hatching from eggs laid early in the spring, deer ticks spend their first year as tiny six-legged larvae which feed just once on the blood of a small mammal or bird, then overwinter and molt the following spring into a slightly larger eight-legged nymph. Nymphs also must take a blood meal before molting to the adult stage at the end of their second summer. Although the white-footed mouse is the most frequent host for tick nymphs, an unwary human is also fair game, and it is at this stage of the tick's life cycle that people are most likely to be bitten. Adult deer ticks, about the size of a match-head, climb onto shrubs or vegetation about three feet off the ground and lie in wait for a deer, human, or other large animal upon which they climb, feed once, drop to the ground, and then mate. Because the tick is so small and inconspicuous, a human victim may not even realize he or she has been bitten until disease symptoms appear, generally several days to a month later.

Three distinct phases of the disease have been described, though not all victims experience each stage. The first and most characteristic feature of Lyme Disease is a spreading red rash (*erythema chronica migrans*) which begins as a small red bump but expands outward in a circular pattern, 4–20 inches in diameter, resembling a rosy "bull's eye" because of the pale area of skin in the center. Most often occurring on the back, buttocks, chest, or stomach, this rash is frequently accompanied by a splitting headache, fever, chills, back-ache, and a feeling of extreme fatigue. The second stage manifests itself primarily as nervous system dysfunction and muscular pains. Some sufferers experience heart problems which may require temporary use of cardiac pacemakers, while others occasionally develop such serious neurological disorders as meningitis or Bell's palsy. The onset of arthritis, usually in the knees or other large joints, typifies the third stage of the disease; attacks generally persist for a few days to several weeks at a time and can be extremely painful. Luckily, since the pathogen causing Lyme Disease is a bacterium, once diagnosed the ailment can be treated by oral administration of an antibiotic such as amoxicillin or deoxycycline. When given early during the rash stage of the disease, such medication generally leads to a quick and complete cure. When used to treat later stages of the disease, antibiotics may or may not be effective—perhaps as many as 50% of patients who have developed chronic symptoms don't respond.

Since surveillance for Lyme Disease was first initiated in 1982, almost 50,000 cases have been reported to CDC. By the early 1990s, nearly 10,000 cases a year were being tallied—a 19-fold increase over the 497 cases from 11 states reported in 1982. The startling rise in incidence may be accounted for in part by heightened awareness of the disease among both patients and physicians, increased reliance on laboratory testing for accurate diagnosis, and more effective surveillance and reporting procedures (49 states and the District of Columbia now require that diagnosed cases of Lyme Disease be reported to the appropriate authorities). A number of medical authorities feel that in certain regions of the country, particularly in the northeast where incidence rates are markedly higher than elsewhere, some of the increase is due to inaccurate over-diagnosis (not long ago, a study published in a leading medical journal reported that only 23% of the patients at a Boston clinic for difficult Lyme cases were actually infected with the causative bacterium!) Nevertheless, most authorities would agree that the number of true cases is indeed increasing. Lyme Disease continues to extend its geographic range (the hypothesis is that birds are carrying *I. scapularis* from one region of the country to another, since tick larvae frequently feed on avian hosts) and to increase in frequency within the areas where it is already well-established.

Clinical trials of a vaccine against Lyme Disease were undertaken on a small group of volunteers in the spring of 1994, offering hope that a preventative approach to combatting the ailment will eventually be available (an anti-Lyme vaccine for dogs has been commercially available for several years but is of limited effectiveness). In the meantime, for hikers, campers, or suburbanites visiting or living in tick-infested areas the advice is to be wary, wear protective clothing, promptly remove any ticks discovered on the body, and contact a physician immediately if mysterious problems arise after a walk in the woods.

References

CDC, 1993. "Lyme Disease—United States, 1991–92." *MMWR* 42, no. 18 (May 14).

Habicht, Gail, Gregory Beck, and Jorge L. Benach. 1987. "Lyme Disease." *Scientific American* 257 (July).

During the peak of Greek civilization, records indicate that some of the wealthier citizens used mosquito nets and built high sleeping towers to evade mosquitoes. They also used oil sprays and sulfur bitumen ointments to deter insects. The Romans designed ratproof granaries, but relied largely on superstitious practices such as nailing up crayfish in different parts of the garden to keep away caterpillars.

In medieval Europe people increasingly relied on religious faith to protect them from pest depredations; as late as 1476, during an outbreak of cutworms in Switzerland, several of the offending insects were hauled into court, proclaimed guilty, excommunicated by the archbishop, and banished from the land!

Not until the 18th and 19th centuries did efforts at pest control make any meaningful progress. This was a time when European farming practices were becoming more productive and scientific and help in combatting agricultural pests was eagerly sought. Botanical insecticides such as pyrethrum, derris (rotenone), and nicotine were introduced at this time. Heightened interest in improved pest control methods was generated during the mid-19th century by several of the worst agricultural disasters ever recorded—the potato late blight in Ireland, England, and Belgium in 1848, caused by a fungal disease; the fungus leaf spot disease of coffee in Ceylon which completely wiped out coffee cultivation on the island; and the outbreak of both powdery mildew and an insect pest, grape phylloxera, which nearly destroyed the wine industry in Europe. Such problems led to the development of new chemical pesticides and ushered in a whole new era of pest control. Two of the first such compounds, Bordeaux mixture (copper sulfate and lime) and Paris Green (copper acetoarsenite), were originally employed as fungicides but were subsequently found to be effective insecticides as well. Paris Green became one of the most widely used insecticides in the late 19th century and Bordeaux mixture even today is the most widely used fungicide in the world. Early in the 1900s arsenic-containing compounds such as lead arsenate, highly toxic to both insects and humans, became the most widely sold insecticides in the United States and retained their leading position until the advent of DDT after World War II (Flint and VandenBosch, 1981).

In 1939, Paul Müller, a Swiss chemist working for the Geigy Corporation, discovered that the synthetic compound dichlorodiphenyltrichloroethane (referred to as DDT for obvious reasons!) was extremely effective in killing insects on contact and retained its lethal character for a long time after application. Müller had simply been looking for a better product to be used against clothes moths, but the outbreak of war in Europe which coincided with Müller's discovery gave far wider significance to the new chemical. Military authorities, recognizing that extensive campaigns would be carried out in the tropics where insect-borne disease threatened high troop losses, made the search for better insecticides a top priority. DDT, highly lethal to every kind of insect yet harmless to humans when applied as a powder, was just what the military needed. Initially, production of DDT was exclusively for use in the armed forces where it was employed first as a louse powder and later for mosquito control. At the end of the war DDT was released for civilian use, both in agriculture and for public health purposes. Its use quickly spread worldwide, amidst high expectations of complete eradication of many diseases and greatly reduced crop losses due to insects. Müller was awarded the 1948 Nobel Prize in Physiology and Medicine in recognition of his contribution. The enthusiastic reception given to DDT encouraged chemical companies in their search for new and even more effective synthetic pesticides. By the mid-1950s at least 25 new products which would revolutionize insect control practices were put on the market, among the more important of which were chlordane, heptachlor, toxaphene, aldrin, endrin, dieldrin, and parathion (Perkins, 1982). The age of chemical warfare against pests had begun.

Types of Pesticides

Pesticides, substances which kill pests, are subdivided into groups according to target organism. For example, insecticides kill insects, herbicides kill weeds, rodenticides kill rats and mice, nematicides kill nematodes, and so forth. Within each of these groups there may be further subdivisions based on such characteristics as route of intake of the poison or physiological effect on the target organism. A brief survey of some of the most common groups of pesticides currently in use would include the following.

Insecticides.   The largest number of pesticides are employed against a wide variety of insects and include **stomach poisons** (taken into the body through the mouth; effective against insects with biting or chewing mouthparts, such as caterpillars); **contact poisons** (penetrate through the body wall); and **fumigants** (enter insect through its respiratory system). Representative types include:

Inorganic insecticides. Most of these compounds, such as lead arsenate, Paris Green, and a number of other products containing copper, zinc, mercury, chlorine, or sulfur, act as stomach poisons and were the most commonly used insecticides until after World War II. Many of these products are quite toxic to humans as well as to insects and their heavy use left significant concentrations of toxic metals in some fields and orchards. In addition to these compounds, some petroleum derivatives such as kerosene, diesel oil, and #2 fuel oil have been sprayed on water surfaces to suffocate mosquito larvae.

Chlorinated hydrocarbons. DDT and its chemical relatives (chlordane, heptachlor, lindane, BHC, endrin, aldrin, mirex, kepone, toxaphene, etc.) are all contact poisons. They act primarily on the central nervous system, causing the insect to go through a series of convulsions prior to death. Members of this group are **broad-spectrum** insecticides, meaning that they kill a wide range of insects and other arthropods, and are also **persistent** in the environment, breaking down very slowly and therefore retaining their effectiveness for a relatively long period after application. Because the chlorinated hydrocarbons are not water-soluble, they tend to accumulate in fatty tissues when taken up by living organisms and may remain in the body indefinitely. Since the 1970s, many of the chlorinated hydrocarbons have been banned for most uses in the United States because animal testing has shown them to be carcinogenic.

Organophosphates. Developed first by the Germans for possible wartime use as nerve gases, this group includes some of the most deadly insecticides such as methyl parathion, ranked in the "super toxic" category of pesticides. Organophosphates, like chlorinated hydrocarbons, are broad-spectrum contact poisons, but unlike the chlorinated hydrocarbons they are not persistent, usually breaking down two weeks or less after application. Thus they present far less danger to non-target organisms. Organophosphates are nerve poisons which act to inhibit the enzyme cholinesterase, causing the insect to lose coordination and go into convulsions. Members of this group range in terms of human toxicity from the extremely deadly parathion and phosdrin (one drop of these in the eye is fatal to an adult) to the moderately toxic diazinon and dichlorvos (the volatile compound used in some pet flea collars), to the slightly toxic malathion, commonly sold for home garden use.

Carbamates. Widely used today in public health work and agriculture because of their rapid knock-down of insects and low toxicity to mammals (a few, however, are quite toxic and their use is restricted to certified applicators), carbamates too are contact poisons which act in a manner similar to the organophosphates. One of the most common of the carbamates, *Sevin,* is widely used as a garden dust and for mosquito control.

Synthetic pyrethroids and other botanicals. Chemical analogs of the natural insecticide, pyrethrum (an extract of chrysanthemum flowers), synthetic pyrethroids such as allethrin, cyfluthrin, resmethrin, permethrin, and fenvalerate are broad spectrum contact poisons widely used in structural pest control, with a growing number of agricultural applications as well. Providing quick knock-down of insects, the pyrethroids are probably the best choice for home or garden use because of their very low toxicity to humans and domestic animals. For this reason, they are among the few insecticides that can be safely used indoors, even in the kitchen. While these products are generally somewhat more expensive than other insecticides, they can be used effectively at much lower rates of application. If it is necessary to use an insecticidal dust, shampoo, or flea collar on young puppies or kittens, a product containing one of the pyrethroids is recommended.

Natural pyrethrum (*Pyrocide*) is still available, as is rotenone (*ChemFish*), a poison derived from a tropical legume. An extremely promising new botanical insecticide recently registered for use in the United States on ornamental plants and vegetables is an extract of the **neem** tree, native to southern Asia. Since ancient times neem has been valued in India for both its insecticidal and medicinal properties. It first attracted the attention of Western scientists in 1959 after a German entomologist reported that billions of locusts swarming over the Sudan devoured everything in their path—except neem trees! Subsequent research has shown that neem seeds and leaves contain nine or more different liminoid compounds that exhibit potent pesticidal properties effective against at least 200 different species of insects. These natural chemicals act primarily by disrupting the hormones that control insect metamorphosis, thus preventing normal development and reproduction. Neem also acts as an insect repellent, as the observation in Sudan amply demonstrated. Because neem products are pesticidal only when consumed, beneficial insects such as pest predators or honeybees are not affected by use of these materials. Neem is quite safe for humans as well—in fact, for centuries South Asians have used neem extensively for dental hygiene and a variety of other medicinal purposes. While much remains to be learned about the plant's many properties, researchers have high hopes that neem may be in the vanguard of a new generation of "soft" pesticides providing environmentally benign methods of insect control (National Research Council, 1992).

Herbicides. Weeds in a field may not appear as threatening as hordes of insects, yet the economic losses caused by these unwanted species can be very high. Weeds compete with crop plants for vital mineral nutrients and water, thus reducing crop yields; they make harvesting more difficult and some species, when consumed, poison livestock.

Widescale application of chemicals for weed control is a relatively new phenomenon. Although a few inorganic compounds such as iron sulfate were used against broad-leaf weeds as long ago as 1896, hand-weeding, mechanical cultivation, tillage, crop rotation, and the use of weed-free seeds were the most common methods of reducing crop losses due to weed infestations. After World War II, the first synthetic herbicide (2,4-D) was introduced and has been followed by a succession of more than a hundred different chemical weed killers during the past four decades. Today herbicide use has considerably surpassed insecticide use in American agriculture, now accounting for about 66% of all pesticides applied. Corn and soybeans are the most herbicide-dependent crops, with 95% of all fields receiving herbicide applications (National Research Council, 1993).

Although herbicides are used most extensively for agricultural purposes, they are also used by public health workers to control weeds that harbor insects and rodents, and to eradicate nuisance plants such as ragweed or poison ivy.

Herbicides may be either selective or nonselective, the former group being by far the more common. Most selective herbicides kill only broad-leafed dicotyledonous plants, a group to which many of the common weed species belong, without harming members of the grass family. Thus they can be used for effective weed control on cereal crops or on home lawns. Examples of some selective herbicides include 2,4-D (the active ingredient in 1500 over-the-counter weed killers), alachlor, and atrazine. Nonselective herbicides kill any plant with which they come into contact and thus have much more limited use, such as spraying railroad and highway right-of-ways. Sulfuric acid and glyphosate (*Roundup, Kleenup*) are examples of nonselective herbicides.

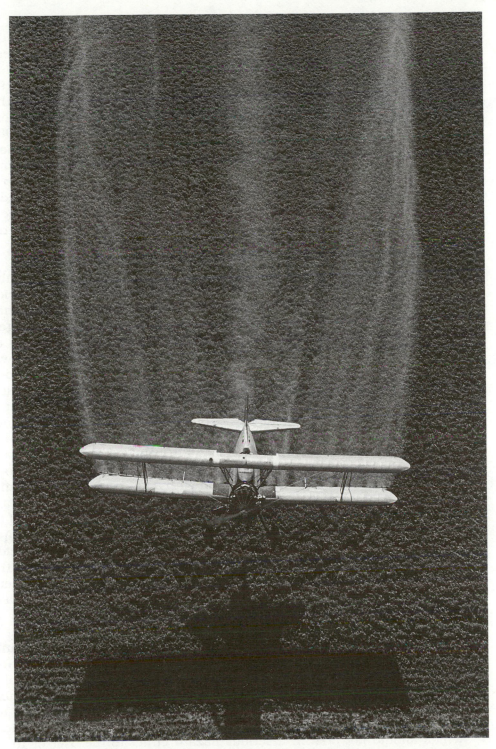

The dusting of agricultural products with pesticides is increasingly being questioned by those concerned with the long-term effects of pesticide exposure on human health and the environment. [U.S. Department of Agriculture]

Although most herbicides are thought to be only slightly toxic to humans, in recent years there have been several studies suggesting that herbicide exposure can cause genetic mutations, cancer, and birth defects. Farm workers occasionally blame health problems such as weight loss, nausea, vomiting, and loss of appetite to contact with herbicides. In 1986 researchers reported that Kansas farmers who used 2,4-D for more than 20 days per year had a six times greater risk of non-Hodgkins lymphoma than did a control group with no exposure to herbicides (Blair et al., 1987). In 1991 the *Journal of the National Cancer Institute* reported that dogs, too, are at risk from 2,4-D. If their owners apply the weed killer four times or more each summer, canines are twice as likely to develop malignant lymphoma as are dogs whose owners abstain from herbicide use. Recognition that some of the most widely used herbicides are known or suspected carcinogens has prompted concerns among some federal regulators that residues of these chemicals on food or in well water may be exposing the American consumer to long-term health risks.

During the late 1970s and early 1980s a great deal of public controversy surrounded the use of 2,4,5-T and silvex, selective herbicides that contained traces of dioxin formed as an unavoidable contaminant during the manufacturing process. Notorious as a component of **Agent Orange**, the chemical defoliant used by U.S. military forces during the Vietnam War, 2,4,5-T (actually, the dioxin contaminating 2,4,5-T) was blamed for a wide range of physical and emotional problems among South Vietnamese living in the target areas, as well as among American servicemen who had come into contact with the herbicide during their tour of duty. Although independent studies of veterans' complaints have never been able to confirm an association between the alleged health effects and Agent Orange exposure, production of 2,4,5-T and silvex was terminated in the early 1980s and in 1984 seven chemical companies agreed to an out-of-court settlement for $180 million with a veterans' group claiming health damage. Antipesticide activists in some communities have also raised a considerable outcry about dangers posed to people, pets, and the environment by chemicals used by the rapidly growing commercial lawn care industry. Making the point that "Dandelions don't kill you, pesticides do!" concerned citizens' groups have been vociferously demanding that lawn care companies post warning signs on treated lawns, inform residents of what pesticides are being used, and provide health and safety data on those chemicals.

Rodenticides.   Although good sanitation and rat-proofing of buildings and food storage facilities provides the only effective long-term control of domestic rodents, use of poisons is an important additional tool in keeping rat populations low. Because some rodenticides used in public health work are extremely toxic to humans as well as to rodents, their use is restricted to certified applicators. General-use rodenticides, chemicals which should not present a serious hazard either to the user or to the environment when used in accordance with instructions, can be purchased by the general public. The rodenticides most commonly recommended for use by householders act as anticoagulants.

Such poisons as warfarin, fumarin, PMP, pival, diphacinone, and chlorophacinone are all multiple-dose poisons which must be consumed over a period of several consecutive days before the rat dies. Thus a child or pet would not be seriously endangered by eating a single portion of bait. Anticoagulants cause internal hemorrhaging, causing the rodents to bleed to death painlessly. These poisons provide excellent control of both rats and mice, although up to two weeks may be required to get an effective kill.

BOX 8-3

To Catch a Mouse

To eliminate the occasional mouse in the pantry, there is probably no more effective device than the old-fashioned snap trap. To use the trap most efficiently, however, one should take the rodent's behavior patterns into consideration. The male mouse, unlike his sociable cousin the rat, is a loner, establishing his own territory with one or more females and seldom venturing beyond its borders. If food is present and the population density of mice in the general area is high, these individual territories may be quite small; it is not uncommon under such circumstances for mice to venture no further than 6–10 feet from their nests. For this reason, effective control requires the use of multiple traps, placed no more than 10–20 feet apart. Mice are most active at night and tend to travel close to walls, between objects, or in runways where they can feel their whiskers in contact with vertical surfaces. For this reason, a trap placed in the middle of a room or at some distance from a wall is unlikely to catch a mouse. For optimum results, a trap should be baited with any type of fresh food (mice like the same types of food people do—peanut butter makes a fine bait since, due to its stickiness, it cannot be easily removed) and placed at a right angle to the side wall across the runway with the baited end of the trap closest to the wall. Concerns that handling the trap could leave a human odor that might frighten the mouse away are unwarranted; mice live in such close association with people that they are constantly surrounded by human smells and pay no heed to such odors.

Environmental Impact of Pesticide Use

In the early 1950s, bird-watchers in both the United States and Western Europe were confronted with a baffling mystery—a sudden, inexplicable decline in the populations of bald eagles, pelicans, and peregrine falcons appeared to threaten the very survival of these well-loved species. Investigations into the reasons behind such an unanticipated population "crash" ultimately revealed that the villain was not a disease, nor overkilling, nor a scarcity of food, but rather was the presence in the tissues of these birds of startlingly high concentrations of the new insecticide DDT. Although DDT did not appear to have a direct lethal effect on the adult birds, it interfered with their ability to metabolize calcium, thereby resulting in the production of eggs with shells so thin that they broke when the nesting parents sat on them. Thus pesticide-induced reproductive failure—the inability of the birds to produce viable offspring—was ultimately shown to be the factor responsible for the ornithologists' distress.

This episode represented one of the first glimmerings of awareness on the part of the scientific community at least, that the advent of the new wonder chemicals was not an unmitigated blessing. The public at large, however, remained largely unaware and unconcerned about such matters until the publication in 1962 of Rachel Carson's literary bombshell, *Silent Spring*. This best-seller represented a scathing indictment of pesticide misuse and for the first time made the average American aware of the havoc which indiscriminate reliance on chemicals could wreak on the environment and on human well-being. In retrospect, the publication of *Silent Spring* made "ecology" a household word and was probably the most important single event in launching what became the environmental movement of the 1970s. Carson and many subsequent researchers clearly demonstrated that extensive use and near-total reliance on chemicals for pest control have been accompanied by unanticipated and undesired side effects, many of which have raised problems serious enough to threaten the continued usefulness of these products. The major environmental effects of pesticide use causing concern today are discussed in the following section.

Development of Resistance

Those who dreamed that the new pesticides held promise of complete eradication of certain insect or other pest species were obviously ignorant of the principles that govern how the forces of natural selection act upon chance variations occurring within any population—particularly insect populations whose long evolutionary history demonstrates the remarkable ability of these organisms to evolve and adapt rapidly to changing environmental conditions. The widespread, frequent, and intensive application of chemicals such as DDT in the years following the war created a new environmental challenge that was initially successful in drastically reducing pest populations but that eventually was responsible for providing the selective forces which would produce new strains of "super bugs," rendering the original poisons worthless. The mechanism by which this occurs can be visualized by considering a hypothetical population of, say, boll weevils ravaging a field of cotton. Aerial insecticide spraying may kill perhaps 99% of the weevils, but a few will survive, either by chance (perhaps an overhanging leaf shielded them from the spray) or because something in the genetic make-up of a particular individual somehow made it less vulnerable to the poison than were its fellow weevils who promptly died. Such a hereditary trait might be the production of a particular enzyme capable of detoxifying the pesticide, a less permeable type of epidermis which prevented penetration of the contact poison, a behavioral characteristic that allowed the individual to avoid fatal exposure, or some other factor of this nature. In a pesticide-free environment (the type of situation prevailing prior to the introduction of DDT) such a genetic trait would confer no special advantage to the individual carrying it, so the frequency of such a gene within that population would remain low. Once DDT came into widespread use, however, the boll weevils' environment was radically altered and those few individuals possessing the gene for immunity suddenly enjoyed a tremendous selective advantage. As the accompanying diagram indicates, successive sprayings largely eliminated boll weevils susceptible to the insecticide, but promoted the build-up of a population in which the vast majority of individuals now carry the gene (or genes) conferring resistance to the chemical. In order to combat this new situation, those seeking to control pest outbreaks turn to newer and more powerful chemicals, only to witness the same cycle of events repeat itself.

Since pesticide resistance had appeared as a localized problem even with the old-fashioned insecticides, it shouldn't have come as a total surprise when development of resistance to DDT began to appear in the late 1940s and early 1950s. Among the first species to display immunity

Figure 8-4 Cycle of Pesticide Resistance

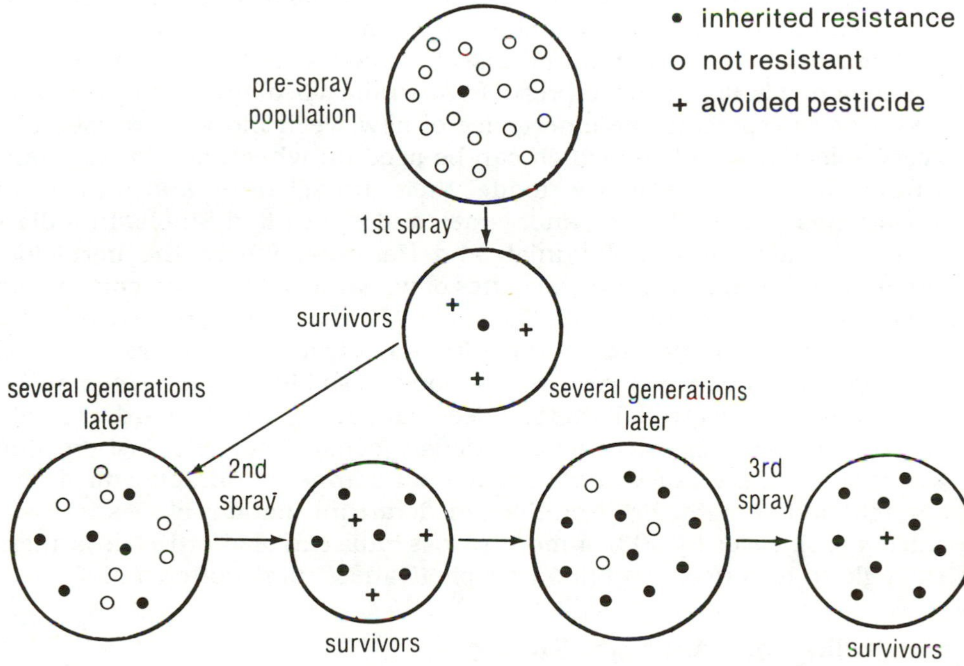

were certain populations of houseflies and mosquitoes which, as early as 1946, could no longer be controlled with DDT. In 1951, during the Korean War, military officials were alarmed to discover that human body lice, vectors of typhus, had become resistant to DDT. Among agricultural pests, spider mites, cabbage loopers, codling moths, and tomato hornworms developed resistance to several of the common insecticides; by the mid-1950s when the boll weevil became resistant to many of the chlorinated hydrocarbons, the need for alternative control methods became obvious (Perkins, 1982). At present, more than 500 species of insects and mites are resistant to common pesticides—more than double the number that were resistant just 20 years ago. Largely due to problems of pesticide resistance, crop losses due to insects are nearly twice as high now as they were when DDT was first brought onto the market, in spite of the fact that American farmers are using ten times more pesticides now than they did in 1945. In the public health field, as in agriculture, growing pesticide resistance is causing serious concern. Worldwide, incidence of malaria is now on a sharp upswing as approximately 64 species of mosquitoes have become resistant to insecticides, according to World Health Organization officials.

Problems of pesticide resistance are not restricted to species of arthropods. Some rat populations, particularly those in cities which have long-established rodent control programs, no longer respond to warfarin, the most extensively used rodenticide in the world. More than 150 species of plant pathogens (fungi and bacteria) are now resistant to at least one pesticide, as are nearly 275 weed species (Mansur, 1994). Although herbicide resistance is a relatively recent development and has received considerably less attention among agricultural experts than has the problem of chemically immune insects, weed scientists warn that the phenomenon is already widespread. In Australia wheat growers by the early 1980s were reporting the emergence of new weed biotypes resistant to every selective herbicide which can be used on wheat; similar resistant strains have subsequently made their unwelcome appearance in wheatfields in Canada, England, Israel, and the United States. In India's "bread basket" states of Punjab and Haryana, where the herbicide-dependent Green Revolution varieties of wheat have received continuous applications of the same weed-killers for 10–15 years, farmers have recently been experiencing increasing difficulty in controlling weed grasses. This problem has fueled worries that serious herbicide resistance may be developing there as well. If this is indeed happening, India's hard-won self-sufficiency in food grains could be seriously jeopardized, since fast-growing weeds like canary grass and wild oats out-compete "miracle wheat" for sunlight and nitrogen fertilizer. Even moderate infestations of these grasses can cut crop yields by 30% or more—a loss India can ill-afford as its farmers struggle to feed nearly a billion people (Ganessi and Puffer, 1993).

Killing of Beneficial Species

Only a small percentage of insect species are considered pests, yet the most widely used synthetic insecticides are broad-spectrum poisons, killing both friend and foe alike. The destruction of many beneficial predator insect species as well as the target pest has led to two related types of problems. The first of these, referred to as **target pest resurgence**, occurs when an insecticide application which initially resulted in a drastic reduction in the pest population is quickly followed by a sudden increase in pest numbers to a level higher than that which existed prior to the spraying. This occurs because the natural enemies of the pest, which formerly kept its numbers under control, were also heavily decimated by the spraying. Since any predators which survived the pesticide would subsequently starve or migrate, the pests would then confront ideal conditions—no natural enemies and an abundance of their favorite food (i.e. the crop that had been sprayed). As a result, their populations can increase in size very rapidly, above and beyond the original level.

A second situation, known as **secondary pest outbreak**, involves the rise to prominence of certain plant-eating species which, prior to the spraying, were unimportant as pests because natural enemies kept their populations below the level at which they could cause significant economic damage. After pesticides eliminated most of their predators, such insects suddenly experience a population explosion and become major pests in their own right. A classic example of this phenomenon was the outbreak of cottony cushion scale in the citrus groves of California after the trees had been sprayed with DDT for control of other citrus pests. The spraying proved devastating to a predator insect, the vedalia beetle, which had been doing such a good job of keeping the scale populations low that the presence of this pest had been largely forgotten. With its natural enemy removed, however, the cottony cushion scale suddenly assumed major importance, causing great economic loss. Only after the adjustment of spraying schedules permitted reestablishment of the beetle population did the scale insect cease to be a problem.

Environmental Contamination

Liberal use of pesticides on a worldwide basis has resulted in a more thorough contamination of the biosphere than anyone in 1945 would have dreamed possible. Today pesticide residues, especially those of the chlorinated hydrocarbons, are found virtually everywhere in the tissues of creatures as diverse as Antarctic penguins, fish in deep ocean trenches, decomposer bacteria, and every human being. Since no one deliberately sprayed pesticides in Antarctica or in the middle of the Pacific, how could this have happened? Because the chlorinated hydrocarbons are persistent pesticides (meaning that they break down very slowly), they can circulate through the ecosystem for a long time, often traveling long distances from their point of origin. When such chemicals are aerially sprayed on forest, field, or pastureland, less than 10% of the pesticide actually hits the target; the remainder is carried off by air currents and is subsequently deposited miles away where it will eventually be washed into waterways or taken up by living organisms in the food they eat. Even when carefully applied according to label directions, pesticides can vaporize into the air, be washed off the land into lakes and streams during heavy rains, or percolate downward through the soil. The results of this unintended contamination include the following.

Direct Killing of Organisms Exposed to Chemicals. Many species of fish, some birds and small mammals, and a number of plants, including phytoplankton, as well as beneficial insect species, are extremely sensitive to chemical pesticides and die immediately after coming into contact with such substances. A dramatic example of this occurred a few years ago when 700 Brant geese died after walking and feeding on a New York golf course which had been treated with the widely used organophosphate insecticide, diazinon. As a result of this and numerous other bird kills linked to the insecticide, EPA cancelled the use of diazinon on golf courses and sod farms, but the insecticide is still widely applied to lawns and gardens throughout the United States. Another insecticide which has caused high mortality among nontarget species is carbofuran, a carbamate pesticide estimated to kill one to two million birds in the United States each year, including bald eagles. Several years ago, in response to a flood of protests from bird lovers, the state of Virginia banned use of carbofuran. The manufacturer agreed to terminate U.S. sales of the granular form of the poison by the fall of 1994 (birds are particularly attracted to the granules which they swallow, presumably mistaking them for grit); *exports* of granular carbofuran will continue, however, and carbofuran sprays—also a cause of wildlife mortality—will remain on the market both here and abroad. Accidents involving pesticides have frequently wrought havoc on wildlife populations. Several massive fish kills made headline news in 1991; a train derailment along the Upper Sacramento River in California spilled 19,000 gallons of metam-sodium into the water, killing virtually every living creature—fish, crustaceans, insect larvae, algae, and plankton—along a 45-mile stretch of the river. That same year an estimated one million fish, along with uncounted numbers of crabs, crawfish, turtles, and alligators, were killed by canefield runoff of the organophosphate insecticide azinphos-methyl (*Guthion*) in southern Louisiana. The following year a similar incident occurred, again due to pesticide runoff from sugarcane fields, this time causing 25,000 fish to go belly-up (Curtis, Profeta, and Mott, 1993; Williams, 1993).

Indirect Killing Via Depletion of Food or Habitat. When pesticides are targeted against insects, plants, or rodents that serve as a major food source for another group of organisms, the long-term effect can be just as devastating as direct poisoning would be. In New Jersey, populations of certain forest bird species declined by 45–55% after carbaryl spraying for gypsy moth control deprived the birds of their supper. Herbicide use similarly reduces both forage and habitat for many plant-eating insects and can have a "domino effect" when plummeting populations of arthropods adversely impact the food supply of insectivorous birds. On the high plains of Wyoming, a population of native sparrows crashed after herbicidal spraying of sagebrush to enlarge pasturelands for grazing. Unfortunately for the sparrows, the sagebrush supplied essential cover and nesting sites without which the birds couldn't survive (Parker, 1994).

Groundwater Contamination. The discovery in 1979 that 96 wells on Long Island were contaminated with a highly toxic carbamate insecticide, aldicarb, came as unwelcome news to a public which assumed that however polluted our rivers and lakes might be, groundwater supplies were safe from chemical contamination. Any hopes that the New York situation might be an isolated aberration were shattered by the revelation that, 3000 miles to the west, more than 2000 wells in the fertile San Joaquin Valley were tainted with the nematicide DBCP, a chlorinated hydrocarbon that had earlier made headlines for causing sterility among male pesticide workers exposed to the chemical. In the late 1980s the EPA launched a nationwide survey to determine the extent of pesticide contamination of groundwater supplies. In 1990 the Agency released a report showing that 14% of all public and private drinking water wells had measurable levels of at least one pesticide. Two years later the Agency reported new results indicating that nearly one-third of rural wells showed unsafe levels of pesticide contamination, with aldicarb and the herbicides atrazine (*Aatrex*) and alachlor (*Lasso*), both suspected human carcinogens, posing the most widespread problems. Agency surveyors reported finding nearly 100 different pesticides in groundwater supplies and concluded that heavy agricultural pesticide use was the main cause of the problem. While the levels of farm chemicals found in well water are too low to cause *acute* pesticide poisoning, they raise concerns about *chronic* health effects among those dependent on such supplies. Since most of the data on groundwater quality has been derived from shallow wells which are presumably more subject to contamination, the full extent of pesticide pollution of groundwater cannot yet be adequately assessed. In addition, because plumes of contamination move so slowly in aquifers, concentrations measured today indicate the impact of agricultural practices years or even decades ago. The fact that total pesticide usage is still increasing (up by 17% two decades after the publication of *Silent Spring*) suggests that pesticide-polluted well water may pose even more serious concerns in the years ahead. In the developing nations, where the rate of pesticide use is increasing even faster than in the industrialized world, virtually no groundwater monitoring is being carried out at present; it is quite likely that current agricultural activities may be seriously degrading underground water supplies over vast areas without anyone recognizing the potential threat to future generations (Nash, 1993; "EPA Study," 1992; Curtis et al., 1993).

Indirect Contamination Via Food Chains. Since the chlorinated hydrocarbons are not water-soluble they are not excreted from the body when ingested but instead are stored in fatty tissues such as liver, kidneys, and fat around the intestines. Toxic substances present in minute amounts in the general environment can thus become quite concentrated as they move along a food chain, sometimes reaching lethal doses in organisms at the highest trophic levels. This process, known as **biomagnification**, was the phenomenon responsible for the reproductive failure in the various birds of prey referred to earlier in this chapter. Eagles, pelicans, and falcons are all top carnivores, fish-eaters, at the end of relatively long food chains. As such, they had accumulated amounts of DDT sufficiently high to interfere with important bodily processes, with the results already described.

The classic example of biomagnification can be seen in the case of Clear Lake, California—a favorite fishing spot about 90 miles north of San Francisco. Recreational anglers had long been annoyed by the swarms of nonbiting gnats which were frequently present at Clear Lake. The new synthetic pesticides offered what appeared to be an easy way of getting rid of a nuisance, so in 1949 it was decided to spray Clear Lake with a dilute solution of DDD (a chemical cousin of DDT which is less toxic to fish). After the first spraying, gnat populations dropped to barely detectable levels, but by 1951 the pesky insects were back in bothersome numbers, so the spraying was repeated. Several more sprayings followed in succeeding years as the gnat populations displayed increasing resistance to the poison. Then some strange side effects became apparent. By 1954 visitors to Clear Lake began reporting significant numbers of carcasses of the Western grebe, a type of water fowl, around the lake. By the early 1960s, the grebe population at Clear Lake had plummeted from 1000 nesting pairs to almost none. Suspecting that the repeated pesticide applications might somehow be related to the birds' demise, biologists began to measure DDD concentrations in various components of the lake ecosystem. Although the lake water itself contained traces of DDD in barely detectable amounts (0.02 ppm), concentrations of the pesticide increased dramatically when the tissues of living organisms were examined. The facts they uncovered are entirely consistent with the basic principles of a food chain:

Organism	DDD Concentration in Tissues (ppm)
Phytoplankton (producers)	5
Herbivorous fish (primary consumers)	40–300
Carnivorous fish (secondary consumers)	up to 2500
Western grebes (secondary consumers)	1600

The pesticide which had been sprayed on the lake in what everybody at the time assumed was a safely dilute amount was absorbed and concentrated by the plankton which were the producer organisms of Clear Lake. When these were consumed by the herbivorous fish (primary consumers), the DDD became more concentrated. By the time these fish were eaten by grebes or by bullheads, the DDD had become sufficiently concentrated to cause the death of the birds.

By the late 1960s the futility of spraying to control the now-resistant gnats became obvious and a gnat-eating fish was introduced into the lake in what subsequently proved to be a very successful method of biological control. As pesticide levels gradually dropped, the grebes returned to Clear Lake and today are once again thriving at approximately their pre-1954 population levels. Numerous other examples of biomagnification involving other chlorinated hydrocarbons and heavy metals (methyl mercury at

Minamata, for example) have since been described and illustrate the unanticipated effects which toxic substances can have as they move through ecosystems.

Hazards to Human Health

Although pesticides are used specifically to kill pests, many of them are quite toxic to humans as well. Acute pesticide poisoning may account for as many as 300,000 illnesses among American farm workers every year, most of them due to contact with organophosphate insecticides. On a global basis, pesticides take a much higher toll: The World Health Organization (WHO) recently estimated that in the Third World alone, acute poisonings among agricultural workers may be as high as 25 million annually (3% of the work force), with 1% dying as a result of their exposure (Jeyaratnam, 1990). Even these figures may be overly conservative, since field laborers in developing countries seldom seek medical treatment when they feel ill on the job and thus many cases of pesticide poisoning go unreported. While increased emphasis on pesticide safety and improved application equipment has contributed to a marked decline in acute pesticide-related deaths and serious illness in the industrialized nations, such is not the case in most developing countries. Few Third World farm workers receive any training in proper use of farm chemicals, which are commonly misused and overapplied. Adequate protective gear is seldom worn or even provided. Most pesticides in developing countries are applied manually (sometimes by reaching bare-handed into a container of pesticidal dust and broadcasting it onto the target area) or by tractor, affording ample opportunity for dusts, mists, or vapors to be inhaled or absorbed through the exposed skin of the applicator. Since field workers seldom have access to running water while working, quick removal of pesticides spilled on garments or on the skin is not possible and workers frequently wear contaminated clothing home, exposing their children, pregnant wives, or elderly parents who are particularly susceptible to health damage from these poisons. Additional exposure to family members may occur when workers, unaware of the danger, bring home empty pesticide containers to use for storing food or water. Although strict adherence to label directions could prevent some of the problems associated with improper handling, storage, and application practices, in fact Third World farm workers seldom read the label instructions, either because they are illiterate or because labels are printed in a language which they don't understand (the latter situation poses a safety concern even in the United States where many agricultural laborers read only Spanish and are thus unable to heed warnings printed in English). Even worse, in many developing countries pesticides are often transferred from the original container to another unlabeled receptacle so that the user, even if literate and multilingual, has no way of knowing what hazards the material might present—or even its identity. Finally, a future threat that hasn't received the attention it deserves is the question of what to do with sizeable stocks of outdated or unusable pesticides—many of them

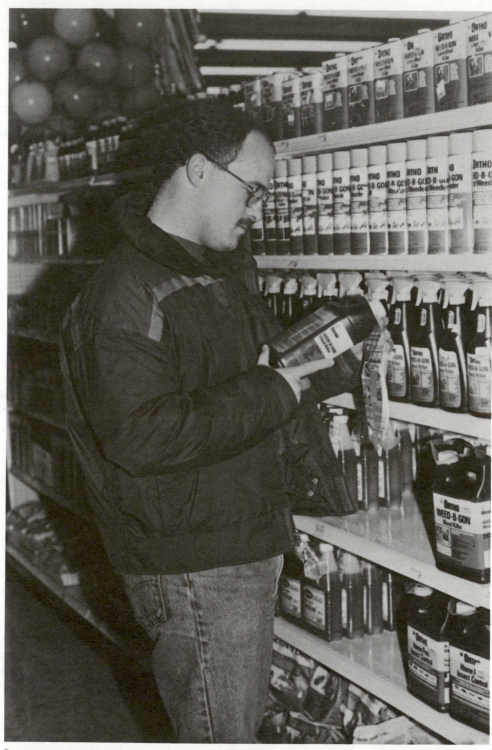

Consumers purchasing pesticides should read label information carefully before using the product. Many human health and environmental problems have been caused by overuse or misuse of these toxic chemicals. [Author's photo]

persistent chlorinated hydrocarbons such as dieldrin and DDT—more than 15 million pounds (7 million kg.) of which have accumulated in 35 developing countries. In many cases the containers in which these are stored are unlabeled, corroded, and leaking, posing serious problems of environmental pollution and future health problems. Yet, the countries involved have no proper means for disposing of such toxins nor the resources for cleaning up contamination that has already occurred (World Resources Institute, 1994).

To cause harm, a pesticide must be taken internally through the mouth, skin, or respiratory system. Most oral exposure is due to carelessness; for example, leaving poisons within reach of young children, smoking or eating without washing hands after handling pesticides, using the mouth to start siphoning liquid pesticide concentrates, eating unwashed fruit that was recently sprayed, or accidentally drinking pesticides that were poured into an unlabelled container. Exposure through the skin can occur when pesticides are spilled on the body or when wind-blown sprays or dusts come into contact with skin.

Reentering a field too soon after pesticide application or careless handling of discarded containers can also result in absorption of pesticides through the skin. The larger the skin area contaminated and the longer the duration of contact, the more serious the results of such exposure will be. Theoretically, dermal exposure could be reduced significantly through the use of protective clothing and equipment. In practice, however, such precautions are frequently ignored. Such gear is often expensive, cumbersome, and uncomfortable, especially during hot weather. All too often, applicators who know better fail to comply with safety recommendations and have been observed, in some instances, to ply their trade wearing little more than bathing suits! Poisoning due to inhalation is most common in enclosed areas such as greenhouses but can also occur outside when pesticide mists or fumes are inhaled during application or if the applicator is smoking.

Symptoms of acute exposure (i.e. "one-time" cases) include headache, weakness, fatigue, or dizziness. If poisoning is due to one of the organophosphate insecticides, the victim may experience severe abdominal pain, vomiting, diarrhea, difficulty in breathing, excessive sweating, and sometimes convulsions, coma, and death.

In contrast, chronic pesticide poisoning (low-level exposure over an extended time period) is characterized by vague symptoms which are difficult to pinpoint as having been caused by pesticide exposure (Bever et al., 1975). The greatest concern regarding chronic pesticide exposure, particularly to chlorinated hydrocarbons, is their potential for causing cancer or reproductive problems.

For many years carcinogenicity was the prime focus of concern regarding chronic effects of pesticide exposure. Beginning with its prohibition on the use of DDT in 1972, the EPA has gradually banned or restricted most of the chlorinated hydrocarbon pesticides, including endrin, aldrin, dieldrin, mirex, heptachlor, chlordane, and so on, largely because tests showed them to be carcinogenic to laboratory animals (however, few other countries followed the U.S. example; most of these chemicals are still

Figure 8-5 Dermal Absorption Rates As Compared with the Forearm

The seriousness of absorbing pesticide through the skin depends on the dermal toxicity of the chemical, the size of the con- taminated skin area, the length of time the material is in contact with the skin, and the rate of absorption through the skin. As the diagram indicates, different parts of the body have very different rates of skin absorption.

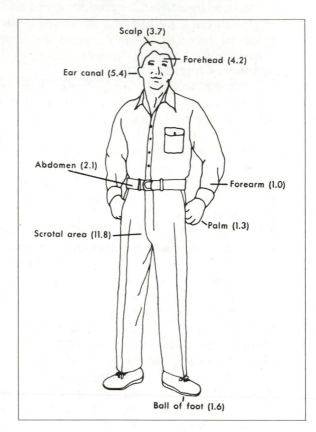

Source: *Illinois Pesticide Applicator Study Guide*, University of Illinois Cooperative Extension Service.

legal elsewhere and continue to be used extensively in Third World countries). The environmental consequences of this phaseout have been dramatic. In the United States, concentrations of these persistent pesticides in animal tissues have been steadily declining since the 1970s; certain bird populations which had nearly vanished by the late 1960s due to bioaccumulation of chlorinated pesticides have now largely rebounded. DDT levels in human breast milk also have plummeted by 90% since the EPA ban took effect (Schneider, 1994).

While the impact of pesticide exposure on cancer incidence is still provoking debate among the experts (in California, the largest case-control study to date, published in April 1994, contradicted results of previous research by finding no association between breast cancer and DDT exposure), a growing body of evidence supports the contention that *disruption of the endocrine and immune systems*, not cancer, constitutes the most serious long-term pesticide-related health concern. Since the endocrine hormones regulate a wide spectrum of bodily functions, including fertility and fetal development, compounds which interfere with such hormones have the potential for serious reproductive effects even at low levels of exposure. Scientists have now identified a number of pesticides, including many of the chlorinated hydrocarbons, as well as some synthetic pyrethroids and triazine herbicides, as potent hormone disruptors. Studies of wildlife populations have shown that exposure to these compounds can lead to abnormal sexual behavior (especially feminization of males), birth defects, and impaired fertility among the offspring of pesticide-exposed parents (Curtis et al., 1993). Several of the more notorious pesticide-related tragedies have involved problems caused by the reproductive effects of chronic pesticide exposure. The nematicide DBCP (1,2-dibromo-3-chloropropane), for example, is known to have caused sterility among men in the California factory where it was manufactured, as well as among 1500 male banana plantation workers in Costa Rica occupationally exposed to the chemical.

Immune system dysfunction can be provoked by either acute or subchronic exposure to many commonly used pesticides, including the herbicide 2,4-D and the insecticides malathion, parathion, aldicarb, carbofuran, and most of the chlorinated hydrocarbons (though most of these are no longer used in the United States, their residues persist in the environment). Young children, especially when malnourished, as well as elderly adults appear most vulnerable to pesticides' immuno-suppressive effects and tend to contract infectious diseases more frequently than individuals not exposed to pesticidal compounds. Pesticide-induced immunotoxicity may also be manifested as allergic contact dermatitis, a skin inflammation caused by immune system response to a foreign substance—in this case to pesticide exposure. Allergic reactions to contact with even minute amounts of pesticides can become chronic and in some cases have resulted in farm workers becoming permanently disabled due to chemical intolerance.

Concerns about pesticide-induced allergies among flight attendants and passengers on jet aircraft recently prompted a request by the U.S. Department of Transportation to 28 foreign governments that they stop requiring the insecticidal spraying of passenger compartments of planes arriving from outside their borders prior to landing. Although the pesticide employed (d-phenothrin, a synthetic pyrethroid commercially sold as *Black Knight Roach Killer*) is characterized by EPA as exhibiting low human toxicity and is approved by the World Health Organization, some chemically sensitive passengers have complained of breathing difficulties, headaches, nausea, seizures, or other health problems after being forced to inhale the spray mist. A few passengers claim far more serious problems than temporary discomfort: one woman alleged that involuntary exposure to d-phenothrin during flight resulted in reactivation of her leukemia (research at the National Cancer Institute has linked pyrethrin exposure to a quadrupling of leukemia risk among farmers): 18 hours after landing in Sydney, Australia, a British traveler suffering from emphysema died of

---

Figure 8-6 Governments Requiring Insecticidal Spraying of Passenger Compartments of Arriving International Aircraft

American Samoa	Dominican Republic	New Caledonia
Antigua	El Salvador	*New Zealand
Argentina	Grenada	Nicaragua
*Australia	India	*Panama
Barbados	Jamaica	Seychelles
Belize	Kenya	St. Lucia
Cape Verde	Madagascar	Trinidad and Tobago
Chile	Mauritius	Yemen
Congo	Mexico	
Costa Rica	Mozambique	

*Require spraying, but leave it up to the airline whether to spray while passengers are on board.

Source: Air Transportation Association, 1994.

---

chronic airway obstruction, fatally exacerbated by inhalation of insecticide mist, after his wife had vainly pleaded with flight attendants to permit her sick husband to exit the plane before spraying commenced. Although at one time the United States was among the nations requiring insecticidal spraying of incoming flights, the practice was terminated in 1979 after the Centers for Disease Control and Prevention argued convincingly that health risks to passengers outweighed any presumed pest control benefits. Such benefits, according to an EPA entomologist, are largely nonexistent: "The spray may get the occasional flying medfly or melon fly, but it lacks the vapor pressure to penetrate luggage or briefcases. It's a token spray to mollify the [overseas governments'] agriculture departments." In the absence of a favorable response from foreign governments to U.S. Transportation Secretary Federico Peña's request that in-flight spraying requirements be discontinued, chemically sensitive fliers can do little more than attempt to avoid air travel to those countries which still insist on zapping arriving visitors with a poison whose full spectrum of health effects is still undocumented (Winegar, 1994; "Warning About," 1994; Tolchin, 1994).

The human health impact of dietary exposure to pesticides via residues on food has attracted intense public scrutiny since the 1987 publication of a study by the National Academy of Sciences, estimating that traces of carcinogenic fungicides, insecticides, and herbicides on the nation's fruits, vegetables, and meat could result in an additional 20,000 cancer deaths per year in the United States. These findings were hotly disputed by agrichemical interests but generated intense public concern over how pesticides are regulated. Demands for reform received added

BOX 8-4

Read That Label!

While most of the controversy regarding pesticidal applications has focused on agricultural use of these chemicals, a substantial portion of total U.S. sales of insecticides, herbicides, and fungicides is to homeowners who use prodigious amounts of these toxic products to zap dandelions in their lawns, banish aphids from their rose bushes, or annihilate roaches in the cupboard. Acre for acre, city dwellers apply considerably larger amounts of pesticides to their lawns and gardens, or inside their homes, than do farmers—and they frequently do so with far less knowledge of safe storage, handling, and application practices. Thus it should not be too surprising when horror stories of chemical-related illnesses and environmental damage surface in local newspapers.

In some cases, reported problems are simply due to unknown inherent hazards of certain pesticidal products. Unfortunately, the fact that a chemical is EPA-registered and legally available to the general public does not necessarily guarantee its safety. Many older chemicals already on the market before passage of the 1972 federal law requiring safety data on new pesticides submitted for registration have still not been tested for their chronic health effects and have been liberally used by unsuspecting consumers for years. Nevertheless, the majority of pesticide-related health problems experienced by nonprofessionals, particularly cases of acute poisonings, are due to careless or ignorant misuse of these products. Take, for example, the case of an Illinois couple who became quite ill from inhalation of chlordane vapors after dousing their living room carpet with the undiluted concentrate in order to eliminate a flea problem! Not only were they acting foolishly, they were breaking the law since at the time of the incident chlordane was registered solely for termite control, had to be properly diluted, and could only be applied by rodding or trenching into the soil. Examples such as this, multiplied by the thousands, constitute our most serious pesticide poisoning threat.

Some rules of safe pesticide use are plain common-sensical: keep pesticides in their original containers, keep them out of reach of children and pets, always wear protective clothing when applying chemicals, avoid spraying when conditions are windy. However, for all users of these explicitly toxic chemicals (obviously we wouldn't be using them if they weren't poisonous), the #1 safety rule—and the one most often ignored—is: READ THE LABEL! The label on a pesticide container, along with any accompanying fliers or brochures, constitutes a legal document; anyone using the product in a manner contrary to label directions is in violation of the law. Simply from the standpoint of concern about one's own personal welfare and getting optimum use out of the product, careful reading of the label directions makes good sense, for the information they contain cost millions of dollars to acquire and represents the most extensive data available for that chemical. The label tells the concentration at which the pesticide should be used (contrary to popular myth, mixing a solution stronger than recommended does not enhance the killing power of a pesticide; at best it is a waste of money, at worst it can be environmentally damaging and diminish the effectiveness of the chemical), lists the pests that the product may be used to control, recommends frequency of spraying and the appropriate interval between applications, gives directions for safe use, supplies antidote information in case of accidental poisoning, classifies the chemical as to its degree of toxicity, describes any special environmental hazards the product may present, and lists the names and amounts of active ingredients. Since the so-called "general use" pesticides available to the public are those considered safe when used according to directions, the incidence of pesticide poisonings could be sharply reduced if all users would conscientiously read all label information prior to hauling out the spray equipment or grabbing that aerosol "bug bomb"!

impetus following publication in June 1993, of a long-awaited study by the National Academy of Sciences on pesticides in the diets of infants and small children. Critical of the EPA's outmoded approach for setting pesticide tolerance levels on agricultural produce (a system based on the estimated amount of any given pesticide the "average person"—i.e. an adult—is likely to consume as part of a typical American diet), NAS scientists concluded that the youngest members of society are at enhanced risk because they consume more calories per unit of body weight and because their diet is less varied than that of adults. Immediately after publication of the NAS report, a second study dealing with the same issue was released by the Environmental Working Group, a nonprofit research organization, stating that up to 35% of an individual's lifetime dose of dietary pesticides occurs before the age of 5, largely because young children consume proportionately far more residue-laden fruits and vegetables than do adults. Preschoolers, for example, eat 6 times the amount of fruit consumed by their parents and drink 31 times more apple juice in relation to their body weight than do adults. Thus pesticide residue safety levels based on presumed "average" diets may greatly underestimate the actual amount of exposure received by a young child. These reports also emphasized the fact that most foods contain residues of several different pesticides (a laboratory analysis performed on one pear identified 11 different pesticidal compounds), not just one, and that the sources of pesticide exposure are not restricted to food, but frequently include drinking water, lawn chemicals, and household insecticides as well. All of these factors suggest that the present regulatory framework for ensuring food safety is inadequate in terms of protecting society's most vulnerable members—infants and children (National Research Council, 1993; Curtis et al., 1993). Such findings have prompted recommendations from the NAS that pesticide tolerance levels on food should be based on anticipated effects on *children* rather than adults and that the EPA take multiple pesticide exposures into account when establishing the upper limit of pesticide residues allowable on any given food product. Major changes in existing federal pesticide legislation are likely within the next several years, spurred in part by the conviction that consumer safety should take precedence over economic benefits to agribusiness.

Alternatives to Chemical Pest Control

As increasing numbers of pest species become resistant to available chemicals and as doubts concerning the long-range effects of pesticide exposure on human health and the environment continue to grow, the advisability of continuing to rely exclusively on chemicals for pest control is increasingly being questioned. In recent years a different philosophy of pest control has gained support, a strategy known as **Integrated Pest Management (IPM)**, also referred to as "Low Impact Pest Control" or "Low Impact Sustainable Agriculture." After ascertaining that a pest problem does indeed exist, IPM practitioners combine various compatible methods to obtain the best control with the least possible environmental disruption. While the emphasis in IPM is on utilizing natural controls such as predators, food deprivation, or weather to increase pest mortality, it can include pesticide application also, but only after careful monitoring of pest populations indicate a need. Unlike the total chemical control approach, IPM recognizes the extraordinary adaptability of insects and does not attempt to eradicate a particular pest entirely, but rather is aimed at keeping pest populations below the threshold level at which they can cause significant economic loss. Among the methods which could be included in an IPM strategy are the following.

Natural Enemies

Many of our most serious insect and weed pests (such as Japanese beetle, gypsy moth, fire ant, kudzu, water hyacinth, and so on) are foreign imports which rapidly multiplied here in the absence of their natural enemies. Other native pests have caused serious problems only after their predators were eliminated by indiscriminate use of pesticides. Over the past several decades the government has imported more than 500 insect predators in an attempt to control alien species; about 20 of these are now providing significant control of several important pests. Laboratory breeding of large populations of insect predators in hopes of overwhelming certain pests is also being attempted. Great success in controlling scale insects and mealybugs in citrus orchards was obtained by mass-rearing and release of vedalia beetles and certain parasitic wasps. Home gardeners and organic farmers are urged to purchase praying mantis egg cases or containers full or ladybird beetles to achieve effective non-chemical insect control.

Pathogens and Parasites

A further step in biological warfare against insects involves introducing various disease agents into a pest population. About a dozen such microbial pathogens are now being commercially developed or produced in various parts of the world. Two kinds of bacteria have been approved for commercial pest-control in the United States—*Bacillus popilliae*, which causes the milky spore disease of Japanese beetles, and the widely used *Bacillus thuringiensis* (*Bt*), which can be used effectively against more than 100 species of caterpillars, including gypsy moth larvae, currently the target of widescale *Bt* applications (Dotto, 1979). Unfortunately, recent observations indicate that some pests are now developing resistance to the toxin released by *Bt*. Among the more promising new approaches to enlisting pathogens in the war against pests is the use of certain fungi whose spores can penetrate an insect's exoskeleton, growing inside the host and digesting its tissues, resulting in death within a few days. One such fungus, *Metarhizium flavoviride* (referred to simply as "*Mf*"), is being tested for control of grasshoppers and migratory locusts; another, under the trade name *Biopath*, has been formulated as a bait and is now commercially available for cockroach control.

Pathogenic viruses are also being viewed as offering a promising method of pest control, since viral diseases in nature are frequently devastating to pest populations. A commercial preparation of polyhedrosis virus which kills the cotton bollworm is being tried on a limited scale and field experiments on control of corn earworm by one of the baculoviruses have been so encouraging that commercial preparations are now available.

A protozoan, *Nosema locustae*, has been successfully employed to control grasshopper infestations. *Nosema* spores sprayed on a wheat-bran bait are consumed by the grasshoppers, germinate inside the insect's stomach, multiply rapidly, and devour the grasshopper from inside.

Sex Attractants

Certain chemical stimulants (pheromones) control many aspects of insect behavior, including mating. Sex pheromones may be excreted by the female to attract the male, or vice-versa. Some of these female pheromones have been synthesized in the lab and used to bait traps which can attract males from miles around. When the males enter the trap, expecting to encounter a receptive female, they are caught by a sticky substance on the bottom or sides of the trap. A variation on this method of using sex attractants involves the "confusion technique" in which an infested area is sprayed with so much female hormone that the males don't know in which direction to fly ("Where *is* she?!"). Because the use of sex attractants as just described is effective only against adult insects interested in finding a mate, the technique is of limited effectiveness, since much crop damage is caused by insect larvae. In addition, because most pest species concentrate on a single crop, the market demand for any particular pheromone is relatively small. If the prospects for sales profits are not sufficiently attractive, manufacturers have no interest in producing them! Therefore, in recent years the prime strategy regarding sex attractants has shifted from using them to capture or confuse pest insects to one of employing pheromones to lure "good bugs" (i.e. predator species) into

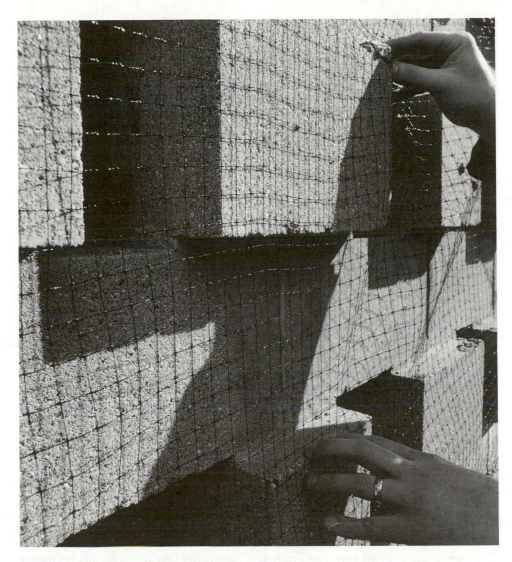

Plastic netting draped on buildings, bridges, and the like is an effective, nonchemical approach to pest bird control. [Internet, Inc.]

problem areas where they will then encounter—and eat—the "bad bugs." Since most predators eat a wide variety of pests, the same predator species could be a useful control agent in many different situations, a fact which significantly enhances the market demand for its pheromone. Conversely, pheromones could be used to entice the beneficial insects to leave a field prior to chemical spraying against crop pests, thereby avoiding such problems as target pest resurgence or secondary pest outbreaks.

Insect Growth Regulators (IGRs)

Sometimes referred to as "biorational" insecticides, IGRs are chemicals which are identical to or closely mimic growth substances

BOX 8-5

IPM for Roach Control

Few creatures inspire more intense emotions of utter loathing than do cockroaches, widely regarded as the most obnoxious of pests. Perhaps such sensations are inspired by the way roaches dart rapidly and unpredictably in every direction when a light is suddenly switched on. It may be due to the foul odor they impart to rooms heavily infested. Such disgust may stem from their propensity to contaminate food or the surfaces they contact with excrement. To many people, cockroach infestations are synonymous with poor housekeeping practices—a cause for shame and embarrassment. Contrary to common belief, cockroaches have *not* been implicated as important vectors of contagious disease, despite the filthy places they often frequent (such as sewers). However, heavy cockroach infestations are known to induce severe allergic reactions among an estimated 10–15 million Americans. Secretions produced by roaches can induce symptoms ranging from skin irritations and runny nose to difficulty breathing or even, in rare instances, life-threatening anaphylactic shock. Among asthma sufferers, exposure to cockroach allergens can provoke severe attacks—an estimated 61% of asthmatics are highly sensitive to roaches (only dust mites cause more widespread distress); among asthmatic children living in heavily infested dwellings, sensitivity to German cockroaches can be as high as 79%.

For all these reasons, the presence of cockroaches within homes, institutions, or workplaces can be psychologically disturbing. As a result, each year Americans spend approximately $2 billion in an effort to banish the bugs to oblivion. The traditional approach to cockroach control has been one of routine spraying or fogging with potent chemical insecticides. In recent years, however, increasing levels of insecticide resistance, especially among German cockroaches (*Blattella germanica*), plus an escalating antipathy toward chemicals among the general public, have led to a growing demand for nonchemical approaches to pest control, not only on the farm but in urban settings as well. Although IPM principles were originally developed for agricultural applications, they can be readily adapted, with minor modifications, to home or institutional settings. Perhaps the greatest difficulty in applying standard IPM concepts at the household level is that of determining the "threshold level" of infestation above which taking action is economically justified. For the average homeowner, the threshold of tolerance for structural pests—especially cockroaches!—is generally "zero to none," meaning that *elimination*, not just reduction in numbers, is usually the goal of cockroach control efforts. Bearing this limitation in mind (meaning that *some* amount of chemical pesticide use will probably be necessary), an environmentally conscious homeowner can devise a strategy which offers far better long-term control with less risk of human pesticide exposure than the standard "spray-the-baseboards-once-a-month" approach. Implementation of an IPM program for control of cockroach infestations requires at least a rudimentary understanding of roach biology and behavior and involves five steps:

1. *monitoring*—there is no point whatsoever in spreading poisons around a home or place of business if

no pests are present. Beware of routine by-the-calendar pesticidal spraying— it's the lazy person's approach to pest control and contributes to a great deal of unnecessary chemical exposure. Strategic placement of sticky traps (available in supermarkets or hardware stores under trade names like *Roach Motel*) in places where roach infestations are suspected—in cupboards, behind refrigerators or sinks, along walls in damp areas such as basements or bathrooms—can give a good indication of whether a problem exists or not. Agricultural Research Service studies conducted in Gainesville, Florida, show that for every roach trapped within a 24-hour period, there are likely to be 600–800 hiding unseen somewhere nearby! Regular monitoring using sticky traps can thus give an indication of the size of an infestation and its approximate location. For example, if traps behind the kitchen stove capture numerous roaches while those in the bathroom are empty, control efforts can be focused on the kitchen, with special emphasis on the problem area. An analysis of the age of individuals trapped can also give helpful clues to the nature of the problem. If all the roaches captured are adults, the infestation may be one of very recent origin involving only a few wayward individuals—perhaps several invaders carried home via infested grocery bags or furniture. On the other hand, the presence of numerous immature roaches ("nymphs") indicates a well-established and hence more difficult-to-eradicate infestation.

2. *proper identification* of the species of cockroach detected (assuming the creature *is* a cockroach—no use getting hysterical over a cricket or June bug!), as well as the source of infestation, is important in order to apply the most effective control measures. The four most common species of cockroaches found within homes throughout the United States— German, American, Oriental, and brown-banded—exhibit differences in food preferences, habitat, reproductive potential, and behavior. Control measures appropriate for one species may be minimally effective against another. Get out that insect ID book or contact an expert to confirm the identity of the unwelcome guests!

3. *environmental alteration* through good sanitation and structural changes that exclude pests is essential. Although good housekeeping alone cannot eliminate a cockroach infestation once it is well-established, removing access to harborage, food, and water will, *in combination with chemical control*, force roaches to spend more time and range farther searching for these necessities of life, thereby increasing their likelihood of coming into contact with residual poisons. Since it takes very little food and water to support a thriving roach population, diligent housekeepers need look beyond such obvious deficiencies as dirty dishes in the sink or spilled foods on countertops and be alert for such nutritional sources as grease build-up on rangetops or ovens, food remaining in pet bowls, crumbs on the floor, empty but unwashed soft drink or beer containers, and so on. In many situations, water is more of a limiting factor to the increase of roach populations than is food, explaining in part why these insects generally congregate in kitchens and bathrooms. Some of the main sources of water to control include: dripping faucets or leaky pipes, drip pan under the refrigerator, condensation on pipes or toilet tanks, pet water bowls, and saucers under houseplants. Removing potential harborage sites can also aid significantly in limiting the size of a cockroach infestation. Indeed, it has been repeatedly

demonstrated that the amount of available shelter is the key factor determining the number of cockroaches which can inhabit any given area. Simply cleaning up clutter (such as cardboard boxes, empty beer cartons, paper bags, overflowing wastebaskets, and so on) within an infested room can greatly reduce the number of roaches present by depriving them of a place to hide. However, even in clutter-free situations, cracks and crevices in walls or baseboards, hollow furniture legs or bedposts, sheltered areas behind mirrors, picture frames, switchplates, or the space inside electrical appliances and computers—all provide excellent roach harborage. Structural alterations such as the use of caulk to seal cracks, application of weatherstripping around door and window frames, and the screening of floor drains thus comprise an important element in an IPM approach by blocking entry to a dwelling or by rendering preferred hiding places inaccessible.

4. *insecticidal applications*— once a roach population is well-established, it is usually necessary to complement the previously cited measures with the use of a residual insecticide. The IPM approach calls for use of the least environmentally disruptive product capable of accomplishing the task at hand (use the "littlest gun"). Homeowners must consider not only which chemical to use, but which *formulation*—dusts, sprays, foggers, baits. All have both advantages and limitations which make each of them more appropriate for some situations than for others. For "do-it-yourself" applications, particularly when infestations are light to moderate, baits can be a very safe and effective method of control. Containerized baits featuring a slow-acting insecticide mixed with a food medium attractive to cockroaches are widely available under a variety of trade names. These should be placed in locations where previous monitoring indicated heavy roach populations. Areas where surfaces intersect—under shelves, behind appliances, in cabinets, or at the back of drawers— are places where roaches travel and are likely to encounter the bait. A number of bait stations should be used, depending on the extent of the infestation, and they must be replaced periodically until the infestation has been eradicated. Baits work most effectively in combination with good sanitation, since the hungrier roaches are, the more appealing the poison bait will be to them. Baits provide an odorless, long-lasting and relatively inexpensive method of chemical control and because many of the products currently on the market employ recently developed insecticidal compounds, no resistance problems have yet been reported. Although determining the most appropriate locations for bait placement and positioning the devices is a bit more time consuming than simply spraying an area, the advantages of using baits considerably outweigh the disadvantages.

5. *evaluation* of the effectiveness of control efforts is the final step in any IPM program and involves routine monitoring for pest presence after control measures have been implemented. Here again, sticky traps are very useful for detecting any remaining focal points of roach activity. If after-the-fact monitoring indicates a continuing problem, a determination of the cause for that problem (lapse in sanitation? uncaulked gap along a door frame?) must be made and appropriate measures then reapplied.

While any one of these control elements, by itself, is unlikely to eliminate a cockroach problem, combining such methods in a total IPM program offers the best approach to reducing the amount of toxic chemicals used around the home while simultaneously achieving long-lasting and

environmentally responsible results.

Reference

Moreland, Dan, ed. 1994. "Cockroach Control: The Best of PCT." Vol. 1, *Pest Control Technology*.

produced by the target pest. IGRs act either as **chitin inhibitors**, preventing proper development of the exoskeleton after molting, or, more commonly, as **juvenoids**. When the larvae of insects with a complete metamorphosis (fleas or mosquitoes, for example) contact or ingest juvenoids, these synthetic analogs of natural insect hormones prevent them from emerging as adults after pupating, thus effectively disrupting their life cycle. For insects characterized by a gradual metamorphosis (such as cockroaches) in which there is no pupal stage, nymphs may progress to adulthood but are abnormal in appearance and incapable of reproducing. Several IGRs are now widely used in structural and public health pest control operations (usually in combination with standard insecticidal formulations to provide a "double whammy") offering long-term control of such troublesome pests as cockroaches, fleas, ants, and floodwater mosquitoes. An obvious limitation to the use of insect growth regulators is that they are only useful against insects which cause damage as adults; many of the worst agricultural pests are larvae (such as caterpillars and grubs) against which IGRs are ineffective.

Sterile Male Technique

This method relies on the mass-rearing and release of huge numbers of male insects which have been sterilized by X-rays or chemicals. Mating of a normal female with a sterile male naturally results in the production of infertile eggs. If the ratio of sterilized to normal males is sufficiently large, most matings will be unsuccessful and pest populations will fall rapidly. This method, which was very successful in eliminating the screw-worm fly from the island of Curacao and from Florida, is most effective when the pest population is geographically isolated, making re-invasion of the area with normal males unlikely.

Development of Resistant Host Plants

Probably the most ecologically sound method of reducing crop damage due to microbial pathogens and nematodes, host resistance has also been successfully employed against such insect pests as the Hessian fly, grape phylloxera, spotted alfalfa aphid, rice stem borer, and corn earworm. In recent years genetic engineering has provided a valuable new tool for introducing desired characteristics from one species to another. In 1993, CibaSeeds received EPA permission to undertake major field trials in Illinois of the first transgenic corn variety engineered for resistance to the European corn borer (ECB), a moth whose larvae cause significant yield reductions throughout the Corn Belt each year. Ciba scientists spliced a gene for toxin production from the bacterium *Bt* into the DNA of corn, creating a hybrid plant that can poison an invading corn borer larva on the first bite. Since corn borers are extremely difficult to control with traditional chemical insecticides, a corn plant that "fights back," killing its enemy before incurring any damage itself, offers big benefits in terms of reduced environmental exposure to pesticides and increased corn yields for farmers. If results of the field testing required for EPA registration of the product are successful, as expected, ECB-resistant corn seed may be commercially available by the late 1990s.

Crop Rotation

Well-known but often neglected, crop rotation is an effective way to control pests that can't survive prolonged periods without contact with the preferred host. In the midwestern Corn Belt, corn rootworm populations were formerly kept at low levels by rotating corn, oats, and clover. As the price of corn relative to other crops has increased, farmers have largely abandoned crop rotation and are now growing corn year after year on the same land. As a result, the corn rootworm has spread from a small area in southern Nebraska to assume major pest status in 18 western and midwestern states.

Sanitation

For control of insect and rodent pests in residential areas or business establishments, the most effective way to reduce pest numbers and keep them low is to apply the basic principles of sanitation. To survive and multiply, pests need a source of food, water, and harborage. If these are in short supply, large pest populations cannot be maintained. Strict observance of the rules of good housekeeping—promptly cleaning up spilled food, storing foods in tightly sealed containers, keeping garbage cans covered, avoiding use of mulch immediately adjacent to building foundations, mowing tall grass or weeds near structures, locating woodpiles at some distance from dwellings, regularly collecting and disposing of animal feces—will be far more effective in eliminating flies, rodents, and roaches over the long term than is the temporary palliative of pesticidal spraying. Similarly, structural alterations such as screens, metal or cement barriers, and caulk applied to cracks and crevices can assist in "building out" certain household pests. Habitat modification such as changing water in birdbaths frequently, keeping roof gutters free of twigs and leaves to permit complete drainage of rainwater, and maintaining premises free of discarded articles which could collect water can be very effective in reducing mosquito breeding. Pesticide use can provide a "quick fix," but without adherence to good sanitary practices, control will be temporary at best.

None of the above methods alone is the total answer to effective pest management. However, in the proper combination after an accurate assessment of a specific pest situation, IPM techniques promise a safer, more ecologically sound, and ultimately more successful approach to limiting pest damage than does the total reliance on chemicals that has characterized U.S. pest control efforts during the past 50 years.

References

Akre, Roger D., and Elizabeth A. Myhre. 1994. "The Great Spider Whodunit." *Pest Control Technology* 22, no. 4 (April).

Bever, Wayne, et al. 1975. *Illinois Pesticide Applicator Study Guide*. Cooperative Extension Service, University of Illinois College of Agriculture, Special Publication 39.

Blair, Aaron, et al. 1987. "Cancer and Pesticides Among Farmers." *Pesticides and Groundwater: A Health Concern for the Midwest*. The Freshwater Foundation.

Centers for Disease Control. 1994. "Human Plague—United States, 1993–1994." *Morbidity & Mortality Weekly Report* 43, no. 13 (April 8).

Curtis, Jennifer, Tim Profeta, and Laurie Mott. 1993. *After Silent Spring: The Unresolved Problems of Pesticide Use in the United States*. Natural Resources Defense Council.

Dotto, Sydia. 1979. "Battling the Bugs." *Science Forum* (March/April).

"EPA Study Links Pesticide Use with Ground Water Contamination." 1992. *Environmental Health Letter*, Jan. 28.

Flint, M. L., and R. vanden Bosch. 1981. *Introduction to Integrated Pest Management*. Plenum Press.

Ganessi, Leonard P., and Cynthia A. Puffer. 1993. "Herbicide-Resistant Weeds May Threaten Wheat Production in India." *Resources*, no. 111 (Spring). Resources for the Future.

Jeyaratnam, J. 1990. "Acute Pesticide Poisoning: A Major Global Health Problem." *World Health Statistics Quarterly* 43.

Mansur, Mike. 1994. "The Food Chain." In *The 1994 Information Please Environmental Almanac*. World Resources Institute, Houghton Mifflin Co.

Nash, Linda. 1993. "Water Quality and Health." In *Water in Crisis: A Guide to the World's Fresh Water Resources*, edited by Peter H. Gleick. Oxford University Press.

National Research Council. 1993. *Pesticides in the Diets of Infants and Children*. National Academy Press, Washington, DC.

National Research Council. 1992. *Neem: A Tree for Solving World Problems*. National Academy Press, Washington, DC.

Parker, Tracey. 1994. "Recent Studies Document the Complex Ways Pesticides Affect Birds." *Journal of Pesticide Reform* 14, no. 1 (Spring).

Perkins, John H. 1982. *Insects, Experts, and the Insecticide Crisis*. Plenum Press.

Pimental, David, et al. 1991. "Environmental and Economic Impacts of Reducing U.S. Agricultural Pesticide Use." *Handbook of Pest Management in Agriculture*. CRC Press.

Pratt, Harry, B. F. Gjornson, and K. S. Littig. 1977. *Control of Domestic Rats and Mice*. Centers for Disease Control, HEW publication no. 77–8141.

Schneider, Keith. 1994. "Progress, Not Victory, on Great Lakes Pollution." *New York Times*, May 7.

Tolchin, Martin. 1994. "20 Countries Urged to Stop Spraying Insecticide in Jets." *New York Times*, April 17.

"Warning About Pesticide Spraying Looms for International Flyers." 1994. *Environmental Health Letter*, Feb. 2.

Williams, Ted. 1993. "Hard News on 'Soft' Pesticides." *Audubon* (March/April).

Winegar, Karin. 1994. "Pesticides in Planes: How Long Before Toxic Sprays Are Banned?" *Conde Nast Traveler*.

World Resources Institute. 1994. *World Resources 1994–1995*. Oxford University Press.

CHAPTER 9

Food Quality

> *There was never the least attention paid to what was cut up for sausage; there would come all the way back from Europe old sausage that had been rejected, and that was moldy and white—it would be doused with borax and glycerine, and dumped into the hoppers, and made over again for home consumption. There would be meat that had tumbled out on the floor, in the dirt and sawdust, where the workers had tramped and spit uncounted billions of consumption germs. There would be meat stored in great piles in rooms; and the water from leaky roofs would drip over it, and thousands of rats would race about on it. . . . These rats were nuisances, and the packers would put poisoned bread out for them; they would die, and then rats, bread, and meat would go into the hoppers together . . . the meat would be shoveled into carts, and the man who did the shoveling would not trouble to lift out a rat even when he saw one—there were things that went into the sausage in comparison with which a poisoned rat was a tidbit.*
>
> —*The Jungle* by Upton Sinclair (1904)

The overwhelming sense of revulsion experienced by the American public upon reading Upton Sinclair's blockbusting exposé of conditions in Chicago's meat-packing industry at the turn of the century was a major factor leading to the passage in 1906 of this nation's First Food and Drug Act (Wiley Act). Although Sinclair's stated purpose in writing the novel was to obtain social justice for the downtrodden worker of the day, the most immediate impact of *The Jungle* was the introduction of new regulations to protect the quality of food consumed by Americans. Sinclair himself made the wry observation that "I aimed at the public's heart and by accident I hit it in the stomach."

From colonial days until the mid-1800s, problems relating to food quality were relatively rare, since most Americans raised their food at home or at least knew from whence it came. Consumers carefully inspected purchased items for signs of insect infestation, sniffed meat and fish to detect spoilage, and in general served as their own food inspectors. Government regulation of food quality prior to the 20th century was extremely limited, focusing primarily on commercially baked bread. Early bread laws were designed to standardize the weight of loaves in relation to the price of wheat; i.e. they were essentially price-fixing laws. Other regulations prohibited adding foreign substances such as ground chalk or powdered beans to flour. Subsequent laws provided for inspection of weights and flour quality (Janssen, 1975).

The growth of cities and the expansion of transportation networks which characterized the years immediately following the Civil War gave birth to an organized food industry whose rapid development was marred by unhygienic conditions (such as those described in *The Jungle*) and frequently unethical practices. The biggest scandal of 19th century food establishments involved the widespread practice of **adulteration**—the deliberate addition of inferior or cheaper material to a supposedly pure food product in order to stretch out supplies and increase profits. Adulteration has undoubtedly been practiced on a small scale for millennia by unscrupulous merchants when they thought they could get away with it, but the anonymity of large, unregulated corporations selling foodstuffs to faceless consumers hundreds of miles away gave great impetus to the proliferation of this age-old practice. Substances used as adulterants in some cases were harmless ingredients, cheating consumers only in a financial sense; in other instances, the adulterants consisted of toxic substances which posed a serious health threat to those consuming the adulterated products. Some foods commonly adulterated during the 18th and 19th centuries included: 1) black pepper commonly mixed with such materials as mustard seed husks, pea flour, juniper berries, or floor sweepings; 2) tea, adulterated on a large scale with leaves of the ash tree which were dried, curled, and sold to tea merchants for a few cents per pound. Green China tea was often adulterated with dried thorn leaves, tinted green with a toxic dye; black Indian tea was more easily adulterated by collecting used tea leaves from restaurants, drying and stiffening them with gum and then tinting them with black lead, also toxic, to make them look fresh; 3) cocoa powder "enriched" with brick dust; 4) milk supplies extended with water; 5) coffee blended with ground acorns or chicory.

Perhaps even more alarming were revelations in the late-19th century that many of the food colors and flavorings in widespread use were poisonous, e.g. pickles colored bright green with copper, candies and sweets brightly tinted with lead and copper salts, commercially-baked bread whitened with alum, beer froth produced by iron sulfate. By the turn of the century, over 80 synthetic agents were being used to color foods as diverse as mustard, jellies, and wine. Many had never been tested for adverse health effects and all were being used without any monitoring or regulatory controls; amazingly, some of these chemical additives had been developed as textile dyes and were never intended to be used in food products! Not surprisingly, contemporary accounts document a number of human illnesses and a few deaths attributable to consumption of toxic food colorants in those years (Tannahill, 1973; Henkel, 1993).

The 1906 Federal Food and Drug Act referred to previously reflected growing awareness of such problems and dealt largely with consumer protection against adulteration, mislabeling of foods, and harmful ingredients in foods. As a result of this act and of subsequent food quality legislation, instances of adulteration in the United States are now much rarer than they were in former years, though regulations have had to be instituted from time to time to prevent the gradual degradation of foods, such as the increase in fat or ground bone content of hot dogs or the decrease in fruit content of jams or fruit pies. However, occasionally flagrant abuses still do occur. In the fall of 1993 the Flavor Fresh Foods Corporation of Chicago, as well as 11 of its corporate officials, pled guilty to charges of defrauding consumers of more than $40 million through sales of adulterated orange juice. For 12 years Flavor Fresh had been marketing a product labeled as "100% pure orange juice from concentrate," selling it widely throughout the Midwest. In reality, the juice contained 55–75% beet sugar, along with other adulterants added to conceal the substitution. The two-year investigation, which culminated in the convictions of those responsible, revealed one of the most extensive and complex fraud cases ever handled by the FDA district office involved, demonstrating that unscrupulous attempts to make a quick dollar at the public's expense are alive and well a century after the adulteration scandals of the late 1800s (Ropp, 1994).

Within recent years the focus of public attention regarding food quality has shifted from adulteration to a concern over the presence of contaminants and additives in our modern food supply. The fact that few Americans today produce their own foods at home means that almost all of us, to a greater or lesser degree, have no choice but to rely on foodstuffs produced by a massive food industry—foods which contain many kinds of additives and, in some cases, contaminants over which we have very little control. The rising interest in "health foods" is due, in no small measure, to the feeling of many people that industrially produced food is somehow less safe and less nutritious than the "natural" foods of yesteryear. Representatives of the food industry and, indeed, many scientists, counter that chemical additives are both safe and essential to ensure an abundant supply of food at affordable prices to a still-growing population. In an attempt to understand the nature of the debate and the rationale behind existing or proposed regulations, it is helpful to distinguish between those substances accidentally introduced into foods and those deliberately added to prevent deterioration or to enhance taste or attractiveness.

Food Contaminants

Substances accidentally incorporated into foods are called **contaminants**. Such contaminants include dirt, hairs, animal feces, fungal growths, insect fragments, pesticide residues, traces of growth hormones or antibiotics, and so on, that are introduced into food during the harvesting, processing, or packaging stage. They serve no useful purpose in the finished product and are presumed to be harmful unless proven otherwise. (In many cases, however, common food contaminants constitute an aesthetic affront to consumers rather than an actual health threat; for example, the thought of eating a fly wing hidden among the oregano leaves on a frozen pizza may be repugnant, but it won't make you sick—at least not if you don't see it!) Certainly every effort should be made to keep our foods as free from contamination as possible; however, it has never been, and probably never will be, possible to grow, harvest, and process crops that are totally free of natural defects. In order to ensure that foods are never contaminated by even a few insects, rodent hairs or droppings, etc., we would have to use much larger amounts of chemical pesticides and would thus risk exposing consumers to the potentially greater hazard of increased levels of toxic residues. Current philosophy holds that it is wiser to permit aesthetically unpleasant but harmless natural defects rather than pouring on more synthetic chemicals. For this reason, the Food and Drug Administration (FDA) has established what it terms **defect action levels**, specifying the maximum limit of contamination at or above which the agency will take legal action to remove the product from the market. It is important to understand that such defect action levels are not average levels of contamination—the averages are considerably lower—but represent the upper limit of allowable contamination. Defect action levels are set at that point where it is assumed there is no danger to human health. Some examples of existing defect action levels are shown in Figure 9–1.

Several groups of food contaminants that are less visible but more worrisome are the traces of antibiotics and growth hormones in meat products and toxic pesticide residues on fruits and vegetables. Subtherapeutic amounts (i.e. levels lower than those used to treat disease) of antibiotics such as penicillin and tetracycline, both of which are extensively used to treat human illnesses as well, have been incorporated

Figure 9-1 Examples of Food Defect Action Levels

Product	Defect	Action Level
Apricots, canned	Insect filth	Average of 2% or more by count insect-infested or insect-damaged
Beets, canned	Rot	Exceeds average of 5% by weight of pieces with dry rot
Broccoli, frozen	Insects and mites	Average of 60 aphids, thrips, and/or mites per 100 grams
Cherries, maraschino	Insect filth	Average of over 5% rejects due to maggots
Corn, canned	Insect larvae (corn ear worms, corn borers)	Two or more 3 mm or longer larvae, cast skins or cast skin fragments of corn ear worm or corn borer, the aggregate length exceeding 12 mm in 24 pounds
Curry powder	Insect filth	Average of more than 100 insect fragments per 25 grams
	Rodent filth	Average of more than 4 rodent hairs per 25 grams
Olives, pitted	Pits	Average of more than 1.3% by count of olives with whole pits and/or pit fragments 2 mm or longer measured in the longest dimension
Peanut butter	Insect filth	Average of 30 or more insect fragments per 100 grams
	Rodent filth	Average of 1 or more rodent hairs per 100 grams
	Grit	Gritty taste and water insoluble inorganic residue is more than 25 mg per 100 grams
Tomatoes, canned	Drosophila fly	Average of 10 fly eggs per 500 grams; or 5 fly eggs and 1 maggot per 500 grams; or 2 maggots per 500 grams

into livestock and poultry feed to an increasing extent since the early 1950s. While the livestock industry contends that this practice helps to prevent disease, promotes growth, and results in greater weight gain per unit of feed consumed, critics point out that beneficial effects are most pronounced when animals are raised under crowded, unsanitary conditions and are, in effect, germ-killers which would scarcely be necessary in situations where high standards of hygiene existed. Concern about the use of antibiotics centers around the fact that widespread use of these drugs could promote the development of bacterial strains resistant to penicillin, tetracycline, and so on—resistance which it is now known can be genetically transferred from one strain of bacteria to another, human pathogens included. In recent decades an increasing number of bacteria which cause such human ailments as salmonellosis, gonorrhea, and pneumonia have become resistant to one or more kinds of antibiotics and it is suspected that the use of such drugs in animal feed, as well as the

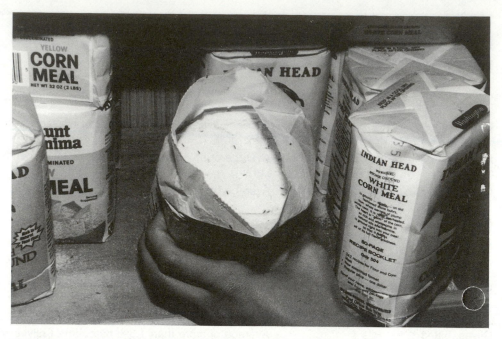

What consumer wouldn't be repulsed by the sight of rodent feces in a package of corn meal? [NYS Department of Agriculture and Markets, Division of Food Safety and Inspection]

overprescription of antibiotics for human use, has played a significant role in the resistance problem. Although it hadn't been conclusively shown that subtherapeutic use of antibiotics in livestock fodder threatens public health, a corresponding lack of proof that their use was safe prompted the FDA in 1977 to propose banning such uses of both penicillin and tetracycline, making feeds containing these drugs available only upon a veterinarian's order—a procedure instituted in Great Britain as early as 1969. Immediate protests from a livestock industry whose economic interests were threatened caused Congress to intercede, halting regulatory action and insisting on further studies (Wirth, 1983). Concerns about acquired antibiotic resistance gained new credibility in the spring of 1985 when the most serious outbreak of salmonellosis on record afflicted more than 16,000 in six Midwestern states and left two people dead. Transmitted through contaminated milk, the strain of bacteria which caused this outbreak demonstrated resistance to tetracycline and all forms of penicillin and was believed to have arisen from the animal population.

Chicken producers initiated use of the sex hormone DES as a feed additive to promote weight gain in poultry in 1947, with cattle raisers following their lead a few years later. Before long, poultry farmers found it more efficient to implant pellets of DES into the necks of chickens, a practice which led to the country's first DES-inspired lawsuit when, in the early 1950s, irate mink farmers went to court after their animals became sterile from eating heads and necks of hormone-treated chickens. When it was discovered that the average DES content of chicken skin fat was higher than the level which induced breast cancer in mice, the FDA suspended the use of this hormone in poultry. Because subsequent testing of beef revealed consistent low-level residues of DES in meat also, the government in 1971 ordered that DES feeding be halted at least one week prior to slaughter, assuming this would be sufficient time for the hormone to be eliminated from the animal's system. Either the original assumption was incorrect or beef producers ignored the mandate, because DES residues continued to be found in beef throughout the 1970s. The link between DES "pregnancy supports" and the development of vaginal cancer in DES daughters generated further concerns about the use of the hormone in cattle feed and by mid-1977 the FDA finally was able to impose a ban against its use. Ironically, the growth promotion aspects of DES use highly touted by the livestock industry bring increased risks but no benefits to the consumer, since the weight gained is almost entirely fat and water, not protein (Norwood, 1980).

BOX 9-1
Is Irradiated Food Safe?

Controversy has raged for years over the pros and cons of utilizing ionizing radiation to kill pests and parasites in food products and to extend the shelf life of fruits, vegetables, meat, and fish. Already employed on a small scale in 36 other countries for the processing of approximately 50 different food items, food irradiation has been vigorously opposed by some U.S. consumer groups fearful of the possible health and environmental implications of "zapping" sizeable portions of the American food supply. Nevertheless, heeding endorsements from groups as diverse as the World Health Organization, the American Council on Safety and Health, the National Food Processors Association, and the American Medical Association, the Food and Drug Administration, after more than 40 years of research and extensive deliberation on the issue, is convinced of the safety of using radiation as a food preservative and is gradually expanding its legal applications.

Employed since the mid-1960s to control insects in wheat and flour, as well as to prevent sprout development in potatoes, irradiation now can be used to kill trichina worms in fresh pork, to control insects and slow ripening in fruits and vegetables, and to kill pests in dry herbs, spices, and tea. In 1990 the FDA approved irradiation for poultry and is reviewing a request to permit seafood irradiation. In 1992 the first U.S. plant built specifically to irradiate a wide variety of foods (the first customer was a strawberry producer) was opened by Vindicator of Florida, Inc., near Tampa. Following numerous recent outbreaks of *E. coli 0157:H7* food poisoning, the U.S. Department of Agriculture is advocating approval of irradiation to kill bacteria in red meat. In permitting such uses, the FDA has specified maximum radiation levels for treating foods and requires that such products on the retail market bear the easily recognizable international logo, indicating to the consumer that the food in question has been irradiated. Food irradiation facilities must adhere to strict safety regulations promulgated by the Nuclear Regulatory Commission and the Occupational Safety and Health Administration (OSHA), and manufacturers must follow prescribed record-keeping requirements.

Some of the objections to food irradiation raised by concerned consumers are based on misinformation about what the process actually entails. The most common irradiation methods employ gamma rays (generally from a cobalt-60 source), X-rays, or electron beams which, unlike pesticides, accomplish the task for which they were intended without leaving any residue and without rendering the food itself radioactive (just as humans receiving dental X-rays or luggage passing through an airport metal detector don't become radioactive themselves as a result). Consumers handling or eating irradiated food are exposed to no radiation whatsoever. Some critics of the process worry that radiation results in certain chemical changes in the food, producing new radiolytic products which may be toxic. The FDA concedes that small amounts of radiolytic chemicals are indeed produced, but insists that 90% of these are natural components of food and the remaining 10% are chemically analogous to naturally occurring substances in food. The FDA disputes any toxic hazard to the public posed by such chemicals, stating that the amounts are far too small to pose any risk. Charges that irradiation can alter the texture, flavor, or nutritional value of foods are countered by observations that cooking, canning, or freezing produce equivalent changes. Studies indicate that irradiation reduces the nutrient value of food by about 10–15%—an amount roughly equivalent to the decrease caused by other processing methods—and is actually less destructive of carbohydrates, fats, proteins, and minerals. Similarly, irradiation destroys smaller amounts of vitamin D, niacin, and riboflavin than would occur with pasteurization. On the other hand, vitamins A, C, E, and K are especially sensitive to irradiation; up to 25% of these nutrients may be destroyed. All things considered, groups such as the United Nations' *Codex Alimentarius Commission* conclude that at radiation levels well in excess of U.S.-permitted dosages, irradiation poses no toxicological hazard to foods nor does it present any special nutritional problems.

In a world where pests and spoilage continue to claim a sizeable share of each year's harvest, and with increasing concerns regarding toxic chemical residues on food, the desirability of expanding the use of irradiation for food preservation deserves careful and dispassionate consideration by the American consumer.

References
Mason, James O. 1992. "Food Irradiation—Promising Technology for Public Health." *Public Health Reports* 107, no. 5 (Sept./Oct.).

Papazian, Ruth. 1992. "Food Irradiation: A Hot Issue." *Harvard Health Letter* 17, no. 10 (Aug.).

Early in 1994 a genetically engineered growth hormone intended to boost milk production was introduced onto the market by Monsanto, a move which provoked an outpouring of concern from some consumer groups (as well as from some dairy farmers worried about milk surpluses and falling prices). The new hormone, alternatively known as **rBGH** (recombinant Bovine Growth Hormone) or **BST** (Bovine Somatotropin), is injected into dairy cows every 14 days, resulting in an almost instant 5% or greater increase in milk production. After extensive studies evaluating the safety and efficacy of the hormone, the Food and Drug Administration approved sale of the hormone, making rBGH the first commercially important product of agricultural biotechnology to be incorporated into the nation's food supply. Fearful of a boycott by consumer activist groups, several large national supermarket chains initially declined to stock dairy products from farms using the engineered hormone, even though milk from hormone-treated cows is indistinguishable from that produced by untreated animals. Critics charged that, by raising milk output per cow, the hormone puts additional stress on the animals, increasing the likelihood of udder infections and thereby necessitating more use of antibiotics and other drugs—thus resulting in more chemical residues in milk. The FDA insists the government has safeguards in place to monitor milk supplies for traces of antibiotics and bacteria and will destroy any milk which is tainted. Dairy farmers who plan to use rBGH acknowledge that herds receiving hormone injections will need additional feed and special care, but are convinced the product is safe for both cows and people (Schneider, 1994; "Lines Drawn," 1994).

Pesticide residues in food can result from direct spraying of crops or from the consumption by livestock of pesticide-contaminated fodder, traces of which can then be translocated into meat, eggs, or milk. EPA has established **tolerance levels** for all pesticides used on food crops representing the maximum quantity of a pesticide residue allowable on a raw agricultural commodity. Such tolerances constitute the federal government's principle means of regulating pesticide residues in food. These levels are based on results of field trials performed by pesticide manufacturers and reflect the maximum residue concentrations likely when farm chemicals are applied properly. In essence, tolerance levels are set on the basis of good agricultural practices and not on considerations of human health. In 1987 the National Research Council of the National Academy of Sciences published an alarming report estimating a significant increase in cancer mortality among American consumers due to ingestion of certain pesticide residues on food, even when the amounts of such chemicals are within the established tolerance levels (National Research Council, 1993, 1987). Of far greater concern than chemical residues on U.S. agricultural commodities, however, is the health threat posed by toxins on imported foods. Since the mid-1970s when the Environmental Protection Agency banned such pesticides as DDT, endrin, dieldrin, aldrin, heptachlor, and Kepone due to test results showing them to be carcinogenic, many consumers have assumed their exposure to the toxins has ceased. Recent revelations, however, indicate that the food Americans eat still contains potentially dangerous pesticide residues because of pesticide use overseas. Many of the chemicals now banned in the United States are sold to developing nations who use them extensively in producing crops for export to the American market. Government estimates indicate that at least 10% of all imported food is contaminated, mostly with pesticides no longer permitted for use in this country. For example, a 1977 FDA study revealed that 45% of unroasted coffee beans tested contained illegal pesticide residues (Weir, 1979); tea and sugar from India as well as cocoa from Ecuador are imported bearing residues of highly toxic

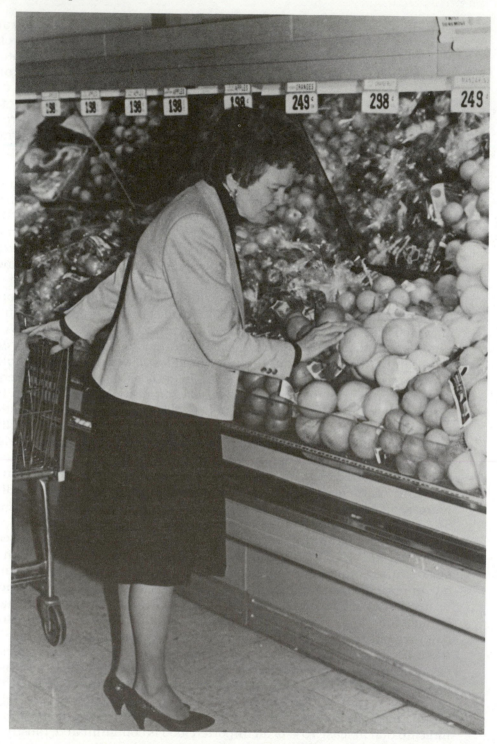

Consumer concerns about pesticide residues on food have been heightened by reports from such groups as the National Academy of Sciences and the Natural Resources Defense Council, warning that many fruits and vegetables in the marketplace bear traces of cancer-causing agrichemicals. [Author's photo]

Figure 9-2 Percent of Various Fruits and Vegetables Found to Contain Residues of One or More Pesticides

	%	Samples Tested
Strawberries	82	168
Cherries	80	90
Oranges	80	237
Peaches	79	246
Apples	78	542
Celery	75	114
Pears	73	328
Lettuce	68	201
Spinach	54	163
Carrots	50	252
Entire Sample	59	4,468

Source: U.S. Environmental Protection Agency, 1990–1992 data.

chlorinated hydrocarbon pesticides. Bananas are repeatedly sprayed with dieldrin, Kepone, and DDT—all banned in the United States; fortunately, such residues are largely discarded with the banana peel (Hornblower, 1980).

Such facts and figures may represent but the tip of the iceberg, since the General Accounting Office (GAO) found that the methods used by the FDA for testing food imports for pesticide contamination are highly ineffective, capable at best of detecting only 90 of the 268 pesticides for which the government has set tolerance levels. Even these are seldom found, since less than 1% of all the food shipments entering the United States are tested at all. When illegal pesticide residues are detected, it is usually too late to prevent marketing and consumption of the product because the shipment isn't detained at the port of entry while a sample is being analyzed ("Better Regulation," 1979). Indeed, the GAO reports that during one 15-month period, half of all the food identified by the FDA as being contaminated was subsequently marketed to consumers without any warning announcements, nor were the importers penalized in any way (Weir and Schapiro, 1980). In light of the extent to which pesticide residues are commonly present as contaminants on fresh produce, the oft-ignored motherly admonition to wash fruits and vegetables well, or to peel them, before eating takes on new significance.

Food Additives

More controversial than the accidental, often unavoidable, food contaminants are the approximately 2800 food **additives**, substances intentionally added to food to modify its taste, color, texture, nutritive value, appearance, resistance to deterioration, and so forth. The years since the end of World War II have witnessed explosive growth of the food chemical industry, as food processors responded to public demand (or occasionally created public demand) by promoting a host of new products—convenience foods, frozen foods, dehydrated foods, ethnic foods, low-calorie foods. Many of these products could not exist in a world free of additives. Nevertheless, a great many people are automatically suspicious of additives with long, unfamiliar, often unpronounceable names; reading the list of ingredients on virtually any supermarket package, can, or bottle seems a bit like a quick tour of a chemical factory. However, there's nothing inherently evil about using additives, provided that the chemical in question has no adverse effect on human health and performs a useful function. Many substances that can technically be termed "additives" have been in use for thousands of years—sugar, salt, and spices constitute just a few examples. Some additives come from natural sources; lecithin, derived from soybeans or corn, is used as an emulsifier to achieve the desired consistency in products such as cake mixes, non-dairy creamers, salad dressings, ice cream, and chocolate milk. Other food additives are factory-made but are chemically the same as their natural analogs. The synthetic vitamins and minerals added to foods to improve nutritive value are examples of these; identical in chemical composition to natural vitamins and minerals found in food, they are preferentially used because they are less expensive and more readily available. Such synthetic additives frequently are more concentrated, more pure, and of a more consistent quality than some of their counterparts in the natural world. The use of synthetic vitamins and minerals in food over the past half century has had a profound impact on public health in the United States, virtually eliminating certain deficiency diseases that in former years afflicted large numbers of Americans. The addition of vitamin D to milk, iodine to table salt, and niacin to bread has relegated rickets, goiter, and pellagra, respectively, to nearly non-existent status in this country. Other additives perform such useful functions as retarding spoilage, preventing fats from turning rancid, retaining moisture in some foods and keeping it out of others.

Most people don't quarrel about additives used for these purposes. What does concern many scientists and laypersons alike is that a not-insignificant number of chemicals are used as food additives for purely cosmetic purposes—and many of these have been shown to be toxic, carcinogenic, or both.

Until 1958, food processors wishing to use a new additive were free to do so unless the FDA could prove that the additive in question was harmful to human health. With the passage of the Food Additives Amendment to the Food, Drug, and Cosmetic Act in that year, the situation

Figure 9-3   Common Types of Food Additives

Group	Purpose	Examples
Antioxidants	prevent fats from turning rancid and fresh fruits from darkening during processing; minimize damage to some amino acids and loss of some vitamins	BHA, BHT, propylgallate
Bleaching agents	whiten and age flour	benzoyl peroxide, chlorine, nitrosyl chloride
Emulsifiers	to disperse one liquid in another; to improve quality and uniformity of texture	lecithin, mono- and diglycerides, sorbitan monostearate, polysorbates
Acidulants	maintain acid-alkali balance in jams, soft drinks, vegetables, etc., to keep them from being too sour	sodium bicarbonate, citric acid, lactic acid, phosphoric acid
Humectants	maintain moisture in foods such as shredded coconut, marshmallows, and candies	sorbitol, glycerol, propylene glycol
Anti-caking compounds	keep salts and powdered foods free-flowing	calcium or magnesium silicate, magnesium carbonate, tricalcium phosphate, sodium aluminosilicate
Preservatives	control growth of spoilage organisms	sodium propionate, sodium benzoate, propionic acid
Stabilizers	provide proper texture and consistency to ice cream, cheese spreads, salad dressings, syrups	gum arabic, guar gum, carrageenan, methyl cellulose, agar-agar

was reversed: the manufacturer of any proposed food additive now has to satisfy the FDA that the product is safe before it can be approved for use. Proof of safety must include such considerations as: 1) the amount of the additive that is likely to be consumed along with the food product; 2) the cumulative effect of ingesting small amounts of the additive over a long period of time; and 3) the potential for the additive to act as a toxin or a carcinogen when consumed by humans or animals (Foulke, 1993). Approval can be rescinded at any time if new information indicates that the additive is unsafe.

While protection of public health is the main intent of the Food Additives Amendment, the law is also designed to prevent consumer fraud by prohibiting the use of preservatives that make foods look fresher than they really are. A case in point is the regulation forbidding the use of sulfites on meats, since these restore the red color, deceptively lending a just-slaughtered appearance to a variety of meat products. On the other hand, sodium nitrite, another additive recognized for its ability to "fix" the red color of fresh meats, *can* legally be added to meat, fish, and poultry because its primary purpose is to act as a preservative, deterring both spoilage and botulism, a deadly disease caused by the presence of a bacterial toxin. Because it is now known that nitrites can react with other compounds in food to produce **nitrosamines**, substances known to be carcinogenic, food processors wishing to use the additive must take precautionary measures to severely limit nitrosamine formation (Foulke, 1993).

Undoubtedly the section of the Food Additives Amendment that has generated the most heated controversy in recent years is the **Delaney Clause**, which flatly prohibits the use in food of any ingredient shown to cause cancer in animals or humans (people who question why the FDA bans certain moderately carcinogenic food dyes yet takes no action against cigarettes have to be reminded that the Delaney Clause pertains solely to carcinogenic food additives, not to carcinogens in general; if a food processor should propose to add cigarette smoke as a flavoring to, say, cured meats, this would undoubtedly be prohibited under the Delaney Clause). While many environmental groups feel that the Delaney Clause constitutes the public's sole line of defense against the deliberate addition of carcinogens to the nation's food supply, critics charge that the "zero tolerance" standard implicit in this mandate is unrealistic and an example of regulatory overkill which fails to recognize enormous advances in analytical techniques since the Delaney Clause was enacted in 1958. Whereas the best efforts at chemical analysis during the 1950s yielded results in the parts per million range, today's monitoring devices routinely detect the presence of chemical residues in the parts per trillion. Whether a carcinogen which presents a health hazard at doses measured in parts per *million* is equally threatening at concentrations of parts per *trillion* is currently the topic of a bitter, as-yet unresolved, debate.

Since many hundreds of food additives were already in widespread use at the time the 1958 amendment was passed, a portion of this legislation exempted such substances from the rigorous safety testing demanded for new additives. Instead, additives already in common usage were designated "generally regarded as safe" and placed on what is referred to as the **GRAS list**. In order to remove a food additive from the GRAS list, the FDA must demonstrate that the substance in question is harmful. Original screening of existing food additives to determine whether they should be placed on the GRAS list was done rather haphazardly, and by the 1970s it was recognized that long-time usage is no firm guarantee of safety. Recently more thorough studies of certain substances included on the GRAS list have resulted in withdrawal of approval for their use. Some of the once-common food additives subsequently removed from the GRAS list include:

- *Cyclamates*—artificial sweeteners banned in 1970 because animal testing indicated they could induce bladder cancer and birth defects.
- *Cobaltous salts*—used from 1963–1966 to improve the stability of beer foam; associated with fatal heart attacks among heavy beer drinkers in the United States and Canada.

- *Polyvinyl chloride*—in plastic liquor bottles, banned in 1973 when carcinogenic vinyl chloride was detected in liquor.
- *Safrole*—carcinogenic, mutagenic extract of sassafras root, formerly used to give root beer its characteristic flavor.
- *Food colors*—a number of coal-tar dyes such as Red Dye No. 2, Orange No. 1 and 2, Violet No. 1, Yellow No. 1, 2, and 4 have been delisted because they were shown to be carcinogenic or to cause organ damage.

Numerous other additives still on the GRAS list are considered of dubious safety by many researchers, yet remain in use due to lack of conclusive evidence or because of industry pressure on FDA regulators. Critics of current policy insist that food additives require a higher standard of care than other environmental chemicals and shouldn't be used if they present a health risk. They base this judgment on the fact that everyone is exposed to chemicals in food, not only those who voluntarily assume the risk. Varying levels of susceptibility among individuals and the effects of simultaneous exposure to other chemicals, including synergistic effects, have to be taken into consideration. Both MSG (monosodium glutamate), a flavor enhancer which can cause the headache, dizziness, nausea, and facial flushing sometimes referred to as "Chinese Restaurant Syndrome," and a group of sulfur-containing compounds known collectively as "sulfites" or "sulfiting agents" (see Box 9–2) are examples of food additives that serve a useful purpose and pose no danger to the majority of consumers but which can provoke severe allergic reactions among a sizeable minority of sensitive individuals. Because of the vast processed food market, any miscalculation of risk can have far-reaching implications on a public which assumes and expects that special care is being taken with the nation's food supply. Nevertheless, although some health authorities recommend avoiding foods containing nonessential additives (such as artificial colors and flavorings) wherever possible, little evidence exists at present to indicate that the health of Americans is suffering due to the chemical food additives currently in use.

Foodborne Disease

Ironically, while questions dealing with the safety of chemical additives generate most of the public's concern regarding food quality these days, most cases of illness or death due to food involve a number of old-fashioned foodborne diseases commonly referred to as "food poisoning." Food poisoning can result from a variety of causes, including the following.

Natural Toxins in Food

The widely prevalent notion that all "natural" foods are safe and nutritious is a dangerous misconception. The faddish trend toward "living off the land" by collecting and eating various types of wild plants has led

BOX 9-2
Sulfites and Salad Bars

Until an FDA-imposed ban on the addition of sulfiting compounds to raw fruits and vegetables took effect in 1986, the trendy salad bar posed a temptation best avoided by up to one million Americans whose reactions to the chemicals can range from the unpleasant to the deadly: difficulty in breathing is the most common reaction among those allergic to sulfites, but some victims may experience nausea, flushing, fainting, diarrhea, hives, difficulty in swallowing, anaphylactic shock, even death. At greatest risk are the 10 million asthma sufferers, 5–10% of whom experts estimate are sensitive to sulfites.

Sulfites, a general term used to describe a number of sulfur-containing compounds such as sodium sulfite, sodium and potassium bisulfite, sodium and potassium metabisulfite, and sulfur dioxide, have been used for many years in foods, wines, and drugs to prevent discoloration and spoilage. Long considered safe, sulfites seemed a logical choice for food service managers who sprayed or dipped cut foods in sulfite solutions to keep salad greens crisp, mushrooms light, and fruits unbrowned while sitting for hours on display. Unfortunately, although sulfiting compounds pose no hazard to most people, a not-insignificant minority of the population lacks the enzyme to metabolize sulfites and hence may experience a severe allergic response to the chemical. After receiving more than 700 reports of adverse sulfite reactions, including several deaths, the FDA banned use of the additive on raw cut fruits and vegetables—a move aimed primarily at salad bars and supermarkets which were the sources of most reported illnesses.

While restaurants can turn to alternatives such as citric acid and lemon juice to maintain an attractive buffet, other sectors of the food and drug industry have few replacement options. Winemakers, who use sulfites to halt bacterial growth in wine, have no substitute for the chemical. In spite of complaints from some consumer groups, the FDA has refused to restrict the use of sulfites in packaged and canned foods, pickles, dried fruits, and potato and shrimp salad, arguing that few illnesses have been related to these sources and that the use of sulfites in such foods confers benefits far out of proportion to the risks. Instead, the agency now requires that if these foods contain at least 10 ppm sulfites, this information must be specifically included among the ingredients listed on the label. Certain medications present a more troublesome situation; over 1000 commonly used prescription drugs rely on sulfites to maintain their stability and potency. Many of these products are used by potentially sensitive asthmatics, but at present there is no effective substitute for sulfur compounds in pharmaceuticals. The best the FDA can do in this case is to require that sulfite-containing prescription drugs carry a warning to advise sensitive persons of the possibility of serious allergic reaction to the medication. It is hoped that the current regulatory approach, combining a selective ban, warning labels, and efforts at consumer education will permit the continued use of an additive which, though hazardous to some, presents no health threat to the majority of consumers and performs a valuable role in a wide variety of products.

References

Foulke, Judith E. 1993. "A Fresh Look at Food Preservatives." *FDA Consumer* (Oct.).

Lecos, Chris W. 1986. "Sulfites: FDA Limits Uses, Broadens Labeling." *FDA Consumer* (Oct.).

to a surge in food poisoning cases, according to some local public health officials. The fact is that there are many common plants, both wild and cultivated, that are poisonous, capable of causing ailments ranging from mild stomach disorders to a quick and painful death if consumed by the unwary. In addition, certain marine fish and shellfish species may contain toxins that induce severe illness or death. Some examples of plants or animals capable of causing a toxic reaction if eaten include the following.

Mushrooms. Mushrooms constitute a gourmet's delight, provided, of course, that the item in question is a nonpoisonous variety. The problem is that there is no simple rule of thumb for distinguishing between those wild forms which are safe and those which are not. Although only a relatively few of the thousands of species found in North America are poisonous, they may look very much like nonpoisonous species and frequently even grow together. One of the most poisonous types, the amanitas (one species of which is called the "Death Angel"), grow commonly in "fairy rings" in woods and on lawns. Just one or two bites of these alkaloid-containing amanitas can be fatal to an adult and, in fact, the vast majority of deaths due to mushroom poisoning are caused by these.

Water Hemlock (*Cicuta maculata*). Sweet-tasting but deadly, this relative of carrots, parsley, celery, and parsnips (to which it bears a strong resemblance) is the most toxic of all native North American plants. Because it is found throughout the continent, since it is quite similar in appearance to edible plants for which it is commonly mistaken, and because it is lethal even in small amounts, water hemlock is responsible for more deaths due to misidentification than is any other plant species. **Cicutoxin**, the poisonous substance in water hemlock, is a neurotoxin present in all parts of the plant and at every stage of development. Concentrations of the toxin are at peak levels in springtime and are highest in the root. In the fall of 1992 a 23-year-old Maine resident died three hours after taking just three bites from the root of a water hemlock plant he had collected in the woods (Centers for Disease Control, 1994). Children have occasionally suffered fatal poisonings after playing with toy whistles made from the hollow stems of water hemlock. Since there is no antidote for cicutoxin, about 30% of reported poisonings have resulted in the death of the victim.

Castor Bean (*Ricinus communis*). This attractive shrub-like plant is commonly grown as an ornamental foundation planting as well as commercially for its oil. The leaves of the plant are only slightly toxic, but the colorful mottled seeds can be deadly, containing a toxin called **ricin**. Children who chew on the seeds experience intense irritation of the mouth and throat, gastroenteritis, extreme thirst, dullness of vision, convulsions, uremia, and death. Only one to three seeds can kill a child; four to eight are generally required to cause fatality in adults.

Jimsonweed (*Datura stramonium*). This common weed contains toxic alkaloids in all parts of the plant. The seeds and leaves are especially dangerous; children have been poisoned by sucking nectar from the

BOX 9-3
Risk/Benefit Analyses: Who Benefits, Who Takes the Risk?

Is a pretty orange worth the threat of cancer? Should diet soda devotees be more worried about obesity or malignancy? Such controversial questions regarding the pros and cons of food additives are part of a wider debate over the extent to which government regulation can, or ought, to protect the public from environmental contaminants.

Desirable though it might be, elimination of all hazards faced by humankind is an impossibility—there is no such thing as absolute safety. Many, if not most, of the hazardous substances discussed in this book are either intrinsically useful themselves or are the unintended by-products of desirable goods or manufacturing processes. Rather than completely doing away with such substances, thereby losing the benefits they confer, society has attempted to reduce the risk by lowering exposure levels, at the same time permitting the chemical to remain in use. The difficulty in this approach, of course—and perhaps the key problem in environmental health—is to determine what level of risk is acceptable.

In recent years it has become fashionable in government circles, particularly among those wishing to undercut environmental protection laws, to resort to a procedure called risk (or cost)/benefit analysis—an effort that attempts to assign a monetary figure to all costs and benefits of a project or product (e.g. dam on a river, mosquito abatement program, installation of filters to reduce dust in an asbestos factory, etc.). The figures are then tallied and, depending on which side of the balance sheet the total is larger, the project is either killed or given the go-ahead. Of course the accuracy of original risk/benefit assumptions is crucial in arriving at a correct decision, as became quite obvious during the debate over whether the use of saccharin as a food additive should be revoked, per Delaney Clause mandate. Opponents of the ban belittled the cancer threat, citing the unreliability of animal testing and warning that millions of diabetics and overweight persons would, in the absence of diet colas, drink sugared beverages and thereby suffer even greater health risk. Supporters of the ban countered with evidence that consumption of saccharin has no positive effect on dieting but rather makes it harder to lose weight. They also cited diabetic experts who felt that victims of this condition have no intrinsic need for saccharin. Obviously there was no consensus on risks and benefits in this case.

Risk/benefit critics have long pointed out an obvious drawback to this exercise: it is virtually impossible to attribute monetary value to a human life or to abstract concepts such as scenic beauty, peace of mind, happiness, quality of life, and so forth. Thus many such studies undervalue risks, giving a false impression of the magnitude of benefits in undertaking environmentally questionable projects. Less discussed but equally relevant are the questions, "Benefits to whom?" "Risks to whom?" Although it's a common assumption that risks versus benefits are but opposite sides of the same coin, this is not always true. The case of food colorings is a prime example of the frequent divergence in risks and benefits. Few dispute the fact that this class of food additives serves no beneficial purpose in terms of making the food more nutritious, extending its shelf life, and so on. Food colors are used solely for cosmetic purposes—to make the food more attractive to the buyer, thereby promoting sales. Consumers have come to expect bright orange oranges (the natural color is slightly greenish), reddish hot dogs, and tinted dog food (obviously for the sake of the owner, since dogs are color-blind), even though the natural articles, while less eye-appealing to some, are just as tasty. In fact, the use of colors has aided manufacturers in subtly degrading the quality of their products. Dyes which make devil's food cake mix a dark, appetizing brown permit the producer to add less chocolate; yellow dye in ''egg'' bread makes it possible for the baker to reduce egg content—but not the price, of course; bright pink in strawberry or cherry-flavored ice cream substitutes for the lighter pink which use of the real, and more expensive, fruit would confer.

Thus the consumer obtains no real benefit from the use of food colors but does incur a certain degree of risk; a number of leading food colors have been removed from the GRAS list due to their proven carcinogenicity, while many others still in use are similarly suspect. For industry, however, the situation is the reverse. Eye-appealing products boost sales and tinting with synthetic chemicals is far cheaper than using real fruits, vegetables, and chocolate. The end result—enormous profits—make the use of artificial food colors extremely beneficial to industry with few, if any, risks. Risks and no benefits to the consumer, huge benefits and no risk to the food industry—this dichotomy exemplifies one of the most serious limitations in making equitable risk/benefit analyses.

flowers, eating the seeds, or drinking liquid in which the leaves have been soaked. A very small amount can be fatal to a child.

Ergot (*Claviceps purpurea*).   This fungus which frequently infects cereal grains, especially rye, produces a toxic alkaloid, ergotamine, responsible for the serious type of food poisoning known as ergotism or ''St. Anthony's Fire.'' When the fungal sclerotia growing on the rye grain are ground up with flour and subsequently consumed in bread, violent muscle contractions, excruciating pain, vomiting, deafness, blindness, and hallucinations can follow. One type of ergotism is characterized by severe constriction of the blood vessels, development of gangrene, and a painful death. Outbreaks of ergotism resulting in thousands of deaths were common until the 20th century when the decrease in home milling and institution of quality control in commercial mills reduced the level of flour contamination. Even so, small outbreaks of ergotism are still reported from time to time. Interestingly, federal controls do not apply to rye grown for the organic foods market (Klein, 1979).

Aflatoxin.   Another mycotoxin (fungal poison) already discussed in chapter 6, aflatoxins are produced by the mold *Aspergillus flavus* which grows on a wide variety of nuts, grains, and peanuts. When consumed, they can cause serious liver damage and are some of the most potent carcinogens known.

Certain Fish and Shellfish. Several different types of food poisoning are associated with eating various marine organisms. **Ciguatoxin**, a poison associated with certain fish living near reefs or rocky bottoms, has accounted for many food poisoning outbreaks in Florida and Hawaii (see Box 9–4). **Scombroid poisoning**, generally associated with deep-sea fish such as tuna and mackerel, is caused by ingestion of a toxin produced by certain bacteria acting on the flesh of fish which aren't handled properly after catching. Onset of symptoms such as a flushing of the skin, headache, dizziness, a burning sensation in the mouth, hives, and the usual gastrointestinal discomfort, generally occurs very quickly, averaging 1/2 hour after eating. **Paralytic Shellfish Poisoning (PSP)** results from eating shellfish such as oysters, clams, or scallops contaminated with saxitoxin, a nerve poison produced by microscopic dinoflagellates (algae). PSP is characterized by numbness in the mouth and extremities, gastroenteritis, and in severe cases, difficulty in speaking and walking; such symptoms occur within 30 minutes to 3 hours after eating. In a small percentage of cases death may result. Protection of the public against PSP depends on effective shellfish sanitation and inspection programs in the states where harvesting occurs.

Microbial Contamination

Microbial pathogens are responsible for the vast majority of food poisoning incidents; in the United States alone, estimates on the frequency of foodborne illness range from 12.6 million to 81 million cases each year, with an economic impact ranging from $1.9 to $8.4 billion (Pierson and Corlett, 1992). While the toll in human suffering is immense, food poisoning cases are often misdiagnosed by victims ("I just had a touch of 24-hour flu"), stoically endured (". . . it'll pass in a day or two"), and, due to the nature of symptoms, often not reported (who wants to discuss the details of a bout with diarrhea?!). As a result, this entirely preventable malady fails to arouse the public attention it deserves and is perpetuated by widespread carelessness and ignorance of safe food handling principles. Although food poisoning can, and frequently does, occur with foods prepared and consumed at home, public health officials are most concerned with the potential for large-scale poisoning inherent in the current trend towards more frequent eating outside the home and with the rapid growth and sheer size of the food service industry in the United States today. As the number of meals eaten away from home increases, the task of preventing foodborne disease grows more challenging.

It should be noted in passing that food *spoilage* is not the same thing as food poisoning. Spoilage involves the decomposition of foods due to the action of natural enzymes within food, to chemical reactions between food and containers, or to the activities of certain types of bacteria, fungi, or

BOX 9-4

Barracuda Blues

Eagerly contemplating a week or two of "fun in the sun," winter-weary tourists bound for the beaches of Florida or Hawaii seldom expect to encounter any health problems more serious than the occasional painful sunburn. Nevertheless, with growing frequency those living in or traveling to the tropics or subtropics have been falling victim to a bizarre foodborne ailment called **ciguatera fish poisoning**. This affliction, which experts claim is now the most common of all seafood-related illnesses in the United States, accounts for over half the cases of foodborne disease traced to fish consumption.

The active agent in ciguatera poisoning is *ciguatoxin*, produced by a marine dinoflagellate, the free-swimming unicellular alga *Gambiendiscus toxicus*, which lives in association with other algae growing on coral reefs in warm ocean waters. As small herbivorous fish browse on the algae and are, in turn, eaten by larger carnivorous fish, the fat-soluble dinoflagellate toxin is transferred up the food chain, becoming more concentrated at each higher trophic level. Biomagnification of ciguatoxin explains why most cases of ciguatera poisoning are linked to consumption of large reef-dwelling fish. In waters off the Florida coast, red snapper, grouper, and especially barracuda have been identified as the chief culprits; in Hawaii, amberjack is the fish most frequently implicated, while throughout the Pacific region red snapper is the leading cause of reported cases.

Since few physicians are familiar with ciguatera poisoning, when the illness does occur it is often misidentified—not surprising since there is no diagnostic test for the ailment and symptoms can be confused with those indicating brain tumors, multiple sclerosis, or chronic fatigue syndrome. Just as there is no definitive test for diagnosis, similarly there is no cure at present (a recently developed treatment utilizing large intravenous doses of mannitol can significantly reduce the severity and duration of symptoms *if* it is administered within 48 hours after the toxin is consumed).

The best safeguard against ciguatera poisoning, as with all food-borne diseases, is prevention—something more easily said than done, since currently there is no commercially available test for determining whether or not fish are contaminated prior to sale. Nor can one rely on thorough cooking or other food processing methods as an assurance of safety, since ciguatoxin is not broken down by high temperatures, freezing, smoking, drying, or marinating. Therefore, about the only precaution a wary diner can take is to avoid eating large red snappers, groupers, or dishes containing unspecified ocean fish species (ciguatera is *not* associated with freshwater fish). Experts advise consumers *never* to eat barracuda; Dade County, Florida, has banned commercial sales of this fish, since more than a third contain dangerous levels of ciguatoxin (notwithstanding this prohibition, authorities worry that unwary customers may still be purchasing barracuda at dockside from independent fishermen). Fish *livers* should be uniformly avoided as well, since the poison accumulates in that organ. Because illness occurs only when concentrations of the toxin exceed a certain level, authorities concede that red snappers or groupers under five pounds are probably safe to eat; nevertheless, they recommend that other species such as mahi-mahi or yellowtail snapper might be a less risky choice.

While those living in northern climes, far from warm coastal waters, may feel smugly secure from the threat of ciguatera poisoning, in this era of rapidly expanding travel for both business and pleasure it's no longer unusual for a person to dine in Tampa, Honolulu, or Tahiti one day and be back home in Seattle, Chicago, or Pittsburgh the next. Consumers (and their physicians) must recognize that their culinary choices can have unexpected consequences and, should they choose to indulge in high-risk foods, be prepared to recognize the symptoms of once-exotic ailments and to seek prompt treatment.

Reference

Brody, Jane E. 1993. "Insidious Poison Lurks in Some Fish." *New York Times*, Sept. 8.

insects, resulting in unpleasant odors, taste, or appearance of the food. However, spoilage organisms do not produce toxins that would cause human illness if they were consumed, nor does eating food containing such live organisms induce sickness. The same cannot be said of food poisoning bacteria, whose presence is not betrayed by the appearance, smell, or taste of the food. The old term "ptomaine poisoning" often used in reference to food poisoning is a misnomer—there is no such thing. Ptomaines are foul-smelling chemical compounds produced by bacterial decomposition of proteins. Eating food containing ptomaines will not produce any illness.

The microbial culprits responsible for food poisoning can be grouped into three general categories: bacteria, viruses, and parasites.

Bacteria.   Of the various foodborne diseases, the greatest number of outbreaks can be traced to ingestion of food containing certain pathogenic bacteria or bacterial toxins preformed in the food before it was eaten. Bacterial foodborne diseases are classified either as **infections** or **intoxications**, depending on whether illness is caused by consumption of large numbers of live organisms or by ingestion of preformed bacterial toxins, respectively. The more common types of bacterial food poisoning have rather similar symptoms—symptoms which almost everyone has experienced at one time or another: diarrhea, abdominal pain, vomiting, dehydration, prostration, and often fever and chills in the case of bacterial infections (not, however, with intoxications). Onset of such symptoms usually occurs within 1–24 hours after eating the contaminated food, depending on the type of bacteria involved and the amount of food ingested. Examples of foodborne bacterial infections include:

Salmonellosis.   Often referred to by more descriptive appellations such as "Delhi Belly" or "The Tropical Trots," salmonellosis is the most common bacterial foodborne disease in the United States, estimated in recent years to afflict about four million Americans annually. Thanks in part to changes in life-style and to the way in which livestock is raised and processed, the incidence of this foodborne illness is steadily increasing. Caused by a number of species of the genus *Salmonella*, the disease is typically associated with eating poultry, meat, or eggs harboring large numbers of the rod-shaped bacterium. Nevertheless, numerous outbreaks have been traced to foods not generally associated with the disease: the largest salmonellosis outbreak in U.S. history, affecting an estimated 200,000 persons (16,000 laboratory-confirmed cases; many more unreported) in Illinois and several other Midwest states in the spring of 1985, was traced to milk. (Although potentially an excellent medium for the growth of *Salmonella* and other foodborne pathogens, milk today is considered one of our safest foods due to pasteurization and high standards of sanitation in the dairy industry; less than 1% of all foodborne disease outbreaks in recent years have been traced to contaminated milk.) Other unusual sources have included cocoa beans and marijuana (both were contaminated with animal feces harboring the pathogen).

Inside the small intestine, colonies of *Salmonella* continue to grow and invade the host tissue, irritating the mucosal lining. Sudden onset of disease symptoms most commonly occurs within 12–24 hours after eating the contaminated food, with 18 hours being the most common time interval; discomfort may persist for several days and some victims may remain carriers for months after all outward symptoms have disappeared, shedding bacteria in their feces and remaining capable of infecting others. Severity of the disease ranges from very mild to very severe, with young children, the elderly, and travelers often the most adversely affected. Among otherwise healthy adults, fatalities due to salmonellosis are rare (victims only *wish* they were dead!) but do occur occasionally—the Illinois outbreak claimed at least two lives, possibly several more. In addition to the obvious short-term effects of the ailment, salmonellosis sufferers may also develop serious chronic disorders as a result of their infection. About 2–3% of victims later contract chronic arthritis, while a much smaller percentage develop painful septic arthritis when the *Salmonella* bacteria invade the joints. Outbreaks of salmonellosis are of particular concern in hospitals or nursing homes where victims are already in a weakened state and where the consequences of an infection are most severe.

Listeriosis. Caused by *Listeria monocytogenes*, a pathogen associated with an extremely wide range of hosts (mammals, birds, fish, ticks, crustaceans) and commonly found in food-processing environments, this disease, once considered rare in human populations, has become a subject of increasing concern in recent years. Listeriosis outbreaks have most frequently been associated with contaminated dairy products such as milk and soft-ripened cheese and often result in tragic consequences; in one California outbreak, *Listeria*-contaminated cheese was blamed for 29 deaths. Listeriosis is particularly dangerous in pregnant women, where infection often results in septicemia, miscarriage, or stillbirth. Apparently healthy babies born to infected mothers may develop meningitis within a few days or weeks after birth. Newborns infected with *Listeria* have high

BOX 9-5
Hazardous Hamburgers

It just blows my mind that a cheeseburger can kill you.
—Diana Nole, mother of food poisoning victim

The anguish and dismay expressed by Diana Nole upon the death of her 2-year-old son Michael was mirrored by a nation horrified that one of America's favorite foods could cause widespread personal tragedy. Enjoying a quick meal at one of the thousands of hamburger restaurants dotting the urban landscape has become an integral part of our modern life-style. Nevertheless, as a serious outbreak of food poisoning in several western states in 1993 vividly reminded us, ground beef remains a potentially hazardous food, regardless of the clean, attractive environment in which it is served. Nearly 500 patrons of local restaurants operated by Jack-in-the-Box, the nation's fifth-largest fast-food chain, learned this lesson the hard way when they fell victim to the ravages of a recently-recognized foodborne pathogen known as **E. coli 0157:H7**.

A physician in the state of Washington was the first to sound the alarm in January, 1993, when he reported a cluster of children afflicted with **hemolytic uremic syndrome (HUS)**, a serious ailment in which red blood cells are destroyed, leading to kidney failure and possible death. He also noted a significant increase in emergency room visits by patients reporting bloody diarrhea. Stool cultures identified *E. coli 0157:H7* as the cause of these illnesses and case histories revealed that the majority of victims had eaten hamburgers at a Jack-in-the-Box restaurant during the week prior to onset of symptoms. Within days a multi-state recall of unused hamburger patties was put into effect; extensive publicity about the situation resulted in the identification of hundreds of additional cases, including one fatality, in Washington, California, Idaho, and

Nevada. In subsequent months, 22 deaths in 16 additional major outbreaks unrelated to the Jack-in-the-Box episode were reported, emphasizing the widespread nature of the problem and demonstrating that home-cooked hamburgers are as likely to harbor pathogenic bacteria as are those in fast-food restaurants. As investigations into the cause of the problem widened, *E. coli 0157:H7*'s importance as an emerging foodborne disease menace became increasingly apparent.

A nasty relative of the harmless *E. coli* strains which are normal inhabitants of the human gut, *E. coli 0157:H7* was first isolated in 1975; not until 1982 was it identified as the cause of human illness, blamed for two foodborne disease outbreaks in Michigan and Oregon. Today the pathogen is recognized as the causative agent of an estimated 10,000–20,000 foodborne infections in the United States each year and as many as 400 fatalities. Some medical authorities suspect the actual incidence may be even higher than reported data indicate, since clinical laboratories have not routinely cultured the stools of diarrhea victims for the presence of *E. coli 0157:H7*. One study conducted over a two-year period at several medical centers revealed that among patients afflicted with bloody diarrhea, *E. coli 0157:H7* is more frequently isolated from stool cultures than any other pathogen, including *Shigella* (i.e. the dysentery bacterium). In the aftermath of the 1993 western states outbreak, such results have prompted recommendations that culturing stool specimens for the presence of *E. coli 0157:H7* should become standard laboratory procedure.

A gram-negative rod-shaped bacterium, *E. coli 0157:H7* normally inhabits the intestinal tract of healthy cattle and is excreted with fecal material. It frequently is found on the udders of cows and thus can be readily transferred to raw milk or to milking equipment. Although the number of bacteria which must be ingested to cause illness isn't known with certainty, most researchers suspect it is quite low—certainly lower than the dose required to cause salmonellosis.

Most reported cases of poisoning with *E. coli 0157:H7* have been traced to consumption of hamburgers. Ground beef is particularly susceptible to contamination with any type of foodborne pathogen because microbes on the surface of the meat are transferred throughout the interior of the product by the process of grinding; similarly, ground meat provides a much more extensive surface area for bacterial growth than does a solid slab of meat. Nevertheless, some cases have been linked to raw milk and to unpasteurized apple cider. In 1991, 21 people in Massachusetts fell sick after drinking cider pressed from unwashed apples which had dropped off the trees onto ground contaminated with cow manure. While direct consumption of tainted food is responsible for most cases of *E. coli 0157:H7* poisoning, person-to-person transmission can also occur; one of the fatalities in the 1993 outbreak was a 17-month-old boy who contracted the disease at a day care center, presumably via fecal-oral contact with another child who had eaten at Jack-in-the-Box (ironically, the child who died had never even tasted a hamburger during his brief life). Since young children recovering from diarrhea remain infectious for one to two weeks after disease symptoms have disappeared, shedding pathogenic bacteria with their feces, strict hygienic precautions must be continuously observed when diapering or toileting youngsters.

Once ingested, *E. coli 0157:H7* multiplies inside the human digestive tract, producing a potent toxin which damages cells of the intestinal lining. These lesions permit blood to leak into the intestines, thus giving rise to the bloody diarrhea which generally develops within several days of eating contaminated food and is one of the characteristic symptoms of infection with this pathogen. Sufferers may also experience abdominal pains, vomiting, and nausea; only rarely will fever be present, however. In most cases the disease runs its course in 5–10 days and the victim recovers completely without treatment. Administration of antibiotics does nothing to improve a patient's condition and may cause kidney problems; similarly, with *E. coli 0157:H7* infections the use of antidiarrheal medicine is not advisable. For 2–7% of victims the consequences of infection are much more serious. In some patients, bacterial toxins pass through the damaged intestinal wall and enter the bloodstream, traveling to the kidneys where they cause severe renal damage, often necessitating blood transfusions and kidney dialysis. Even with intensive care, 3–5% of patients who develop HUS die. The disease takes its heaviest toll among the very young and the very old; the median age of the 477 patients in Washington state during the 1993 outbreak was 7½. The pathogen is now regarded as the leading cause of acute kidney failure in children—a fact which should prompt parents to be particularly vigilant about ground beef fed to toddlers.

Spurred by this tragedy, during the months following the outbreak personnel from public health agencies and the U.S. Department of Agriculture (USDA) launched a full-scale investigation of U.S. meat-handling practices and of the federal regulatory programs which are supposed to ensure food safety. The *E. coli*-tainted hamburger patties identified as the ultimate source of the problem were eventually traced to a number of meat-packing plants in the western United States and Canada. The fact that no glaring lapses in proscribed sanitary procedures were identified at these facilities emphasized the reality that current inspection practices—originally developed to guard against such early 20th century hazards as obviously diseased, rotted, or discolored meat—are incapable of protecting consumers against the invisible dangers posed by bacterial contamination or chemical residues. Until more modern methods for quickly and effectively detecting the presence of microbial pathogens can be perfected (and research efforts are underway to achieve this goal), it should be assumed by those who purchase and prepare meats that *some* level of bacterial contamination is likely to exist. This being the case, the immediate cause of the Jack-in-the-Box outbreak was failure of food service personnel to cook the meat thoroughly enough to kill any pathogens present. Perhaps the most useful information to emerge from this sad incident is the fact that previous recommendations that beef be cooked to an internal temperature of 140°F in order to kill *Salmonella* were insufficiently protective of public health regarding *E. coli 0157:H7*. As a result of the outbreak, the FDA now advises that hamburgers be cooked to at least **155°F** and held at that temperature for 15 seconds until no traces of pink remain in the center and juices run clear. For those cooking ground beef at home without benefit of the precise temperature-control equipment possessed by food service establishments, FDA recommends the higher temperature of **160°F** to ensure food safety. As consumer advocate Jeremy Rifkin remarked shortly after the 1993 incident, "The days of rare hamburgers are over." Liability-conscious food service managers in increasing numbers are refusing to accommodate those who request bloody burgers—thanks to *E. coli*, "well-done" or "burned" may be a diner's only choice in hamburgers from now on.

Moving beyond precautions in the kitchen, government agencies are currently striving to improve regulatory efforts to keep pathogens out of our meat supply. The Centers for Disease Control and Prevention (CDC) is assisting USDA's Food Safety and Inspection Service in its recently developed Pathogen Reduction Program, helping to identify critical control points, both on the farm and in meat processing plants, where bacterial contamination might occur. In March 1994, USDA announced new regulations to help consumers avoid foodborne problems by requiring meat processors to include safe handling information on all raw meat and poultry labels. Concurrently, research efforts have been initiated to determine the feasibility of developing a vaccine against *E. coli 0157:H7* for cattle. Some observers speculate that the most practical approach to preventing microbial contamination of meat is irradiation, a procedure whose effectiveness is now being scrutinized.

In the meantime, consumers would do well to heed CDC's precautionary advice on avoiding *E. coli 0157:H7* infection: cook all ground beef or hamburger thoroughly; if served an undercooked hamburger in a restaurant, send it back for further cooking; consume only pasteurized milk and milk products—avoid raw milk; make sure that infected persons, especially children, wash hands carefully and often with soap to reduce the risk of spreading infection.

References

Foulke, Judith E. 1994. "How to Outsmart Dangerous E. coli Strain." *FDA Consumer* (Jan./Feb.); CDC/NCIU. 1993.

Preventing Foodborne Illness: Escherichia coli 0157:H7. U.S. Dept. of Health and Human Services, Public Health Services (April).

fatality rates, as do older victims suffering from diabetes or compromised immune systems (AIDS victims or persons receiving corticosteroids, chemotherapy, radiation therapy, etc.). In the absence of antibiotic treatment, fatality rates due to listeriosis can be as high as 70%, though a 25%–35% fatality rate is more common. Recognition that *Listeria*, unlike other microbial pathogens, grows vigorously at low temperatures, makes this organism a subject of serious concern to regulatory agencies and to the food industry in general, since refrigeration provides no assurance against bacterial multiplication. The FDA has set a "zero tolerance" requirement for presence of *Listeria* in foods; as a result, 28% of all food recalls in recent years have been due to *L. monocytogenes* contamination (Pierson and Corlett, 1992).

Exhibiting characteristics of both an infection and an intoxication is:

Clostridium perfringens.   Because outbreaks of this foodborne ailment are usually associated with quantity food preparation in restaurants or institutions, *Clostridium perfringens* is often referred to as the "cafeteria germ." This illness is sometimes categorized as a foodborne infection because live bacteria multiply within the host; alternatively, it may be classified as an intoxication because the disease symptoms are caused by a toxin which is either produced by live bacteria inside the body or is already present in the food at the time of consumption. In either case, very large numbers of bacteria or large amounts of toxin must be ingested to produce *C. perfringens* food poisoning. Cooked meat and poultry that have been left unrefrigerated for several hours have frequently been traced as the source of an outbreak, as have meat pies, stew, and gravies. Disease symptoms generally become evident 8–22 hours after eating; fortunately, *C. perfringens* poisonings are relatively mild and of brief duration, discomfort generally lasting only a day or two. This type of food poisoning is becoming increasingly common as more and more meals are eaten outside the home.

Among bacterial foodborne intoxications the most important are:

Staphylococcus aureus. Sometimes known as "Roto-Rooter Disease" because of its violent onset, *Staphylococcus* intoxication is estimated to account for between 20–40% of all food poisoning cases. The causative bacteria are present in pimples, boils, hang-nails, wound infections, sputum, and sneeze droplets. People thus constitute the prime source of these organisms which flourish in such proteinaceous foods as cooked ham, sauces and gravies, chicken salad, egg salad, cream pies and pastries, and so on. Growth of the bacteria within the food medium results in production of an enterotoxin (poison of the intestinal tract) which is not destroyed when the food is cooked. When consumed, the toxin causes irritation and inflammation of the stomach and intestine, resulting in vomiting and diarrhea. Since illness is produced by a poison already in the food at the time of eating rather than by bacterial growth within the victim's intestine, the effects of bacterial intoxication appear more rapidly than do those of an infection. People consuming *Staphylococcus* toxin may experience the sudden onset of vomiting and diarrhea within as little as

30 minutes after eating, although a period of 2–4 hours is more common. As is the case with most foodborne illness, individual differences in susceptibility will result in some people becoming quite ill after eating the tainted food, while others may not be affected whatsoever (Koren, 1980). Due to the nature of the symptoms and to the fact that duration of the illness is relatively brief, seldom persisting for more than a day or two, sufferers of staph intoxication frequently blame their miseries on "the 24-hour flu" rather than on the true culprit—contaminated food. Deaths from this foodborne disease are extremely rare and most victims recover quickly without any complications developing.

Botulism. The most serious of all bacterial foodborne diseases, botulism is caused by the spore-forming soil bacterium *Clostridium botulinum* which, growing under anaerobic conditions, produces a deadly neurotoxin, the most poisonous substance known. Outbreaks of botulism have been most frequently associated with home-canned, low-acid foods such as beans, corn, beets, spinach, and mushrooms. This is because many home canners fail to realize that a long processing time (or a shorter time at high pressure in a pressure cooker) is necessary in order to kill the heat-resistant bacterial spores. If the spores survive, they can germinate and, in the absence of oxygen, multiply within the food medium, producing the deadly poison. If food contaminated with the botulism toxin is boiled for 15–20 minutes, the poison will be destroyed, but all too frequently such food is eaten uncooked or only briefly warmed, with disastrous results. In recent years a number of botulism outbreaks have been traced to commercially processed foods as well, mostly smoked fish or vacuum-packed items. Some recent botulism outbreaks have been traced to highly atypical sources, indicating a need for caution in situations where the causative bacteria encounter a warm, oxygen-free environment. In the fall of 1983, one of the worst botulism outbreaks in U.S. history resulted in the hospitalization of 28 victims (one of whom subsequently died) who had eaten "patty melt" sandwiches at a restaurant in Peoria, Illinois. Surprised investigators ultimately identified sauteed onions as the cause of the problem. Contaminated with *C. botulinum* spores from the soil in which they grew, the onions were fried in margarine which provided a protective air-free shield for germinating bacteria which proceeded to multiply in the incubating temperatures provided by the warming tray in the restaurant kitchen. By the time the onions were consumed many hours later, enough of the deadly botulinum toxin had been formed to cause the disease outbreak. In an unrelated incident in Baton Rouge, Louisiana, the following year, a restaurant patron was stricken with botulism after eating a foil-wrapped baked potato, warmed up from the previous day. The foil wrapping had provided the anaerobic conditions which permitted growth of bacterial spores on the potato skin, while remaining at room temperature overnight allowed multiplication of the organism and production of the toxin (Miller, 1984). Botulism is first evidenced by the usual gastrointestinal distress which generally appears within 12–36 hours, followed by the onset of neurological symptoms—double vision, difficulty in swallowing and breathing, stammering, and respiratory paralysis leading to death. Prior

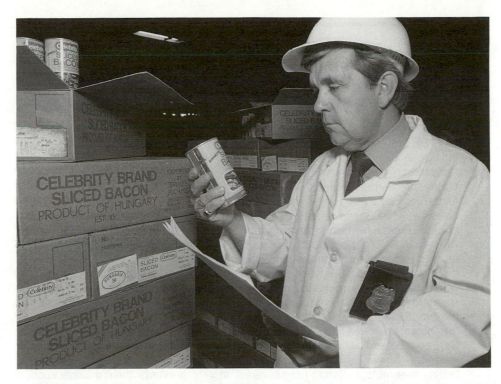

An inspector with the USDA checks a container of Hungarian bacon to verify its eligibility for importation into the United States. [U.S. Department of Agriculture]

to the 1950s, the fatality rate among botulism victims stood at about 60%; more recently, thanks to prompt administration of antitoxin and to improvements in respiratory therapy, death rates have dropped to 15% or less—still high in comparison with other bacterial foodborne diseases (Gunn, 1979).

Viruses.   Since viruses are unable to multiply outside a living host cell, these pathogens do not increase in number when they are introduced into food materials. Virus-contaminated foods simply serve as a route of transmission—a means by which virus particles can be transported from one host to another. Nevertheless, because the infectious dose needed to cause a viral disease is thought to be quite small, perhaps as low as 10–100 particles, viruses should never be allowed to contaminate food in the first place. Because the viruses associated with foodborne illness are of fecal origin, poor hygienic practices on the part of food handlers or food contact with sewage-polluted water are the most frequent causes of outbreaks. Since viruses are not utilizing the food as a growth medium, *any* type of food is a potential reservoir (i.e. pathogenic foodborne viruses, unlike bacteria, do not have any particular nutritional requirements for survival and hence are not restricted to certain "potentially hazardous foods"). Two of the more prevalent foodborne illnesses of viral origin are:

BOX 9-6

"It Must Have Been Something I Ate—But What?"

Scenario:

Concluding that they deserved a treat after completing mid-term exams, Susan and her roommate Amy decided to indulge in dinner out at an off-campus restaurant Friday evening. After pondering the menu selections, Amy opted for the seafood platter, baked potato, and coleslaw, while Susan chose barbecued chicken, French fries, and a tossed salad with Italian dressing. Both women ordered diet colas and German chocolate cake for dessert. Everything tasted delicious—a welcome change from the standard fare in the dorm cafeteria—and the two friends returned to their room a few hours later well-filled and content. Between 3 and 4 o'clock the next morning, however, Susan woke up feeling miserable, suffering from severe stomach cramps and nausea. She staggered down the hall to the bathroom where she promptly vomited. Shortly afterwards she began to pay repeated return visits to that facility as diarrhea began to take its toll. Susan spent the remainder of the weekend traveling between bedroom and bathroom, but by Monday morning she was beginning to feel human again and was able to make it to her 10 A.M. class. Some friends who had heard she was ill inquired as to the nature of her problem, to which she replied, *"It must have been something I ate!"*

Can *You* Identify the Cause of Susan's Problem More Precisely?

Theoretically, *any* food could be a route of transmission for foodborne disease. Nevertheless, some foods are implicated in food poisoning outbreaks much more frequently than others and are therefore designated by the U.S. Public Health Service as **potentially hazardous foods**—those which are capable of supporting rapid and progressive growth of infectious or toxigenic microorganisms.

For the most part, potentially hazardous foods are high protein animal products such as poultry, meat, fish, dairy products, and eggs—pathogenic microbes thrive on the same nutritious fare that humans prefer! They also grow well in cooked rice or beans, baked or boiled potatoes, and tofu. Because bacteria must obtain their nutrients in dissolved form, they can only multiply on moist food media, explaining why *cooked* rice, for example, is designated as "potentially hazardous" while raw rice is not. This inability of bacteria to grow in foods with very low water content is the basis for preservation of such food products as beef jerky or dried apricots. Drying foods does not *kill* microbes, however—it merely prevents their multiplication. If these foods become wet, bacterial growth will resume and their consumption could result in foodborne disease. Certain types of moist foods, peanut butter for example, are not considered potentially hazardous because the sugar and salt they contain tie up the water through chemical bonding, making it unavailable to support microbial growth. Food poisoning bacteria also have specific pH requirements. Most species grow best at pH levels ranging from 4.6 to 9; highly acidic foods such as citrus fruits, tomatoes, most fresh fruits, and pickles are seldom implicated in bacterial foodborne disease outbreaks.

Given this information, a sleuth attempting to discover what menu item was the likely cause of Susan's foodborne illness would, in all probability, zero in on the barbecued chicken; the acidic nature of salad ingredients and the fact that the potatoes were fried at high temperature and served immediately make them less suspect. Although chocolate cake could possibly be a vehicle for disease transmission if the eggs used in making it were contaminated, such an eventuality is uncommon (and the fact that Amy also ate the cake yet remained perfectly healthy further discredits the cake as a plausible suspect). Cola drinks are too acidic to support food poisoning bacteria, leaving the chicken as the only likely candidate—not surprising, since chicken and turkey are more often implicated in foodborne disease outbreaks than any other single food item. To confirm this suspicion it would be necessary to culture both a sample of Susan's stool and some of the leftover chicken from the restaurant and to show that bacterial isolates from the two are identical. Until such positive laboratory confirmation is obtained, the official cause of the illness can only be termed as "suspected." However, knowledge of which foods are potentially hazardous can prompt both food handlers and consumers to take special precautions with such items to avoid the situations which contribute to food poisoning outbreaks.

Reference
Educational Foundation of the National Restaurant Association. 1985. *Applied Foodservice Sanitation*. John Wiley & Sons.

Hepatitis A (HAV).   Most commonly associated with the consumption of raw clams or oysters harvested from sewage-tainted coastal waters, hepatitis A outbreaks have also been traced to foods as diverse as glazed doughnuts, strawberry sauce, sandwiches, orange juice, and salads. Symptoms of the disease, which include jaundice (an indication of liver infection) as well as the usual gastrointestinal distress, generally don't appear until 10–50 days after eating the contaminated food. An infection typically persists for weeks or even months, depending on its severity. An individual suffering from HAV can easily transmit the virus to others if he or she isn't conscientious about good hygienic practices, since the virus is shed in urine and feces. A victim is most contagious 10–14 days before the onset of disease symptoms and remains infectious until about a week after jaundice appears; thus rigorous adherence to routine handwashing practices at all times is of critical importance in preventing the transmission of HAV. A number of hepatitis A outbreaks have been attributed to direct person-food-person transmission, when an infected foodhandler failed to wash his/her hands after using the toilet, subsequently touched food which received no further cooking, and then served it to a customer. Since HAV can lead to permanent liver damage, extreme care should be taken to ensure that shellfish are obtained only from safe sources and are thoroughly cooked; similarly, it is essential that foodhandlers consistently maintain high standards of personal hygiene (Applied Foodservice Sanitation, 1985).

Norwalk virus.   A milder affliction than HAV, Norwalk virus causes an infection characterized by nausea, vomiting, abdominal pains, and diarrhea, with headache or slight fever experienced by some victims. The means of transmission (fecal contamination of water or foods) is the same as for HAV. Salads and shellfish are the foods most often implicated in outbreaks, particularly when consumed raw or undercooked (Pierson and Corlett, 1992).

Parasites. Certain parasitic protozoan diseases such as amoebic dysentery or giardiasis are typically associated with ingestion of sewage-contaminated drinking water but have been known to occur when infected food service workers transmitted the microbes to food as a result of faulty handwashing practices. Certain parasitic roundworm infections can occur when untreated sewage (''nightsoil'') containing worm eggs is used to fertilize certain vegetable crops. If such produce is consumed raw, the eggs subsequently hatch inside the human host and perpetuate the cycle of infection. Other sources of helminthic (i.e. worm) foodborne ailments include the consumption of raw or undercooked fish preparations. In recent years the United States has witnessed a small but increasing number of foodborne helminthic ailments traced to the growing popularity of ethnic specialties such as *sushi* or *ceviche*. Tapeworm infections are the most commonly reported problems, occurring predominantly along the West Coast where most victims admit to having eaten raw fish, mainly salmon. Symptoms of tapeworm infections, as well as time of onset, vary greatly from one person to another: some victims report experiencing severe cramps, nausea, and diarrhea almost immediately after eating; others may not develop symptoms for weeks or months. However, the majority of victims have no symptoms at all and only discover their infection when they pass the tapeworm, or segments of it, in their stool. Tapeworm infections can be eradicated with drugs, but roundworm infections (anisakiasis) are much more serious since there is no effective medication available. Such infections are very painful and may require surgery to remove the parasite. Consumers can easily avoid such problems simply by thoroughly cooking fish until it is flaky (internal temperature should be at 145°F for five minutes) or by freezing it at -4°F for 3–5 days before eating in order to kill the worms. Trichinosis, another foodborne illness caused by a parasitic roundworm, results primarily from the consumption of undercooked pork products (occasionally outbreaks are traced to bear meat or other wild game) which may harbor the larvae of the pathogen, *Trichinella spiralis*. Inside the human host, larvae mature into adult worms and burrow into the intestinal wall, producing new larvae which travel via the circulatory system to muscle tissue. There they embed themselves and produce the typical symptoms of foodborne disease. Although the presence of *Trichinella* in pork is considerably lower today than in past decades (thanks, in part, to prohibitions on feeding uncooked garbage to hogs—a practice which in years past perpetuated the cycle of reinfection), a potential for infection remains nevertheless. Because *Trichinella* larvae are killed by high temperatures, the surest way to prevent trichinosis *is always* to cook pork until well done. *Trichinella* is also cold-sensitive and will die if exposed to a temperature of 5°F (-15°C) for 30 days.

Preventing Foodborne Disease

Microbial contamination of foods can occur at any time from the production of food in field or feedlot right up to preparation and serving of the meal. Thus strict adherence to principles of food sanitation are essential at every step from production to processing, transportation, storage, preparation, and service if food poisoning outbreaks are to be avoided. The bacterial pathogens that cause foodborne disease are common inhabitants of the intestinal tracts of humans and domestic animals, present in healthy and sick individuals alike; some are naturally present in soils as well. When discharged in fecal material, these organisms can survive for long periods in litter, feces, trough water, and soil. Livestock feed is often contaminated with *Salmonella* organisms introduced when infected animal by-products are rendered and added to the feed mixture. Animals can become infected from any of these sources and thus bring such pathogens into slaughterhouses and poultry processing plants. Just one infected organ or carcass or animal feces can contaminate cutting equipment or workers' hands and thereby can transfer the bacteria to other carcasses or foods, a process referred to as **cross-contamination**. Once in a processing plant or food establishment, pathogenic organisms can survive on the surface of equipment for long periods and thus constitute sources of food contamination over an extended time period. For this reason, cleaning and sanitizing of grinders, choppers, slicers, and other equipment after each use and frequent washing of workers' hands are important measures in preventing cross-contamination.

Foods, particularly those of animal origin, often contain pathogens such as *Salmonella* and *Clostridium perfringens* when they enter the kitchen. *Salmonella* is present in 15–30% of commercial egg products and of raw dressed poultry. A worrisome development since the mid-1980s has been the recognition that even whole, uncracked eggs can harbor *Salmonella* organisms transmitted from infected hens via their ovaries into the developing egg. An increasing number of egg-related outbreaks of salmonellosis have been reported from the Northeast and Middle Atlantic regions of the United States since 1985. For this reason, much to the dismay of Caesar salad and homemade eggnog lovers, health agencies are now strongly advising against the consumption of raw or undercooked eggs. Such warnings should be regarded with special seriousness by nursing home administrators, since the elderly are especially susceptible to the ravages of salmonellosis (during the first 10 months of 1989, 12 of the 13 U.S. deaths associated with *Salmonella*-tainted eggs occurred among nursing home residents). In situations involving high-risk populations, only pasteurized or hard-boiled eggs can be considered entirely safe (Bennett, 1993).

Once in the kitchen, additional opportunity for contamination of food is presented by the food handlers themselves. The primary reservoir of the *Staphylococcus* organism is the human nose; if kitchen workers cough or sneeze near foods, the bacteria are readily transferred to an appropriate growth medium. If food handlers have infected cuts on their hands, boils, bad cases of acne or other skin eruptions, *Staphylococcus* bacteria likewise can be transferred to food. Similarly, since approximately 40% of all healthy people carry *Salmonella* organisms in their gastrointestinal tract and regularly shed the live bacteria when they defecate, failure of kitchen workers to wash their hands thoroughly after using the bathroom can result in contamination of foods with this pathogen.

Since so many foods contain at least *some* disease-causing bacteria, it is fortunate that the number of bacterial cells or concentration of bacterial toxins within the ingested food must be relatively high to induce the symptoms of most bacterial foodborne diseases (listeriosis and *E. coli 0157:H7* food poisoning are exceptions to this general rule). Thus the approach to preventing foodborne disease outbreaks must be two-pronged: 1) to the greatest extent possible, avoid microbial contamination of food in the first place through rigorous adherence to rules of good sanitation and hygiene; and 2) maintain environmental conditions that inhibit the multiplication of bacteria which may be present in small numbers within the food medium.

Sanitation

The importance of high standards of cleanliness and personal hygiene for protecting food quality has been given added emphasis in FDA's most recent (1993) revision of its model Food Code, a compilation of recommendations which local and state regulatory agencies can use to develop or update the mandatory regulations they impose on the more than one million retail food establishments in the United States (although the Code recommendations were designed specifically for application to the food service industry, the principles they embody pertain with equal relevance to food handling and preparation practices in the home). Under the new Code, issues related to personal health, hygiene, and handwashing practices of food service personnel have been assigned primary importance by placing them at the front of the book, ahead of all other requirements. For the first time ever, the Code holds the food service *worker* (as opposed to the facility owner or manager only) accountable for lapses in maintaining acceptable standards of personal hygiene. In an effort to forestall outbreaks of the "fearsome four"—the serious foodborne ailments most frequently transmitted by food workers (i.e. *Shigella*, *E. coli 0157:H7*, typhoid fever, and hepatitis A)—the new Code places a special obligation on employees to notify the person in charge if they are experiencing any symptoms of gastrointestinal illness or if they are suffering from boils, dermatitis, or other infections on the hands, wrists, exposed portions of the arms, or other parts of the body unless covered by a proper bandage (such infections are prime sources of *Staphylococcus* bacteria). Thus informed, the person in charge is required to restrict sick employees from direct contact with food or to exclude them from the establishment altogether until health problems have been resolved. Another prominent issue pertaining to personal hygiene under the new recommendations is handwashing. Justifying the strictest handwashing standards ever incorporated into a code, FDA cites

BOX 9-7

HACCP—Preventive Approach to Food Safety

In confronting the challenge of how best to ensure the safety of food supplies from biological, chemical, or physical hazards, government regulators and food industry quality assurance personnel alike have traditionally relied on an approach that involved periodic inspections of food processing facilities (e.g. mills, slaughterhouses, canneries, bakeries, supermarkets, restaurants, etc.) and random end-product analyses. The ineffectiveness of trying to protect public health in this manner through sole reliance on efforts to detect problems after-the-fact is attested by the continued prevalence of foodborne disease, prompting efforts to find a better way of ensuring food safety.

In recent years a concept known as the **HACCP** (pronounced "hassip"— **Hazard Analysis and Critical Control Point**) system has been winning enthusiastic converts among government regulators, food industry executives, and scientific organizations alike. Its endorsement by the National Advisory Committee on Microbiological Criteria for Foods and the 1992 publication by that group of a document defining HACCP terminology and describing HACCP principles promises to give a further boost to widespread implementation of HACCP programs throughout the United States and abroad. Indeed, promoters envision HACCP as contributing ultimately to a universal system of food safety which will facilitate international trade in food products while providing consumers with a high level of confidence that the products they purchase are safe.

So what *is* this radical new approach? Essentially HACCP is a preventive system of quality control which, when properly applied, can be used to control any point in the food system which might contribute to a hazardous situation—anywhere from a farmer's field to the consumer's table. The concept, like so many other innovations to late 20th-century American life, originated with the space program. In the late 1950s, NASA asked the Pillsbury Company to produce a food that could be eaten by astronauts in orbit. Such an undertaking presented a number of challenges, none more daunting than the imperative of ensuring that any food developed be 100% free of microbial, chemical, or physical contamination. The potentially disastrous consequences of a food poisoning outbreak inside a space capsule had to be avoided at any cost. Pillsbury scientists realized that only a proactive preventive system could provide the high degree of safety assurance required. Pillsbury spent the following decade developing and refining its concept and in 1971 adopted the HACCP approach in its own facilities. That same year the Food and Drug Administration awarded Pillsbury a contract to conduct classes for FDA employees on the HACCP system and in 1973 the company published the first comprehensive document on HACCP principles as a training manual for FDA personnel. By the early 1980s a number of U.S. food companies, following Pillsbury's example, had established their own HACCP programs, but HACCP's wider application in the public sector remained extremely limited. In 1980, several federal agencies requested that the National Academy of Sciences (NAS) examine the potential applications for microbiological criteria in food.

The result of that study was a 1985 NAS publication that strongly recommended the application of HACCP in regulatory programs, stating that HACCP "provides a more specific and critical approach to the control of microbiological hazards in foods than that provided by traditional inspection and quality control approaches."

Following this ringing endorsement by NAS, an increasing number of federal, state, and local agencies have been redesigning their regulatory approach in conformance with HACCP principles. Elements of the HACCP approach are now being used in the FDA's Seafood Inspection Program and by the USDA's Food Safety and Inspection Service. While food producers must develop individualized HACCP systems tailored to their own processing and distribution conditions, each HACCP program consists of seven basic steps:

1. *Analyze hazard*, identifying potential hazards associated with the food in question, based on close observation of how the food is grown, processed, and distributed—right up to the point of consumption; an assessment is then made of the likelihood of those hazards occurring and preventive measures for controlling such hazards are identified.

2. *Determine critical control points (CCPs)* to minimize or eliminate the hazards identified; CCPs comprise operational steps or procedures such as cooking, chilling, sanitizing, employee hygiene, etc.

3. *Establish critical limits or tolerances* which must be met to ensure that the CCP is under control; some of the criteria most often used as critical limits include temperature, time, pH, humidity, salt concentration, etc.

4. *Establish a monitoring system* through scheduled testing or observa-tion to ensure that CCP is being controlled.

5. *Establish the corrective action* to be taken when monitoring indicates a deviation from appropriate controls; because of the wide range of possible critical control points, a specific corrective action plan must be developed for each one.

6. *Establish effective record-keeping systems* that document the HACCP plan.

7. *Establish verification procedures* which demonstrate that HACCP is working correctly; such procedures require minimal end-product sampling (due to safeguards built into the system), relying instead on frequent reviews of plan procedure and affirmation that the plan is being followed correctly. Both the food producer and the appropriate regulatory agencies have a role to play in verifying HACCP plan performance.

Implementing a HACCP program in any given setting is neither quick nor easy. HACCP is a technically sophisticated system requiring extensive site-specific research, discussion, and preparation prior to application. Intensive training of both in-plant personnel and regulatory agency inspectors, as well as a high degree of cooperative interaction between government and industry are essential prerequisites to the success of any HACCP plan. Nevertheless, ultimate results are well worth the effort. According to the National Academy of Sciences analysis, effective use of HACCP in food protection systems is the one approach by which meaningful reductions in the incidence of foodborne disease can be achieved.

Reference

Pierson, Merle D., and Donald A. Corlett, Jr., eds. 1992. *HACCP: Principles and Applications*. Chapman & Hall.

germ-laden hands as a major vehicle of disease transmission in the food service industry, a situation resulting largely from negligence on the part of food handlers. The new Food Code calls on food service managers to monitor their employees' handwashing practices and describes what FDA considers effective handwashing: a vigorous 20-second scrub using soap and running water, followed by thorough rinsing under clean water; after using the toilet, employees must scrub *twice*, using a fingernail brush during the first wash to clean fingertips, under the nails, and between the fingers. In spite of the fact that food service employees are required to wear disposable gloves and to use tongs or deli tissue to handle exposed food, *rigorous handwashing practices represent the single most effective means for breaking the chain of infection.*

The new Code recommends that food service employees wash hands appropriately in each of the following situations (Foulke, 1994):

- immediately before preparing food
- during food preparation, as often as necessary to remove soil and contamination and to prevent cross-contamination when changing tasks
- when switching between raw foods and ready-to-eat foods
- after handling soiled equipment or utensils
- after using the toilet
- after touching bare human body parts
- after coughing, sneezing, using a handkerchief or tissue, smoking, eating, or drinking

Good sanitation of course involves attention to more than employee health and hygiene. General cleanliness of the facility, routine sanitization of cutting tools and food preparation equipment, safe food storage practices, effective dishwashing procedures, proper waste disposal and trash storage—all are important for ensuring that dangerous microbes and food never have a chance to meet.

Time-Temperature Control

When certain environmental preconditions such as optimum pH, moisture, essential nutrients, and temperature are met, populations of pathogenic bacteria in food multiply in accordance with the sigmoidal growth pattern described in chapter 2: after an initial lag phase of about one hour, during which there is negligible increase in numbers while the organisms adjust to new conditions, a period of extremely rapid increase in population size continues until the supply of essential nutrients diminishes and toxic by-products accumulate. At this stage, growth levels off and the number of organisms remains relatively constant until eventually a progressive die-off of cells occurs. Perhaps the most crucial element in determining the rate of bacterial multiplication during this sequence of events is *temperature*. The bacteria responsible for the majority of foodborne disease outbreaks multiply most rapidly within a temperature range referred to as the **Danger Zone,** defined under the FDA's new Food Code as **41°–140°F (5°–60°C).** Temperatures above 140°F will kill most actively growing bacteria, though bacterial spores and a few thermophilic species may survive. At temperatures below 41°F, growth of the bacterial populations associated with common foodborne illnesses either ceases entirely or is extremely slow; however, the organisms are not killed by cold temperatures and can remain viable for long periods of time, resuming multiplication when temperatures rise. Therefore, the most effective way to prevent buildup of bacterial numbers is to keep foods refrigerated, especially those proteinaceous foods that most frequently harbor pathogenic bacteria. Heating such foods thoroughly will kill bacteria that may be present in the food; the higher the temperature above 140°, the shorter the time the bacterial population will be able to survive (normal cooking times and temperatures are not sufficient, however, to break down *Staphylococcus* toxin).

To ensure complete heat penetration throughout the item being cooked, it is advised that internal temperatures reach the following FDA-recommended minimum levels to guarantee that any pathogens present within the food are killed:

Poultry and stuffed meats	165°F for 15 sec.
Pork	155°F for 15 sec.
Ground beef	155°F for 15 sec.
Other potentially hazardous foods	145°F for 15 sec.

It should be noted that the internal temperature of the item being cooked, rather than the temperature of the oven or burner, is the crucial factor. In many instances, large roasts of beef, ham, or turkey still harbor viable pathogens after cooking because they weren't in the oven long enough for temperatures at the center of the roast to reach the recommended 140° level. In the same way, large pieces of cooked meat held in the refrigerator for cooling frequently have internal temperatures well within the growth range, even though the refrigerator thermostat registers at or below 41°F as advised. To promote rapid cooling, cooked meat should be sliced into thin layers and placed in shallow pans before being refrigerated.

The most effective methods that food handlers can follow to prevent foodborne disease, be it in the home, in restaurants, or at large public gatherings, is to complete the processing of food within an hour or two while the bacteria remain in the lag phase of growth and to cool foods rapidly if they are not to be consumed immediately. Bearing these principles in mind, it should come as no surprise that an analysis of food poisoning outbreaks revealed that five out of the six factors which most frequently contribute to such illness are related to time-temperature control. The six factors most often implicated in bacterial food poisoning outbreaks are, in order of importance:

1. failure to refrigerate foods properly
2. preparing and cooking foods a day or more before they are to be served
3. failure to cook foods thoroughly

4. infected food handlers who practice poor personal hygiene
5. improper hot holding (keeping foods in heating trays at temperatures under 140°F)
6. inadequate reheating of cooked foods

Unfortunately, although good sanitation and proper time-temperature controls are relatively simple preventive concepts, they are all-too-frequently neglected by homemakers and commercial food establishments alike. Thus bacterial food poisoning, which fundamentally is a result of improper food handling practices and should not even exist in affluent modern societies, will undoubtedly remain our most prevalent food-related health problem.

References

Applied Foodservice Sanitation. 1985. John Wiley & Sons in cooperation with the Educational Foundation of the National Restaurant Association.

Bennett, Richard G. 1993. "Diarrhea Among Residents of Long-Term Care Facilities." *Infection Control and Hospital Epidemiology* 14, no. 7 (July).

"Better Regulation of Pesticide Exports and Pesticide Residues in Imported Food is Essential." 1979. U.S. General Accounting Office, Washington, DC, June 22.

Centers for Disease Control and Prevention. 1994. "Water Hemlock Poisoning—Maine, 1992." *Morbidity and Mortality Weekly Report* 43, no. 13 (April 8).

Foulke, Judith E. 1994. "New Food Code." *FDA Consumer* 28, no. 3 (April).

Foulke, Judith E. 1993. "A Fresh Look at Food Preservatives." *FDA Consumer* (Oct.).

Gunn, Robert A., ed. 1979. *Botulism in the United States, 1899–1977*, U.S. Department of Health, Education, and Welfare, Public Health Service (May).

Henkel, John. 1993. "From Shampoo to Cereal: Seeing to the Safety of Color Additives." *FDA Consumer* (Dec.).

Hornblower, Margot. 1980. "U.S. Firms Export Products Banned Here As Health Risks." *The Washington Post*, Feb. 25.

Janssen, Wallace F. 1975. "America's First Food and Drug Laws." *FDA Consumer* (June).

Klein, Richard M. 1979. *The Green World: An Introduction to Plants and People*. Harper & Row.

Koren, Herman. 1980. *Handbook of Environmental Health and Safety*. Vol. 1. Pergamon Press.

"Lines Drawn in a War Over a Milk Hormone." 1994. *New York Times*, March 9.

Miller, Roger W. 1984. "How Onions and a Baked Potato Became Sources of Botulism Poisoning." *FDA Consumer* (Oct.).

National Research Council. 1993. *Pesticides in the Diets of Infants and Children*. National Academy Press, Washington, DC.

National Research Council. 1987. *Regulating Pesticides in Food: The Delaney Paradox*. National Academy Press, Washington, DC.

Norwood, Christopher. 1980. *At Highest Risk*. Penguin Books.

Pierson, Merle D., and Donald A. Corlett, Jr., eds. 1992. *HACCP: Principles and Applications*. Chapman & Hall.

Ropp, Kevin L. 1994. "Juice Maker Cheats Consumers of $40 Million." *FDA Consumer* (Jan./Feb.).

Schneider, Keith. 1994. "Cow Drug Is Viewed As a Tool." *New York Times*, Feb. 5.

Tannahill, Reay. 1973. *Food in History*. Stein and Day.

Weir, David. 1979. "The Boomerang Crime." *Mother Jones* (Nov.).

Weir, David, and Mark Schapiro. 1980. "The Circle of Poison." *The Nation* (Nov. 15).

Wirth, David A. 1983. "FDA Flip-Flops on Antibiotic Hazard." *Environment* 25, no. 5 (June).

CHAPTER 10

Radiation

> The unleashed power of the atom has changed everything save our modes of thinking, and we thus drift toward unparalleled catastrophes.
>
> —Albert Einstein
>
> The most fundamental lesson of Three Mile Island, and one that must be continually emphasized, is that accidents can happen.
>
> —Report of Congressional Subcommittee
> on Energy Research and Production (1980)

Late in the autumn of 1895, a German physics professor, Wilhelm Roentgen, was busily pursuing a line of research which would soon revolutionize medical science and transform our understanding of the nature of matter and energy. Roentgen was experimenting with a cathode-ray tube, a device perfected by the English scientist Crookes two decades earlier which consisted of a glass vacuum tube through which flowed a high voltage electric current. By chance, Roentgen noticed that emissions from the tube caused a nearby sheet of paper coated with a fluorescent chemical to glow, and he observed that these emanations could be blocked to varying degrees by materials of different densities. Calling his wife to place her hand on a photographic plate, Roentgen turned on the cathode ray tube; when the plate was subsequently developed, Roentgen amazed the world with a picture of his wife's bones inside her hand. Realizing that he had stumbled upon a form of radiation whose existence was hitherto completely unsuspected, Roentgen appropriated the Greek symbol for the unknown and called his discovery "X-rays." Within a few days after publication of his findings, the medical profession put the fluoroscope and "roentgenogram" to use—the shortest time gap between announcement of a major medical discovery and its practical application yet recorded.

The implications of Roentgen's announcement far transcended the field of medicine, however. Upon hearing of Roentgen's findings, the noted French scientist Henri Becquerel became intrigued by the relationship between X-rays and fluorescence and thereupon directed his attention to naturally phosphorescent minerals. In February of 1896, just two months after publication of Roentgen's report, Becquerel placed some crystals of a uranium compound on a photographic plate wrapped in black paper and demonstrated that the emanations from the uranium exhibited the same characteristics as Roentgen's X-rays. Becquerel's work was quickly picked up by Marie and Pierre Curie who termed the mysterious phenomenon "radioactivity" and who soon succeeded in isolating two new radioactive substances, polonium and radium, from uranium ore (Cooper, 1973). Thus the independent discovery of both artificial and natural radioactivity within a three-month time span quickly led to the birth of a whole new field of scientific inquiry with far-reaching implications in physics, biology, medicine, and, unfortunately, warfare.

Ionizing Radiation

Early investigations of radioactivity quickly revealed that the observed emissions were of several different kinds. Some consisted of subatomic particles—protons, neutrons, or electrons—released when atoms spontaneously decay; these came to be known as **particulate radiation**,

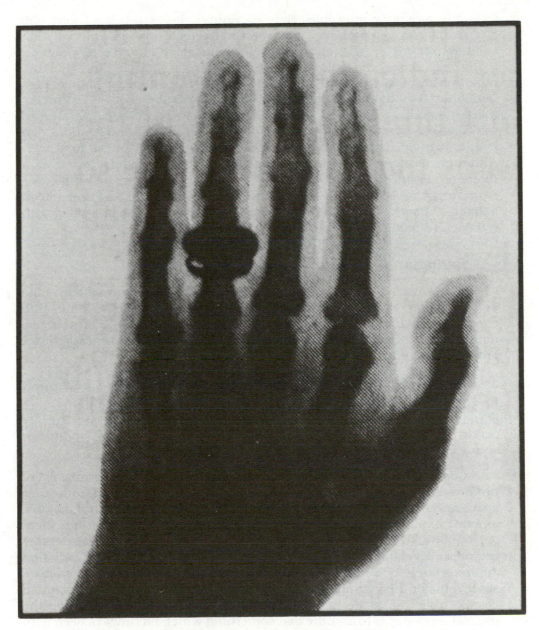

World's first X-ray: this is the "roentgenogram" that Wilhelm Roentgen took of his wife's hand thereby demonstrating the existence of the mysterious emanations that he named "X-rays."

a group which includes **alpha** and **beta particles**. Other emissions, such as Roentgen's X-rays and naturally occurring **gamma rays**, were shown to consist of highly energetic short wavelengths of electromagnetic radiation, a form of energy which also includes ultraviolet light, visible light, infrared waves, and microwaves. Alpha and beta particles, as well as X-rays and gamma rays, are today referred to as **ionizing radiation** because the particles or rays involved are sufficiently energetic to dislodge electrons from the atoms or molecules they encounter, leaving behind ions, i.e. electrically-charged particles. While certain forms of non-ionizing radiation such as ultraviolet light and microwaves can have an adverse effect on living organisms and will be discussed later in this chapter, ionizing radiation's ability to destroy chemical bonds gives it special significance in relation to both human health and environmental pollution. It is recognized today that when certain particularly vulnerable cells (e.g. fetal cells, sex cells) are exposed to ionizing radiation, birth defects or mutations can result; in any cell, radiation-induced alteration of DNA can lead to cancer. Although discovery of ionizing radiation was immediately hailed as a momentous medical and scientific event, subsequent investigations regarding what is frequently called our "most studied and best understood pollutant" have revealed the importance of extreme caution in dealing with radioactive materials.

Radiation Exposure

Exposure to ionizing radiation is an inescapable circumstance of life on this planet. Every individual, to a greater or lesser extent, comes into contact with ionizing radiation from three general types of sources: naturally occurring, naturally occurring but enhanced by human actions, and human generated.

Natural Sources. Although the fact was not realized until Becquerel's discovery in 1896, earth, air, water, and food all contain traces of radioactive materials which constitute a ubiquitous source of naturally occurring, or "background," radiation. Some of the more significant sources of background radiation include the following:

Cosmic radiation. High energy particles composed primarily of protons and electrons continually stream toward the earth both from outer space and from the sun following episodes of solar flares. An appreciable amount of such cosmic radiation is blocked by the layer of atmosphere surrounding the globe, so that exposure to cosmic radiation is considerably less at sea level than at high altitudes (annual exposure to cosmic radiation approximately doubles with each 2000 meter increase in altitude above sea level). For this reason, residents of Denver receive about twice as much cosmic radiation as do inhabitants of Los Angeles or Miami. While the natural tendency is to assume that something which has always been with us must be harmless, some biologists assert that perhaps 25% of all spontaneous mutations are caused by cosmic radiation.

Radioactive minerals in the earth's crust. Radioactive compounds of uranium, thorium, potassium, and radium are found in soils and rocks in many parts of the world. People living in areas such as the Rocky Mountain region of the United States are exposed to background levels of radiation several times higher than are inhabitants of areas such as the Midwest or East Coast where radioactive minerals are much less abundant. Such an advantage may be lost, however, if easterners or midwesterners choose to live in homes or work in buildings constructed of granite, which

BOX 10-1

Types of Ionizing Radiation

Although any exposure to ionizing radiation is potentially dangerous, the degree and nature of harm varies depending on the type of radiation involved. Early studies of radioactivity revealed that ionizing radiation comprises several different types of emissions, the most biologically significant of which include:

Alpha particles, basically helium nuclei consisting of 2 protons and 2 neutrons, are relatively massive particles which, although the most energetic type of radiation, are the least penetrating. Such flimsy barriers as a sheet of paper, clothing, or even human skin can stop them. The greatest threat to health involving alpha radiation occurs when alpha-emitting particles (e.g. plutonium, radium, radon) are inhaled, ingested with food or water, or taken into the body through a cut or wound. Once in contact with delicate internal tissues, alpha radiation can cause intense damage within a localized area. Theoretical projections of large numbers of lung cancer deaths following a nuclear power plant meltdown are based on assumptions of pulmonary damage caused by inhalation of alpha-emitting plutonium dust.

Beta particles, consisting of single electrons, are more penetrating than alphas, capable of passing through the skin to a depth of about a half-inch. Like alphas, however they are most dangerous when ingested. Since several beta-emitters (e.g. strontium-90, iodine-131) are chemically similar to naturally occurring bodily constituents, they may substitute for those elements and concentrate in living tissues (e.g. bones, thyroid), where they continue to emit radiation for an extended period of time, increasing the risk of cancer or mutations. Most fission products in spent fuel rods or in reprocessed nuclear wastes are beta-emitters.

Gamma rays are the most penetrating form of ionizing radiation and generally accompany beta radiation. Shielding with a dense material such as lead is necessary to prevent gamma radiation from penetrating the body and harming vital organs. Short-lived beta emitters such as krypton-85 generally exhibit the highest levels of gamma radiation.

X-rays, thought slightly less penetrating, have basically the same characteristics as gamma rays.

gives off a considerable amount of radiation. Brick, too, is a source of radiation exposure due to its radioactive mineral content—a person living in a brick house experiences double the level of background radiation as does a person in a home built of wood (Spiers, 1957). Because of the extensive use of stone for streets and buildings, cities in Europe generally have significantly higher levels of background radiation than do their counterparts in the eastern United States.

Coal deposits frequently contain a number of radioactive elements that are released into the atmosphere when the coal is burned. At a time when many large coal users are contemplating switching to low-sulfur western coal as a means of reducing sulfur emissions, it is interesting to note that western coal contains about 10 times more radionuclides than do eastern or midwestern deposits (Carter, 1977).

Radionuclides in the body.   A number of radioactive substances enter the body by ingestion of food, milk, water, or by inhalation and are incorporated into body tissues where their concentration may be maintained at a steady state or gradually increase with age. Plants growing in soil containing radioactive minerals readily take up such isotopes as radium and potassium-40, and in areas where people live on radioactive soils, consuming locally grown foods further increases radiation exposure. In regions where groundwater is in contact with radioactive rock strata, well water used for domestic drinking supplies may constitute a significant source of indoor exposure to the radioactive gas radon. Another unavoidable source of radiation exposure is carbon-14, a naturally occurring isotope of carbon, which is inhaled with the air we breathe and is incorporated into the tissues of all living organisms (a fact which has useful implications for scientists who employ C-14 dating techniques to ascertain the age of ancient plant and animal remains).

Enhanced Natural Sources.   This category of sources, while not fundamentally different from the group discussed above, is considered separately because of the impact human activities have on levels of exposure which would, under other conditions, be much lower. Examples of enhanced natural sources include uranium mill tailings, phosphate mining, and jet airline travel (due to increased exposure to cosmic radiation at high altitudes). Recently, national attention has focused on what experts consider our single most significant source of radiation exposure–radon gas which, though naturally occurring, can be considered an "enhanced natural source" because it reaches potentially dangerous concentrations only in enclosed environments such as houses and mine shafts ("Ionizing Radiation," 1987). For more information on radon, see the section on "Indoor Air Pollutants" in chapter 12.

Human-Generated Sources.   Human beings have evolved and multiplied in an environment where constant exposure to low levels of ionizing radiation was a universal experience. With the exception of indoor radon concerns which are currently the subject of a great deal of attention and remedial action, most naturally occurring radiation is relatively constant and cannot be controlled or reduced in any feasible way. However, human-created sources of ionizing radiation have multiplied at exponential rates during the years since Roentgen first exhibited the X-ray of his wife's hand to an astonished world. It is these artificial sources,which can be controlled, that constitute the focus of a growing concern today about the impact of ionizing radiation on human health.

Medical applications.   By far the greatest source of exposure to artificial ionizing radiation for the average American comes from the use of medical X-rays and radiopharmaceuticals for both diagnostic and therapeutic purposes. Today approximately 75% of all Americans receive one or more medical or dental X-rays annually. Radioactive isotopes of phosphorus, technicium, iodine, iron, chromium, cobalt, and selenium are widely employed in hospitals for therapy and diagnosis, with as many as one-fourth of all patients in some hospitals receiving applications of some form of nuclear medicine. In addition to X-ray machines and radionuclides, the health professions utilize other such radiation-producing devices as teleradioisotope units and accelerators (e.g. cyclotrons, linear accelerators) to generate subatomic particles for radiotherapy. While radiation has provided medical science with an extremely valuable tool, its occasional misuse has been accompanied by some serious health problems; thus a thoughtful weighing of risks versus benefits should precede any decision regarding the application of ionizing radiation for medical purposes.

   Nuclear weapons fallout.   Since the explosion of the first atomic bomb in 1945 until the signing of the Limited Test-Ban Treaty in 1963, atmospheric testing of nuclear weapons by several of the major powers, primarily the United States and the former Soviet Union, resulted in significant amounts of radioactive fallout worldwide. Such fallout consists of a number of atomic fission products, including strontium-90, iodine-131, cesium-137, and radioactive krypton. Weapons fallout is not always evenly distributed, however. Local fallout close to the test site can be quite intense for about a day following the explosion, a fact which became obvious after the March 1, 1954, detonation of a multimegaton U.S. bomb over Bikini Atoll in the Pacific. Heavy fallout of large radioactive particles and dust contaminated several inhabited islands nearby, as well as a Japanese fishing boat sailing in the vicinity. Many of the Marshall Islanders and the fishermen developed burns, skin lesions, and loss of hair as a result of radiation exposure, and one of the islands, Rongelap, had to be evacuated and remained unoccupied for a number of years following the incident. In some cases air currents or rainstorms can cause radioactive particles and gases to precipitate unevenly. The greatest concern about weapons fallout is focused on those isotopes which enter the human system in food and are incorporated into body tissues. Strontium-90 and iodine-131 enter the food chain when contaminated plant material is consumed by cows and passed on to humans in milk. Strontium tends to displace calcium, being incorporated into bones, while iodine localizes in the thyroid gland; both thereby constitute internal sources of exposure, continuing to emit radioactive particles inside the body over a period of weeks or months in close proximity to vital organs. Radioactive cesium also is ingested in both meat and milk and remains in the body for several months before being metabolized (Hall, 1976). During the peak period of weapons testing, an average individual's radiation exposure due to bomb fallout was 13 millirems annually, a figure which has been steadily falling since 1963 (Eisenbud, 1973). According to a recent report by the National Council on Radiation Protection and Measurements, annual fallout exposure currently averages less than 0.01 mSv (1 mrem) and, barring a resumption of atmospheric testing of nuclear weapons, will continue to decline. Having reached such negligible levels, nuclear weapons fallout need no longer be taken into account in calculating total human radiation exposure.

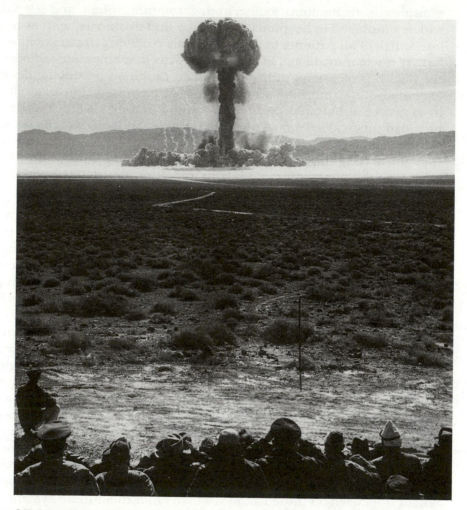

Official military observers watch the mushroom cloud form after an atomic artillery shell was fired in the Nevada desert in 1953. Such tests resulted in significant amounts of radioactive fallout. [AP/Wide World Photos]

Nuclear power plant emissions.   Public opposition to construction of nuclear power plants often centers around fears concerning radioactive emissions both to the air and in wastewater released from such plants. Radioisotopes such as tritium (H3), iodine-131, cesium-137, strontium-90, krypton, and others are indeed released into the environment during routine operation of a nuclear power generator, but the quantities involved are extremely minute—the average dose to individuals living within a 10-mile radius of the plant being 0.8 mSv (8 mrem), an amount considerably lower than that received from background radiation ("Ionizing Radiation," 1987).

Consumer products.   In addition to the sources mentioned above, very small amounts of exposure are received from luminous instrument dials (radium, tritium), home smoke detectors (americium), static eliminators (polonium), airport security checks (X-rays), TV receivers (low energy X-rays), gas lantern mantles (thorium), and tobacco products (polonium). Of these sources, the most significant is tobacco; the radioactive polonium particles in cigarette smoke lodge primarily in the bronchial epithelium of the upper airways—the site of most lung cancers—thereby further contributing to the health risk posed by other carcinogenic and toxic substances in tobacco smoke ("Ionizing Radiation," 1987).

Until recently it was estimated that the average American receives approximately half of his or her annual radiation exposure from naturally occurring background radiation and half from artificial sources, primarily medical applications. However, a growing realization of the extent to which citizens everywhere are exposed to radon in their homes has prompted a drastic revision in calculations of the contributions of various radiation sources to total average exposures. Due to estimates that as much as 55% of our annual radiation burden results from radon exposure alone, it is now believed that fully 82% of the average American's exposure originates from background (including enhanced) radiation, only 18% from artificial sources ("Ionizing Radiation," 1987). For any one individual, of course,

Figure 10-1 The Percentage Contribution of Various Radiation Sources to the Total Average Effective Dose Equivalent in the U.S. Population

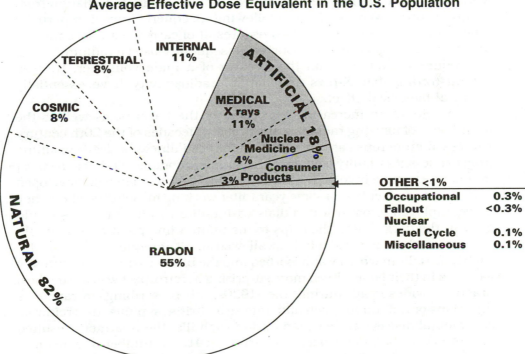

Source: National Council on Radiation Protection and Measurements Report No. 93.

the ratio can vary widely. A person living in an area of unusually highnatural radioactivity (e.g. Salt Lake City, Denver) or sleeping in a basement bedroom where radon levels are exceptionally high might receive an even larger portion of his or her total exposure from background sources, while a person undergoing radiation therapy or working inside a nuclear power plant would receive a disproportionate share from artificial sources.

Health Impacts of Ionizing Radiation

The advent of X-ray technology for diagnosing and treating human maladies, so eagerly and immediately seized upon by the medical profession, was soon shown to be a double-edged sword so far as its impact on human health was concerned. The first reported case of X-ray induced illness involved an American physician, Grubbe, who also manufactured cathode-ray tubes and who had been using them to study chemical fluorescence. When Grubbe heard of Roentgen's discovery he promptly began self-experimenting with X-rays and within a few weeks reported acute irritation of the skin on his hand. Subsequently the skin began peeling off, cancer developed, and eventually his hand had to be amputated. Grubbe's case was not an isolated one. By 1897, scarcely a year after the new technology came into use, 69 cases of X-ray induced injuries had been documented from various clinics and laboratories in different parts of the world (Eisenbud, 1973). Reports of health damage due to radiation from natural sources were not long in following. Becquerel himself reported a reddening of the skin on his chest as a result of carrying a vial of radium in his vest pocket. He and the Curies subsequently used a radium extract to produce a skin burn on the forearm of a male volunteer, thereby demonstrating that X-rays and natural radioactivity have essentially identical biological effects (Cooper, 1973).

In spite of an increasing awareness of the hazards, as well as the usefulness, of ionizing radiation, the first few decades of the 20th century witnessed numerous cases of radiation-induced illness or death resulting from carelessness, faulty equipment, or simple ignorance. Perhaps the most infamous example involved the approximately 40 women who developed bone cancer and leukemia some years after working in factories where they were employed to paint watch dials with radium so the numbers would glow in the dark. Using their lips to maintain a fine point on the brush, the women thereby accidentally swallowed small amounts of radium with each lick, radium which was absorbed into the bloodstream and eventually localized in their bones. Even more surprising in retrospect was the medical practice, widespread during the 1920s, of prescribing intravenous injections of radium for such ailments as arthritis, syphilis, tuberculosis, and mental disease; rather than curing such ills, the treatment resulted in more cases of bone cancer. As early as 1915, a number of consumer products—candies, liniments, creams, etc.—were being marketed to the public with assurances that the effects of radiation in trace amounts were beneficial to health, perhaps even necessary! One such bogus cure-all,

"Radithor," was advertised as a panacea for impotence, high blood pressure, indigestion, and more than 150 other ills. Sold in the United States for over six years, Radithor was taken off the market only after it had induced fatal cancer in a well-known socialite, a Radithor devotee who was reported to have consumed 1000 to 1500 bottlefuls of the radium solution between 1927 and 1931. The legal restrictions on sales of radio-pharmaceuticals currently prevailing in the United States were a direct result of the outrage provoked by the Radithor scandal more than 60 years ago (Macklis, 1993). To cite another example of a practice which, in retrospect seems inconceivably misguided, starting in about 1925, some doctors began irradiating children's scalps to treat ringworm, their heads and throats for enlarged tonsils and adenoids, and their faces to banish acne. Even as late as the 1960s some physicians used low-voltage X-rays to shrink the thymus gland (located in the neck) of infants in the erroneous belief that such treatments would cure colds. Unfortunately, such X-rays could not be precisely focused. As they spread out they irradiated not only the target tissue but the thyroid gland as well. The thyroid is one of the most radiation-sensitive organs in the body, and about 10 or more years following exposure (19 years seemed to be the peak period) significant numbers of these now-teenagers or young adults developed thyroid cancer as a result of this ill-advised application of radiation therapy (Norwood, 1980).

One segment of the population at special risk during the early years of work with radioactivity was the medical community itself, particularly radiologists whose enthusiastic use of their new machines exposed not only their patients but also themselves to large amounts of radiation on a daily basis. By the mid-1940s, physicians were succumbing to leukemia at double the rate seen in the general population, an incidence researchers attributed to the extent of their exposure to X-rays; an even more revealing statistic was the fact that among physicians, radiologists who regularly worked with X-ray machines exhibited a leukemia mortality rate 10 times that of their medical colleagues (Environmental Defense Fund, 1979).

Observations of radiation-induced health problems such as those just described led to extensive research into safer methods of utilizing this valuable but dangerous tool. Since the early 1940s, improvements in equipment design and increasingly stringent standards relating to allowable exposure have significantly reduced the incidence of overt cases of radiation damage. Nevertheless, concerns regarding unnecessary use of X-rays for diagnostic purposes and new understanding regarding long-term effects of low-level exposure require that individuals must be alert to the dangers implicit in any degree of radiation exposure and take an active role in deciding whether such exposure is justified.

Dosage

Since ionizing radiation can neither be seen nor felt, human exposure is measured in terms of the amount of tissue damage it causes. Under the International System of Units, the term **gray (GY)** is the unit of absorbed

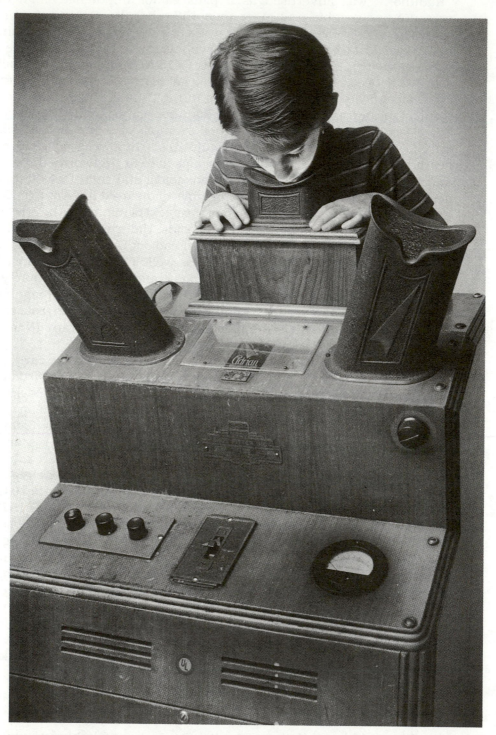

A child looks through a fluoroscopy machine at a shoe store to see if his shoes fit. This and other ill-advised practices were gradually discontinued as the deleterious health effects of radiation exposure became known. [FDA Consumer]

BOX 10-2

Half-Life

Not all radioisotopes are dangerous for the same length of time. Each radioactive element is characterized by its own unique half-life (t1/2)—a period of time during which half of the amount originally present, undergoing radioactive decay, is transformed into something else. The concept of half-life, in essence, is the reverse of exponential growth. Assume, for example, that one has a gram of cesium-137 whose half-life is 30 years. After 30 years, only 1/2 gram would remain; in 60 years, 1/4 gram; in 90 years 1/8 gram, and so forth. Obviously the term half-life is not synonymous with safety—1/2 gram of cesium-137 still presents a hazard. Indeed, highly radioactive substances may have to go through 10 or more half-lives (i.e. 300 years in the case of cesium) before their level of radioactivity is low enough to pose no significant health threat. However, the half-life concept has considerable relevance in assessing relative hazards and in devising waste management strategies.

Isotopes with very short half-lives are intensely radioactive initially; that is, they are experiencing a very high number of transformations at any one point in time. However, within a few days or weeks they go through so many half-lives that they no longer present a significant risk. The best management strategy for such wastes is simply to isolate them from human contact during the brief period when they are dangerous. Isotopes with extremely long half-lives will be radioactive virtually forever, but the level of emissions at any one point in time is relatively low; one can briefly handle a piece of long-lived uranium or thorium ore with little concern for radiation injury. The most difficult management problems involve those isotopes with intermediate-length half-lives, elements such as plutonium which, with a half-life of 24,000 years, remains hazardous for hundreds of thousands of years. Human contact with such radioisotopes must be accompanied by stringent safety precautions and ultimate disposal of such material must be carried out in such a way that it remains isolated from the general environment for extremely long periods of time.

Some representative half-lives

Element	Half-life	Element	Half-life
Radon-222	3.8 days	Cesium-137	30 years
Iodine-131	8.1 days	Radium-226	1600 years
Phosphorus-32	14 days	Carbon-14	5800 years
Krypton-85	11 years	Plutonium-239	24,000 years
Tritium	12 years	Uranium-235	710,000,000 years
Strontium-90	29 years	Thorium-232	14,000,000,000 years

dose, used to quantify the amount of energy from ionizing radiation absorbed per unit mass of material (the gray is replacing the term "rad" which is still in temporary use; a gray is equivalent to 100 rads). The most common unit for measuring radiation damage in humans, however, is the **sievert (Sv)**, a figure obtained by multiplying the absorbed dose in grays by a factor called the **relative biological effectiveness (RBE)**. This measurement reflects the fact that the health impact of radiation depends not only on the amount of energy absorbed, but also on the form of that energy. For example, X-rays and gamma rays which pass through tissue striking only occasional molecules along their path have an RBE of 1; beta particles have RBEs ranging from 1 to 5, depending on their energy level, while the relatively massive alpha particles have an RBE of 10, indicating their greater potential to damage living tissue. For practical purposes, human radiation exposure standards are set in terms of **millisieverts (mSv)**, an amount one-thousandth of a sievert, since these represent levels of exposure most commonly encountered by the average individual. Just as the gray is a relatively new term for what formerly was called the rad, sieverts and millisieverts are gradually replacing units, still used in many references, called "rems" and "millirems" (mrem). Under the new system a sievert is equivalent to 100 rems. The average amount of whole-body radiation exposure for a person in the United States from all sources is estimated to be approximately 3.6 mSv (360 mrem) a year or 0.01 mSv (1 mrem) per day.

There is little evidence that present average levels of exposure to ionizing radiation are having a serious adverse effect on the health of the general public. It is well known, however, that higher doses can be extremely injurious to living tissues. Types of radiation-induced biological damage include mutations, birth defects, impairment of fertility, leukemia and other forms of cancer, infections, hemorrhage, cataracts, and reduced lifespan. Humans, and mammals in general, are far more sensitive to ionizing radiation than are lower forms of life. The same degree of damage which a dose of 0.5 Sv (50 rems) can cause in a mammalian cell requires 1000 Sv (100,000 rems) exposure in an amoeba or 3000 Sv (300,000 rems) in a paramecium. The frequent reference in horror films to cockroaches inheriting the earth in the aftermath of all-out nuclear war is reflective of the fact that insects also have a very high level of tolerance to ionizing radiation.

Dose **rate**, the time span during which a given amount of radiation is delivered, is thought to be very significant in determining the extent of tissue damage incurred, perhaps even more important than total dose. The prevailing view holds that radiation absorbed over an extended period is less harmful than the same amount delivered during a brief time span, due to the existence of bodily repair mechanisms. A contrary conclusion was reached recently by two noted British epidemiologists who argue that, at least in relation to carcinogenesis, numerous small doses of radiation exposure are *more* likely to induce cancer than is a single large dose. Basing their conclusions on a study of health records of 35,000 nuclear bomb production workers at the federal government's Hanford Reservation in Richland, Washington, these researchers hypothesize that large doses of

Figure 10-2 Penetrating Power of Alpha and Beta Particles and Gamma Rays

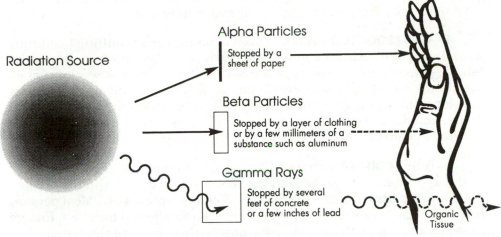

Source: U.S. Environmental Protection Agency.

radiation *kill* cells, while smaller doses simply *damage* the genetic material, giving rise to mutations which increase the likelihood of cancer (Kneale and Stewart, 1993).

Health effects of ionizing radiation can be subdivided into those types of damage caused by high-level and low-level exposure, respectively. High-level radiation exposure is defined as a whole-body dose of 1 Sv (100 rems) or more, delivered within a relatively short period of time—minutes or hours. Such exposure will produce obvious symptoms of radiation sickness within a period ranging from a few hours to several weeks, symptoms ranging in severity from temporary nausea to death, depending on the dosage. Human effects of high-level exposure have been determined from studies of victims of the Hiroshima-Nagasaki atom bomb explosions, from experience with radiation therapy, and from observations of the results of nuclear accident victims. The 135,000 unfortunate Ukrainians and Byelorussians exposed to large amounts of radioactive debris resulting from the 1986 disaster at Chernobyl constitute a particularly valuable study group for radiation biologists because the radiation doses they received were measured at the time of the accident, unlike the wartime situation in Japan where exposures were estimated after the event. As one British radiation specialist remarked, "The human experiment has now been done. At last we can test our hypotheses" (Hawkes et al., 1987). Study results indicate the following consequences of varying levels of acute whole-body radiation exposure:

1–2 Sv (100–200 rems). At this level of exposure, symptoms are generally so mild as to be unnoticeable in ordinary clinical examinations; heartbeat may be more rapid than usual and some nausea and vomiting may be experienced. At levels close to 2 Sv, miscarriages of early pregnancies or temporary sterility of males may occur.

2–4 Sv (200–400 rems). Onset of nausea and vomiting beginning a few hours after exposure and lasting about one day; mild weakness and fatigue persist for a few days to 3 weeks, followed by 3–4 weeks of such symptoms as sore throat, fever, general weakness, and in some cases development of purplish blotches on the skin as the white blood cell count drops. About 3 weeks after radiation exposure, loss of hair occurs. Recovery generally begins around the 5th week and is complete within 3–6 months.

4–6 Sv (400–600 rems). The same sequence of events occurs as in the 2–4 Sv range, except that the onset of specific symptoms is more rapid and the decrease in white blood cell count more severe. Most persons receiving this dosage will die from infections and internal bleeding, though in some individuals bone marrow transplants may save the patient.

6–10 Sv (600–1000 rems). Within a few hours after exposure severe vomiting, stomach cramps, and diarrhea commence, indicative of damage to the gastrointestinal tract. After the first day or two, the exposed person may begin to feel better, but within about one week nausea and vomiting return, progressing to bloody diarrhea, shock, and death within 10–14 days after exposure, due to destruction of the gastrointestinal lining.

10 Sv (1000 rems) and above. Doses of this magnitude have their primary impact on the central nervous system. A burning sensation occurs minutes after exposure, quickly followed by severe nausea and vomiting and occasionally by loss of consciousness. Within the hour the victim experiences loss of muscular coordination, mental confusion, and prostration; a period of seeming improvement may occur for several hours, but 5–6 hours after exposure watery diarrhea commences, together with a bluish discoloration of the skin, resulting from inadequate oxygen in the blood. Shock sets in a few hours later and death occurs approximately 20–38 hours following the acute radiation exposure (Maxfield et al., 1973).

Levels of ionizing radiation capable of inducing the above mentioned effects would most likely occur only in the extreme situations represented by a nuclear bomb explosion, a nuclear power plant melt-down, or in severe industrial accidents involving mishandling of radioactive materials. Such effects are largely reflective of cell death which, if extensive, can be fatal to the entire organism.

At levels of radiation exposure below 1 Sv (100 rems), well within the range experienced by many individuals today, few, if any, harmful effects are readily apparent. Nevertheless, low-level doses of ionizing radiation are the focus of great concern because of their potential to cause cell damage rather than cell death—damage which can eventually lead to genetic defects, congenital abnormalities, or cancer.

BOX 10-3
Cold War Fallout

The "Cold War" tensions which dominated national life in both the United States and the former Soviet Union for more than a generation have now, like the Berlin Wall, crumbled and faded into oblivion. Military leaders no longer debate potential targets for their nuclear-tipped ICBMs but instead ponder the details of how to dismantle and dispose of all those bombs built during decades of super-power rivalry. Nevertheless, the radio-active legacy of those years remains very much with us today, posing immense technological—and moral—dilemmas for which there are no easy answers. Only recently has the dark veil of secrecy, imposed for reasons of "national security" or "defense of the motherland," been lifted, revealing a shocking record of environmental contamination, disease, and death on two continents—the direct result of more than 40 years of nuclear weapons production and testing.

From 1945 when the first atomic bomb was detonated at Alamagordo, New Mexico, until its last tests in 1992, the U.S. conducted 1,051 nuclear explosions: 210 in the atmosphere, 5 underwater, and 836 underground. The vast majority were held in Nevada at Yucca Flats, north of Las Vegas, but over 100 were conducted in the Pacific and a few (underground) in Colorado, New Mexico, Alaska, Mississippi, and at other Nevada sites. The USSR, which exploded its first nuclear bomb in 1949, by 1989 had conducted an estimated 713 tests, including one in 1961 which, at a yield of 58 megatons, ranks as the largest nuclear explosion ever. Most Soviet testing was carried out near Semipalatinsk in Kazakhstan (now an independent republic in Central Asia) and at Novaya Zemlya in the Arctic, but 50 other sites were utilized as well—meaning that radioactive contamination affects far more territory in the former USSR than it does anywhere else in the world. Until both nations signed the 1963 Limited Test Ban Treaty banning atmospheric or underwater testing of nuclear weapons, test explosions invariably generated large amounts of airborne radioactive fission products which, depending on weather conditions and the direction of prevailing winds, settled to the ground at varying distances from the test site. Although about half the fallout generally returned to earth near "Ground Zero" or within a few hundred miles downwind, the remainder was deposited randomly world-wide, often occurring in unpredictable "hotspots" when local rainstorms washed out radioactive particles.

Exercises carried out during the early years of weapons testing betrayed an enormous ignorance—or lack of concern—about the effects of human exposure to fallout. Safety limitations on acceptable radiation doses among test participants were set higher than guidelines for civilian workers, and even those limits were regularly exceeded. In a 1951 test at the Nevada Proving Grounds, hundreds of troops with no protective gear other than helmets were ordered to stand outside in the desert to witness an atomic explosion just seven miles away. To this day, veterans of that event wonder if health problems many of them are experiencing, as well as birth abnormalities among children they subsequently fathered, can be traced to radiation exposure received at that time. Since Yucca Flats is located scarcely over 100 miles from numerous small towns, farms, and ranches downwind in Nevada, Utah, and Arizona, it was predictable that residents of those areas would be at risk from radioactive fallout. Ironically, when the search for a test site got underway in the late 1940s, some experts recommended a location near Cape Hatteras, North Carolina, as the ideal spot, since prevailing westerly winds would ensure that most fallout would be deposited over the Atlantic Ocean; this suggestion was bypassed in favor of the Nevada site because of the latter's proximity to existing laboratory facilities at Los Alamos and because the federal government already owned the land. The decision was a fateful one for "downwinders" living near the test site who, for 12 years of atmospheric testing (1951–1963) endured exposure to clouds of radioactive dust which drifted onto their fields, pastures, and into water supplies. Throughout this period they were reassured by government pamphlets which appealed to their patriotism by such statements as "You are, in a very real sense, active participants in the Nation's atomic test program."

Half a world away on the plains of Kazakhstan, Soviet officials, like their American counterparts, paid little heed to health or environmental considerations in their single-minded push for military superiority. At least 10,000 Kazakhs living downwind of Semipalatinsk received high doses of radiation following tests; although villages near the blast site were evacuated prior to the Soviet Union's first thermonuclear explosion, nine days after the test they were allowed to return home even though lingering levels of radiation remained dangerously high. In the Soviet Union, as in the United States, the fact that the same governmental agencies charged with assessing the health and environmental effects of nuclear fallout were also responsible for manufacturing and testing the bombs created an inherent conflict of interest. It was obvious to officials in both countries that if they candidly warned people living near test sites of the true hazards they faced, public opposition might jeopardize the testing program. Accordingly, a calculated decision was made to trivialize fears, assuring people that as long as they didn't experience overt symptoms of radiation sickness, they had nothing to worry about. A Kazakh witness of the first Soviet H-bomb explosion who had been ordered to remain in his village after most of its residents were evacuated reported that "Afterward they gave us a checkup and the military men gave us some vodka as protection against radiation . . . No one

ever told us that there was any danger."

The ultimate result of this conspiracy of silence, both in the American Southwest and in Kazakhstan, has been an epidemic of cancer, birth defects, and immune system damage which continues to claim victims more than 30 years after above-ground testing came to a halt. In a belated act of redemption, the U.S. Congress in 1990 passed the Radiation Exposure Compensation Act, creating a trust fund to compensate victims (or their survivors) whose cancer was determined to have been caused by radioactive fallout. However, eligibility requirements are strict and dollars are limited, further embittering "downwinders" already made callous by years of sickness, grief, and bureaucratic indifference.

It is now sadly apparent that "downwinder" communities and soldiers exposed on maneuvers are not the Cold War's only radiation victims. In 1993 a visibly shaken U.S. Energy Secretary Hazel O'Leary disclosed information documenting post-World War II radiation experiments carried out from the late 1940s to the early 1970s, without the knowledge or consent of the patients involved. Most of these studies were sponsored or conducted by the Atomic Energy Commission (DOE's predecessor), the same agency that was building bombs and promoting nuclear power. A number of medical experts contend that most of these experiments utilized doses of radiation so small (100 millirems was the common dose in many of the studies) that they presented minimal hazard and justify such experiments by the fact that important medical information was gained as a result. Not all tests were so benign, however. For 11 years at the University of Cincinnati one team of researchers exposed 88 terminally ill cancer patients to whole-body, high-level doses of radiation in an effort to learn how much radiation a soldier could endure before becoming disoriented or disabled. The U.S. government has launched an intensive review of Department of Energy (DOE) records to learn more about the nature and scope of these medical studies and several members of Congress are urging fair and full compensation to any subjects injured by such experiments.

Recognition of the Cold War's civilian health toll continues to expand. It is now apparent that workers employed in the factories where nuclear weapons were produced are now falling ill and dying of occupationally related disease. At Fernald, Ohio, near Cincinnati, employees of a uranium processing facility suffer a higher incidence of lung, colon, liver, blood, and lymphatic cancers than the general population and die at significantly younger ages. Occupational cancers due to radiation exposure have also been experienced by workers at the Hanford nuclear reservation in southeastern Washington State, the oldest and largest facility in the U.S. nuclear weapons complex. Health problems at Hanford are not restricted to production workers, however. Like the fallout from nuclear weapons testing, deliberate radioactive releases from the plant have exposed thousands of people in Washington, Oregon, and Idaho to dangerously high levels of radiation, most of it in the form of radioactive iodine-131 which settled on grass, was eaten by cows, and subsequently entered the milk supply consumed by humans. Radioactive iodine concentrates in the thyroid gland where it can cause various thyroid diseases, including cancer. A panel of government scientists studying radioactive releases at Hanford estimate that children in Eltopia, Washington, immediately downwind of Hanford, may have received radiation exposure to their thyroids as high as 870 rads, adults as much as 350. By comparison, under Federal guidelines, in the event of a *civilian* nuclear accident, evacuation is advised if radiation dose to the thyroid reaches 5–25 rads. The most notorious of the releases at Hanford, referred to as the "Green Run," was conducted over a 12-hour period in 1949 but kept secret until 1986. Ironically, this test was not carried out to obtain radiobiologic information regarding humans but to test aerial monitoring and sampling techniques in order to perfect methods for monitoring Soviet nuclear weapons. Thanks to the declassification of formerly secret DOE documents, it is now known that the United States carried out at least 13 tests releasing radiation into the air during the Cold War years.

Undoubtedly the most lasting environmental legacy of U.S.-Soviet rivalry is the radioactive contamination of soil and water bequeathed to future generations. While atmospheric bomb testing contributed to worldwide radioactive fallout, the underground testing which followed implementation of the Limited Test Ban Treaty created huge volumes of crushed rock and other "hot" debris whose long-term dangers have never been adequately assessed. Equally, if not more, troublesome is the extensive contamination at weapons production sites at numerous locations in both the United States and the former Soviet Union.

There is arguably no place on earth more radioactively polluted than the Chelyabinsk region of Russia where for years the Soviet defense establishment manufactured nuclear weapons with scant regard for the health and safety of nearby residents. From 1951 until at least 1961, the bomb-makers pumped enormous volumes of cesium- and strontium-poisoned wastes onto the bottom of nearby Lake Karachay which became, in effect, a 100-acre holding pond for intensely radioactive liquid wastes, an undetermined amount of which has already migrated into the groundwater underlying the lake. Containing levels of radiation far in excess of amounts released during the Chernobyl accident, Lake Karachay constitutes an acute environmental health hazard today and for centuries to come. In 1990 American observers from the Natural Resources Defense Council found that radiation levels along the lakeshore were so high that a person standing there for an hour would receive a lethal dose!

In the fall of 1957, in what a Russian parliamentary representative from the region has termed "one of the greatest human tragedies of our age," an estimated 437,000 residents of the Chelyabinsk area were exposed to fallout from 70–80 tons of radioactive material blasted into the atmosphere when a storage tank for liquid high-level wastes exploded at Kyshtym, a secret weapons production site in the Ural Mountains. Although the outside world was not told of this event until three decades later, during the year following the accident 11,000 people were evacuated from the area and for a number of years farming was banned on 440 square miles of heavily contaminated land surrounding the site. While Soviet officials denied any subsequent increase in the incidence of health problems, local people speak of numerous cases of leukemia and other cancers among fallout recipients.

News of the Kyshtym explosion should cause some anxiety among managers at DOE's Hanford facility where waste tanks contain many of the same materials responsible for the 1957 Soviet disaster. Of the 17 U.S. bomb plants—all of which exhibit some radioactive pollution problems—only Hanford has been classified in the "most urgent" category due to the threat of explosion and groundwater contamination. Many of the 177 tanks of highly radioactive liquid wastes stored at Hanford, cumulatively containing 57 million gallons, are now in dangerously deteriorating condition, having been constructed for a 25-year lifespan exceeded long ago. Each year several additional tanks begin to leak their contents into the soil—68 are now listed as "assumed leakers"—and DOE admits to the loss of at least one million gallons of liquid radwastes over the years. Hanford is now near the top of the list of worst U.S. "Superfund" sites, slated for cleanup in a project estimated to require 30 years at a cost of $57 billion. Authorized in 1989, by the mid-1990s the project had still not progressed beyond the planning stage, with engineers struggling just to understand the scope of the problem. "We have about every waste form you could ever hope to have," commented a spokesman for Westinghouse, prime contractor for the project. The excruciatingly slow progress of cleanup efforts at Hanford, due not only to the vast extent of contamination but by the lack of known, affordable remediation technologies as well, is a cause for constant worry among those aware of the potential for catastrophe which Hanford's corroding radwaste tanks represent. How ironic that the bitter radioactive fruits of now-obsolete Cold War rivalry persist to poison the future of those very citizens the protagonists were ostensibly protecting.

References

Feshbach, Murray, and Alfred Friendly, Jr. 1992. *Ecocide in the USSR: Health and Nature Under Siege*. Basic Books.

IPPNW and IEER. 1991. *Radioactive Heaven and Earth*. Apex Press and Zed Books.

Schneider, Keith. 1994. "Cold War Radiation Test on Humans to Undergo a Congressional Review." *New York Times*, April 11.

Wald, Matthew. 1993. "At an Old Atomic Waste Site the Only Sure Thing is Peril." *New York Times*, June 21.

Radiation-Induced Mutations

Exposure even to very low levels of ionizing radiation can result in gene mutations; indeed, experiments to date indicate that there is no threshold level below which no mutations would be expected (however, at very low levels of exposure the mutation rate will correspondingly be quite low). There is, rather, a direct linear relationship between increasing radiation dosage and an increased number of mutations, either at the gene or chromosomal level. Both diagnostic X-rays and radioactive isotopes used for treating various ailments have been shown to damage chromosomes. Nuclear power plant workers and medical personnel, particularly radiotherapy nurses, who receive small doses of radiation on a daily basis have been shown to exhibit a marked increase in the frequency of mutations in their chromosomes (these can be observed as breaks or changes in chromosome number when chromosome smears are made from a sampling of white blood cells). The number of such abnormalities is generally highest among individuals who have been occupationally exposed to radiation for a number of years, indicating that the effects of exposure are cumulative.

Of greatest concern from a genetic standpoint, of course, are the mutations which accumulate in the gonadal cells which are the precursors of eggs and sperm. The number of new mutations which an individual passes on to his or her children depends on the amount of radiation the sex organs have absorbed from the time of conception up to the moment each of his or her children are conceived. Most radiation-induced mutations are recessive; hence even though most are of a harmful nature, they are likely to persist in the human gene pool, increasing in frequency over several generations before carriers of the recessive gene mate, producing offspring who exhibit the mutant characteristic.

In addition to inducing mutations in sex cells, X-ray exposure has also been shown to be capable of causing chromosomal damage in developing fetuses. Because the majority of such instances involved diagnostic X-rays of women in the very early stages of pregnancy who were not yet aware of their condition, it is now recommended that irradiation of reproductive-age women be limited to the first ten days after the onset of their last menstrual cycle to prevent exposure of an unsuspected embryo. Males and females alike should insist on being provided with a gonadal shield (e.g. lead apron) to reduce the risk of sex-cell mutations whenever X-rays are administered.

Radiation and Birth Defects

A number of congenital abnormalities, as distinguished from defects caused by mutant parental genes, are known to result from X-ray exposure in utero. Sensitivity to radiation is many times greater during fetal development than at any subsequent period of a person's life, since rapid development and differentiation of tissues is occurring during this time (the more actively cells are dividing, the more vulnerable they are to radiation). The most pronounced impact of fetal irradiation is on the central nervous system, where the developing neurons are extremely radiosensitive. Once injured or killed by ionizing radiation, embryonic nerve cells cannot be regenerated—the damage is permanent. Thus it should not be surprising that some of the most commonly observed birth defects resulting from fetal irradiation are microcephaly (abnormally small head) and mental retardation. In addition to decreased head size, a general stunting of growth frequently results from radiation exposure in the womb, and skeletal malformations, genital abnormalities, and eye problems may occur.

The nature and extent of fetal injury caused by radiation varies widely depending not only on dose but also on the precise stage of development. Because the fetal tissues are constantly growing and differentiating, the developmental response to radiation exposure on any given day may be quite different from what it would have been the day before or the day after. In general, as with other teratogenic agents, ionizing radiation is most harmful to the human fetus from the second week through the sixth week of pregnancy, with peak sensitivity occurring between days 32–37 (from the time of conception through the 10th–12th day, radiation exposure can cause fetal death; if not, the pregnancy will proceed normally, with no teratogenic effect). Overall, the early stage of fetal development is about 10 times more radiosensitive than is the period shortly before birth (Sternglass, 1972). In addition, there are individual genetically controlled differences in sensitivity to radiation which make it unlikely that any two fetuses would respond in precisely the same manner to radiation exposure, even when the doses are identical.

Controversy persists among researchers concerning whether or not a "safe level" of radiation exposure exists in relation to the induction of birth defects (as opposed to mutations for which it is presumed there is no threshold). While acknowledging that some difficult-to-detect damage may occur at exposure levels even below 0.01 Sv (1 rem), most authorities agree that if exposures of 0.15 Sv (15 rem) or above occur during the first six weeks of pregnancy, chances of severe congenital abnormalities are so great that therapeutic abortion is advisable.

Radiation-Induced Cancer

The potential for health damage as a result of radiation exposure was first recognized in connection with the development of skin cancers among early radiologists, of whom nearly 100 fell victim to this disease within 15 years following the discovery of X-rays. Since then other forms of cancer, most notably leukemia, bone cancer, lung cancer, and thyroid cancer, have also been linked to radiation exposure.

Leukemia is perhaps the classic example of X-ray-induced malignancy. As early as 1911 a report of 11 cases of leukemia among radiation workers suggested a connection between the disease and their occupational exposure. Subsequently, epidemiological studies among radiologists, Japanese survivors of Hiroshima and Nagasaki, patients treated with X-ray therapy, and children who were irradiated in the womb when their mothers received diagnostic X-rays, all confirm the association between exposure to ionizing radiation and the induction of leukemia. Leukemia, like other forms of cancer, is characterized by a latency period following the initial exposure, with development of disease symptoms in this case occurring, on the average, after 5–7 years (some as early as just 2 years after irradiation). Although the greatest number of cases have been traced to exposure dosages in the 0.5-10 Sv (50-1000 rem) range (there appears

BOX 10-4

Just Say No

Each year in the United States approximately 600 million medical and dental X-rays are given, about one-third of which federal officials estimate are unnecessary. Since the effects of radiation exposure are cumulative, consumers have both the right and the responsibility to question the overuse of a technology which presents a hazard to their well-being. Fortunately, the degree of risk is small. While the ability of large doses of radiation to kill or injure living cells is well established, the levels absorbed in most diagnostic procedures today are far lower than those which in past decades resulted in radiation-induced cancers and leukemias among patients receiving radiation treatment for problems ranging from ringworm to enlarged thymus glands. In those situations, doses exceeding 1 Sv (100 rems) generally were employed—considerably more than today's average bone marrow dose of 0.1 Sv (100 mrem) from diagnostic use of medical X-rays (dose to the red bone marrow is the most critical radiation-safety consideration because of its relationship to leukemia induction). Even at high dose levels, the incidence of radiation-induced cancer and leukemia is low and is an acceptable risk in situations where the health benefit of X-ray examination to a patient is clear and where the health risk of not having the X-ray is much greater.

Nevertheless, since all radiation exposure is cumulative and since such exposure does present some risk, however small, of causing subsequent cancer or birth defects, the estimate that a significant number of all X-rays administered each year are unnecessary is a situation which merits serious scrutiny on the part of a concerned public. Why are so many Americans receiving excess exposure to X-rays? The finger of blame can be pointed in several directions:

1. physicians' fear of malpractice lawsuits; to avoid charges by patients that they didn't do everything possible to detect the cause of a particular problem, doctors may order X-rays they know will reveal nothing of diagnostic value but which can provide future documentation in court of their thoroughness.

2. equipment malfunction; not all X-ray machines are in peak operating condition. Older models particularly may not tightly focus beams on the area being irradiated. Studies of radiation equipment across the nation have revealed a variation in radiation exposure of more than 200-fold for the same type of examination. Equipment failure can also result in film being over- or underexposed, necessitating retakes.

3. technician or physician error; in three-fourths of the states, no special training is required to administer X-rays and any doctor or dentist can purchase X-ray equipment. Few practicing medical personnel have time to keep abreast of the latest advances in radiology and many received only minimal training during their medical school days. Mistakes by the technician in operating the equipment or in positioning the patient necessitate millions of retakes, resulting in additional radiation exposure to patients, and doctors' initially ordering wrong views account for millions more. Suboptimal use of protective shielding for patients remains a problem in the rush to complete examinations quickly.

With these facts in mind, patients whose physician or dentist orders X-ray examinations have every right to question whether such exposure is really essential and to ask how the information gained thereby will affect treatment; to request protective shielding if the area being X-rayed is near the thyroid gland, breasts, eyes, or reproductive organs; to ask for an additional copy for one's own records, especially when the problem relates to a chronic condition which may require consultation with other doctors; and to refuse to allow routine dental X-rays (especially for children, for whom a cavity in a baby tooth that will soon be lost anyway is less menacing than a dose of radiation) without first having the teeth visually examined and a dental history taken.

A century of experience has amply demonstrated that use of medical X-rays is a double-edged sword: a valuable diagnostic and therapeutic weapon, yet one whose use, in a small percentage of cases, can lead to radiation-induced malignancies or teratogenic effects. Where it is clear that benefits substantially outweigh risks, there should be no hesitation in utilizing such a tool. However it's time for Americans to begin saying "no" to those 200 million X-rays taken each year which confer no benefit to the recipient whatsoever, while increasing their overall radiation burden.

to be a linear relationship between dose and leukemia incidence rates), the fact that even very low doses may be carcinogenic is suggested by evidence that prenatal X-ray exposure to just 0.01-0.05 Sv (1-5 rems) can result in increased risk of childhood leukemia and other cancers. Interestingly, however, studies of Japanese children prenatally exposed to radiation from the 1945 blasts revealed no excess leukemias among that group (Upton, 1973).

Evidence on the amount of radiation required to induce a malignancy is scarce, particularly at doses less than 0.5 Sv (50 rems). Many authorities believe that proportionately fewer cancers are initiated at low doses of radiation exposure than at higher doses, owing to the ability of cells to repair some radiation damage, while other researchers present experimental evidence showing that the risk of radiation-induced leukemias, skin cancer, and thyroid cancer is greater after exposure to low doses of medical irradiation than following high-dose applications. These investigators hypothesize that high doses severely inhibit the irradiated cells' ability to divide and proliferate, whereas lower doses, especially when administered over a time period of several years, do not similarly impede the capability of malignant cells to multiply (Basso-Ricci, 1985). Contradicting conventional wisdom, the previously mentioned epidemiologic study of Hanford nuclear workers conducted by Drs. Alice Stewart and George Kneale found that the cancer risks posed by low levels of radiation exposure were 4–8 times greater than previously recognized; in fact, although workers at the nuclear bomb facility averaged doses equivalent to what most people receive over a 6–7 year period simply from background radiation, Stewart and Kneale estimate an excess of approximately 200 cancer deaths among the 35,000 workers at the facility above what would normally be expected among a group of that size. In another departure from conventional thinking, Stewart and Kneale also contend that, far from being age-neutral, the risk of radiation-induced cancer is far greater for those exposed later in life than among younger individuals whose more vigorous immune system is better able to suppress mutant cells before they can develop into cancer. Results of their study indicate that for the group as a whole (ages ranging from 18–65), cancer risk doubles with every 26 rems of exposure. However, for those aged 58 or older, the risk doubles with just 5 rems of exposure, and after age 62, exposures of *less than 1 rem* result in a doubling of cancer risk! (Kneale and Stewart, 1993).

Whatever the case, for purposes of regulation, federal agencies subscribe to the linear dose-response curve which assumes a directly proportional increase in number of cancer cases with increasing radiation dosage and no threshold level below which cancer incidence would be zero. In the absence of definitive evidence, this approach is considered to provide the most prudent way of safeguarding public health. Currently, federal standards set 1.7 mSv/year (170 mR/year), excluding medical exposure, as the maximum permissible radiation dose for members of the general population as a whole, no more than 0.25 mSv (25mR) of which should come from a nuclear power facility. Individuals may receive up to 5 mSv/year (500 mR/year), while workers in radiation-related occupations are allowed average yearly exposures of 50 mSv (5 rems). Persons under the age of 18 are permitted no occupational exposure whatsoever. Such standards have been set for the intended purpose of protecting human health against the long-term radiation effects of cancer and genetic defects. These standards do not reflect levels of absolute safety but rather attempt to strike a balance between possible adverse effects of low-level exposure and the known benefits of nuclear power and other uses of radioactive materials. Recently the safety of current exposure limits has been called into question by new interpretation of data on exposure received by Japanese survivors at Hiroshima and Nagasaki. Post-war estimates of likely radiation levels at varying distances from ground zero, correlated with observed health effects, have formed the basis for radiation standards since the end of World War II. Results from studies conducted during the 1980s suggested that the original data overestimated the radiation dosage received by persons in the affected area. Some researchers now believe that the observable health damage experienced by survivors was caused by approximately one-half the amount of radiation exposure calculated previously. These findings, if correct, imply that current radiation protection standards should be at least twice as stringent as they are now in order to protect public health. More recent studies conducted in the United Kingdom provide additional basis for doubt regarding the adequacy of existing exposure limits. A large-scale survey of British nuclear plant workers who experienced occupational exposure to low levels of ionizing radiation over a period of many years showed a statistically positive association between leukemia death rates and radiation exposure, with risks rising as dosage increased. These results, along with observations that rates of terminal cancer are higher among A-bomb survivors in Japan than among Japanese not exposed to radiation from those atomic blasts, have led Britain's National Radiological Protection Board (NRPB) to urge the adoption of new radiation protection standards. In place of the present 50 mSv yearly exposure limit for occupational exposure, the NRPB is recommending an upper limit of just 20 mSv, while similarly advocating that the annual dose for members of the general public be reduced from 5 mSv to 1 mSv (Perera, 1993; "New Study," 1992; Hawkes et al., 1987).

It should be noted in passing that the above-mentioned consequences of low-level radiation exposure may also be manifested at higher rates among survivors of high-level radiation doses. Mutations, birth defects among offspring, a significantly heightened risk of leukemia and other cancers, as well as cataracts and a general shortening of life span due to premature aging, are realistic possibilities confronting individuals who have recovered from overt symptoms of radiation sickness.

Radiation and Nuclear Power Generation

While medical uses of X-rays and radioisotopes constitute by far the largest amount of non-background radiation exposure, it is not these sources but rather the perceived health threat from nuclear power plants that has received the lion's share of public attention in recent years. Since 1957 when the first commercial nuclear power plant came on line in Shippingsport, Pennsylvania, the percentage of electricity generated by nuclear energy in the United States grew rapidly until the mid-1970s, much more slowly since then—no new commercial nuclear reactors have been ordered by U.S. utility companies since 1978. In 1994, 107 operating nuclear power plants accounted for approximately 20% of all electrical energy produced in this country. Even before the serious accident in 1979 at the Three Mile Island power plant near Harrisburg, Pennsylvania, and the catastrophe at Chernobyl in the USSR in 1986, concerns about the safety of nuclear power had given rise to an active and vocal antinuclear movement. Chants of "Hell, no, we won't glow!" have been countered by dire warnings from pronuclear power forces that Americans are doomed to "freeze to death in the dark" if we don't proceed full steam ahead to develop the nuclear power option. In all likelihood, with construction costs soaring and demand for electricity declining, economic considerations will be the major factor determining the outcome of this national debate. Nevertheless, the impact of citizen protests and political considerations in shaping nuclear power policy was made evident in the announcement of New York Governor Mario Cuomo, in May 1988, that the recently completed Shoreham nuclear power plant on Long Island would be dismantled before it ever generated a single kilowatt of electricity. This action, taken in response to local concerns about the feasibility of federally required emergency evacuation plans in that densely populated area, represented the first time a U.S. nuclear plant was abandoned before it was ever opened. Given the emotionalism involved, it is important that citizens clearly understand the extent to which nuclear power generation contributes to the overall radiation burden experienced by the general public. Although most attention is focused on the power plants themselves, nuclear power production involves a number of steps, referred to as the **nuclear fuel cycle**, several of which have greater relevance to the public safety issue than others.

Mining.   The uranium which constitutes the fissionable fuel in all U.S. reactors is mined in four western states—New Mexico, Wyoming, Colorado, and Utah. The most significant radiation hazard involved in mining uranium is the increased risk of lung cancer from inhaling alpha-emitting radon gas and radon daughters (radioactive polonium and lead) attached to tiny particles of mine dust. Such exposure in the underground mines from which half of all U.S. uranium ore is extracted (the other half being from open-pit mines) has contributed to a lung cancer mortality among uranium miners (the majority of them Navajos recruited by the government to work for the nuclear weapons industry but never warned about the known health risks) which is four to five times higher than that prevailing among the general population. Closing off unused sections of mines, better mine ventilation, and encouraging miners to wear respirators can reduce, but not entirely eliminate, this hazard ("Health Implications," 1977). Belatedly, after years of litigation, the Navajos in 1990 received a formal apology and promises of compensation from the U.S. Congress for the "hardships" they endured in the form of radiation-induced death and disease. Halfway around the world, on the opposite side of the former "Iron Curtain" which separated the Communist world from the Western democracies, at least 20,000 East German miners, mobilized in the late 1940s and early 1950s to supply uranium for the Soviet Union's nuclear arsenal, have died or are dying of lung diseases caused by occupational exposure to radioactive gases and dust in the underground mines (Kahn, 1993).

Milling.   The crushing and processing of uranium ore to produce the form of uranium oxide known as "yellowcake" leaves behind enormous quantities of sand-like mill tailings. At present more than 140 million tons of radioactive tailings exist at approximately 20 now-abandoned mill sites scattered across seven western states, releasing radon into the air and leaching radium into the subsoil. In 1979 the rupture of an earthen dam at a uranium mine and mill site near Churchrock, New Mexico, released hundreds of tons of tailings sludge into a stream running through the Navajo reservation. Considered one of the worst radwaste spills ever to occur in the United States, this accident resulted in traces of radioactive materials being carried at least 75 miles downstream across the Arizona border. At many unprotected sites, wind has blown the loose material close to buildings and onto grazing land. This is a cause for concern because radioactive mill tailings emit between 0.2–20 millirads of radiation per hour, an amount 40–400 times above normal background radiation levels (IAEA, 1983; League of Women Voters, 1993). In Grand Junction, Colorado, mine tailings were incorporated into cement which was used for foundations of homes, churches, and schools. For nearly 20 years until the problem was recognized, approximately 30,000 people living in these dwellings were exposed to levels of radon up to seven times the maximum allowable level for uranium miners. On a smaller scale, a number of other western communities, including Denver and Salt Lake City, also have used radioactive tailings in constructing roads and the foundations of buildings. Among highly exposed individuals, annual radiation dosage from mill tailings is estimated at about 2.6 mSv or 260 mrem ("Ionizing Radiation," 1987). Many authorities regard uranium mill tailings as the most neglected of all radioactive wastes and the source of greatest public exposure to ionizing radiation related to nuclear power production. In January 1994, a final EPA ruling took effect, requiring that closure of nonoperational mill tailings sites must be achieved by constructing permanent radon barriers which will limit atmospheric releases of the radioactive gas to 20 picocuries per square meter of air per second.

Conversion. Converting yellowcake to gaseous uranium hexafluoride produces some solid or sludge-like wastes containing radium, some uranium and thorium, but presents a negligible health threat. However, extensive environmental contamination due to improper disposal of radwastes has been documented in the vicinity of the Sequoyah Fuels conversion plant at Gore, Oklahoma (one of only two such facilities in the United States), 75 miles southeast of Tulsa. In 1991 this plant was temporarily closed by the Nuclear Regulatory Commission which cited management with safety violations and coverup of serious environmental releases. The plant reopened in 1992 but experienced a major chemical accident later that year and was closed permanently in June 1993. A multimillion dollar environmental cleanup effort is anticipated, as government and company officials wrestle over responsibility for remediation of uranium-contaminated soil and groundwater on the 85-acre site (Beasley, 1994).

Enrichment. Enriching uranium to increase the concentration of the U-235 isotope from its original 0.7% (the bulk of uranium ore is U-238) to about 2–4%, the level necessary to sustain a fission reaction, results in the venting of small quantities of radioactive gases into the atmosphere and some discharge of diluted liquid wastes, but here again the environmental health impact is minimal.

Fuel Fabrication. Converting enriched uranium hexafluoride gas into solid uranium dioxide pellets, which are then loaded into fuel rods, entails virtually no release of radioactive material into the environment; exposure of fabrication plant workers to radioactive emissions likewise is low.

Power Production. Under normal operating conditions, radiation exposure to the general public emanating from nuclear power plants comes primarily from the deliberate release of controlled amounts of radioactive gases to the atmosphere. Gaseous fission products such as tritium and krypton build up in the fuel rods, leak through the cladding into the reactor building, and must be periodically vented. In addition, small amounts of radioactive materials may be discharged with wastewaters. Public exposure to such emissions has been calculated as ranging from a maximum individual dose of less than 1 mSv (100 mrem) to an average of 0.8 mSv (80 mrem) for those living within a 10-mile radius of the plant. Routes of such exposure include inhalation or skin contact with airborne radionuclides and ingestion of radioactive contaminants in food (especially fish from cooling lakes) and water ("Ionizing Radiation," 1987). Quite clearly, the radiation hazard to people living in the vicinity of a normally operating nuclear reactor is minimal, considerably less than that from natural background sources.

The main fear among those opposed to further reliance on nuclear power, of course, is the potential, however remote, of catastrophic release of radioactive materials should a major accident occur. Although most people today realize that it is physically impossible for a nuclear power plant to explode like a bomb (for this to occur the U-235 fuel would have to be enriched to a concentration far above the level necessary to sustain a fission reaction for power production purposes), a **core meltdown**, which represents a worst-type accident scenario, would be nearly as devastating. Overheating of the reactor core, such as might occur if water should cease to circulate among the fuel rods (a "loss-of-coolant" accident), could result in melting of the fuel rods and breaching of the containment vessel. The massive release of highly radioactive isotopes into the atmosphere, such as occurred at Chernobyl (see Box 10–5), or into groundwater supplies could cause widespread human exposure to lethal doses of radiation, contamination of the general environment with radioactive fallout, and would initiate numerous leukemias and other cancers which would be manifested years later. Although physical destruction of buildings and property would not occur, the biological impact of a core meltdown would be nearly as serious as a bomb blast in terms of human health and environmental degradation. The "defense in depth" concept employed in the construction of nuclear plants, characterized by repeated layers of thick shielding materials and multiple safeguards designed to ensure safety even in the event of partial failure, are intended to prevent this situation from ever becoming a reality.

In spite of such precautions, thousands of mishaps have occurred both here and abroad since the advent of commercial nuclear power. Prior to the Three Mile Island incident, two of the most serious U.S. accidents occurred at the Enrico-Fermi experimental fast breeder reactor near Detroit where part of the fuel in the core melted in early October 1966, and at Browns Ferry, Alabama, where in March 1975, a fire ignited by an electrician's candle raged for seven hours, destroying all the emergency cooling systems in one of the reactors at the complex. In both cases, a core meltdown was only narrowly averted. Each major accident has led to a tightening of safety regulations; a recent report issued by the Congressional Office of Technology Assessment (OTA) affirms that safety performance of American commercial nuclear power plants has been generally good. No accidents resulting in damage to the reactor core have occurred since the partial meltdown at Three Mile Island in 1979, nor have any offsite

BOX 10-5

"China Syndrome" in the Ukraine

When Pennsylvania Governor Richard Thornburgh visited the Soviet Union in 1979 to tour nuclear facilities in that country soon after the partial meltdown at Three Mile Island, he was smugly informed that an accident such as the one which had devastated the nuclear power plant near Harrisburg could never happen in the USSR. "Safety is a solved problem in the Soviet Union," Thornburgh was told by one official who suggested that before long it would be possible to operate a reactor without risk in the middle of Red Square. On April 26, 1986, this optimism suddenly evaporated when reactor #4 near the Ukrainian town of Chernobyl experienced a "worst-case" accident which resulted in a breaching of the containment vessel and massive radioactive contamination of the environment with the equivalent of fallout from several dozen Hiroshima-type bombs (by contrast, the near-meltdown at Three Mile Island resulted in negligible amounts of radiation escaping from the containment structure).

The unlikely chain of events leading to this tragedy was initially blamed on human error rather than on facility design, since the Chernobyl power station was among the newest facilities in the Soviet Union and one which boasted the best operating record of any nuclear power plant in the country. On the fateful day, operators at the plant were engaged in a special test to determine how long the station's turbines could continue generating power after the steam supply had been shut off. The technicians shut down one safety system after another, including turning off the emergency core cooling system and pulling out all the control rods (a Soviet investigating team subsequently reported that fully six serious rules violations had been committed). However, follow-up investigations of the accident in the years since 1986 have led many scientists to con-clude that inherent design flaws in the R.B.M.K.-1000 graphite-core reactor were as much, if not more, to blame than human error—a worrisome conclusion since 15 additional reactors of the same design, many in badly deteriorating condition, remain operational in Russia, Ukraine, and Lithuania. In any case, when the operators realized that the reactor was suddenly beginning to run out of control, it was too late to prevent disaster. Power levels soared to 120 times normal levels, rupturing fuel rods within the core and causing the cooling water to vaporize. The resulting steam explosion blasted apart the 1000-ton concrete slab above the reactor, releasing an estimated 185 million curies of radioactivity and sending "hot" fuel particles hurtling into the sky. These flaming fragments kindled 30 separate fires around the power station complex, and the graphite core of reactor #4 began to burn uncontrollably. Soviet firefighters who rushed to the scene performed heroically, neglecting their own safety as they fought desperately to get the fire under control and prevent its spread to nearby reactors. Most of the human fatalities occurring soon after the accident were among these men who knowingly braved fatal doses of radiation, standing their ground even as their boots stuck to the melting tar on the reactor roof. Efforts to extinguish the fire and stem the release of radioactive particles included the use of military helicopters which dropped 5000 tons of sand, clay, limestone, and lead into the burning reactor core. Although the fires were extinguished fairly quickly, it was not until 11 days after the accident, when liquid nitrogen was pumped under the reactor, that the core cooled sufficiently to reduce radiation levels sharply.

By this time the radioactive plume rising from the stricken reactor had spread over much of Europe. Detected first over Sweden, nuclear fallout was carried by shifting winds over most countries of eastern and central Europe, with some radioactive contamination reported from as far away as Scotland. In all, at least 20 countries reported levels of fallout high enough to constitute a potential public health threat (while traces of fallout were detected by monitors in the U.S., levels were so low as to constitute a negligible threat to the health of Americans).

Most directly affected by radiation exposure, of course, were those living in the vicinity of Chernobyl. Thanks to an efficient, if somewhat delayed, evacuation of towns in the region, about 135,000 people within a 19-mile radius of the plant were bussed to resettlement areas. The evacuated region, officially designated the "Scientific Exclusion Zone" (but commonly referred to as the "Dead Zone"), is now being used as a living laboratory by scientists studying the long-term ecological effects of radioactive contamination on biotic communities. Although dangerously high radiation levels are expected to persist in the general area for years, many villagers have returned to their homes, convinced by government assurances that Chernobyl no longer presents a serious threat (two of the reactors at the complex remain in operation, though the Ukrainian government in 1994 made a commitment to close them at an unspecified future date). Estimates place the number of people currently living in heavily contaminated regions at 8–10 million, many of them in Ukraine's neighboring republic of Belarus which received fully 70% of the former USSR's share of radioactive fallout from Chernobyl. Fortunately for the Ukrainians, favorable weather patterns at the time of the accident kept fallout levels in their republic considerably lower than they might otherwise have been. During the periods of most intense radioactivity, winds were blowing away from major population centers. Dry conditions meant that inhabitants were spared exposure to the radioactive pollutants which would have rained down on them if showers had occurred during that time. In addition, the intense fire which raged for more than a week created a "chimney effect" which carried radioactivity high into the atmosphere, ensuring its spread over neighboring countries but lessening the amount of local fallout. Nevertheless, researchers in Russia, Ukraine, and Belarus report a significant rise in birth defects, thyroid cancer, and goiter within contaminated areas, particularly in the Gomel region of Belarus where fallout was heaviest.

While the nuclear accident at Chernobyl was less devastating in terms of immediate health impact than might have been expected, its toll unquestionably represents the most disastrous release of radiation into the human environment since the advent of commercial nuclear power. Shortly after the event, Soviet authorities placed the official death toll at 31. This figure, however, represents only those killed in the original explosion. On-the-scene observers and medical experts reviewing the fate of the coal miners and young army conscripts recruited for cleanup work after the fires were extinguished estimate that as many as 5000–7000 perished soon afterward due to radiation sickness—and predict that thousands more will die in the years ahead due to radiation-induced cancers.

Unfortunately, nearly a decade after the word "Chernobyl" became synonymous with "nuclear disaster," the damaged reactor continues to pose serious health and environmental threats. The concrete "sarcophagus" built to contain further radioactive releases from the molten core was hastily constructed without a structural margin of safety. Experts fear that the sarcophagus, which has already developed dangerous cracks, is likely to collapse if overburdened with heavy snow or hit by one of the 10–14 tornadoes which can be expected in the Chernobyl area each year. The basement of the sarcophagus below the reactor is flooded with 700–900 cubic feet of water; outside burial pits are also flooded and leaking radioactive fission products into the groundwater below. Inside the sarcophagus, high humidity and standing water are dissolving fission products in the radioactive debris, causing it to crumble and leading to fears that a burst of neutrons (a "criticality incident") could result due to the increasing concentration of fission products. While the international scientific community agrees that the damaged reactor is neither safe nor stabilized, no donors have yet come forth with the billions of dollars which an effective remediation effort would require. In the fall of 1993 the government of Ukraine, its economy in shambles, ran out of money to pay scientists and technicians working at the site.

The lethal legacy of Chernobyl—and the threat of death and disease it continues to pose—guarantees that the public's perception of electricity generated by "the friendly atom" will never be quite the same again.

References

Flavin, Christopher. 1987. "Reassessing Nuclear Power: the Fallout from Chernobyl." *Worldwatch Paper 75*, Worldwatch Institute. (March).

Hawkes, Nigel et al. 1987. *Chernobyl: The End of the Nuclear Dream*. Vintage Books.

"Slants & Trends—Chernobyl." 1994. *Nuclear Waste News 14*, no. 14 (April 7).

releases of large amounts of radioactivity taken place. Although hundreds of emergency shutdowns occur annually, OTA asserts that the number of such events in recent years has not been abnormal and few of them were serious enough to pose a threat of core damage. OTA also reported that radiation exposure to nuclear plant workers, already well below the limits established by the Nuclear Regulatory Commission (NRC), continues to decline.

The operating record of nuclear power plants in Japan and the countries of western Europe roughly parallels that of the United States. Major concerns have surfaced over the past few years, however, over what are regarded as highly unsafe conditions prevailing at a number of nuclear power plants operating in the former Soviet empire. Pointing to some 20,000 reported safety violations at Russian reactors during 1993 alone, Russian safety experts, nuclear plant workers, and Western scientists have all concluded that the nuclear power industry throughout the former USSR is on "the verge of disaster." In April 1994, after plant workers picketed in front of the Russian Parliament building to protest deplorable conditions at the country's eight largest nuclear generating facilities, a high-ranking official warned delegates at a government-sponsored conference that "Today the plants work in an emergency regime. It is impossible. It's like a bomb." A recent report jointly compiled by the World Bank and the International Atomic Energy Agency focuses attention on 25 of the most dangerous nuclear power plants currently operating in six nations (Russia, Lithuania, Armenia, Ukraine, Bulgaria, and Slovakia). Fifteen of these are of a Chernobyl-type design which many Western experts believe is inherently hazardous, posing a serious threat not only to plant workers and surrounding communities, but to the rest of Europe as well. Neither the Chernobyl-style reactors nor the older Soviet-version pressurized water reactors are enclosed by the containment structures which are a standard feature of reactor design in other industrialized countries. The lack of such "defense-in-depth" means that any radioactive releases would be vented directly into the atmosphere rather than being captured and contained. The World Bank report called for a multi-billion dollar contribution by Western nations to close the highest-risk nuclear plants as soon as possible, replacing them with gas-fired facilities, and to retrofit the less dangerous plants with modern safety features. While such huge investments by fiscally strapped donor governments appear problematic at best (the World Bank estimates $18 billion would be needed to carry out report recommendations by the year 2000), the countries whose facilities have been targeted for replacement are resistant to such suggestions as well. Denying that their existing plants are as unsafe as Western experts contend, some Russian officials are loathe to substitute gas-fired plants for nuclear power because they view sales of natural gas as a means of obtaining hard currency and want to reserve domestic gas supplies for export. Countries like Armenia and Bulgaria, which lack gas supplies of their own, are equally reluctant to make the switch because they can't afford to import expensive natural gas from abroad. In addition, all six countries worry that closing any of the plants now operating would result in more job losses at a time when rising unemployment is causing serious social and political unrest. In countries like Lithuania and Ukraine, which depend on nuclear power for 60% and 25%, respectively, of their electrical generating capacity, closure of such plants would further undermine already shaky economies. As a result, it is likely that for the foreseeable future these plants will remain in operation, posing a constant threat of disaster to all who live downwind of these facilities (Browne, 1992; Simons, 1993).

Reprocessing.   After a fuel assembly has been in operation for about a year, waste fission products accumulate in the rods to such an extent that the fission reaction can no longer be sustained, necessitating replacement of these "spent" rods with fresh ones. Spent fuel rods, highly radioactive, are initially placed in swimming pool-like cooling tanks where the isotopes with very short half-lives decay within a relatively brief time. The rods are still highly radioactive (and physically hot as well) due to longer-lived fission products still present and also contain appreciable amounts of unused fuel in the form of U-235 and plutonium which formed during the fission process within the fuel rods. To separate these two useful products from the other isotopes which constitute high level radioactive wastes, reprocessing of the material in the spent rods was envisioned as a vital part of the nuclear fuel cycle. In this process the fuel is removed from the rods and dissolved in nitric acid, the solution then being treated chemically to separate it into uranium, plutonium, and waste components. This operation represents a potential public hazard, since volatile radioisotopes, particularly krypton, are released into the atmosphere and other radioisotopes are discharged with liquid wastes. Workers inside the reprocessing plant are also exposed to higher levels of radioactivity than are nuclear power plant workers, though conceivably safeguards could be taken to reduce this risk. Although reprocessing was considered a key part of the nuclear fuel cycle, reducing the amount of what would otherwise be considered waste and extending the fuel supply, a moratorium on commercial reprocessing was imposed by President Ford in 1976 and continued by President Carter due to the concern that reprocessing plants would be tempting targets for attack by terrorists attempting to obtain weapons-grade plutonium. Although President Reagan subsequently lifted the ban, financial considerations have deterred private interests from reentering the reprocessing business and at present no commercial reprocessing facilities exist in this country, despite cries from the nuclear power industry that they will soon have no place to store the spent fuel rods that continue to accumulate on-site. Overseas, both France and the United Kingdom reprocess spent fuel from commercial nuclear reactors; the Japanese have begun construction of a giant reprocessing plant at Rokkasho-mura in northeastern Japan, and India has expressed its intentions to build reprocessing facilities sometime in the future.

Waste Disposal.   Nuclear power production results in the generation of large quantities of both high- and low-level wastes, the former primarily in the form of spent fuel from reactors, the latter consisting of contaminated clothing, clean-up solutions, wiping rags, hand tools, etc. **High-level wastes** are extremely radioactive, highly penetrating, and generate a great deal of heat, hence must be handled without direct human contact. Currently, most high-level commercial wastes are being stored in cooling ponds at the power plants where they were produced; a relatively small percentage is in storage at facilities in Morris, Illinois, and West Valley, New York, once intended as reprocessing plants.

Responding to criticism that the lack of any clear-cut policy for permanent disposal of high-level radioactive waste could prove the Achilles' heel of the nuclear power industry, Congress in 1982 enacted the **Nuclear Waste Policy Act**. This legislation delegated responsibility for high-level radwaste management to the federal government and designated the U.S. Department of Energy as the lead agency to coordinate the effort to site, construct, and operate the nation's first permanent repository for such wastes. The politically sensitive search for a location for this facility is now focused on Yucca Mountain, Nevada, where extensive characterization studies are underway to determine the site's geologic suitability for deep burial of solidified wastes. Since the fission products in spent fuel rods will be dangerously radioactive for tens of thousands of years, suitability of any site chosen for an underground repository will depend on the ability of surrounding geological formations to absorb heat and to prevent radioactive emissions from escaping into the environment. Issues of special concern at the Yucca Mountain site include the long-term potential for earthquakes or volcanic eruptions in an area of known seismic activity and the possibility of groundwater intrusion into storage caverns in the eventuality of future climatic change. The fact that the area contains numerous mineral deposits raises worries that future generations, ignorant of the hazardous materials entombed on the site, might drill into the repository in search of gas or oil. These and numerous other questions must be resolved before the Department of Energy concludes the characterization process, a task which DOE hopes will be completed by the year 2000 or soon thereafter.

If DOE resolves that the site is indeed suitable, it will prepare an environmental impact statement and forward a recommendation to the president that Yucca Mountain be approved as the nation's first permanent repository for high-level radioactive wastes. If the president agrees, Congress must then vote to approve or reject the site. At that point, the State of Nevada has the right to veto the entire project—and will likely do so, given the intense opposition toward the repository being expressed throughout Nevada by public and policymakers fearful of their state's image as a "national sacrifice zone." Such an action could be overturned only by a joint resolution by the U.S. Senate and House of Representatives. Only after congressional approval of the site has been obtained can DOE apply to the Nuclear Regulatory Commission for a license to begin construction of the facility. Since approval of the license request can take up to three years and construction of the repository several years more, it is obvious that utility companies have a long time to wait before the spent fuel rods accumulating at reactor sites can be moved to their final resting place (League of Women Voters, 1993). Although the 1982 Nuclear Waste Policy Act mandates that the facility be operational by 1998, DOE Secretary O'Leary has admitted that the earliest possible date Yucca Mountain could begin accepting radwaste shipments is 2013 (Wald, 1993).

In the meantime, spent fuel rods continue to accumulate on site and some utilities warn that they may have to close down within the next several years for lack of a waste disposal alternative. This situation poses a major problem for the federal government as well as for the nuclear power industry. Under terms of the Nuclear Waste Policy Act, Washington has been collecting a 0.1¢ fee on every kilowatt hour of electricity generated by nuclear power since 1983, with these revenues being deposited in a special fund earmarked for development of the permanent repository. In return, Washington made a contractual commitment to the utility companies that it would begin to move spent fuel from reactor sites in 1998. With this deadline date looming on the horizon and no permanent disposal facility likely to open in the near future, DOE is now attempting to devise an interim solution in the form of a **Monitored Retrievable Storage (MRS)** facility—a "temporary" away-from-reactor site where spent nuclear fuel could be stored in above-ground dry casks for an indefinite period until a permanent repository is ultimately opened (dry cask storage of spent fuel, already being utilized at six power plants around the country, entails sealing radioactive wastes inside huge steel containers with 9-inch thick walls and placing them outdoors on a barbed-wire enclosed concrete pad). While opponents of nuclear power oppose any away-from-reactor storage of spent nuclear fuel due to the potential for accidents in transit, advocates of this option argue that until a final disposal site is operational, it is preferable to store mounting stocks of nuclear waste at one, carefully maintained site rather than at scores of power plants across the nation, many of them located in densely populated or environmentally sensitive areas. The DOE has been trying, with limited success, to attract interest from states, counties, or Indian tribes to host such a facility in return for certain financial benefits. By the spring of 1994, the only group seriously considering such an undertaking was the tribal council of the Mescalero

Apaches. Their 460,000 acre reservation north of Alamagordo, New Mexico, seems to meet DOE criteria for storing several thousand tons of nuclear waste for two or three decades, since it is sparsely settled and not too far from major transportation routes. Although their non-Apache neighbors and New Mexico state politicians are adamantly opposed to the idea, Apache leaders are aggressively pursuing an opportunity which they feel would bring badly needed income and employment opportunities to the 3400 member tribe while posing minimal, if any, risk to human health or to the environment (wastes would arrive in solid form inside sealed containers; since they would no longer be hot enough to require water cooling, there would be no liquid to leak nor any need for reliance on failure-prone pumps, valves, or mechanical systems—casks would simply sit in the open, passively cooled by the surrounding air). Contending that, as a sovereign Indian nation, they are entitled to proceed without state approval, the Mescaleros have entered into negotiations with a Minnesota-based utility, Northern States Power, to provide monitored retrievable storage at a site they believe could be completed by 2001. While such plans are contingent on the partners obtaining a license from the NRC, tribal leaders are hopeful for the eventual success of their efforts and the opportunity to bring a measure of prosperity to their people. As Wendell Chino, president of the Tribal Council, explained to a visiting reporter, "The Navajos make rugs. The Pueblos make pottery. And the Mescaleros make money" (Wald, 1993; "Mescaleros Prepare," 1994).

Controversy over a monitored retrievable storage facility is not the only radioactive waste issue inflaming passions in New Mexico. For over a decade an even more heated debate has focused on the proposed opening of the **Waste Isolation Pilot Plant (WIPP)**, a complex of shafts, tunnels, and rooms excavated more than 2000 feet (655 meters) below ground surface in a deep salt formation near Carlsbad, New Mexico. Intended as a final resting place for up to 6.5 million cubic feet of **transuranic wastes**, plutonium-contaminated debris from nuclear weapons production (no commercial radwastes will be sent to the facility), WIPP's opening has been repeatedly delayed by legal challenges related to technical and safety issues. In the fall of 1993, DOE agreed to postpone placement of contaminated materials in the Carlsbad repository until laboratory tests confirming the site's suitability can be completed. DOE must then obtain EPA certification, based on these lab results, stating that WIPP is in compliance with federal environmental laws. Opening of the facility, which by late 1993 had run up a price tag of $1.5 billion (a figure expected to climb to $3 billion by the turn of the century), is thus unlikely to take place before 1998 at the earliest. In the meantime, about 60,000 cubic meters of dangerous plutonium-contaminated wastes, 70% of which have been in storage for over 10 years, remain in badly deteriorating containers at 10 different national weapons laboratories around the country. These materials have become unwelcome commodities in states like Idaho, whose Idaho National Engineering Laboratory near Idaho Falls houses 60% of all plutonium defense wastes. Resentful of the federal government's failure to provide a permanent disposal site and fearful of being burdened with some of the nation's most dangerous nuclear wastes in perpetuity, Idaho

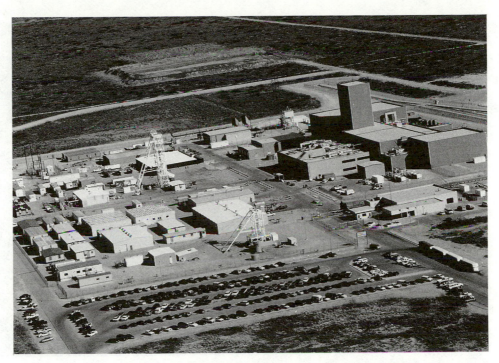

The Waste Isolation Pilot Plant (WIPP) near Carlsbad, New Mexico was built as a permanent disposal site for plutonium-contaminated debris from nuclear weapons production, though legal challenges have delayed its opening until at least 1998. [Courtesy of U.S. Department of Energy]

officials—along with their counterparts in Colorado, Tennessee, South Carolina, and other states where plutonium wastes are now languishing in "interim storage"—eagerly await the long-anticipated opening of WIPP (Cushman, 1993; League of Women Voters, 1993).

Low-level wastes, produced not only by nuclear power plants but also by hospitals, research labs, universities, and industries, exhibit low but sometimes potentially hazardous concentrations of radioisotopes. They differ from high-level wastes in having significantly lower levels of radioactive emissions; they are not physically hot, generally require no shielding, and, unlike high-level wastes which remain dangerous for millennia, decay to harmless levels within 100–300 years. In the United States during the 1950s, many low-level commercial radwastes were buried on military reservations along with defense wastes or were simply dumped into the ocean—a practice which didn't cease entirely until 1970 (as recently as the fall of 1993, Russia defied world public opinion and infuriated the Japanese by brazenly dumping more than 900 tons of low-level radwastes into a prime squid fishing area in the Sea of Japan). Much of this dumping, some of which included plutonium wastes from atomic research labs as well as low-level wastes, occurred in the vicinity of the Gulf of Farallones National Marine Sanctuary, an ocean wildlife preserve 30 miles offshore from San Francisco. Though few studies have been

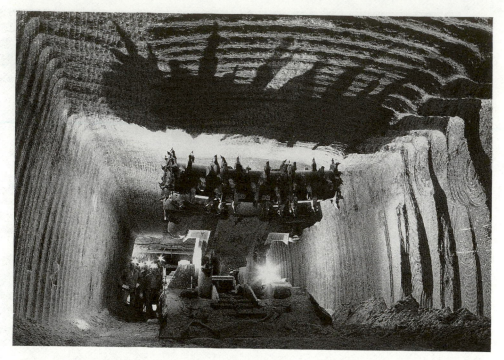

A portion of an underground tunnel at the WIPP facility is shown here, along with a machine used for excavation. [Courtesy of U.S. Department of Energy]

carried out to determine whether the rich sea life in the area has been adversely affected by radiation exposure, it is known that many of the waste barrels have corroded or burst under pressure, leaking their contents into the ocean sediments. By the 1960s, the commercial nuclear industry was relying on shallow land burial for disposal of low-level wastes, utilizing six privately owned facilities specifically licensed for this purpose. By the late 1970s, three of these sites had closed due to migration of radioactive materials from the trenches, though no radioactive contamination was detected outside site boundaries. Because the states in which the three remaining sites were located (South Carolina, Nevada, and Washington) vigorously objected to being the "nuclear dumping ground" of the nation, Congress was persuaded to enact the **1980 Low-Level Radioactive Waste Policy Act**. This legislation placed responsibility for low-level radwaste management on *state* governments (as opposed to *federal* jurisdiction over high-level wastes), which were required to provide a means of safe disposal for all low-level wastes generated within their borders. Any states failing to do so could find their radwastes barred from disposal at existing sites in other states. However, recognizing that construction of 50 separate disposal facilities was neither necessary nor economically feasible, Congress permitted states to negotiate regional "**compact**" agreements among themselves to provide for the establishment, operation, and regulation of low-level radioactive waste facilities within each compact area. By 1994 ten regional compact agreements had been concluded, with five states still unaffiliated. Each regional compact is required to designate one of its members as the "**host state**"—i.e. the state in which the disposal facility is to be located—and to make numerous decisions regarding operational procedures, disposal fees, and type of facility to be constructed. Since shallow land burial has been deemed unacceptable by most host state legislatures, various designs for engineered structures are being considered, all of which offer much greater assurance of environmental safety than trench burial.

The original 1986 deadline date for completion of regional facilities was extended to January 1, 1993, but in every compact area, intense public opposition to siting has stymied efforts to carry out the requirements of the law. At the end of December 1992, the small facility at Beatty, Nevada, closed its gates and the Hanford, Washington, landfill restricted access to all but 11 northwestern and Rocky Mountain states. This left only the Barnwell, South Carolina, facility to accommodate the radwaste disposal needs of the rest of the country. That last remaining option was foreclosed for all but the eight members of the Southeastern Compact on July 1, 1994, when out-of-region radwaste shipments were barred access to Barnwell. Southeasterners themselves have little time for complacency, since under the terms of the Southeastern Compact, the Barnwell site will close permanently in 1996, with host state status being assumed by North Carolina—where the site designated as Barnwell's replacement is being vigorously opposed by protesters demanding the state look "somewhere else." Caught in the middle of the siting controversy are the radwaste generators which now have no place to send their wastes and may have to cease using radioactive materials if a solution to the impasse is not devised soon. While most utility companies have been taking steps to reduce radwaste volume and have the capacity to store wastes on-site for several years, the lack of viable disposal options threatens continued operations at the thousands of hospitals, research laboratories, and industries which utilize radioactive materials. While many observers contend that low-level radioactive wastes, properly managed, pose minimal health or environmental hazards, the public's inability to distinguish between the vastly different risks presented by high-level vs. low-level radwastes contributes to the hysteria surrounding the siting issue and makes it difficult to predict how states will ever resolve the disposal dilemma.

Ultraviolet Radiation

Wavelengths of the electromagnetic spectrum ranging between 40–400 nanometers in length are categorized as ultraviolet (UV) light. Although ultraviolet radiation is not of sufficiently high energy to ionize atoms and molecules, certain portions within this range are strongly absorbed by living tissues, particularly by DNA which constitutes the major target of UV damage. Injury to the hereditary material of cells is the reason for the lethal or mutational effects which excess UV exposure can provoke

BOX 10-6
Radwaste Management Abroad

Engaged in an intense domestic debate over what to do with radioactive wastes, Americans have paid little attention to radwaste management policies being pursued elsewhere in the world. Since there are over 300 nuclear power plants currently operating in 30 other nations, disposal dilemmas pose challenges for policymakers in many countries. Everywhere high-level wastes are proving the thorniest problem. While the United States is finally making at least halting progress toward developing a permanent high-level waste repository, no other countries have anything more than temporary storage facilities for these intensely hazardous by-products of nuclear power. Most national energy planners continue to assume that spent nuclear fuel will be reprocessed and that the remaining wastes will be solidified into a glass-like material and buried in deep geologic strata—very similar in concept to the government's disposal plans for high-level liquid wastes from reprocessing carried out at U.S. nuclear weapons production facilities (spent fuel rods from commercial reactors will be buried intact, since no commercial reprocessing exists in the U.S.). However, such plans have not progressed beyond the research stage in most countries due to political opposition to siting such facilities in those densely populated nations. France currently has two reprocessing plants, handling spent fuel from its own 44 nuclear plants as well as from plants in a number of neighboring countries. The high-level wastes generated by this process are converted into solid glass blocks which the French intend to store in an engineered facility for 50–60 years, after which they plan to bury them in a currently nonexistent repository deep underground (this repository will be used solely for French wastes, however; reprocessed, vitrified wastes from other countries will not be eligible for disposal in the French facility).

Other countries have made somewhat less progress than France in managing their high-level wastes. The United Kingdom has a large reprocessing facility at Sellafield (formerly called Windscale) on the northwest coast. The U.K. intends to store the resulting vitrified wastes until at least 2030 in an engineered facility and has no plans at present for any permanent repository. In Germany, where antinuclear sentiment is running high in the aftermath of Chernobyl, plans for a reprocessing plant in Bavaria have been cancelled; a permanent disposal facility deep in a salt dome in lower Saxony will be developed if studies indicate the site is geologically suitable. Construction of an away-from-reactor facility for temporary storage of high-level radwastes is also planned.

Canada, like the United States, continues to store spent fuel rods at reactor sites while an independent commission studies a government plan to bury spent fuel in a granite formation at a location yet to be determined.

Sweden, which has decided to forego further development of nuclear power and to phase out its 12 existing plants by 2010, will contract with other countries to handle its limited reprocessing needs and is committed to selecting a site for a permanent repository by 1997; studies to evaluate a granite formation at Apso near Sweden's Oskarshamn nuclear complex are now underway.

Densely populated, earthquake-prone Japan has the most ambitious nuclear power program in Asia but faces difficult radwaste disposal problems. Currently Japan is involved in a cooperative program with China to build an underground research facility, possibly in the Gobi Desert.

The government of Argentina has

recently begun testing granite formations in central Patagonia, 900 miles
south of Buenos Aires, as a possible
repository for wastes from its three
nuclear power plants. While many
Argentines are horrified that officials
would consider burying such dangerous material just 30 miles outside the
small town of Gastre, many of the residents of the isolated, economically
depressed community say they would
welcome the jobs, income—and
excitement—such development would
bring.

Low-level radioactive waste disposal
practices overseas are scarcely more
advanced than those in the United
States. France currently boasts a state-
of-the-art engineered structure designed to accept cement-encased low-
level wastes and to prevent any possibility of leachates migrating away from
the facility. Elsewhere, disposal
methods include shallow land burial,
placement in abandoned mine shafts,
and ocean dumping.

in living organisms. Research has shown that the most detrimental effects
to biological systems occur when UV radiation is in the 230–320 nanometer
range (referred to as UVB, as opposed to longer-wavelength UVA), peak
absorption by DNA occurring at 260 nm. Much of the ultraviolet light
naturally present in incoming solar radiation is filtered out by the layer
of atmospheric ozone located about 20 miles above the earth's surface (see
chapter 11). Living organisms have developed various defense mechanisms
to protect themselves against the amounts that do penetrate—shielding
devices such as fur, feathers, shells, or darkly-pigmented skin, as well as
light-avoidance behavior patterns among a variety of species. Of equal
importance has been the evolution of enzymatic mechanisms for repairing
UV-induced damage to DNA when levels of injury are not excessive.
Without this cellular repair ability it is doubtful whether many organisms
could survive existing levels of UV exposure. The importance of such
mechanisms can be seen in the example of individuals suffering from the
genetic disease xeroderma pigmentosum. Lacking the enzyme needed for
repair of radiation-damaged DNA, victims of this ailment have to remain
indoors throughout daylight hours or risk the development of multiple fatal
skin cancers. There appears to be a tenuous balance between continual
UV assault on the hereditary material and its biochemical repair. If the cell's
capacity to deal with such damage is overwhelmed, the cell will die.

Since ultraviolet light cannot penetrate very deeply into living tissues,
the major concern in reference to UV injury to humans involves the
induction of skin cancers, particularly in lighter-skinned individuals who
lack protective melanin granules in their epidermal skin layers.

After World War II, when the tyranny of fashion decreed that pale skin
was "out" and the bronzed look "in," the apparently irresistible urge
among fair-complexioned citizens to spend hours broiling themselves under
the sun or at rapidly proliferating tanning parlors, while at the same time
wearing increasingly skimpy clothes outdoors, has resulted in an alarming

BOX 10-7
Why Johnny Should Wear Sunscreen

For generations, plenty of fresh air and sunshine has been the standard prescription for raising healthy children. Recently, however, the sunshine portion of that formula has been disputed by dermatologists witnessing a dramatic rise in the incidence of skin cancer among young and middle-aged patients. Growing awareness that children are particularly vulnerable to UVB-induced skin damage and the fact that youngsters generally spend much more time outdoors than do adults have prompted warnings that parents should do more to protect their little ones from the hazards of UV exposure—especially in light of findings that fully 80% of the typical American's lifetime exposure to UV radiation occurs before age 20.

Efforts are underway to educate not only mothers and fathers but also teachers, coaches, recreation counselors, and children themselves of sun-protection strategies. Admonitions include not allowing infants or children to become badly sunburned and keeping children indoors between 10 A.M. and 3 P.M. when the summer sun is most intense. Taking such precautions with infants is particularly important; babies under six months of age have very sensitive skin and should be kept in the shade out of direct sun. Conscientious parents will ensure that strollers are fitted with hoods and babies protected with wide-brimmed hats. Baby oil should never be applied to an infant's skin before going outdoors, since it makes the skin more translucent to harmful solar radiation. Toddlers and older children are somewhat less vulnerable than infants, but dermatologists advise that they, too, should wear long-sleeved shirts, slacks, and hats while playing outdoors. From a health protection standpoint, these are undoubtedly sound suggestions, but inconvenience of implementation makes it unlikely that they will attract many adherents.

An alternative recommendation which could have a major impact on reducing a child's risk of developing skin cancer later in life could be adopted with minimal effort, however—insisting that children above the age of six months regularly use sunscreen with an **SPF** (sun protection factor) of 15 or higher. It is well recognized that sunscreens are very effective in preventing sunburn (in addition to the discomfort it produces, sunburn is suspected as being the triggering event in the development of malignant melanoma); animal research results indicate that sunscreens are also instrumental in reducing the risk of basal and squamous cell carcinomas. It has been calculated that regular use of sunscreen with SPF 15 from infancy through age 18 would reduce an individual's lifetime risk of basal and squamous cell carcinomas by fully 78%. Additional benefits would include fewer sunburns, slower aging of the skin, and possibly a lower risk of melanoma. Sunscreens with SPF values lower than 15 are regarded by skin specialists as providing insufficient protection for users of any age, regardless of skin type; experts are unsure whether *higher* SPF sunscreens offer any additional protection. Unfortunately, there are no generally accepted industry-wide standards for determining the SPF of a sunscreen; each manufacturer has its own method for assigning SPF values. For this reason, the actual SPF of any given product could be lower than its advertised SPF. The best sunscreens are those which are most resistant to being washed off by sweating, swimming or bathing—a feature that is largely determined by the product's base material. In general, the most water-resistant sunscreens are those which feel the greasiest (e.g. Vaseline-type ointments);

clear lotions and gels are the most easily washed-off, while creamy lotions rank midway between. For greatest effectiveness, sunscreen should be applied 30 minutes prior to sun exposure so that protective ingredients have time to be absorbed and should be reapplied every two hours or whenever contact with water or sweat removes the original protective layer.

The fact that few children currently use high SPF sunscreens indicates that extensive public education efforts are needed to spread the word that the irreparable skin damage that can be caused both by chronic and acute sun exposure can be prevented by applying a dose of common sense—and sunscreen.

References

Stern, Robert S., et al. 1986. "Risk Reduction for Nonmelanoma Skin Cancer with Childhood Sunscreen Use." *Archives of Dermatology* 12, no. 5 (May).

Robbins, Perry, M.D. *Play it Safe in the Sun.* Skin Cancer Foundation.

increase in the incidence of skin cancer in Western countries. Whereas a child born in the United States in 1930 had about a 1 in 1500 risk of developing skin cancer within his or her lifetime, for a white child born today that risk has soared to 1 in 100 (for blacks the danger is much lower—less than 1 in 1000). The main villain behind these grim statistics is increased exposure to UVB radiation, a known carcinogen and mutagen. Three major types of skin cancer account for over 700,000 new cases of the disease diagnosed in the United States each year. **Basal cell carcinoma** and **squamous cell carcinoma** represent the vast majority of skin cancers, accounting for fully one-third of all cancers occurring in the United States today. Chronic exposure to sunlight (actually the UVB component of sunlight) is recognized as the cause of over 90% of these two cancers. They appear, predictably, on portions of the body receiving the greatest sun exposure—face, neck, ears, back of the hands—and until recently were unusual in people under the age of 50. Now, however, numerous cases have been diagnosed among people in their 20s and 30s and occasionally even in teenagers. Not surprisingly, they are also being found on the legs, chest, and back of victims as the sunbathing mania takes its toll (Schreiber, 1986).

Fortunately, the majority of such cancers can be treated if detected early, but each year several thousand cases prove fatal when their neglect leads to invasion of underlying tissues. **Malignant melanoma** is much less common than basal cell or squamous cell carcinomas, but far more deadly. Each year recently about 32,000 Americans have been diagnosed with malignant melanoma and 6700 annually die of the disease. The incidence of malignant melanoma has been increasing by approximately 4% annually since 1973 and is now the most common form of cancer to strike women under the age of 30. Americans born during the 1990s are at 12 times the risk of eventually developing malignant melanoma as are those born 50 years ago and twice as likely as those born just 10 years ago (DeLeo, 1992). Unlike the nonmelanoma skin cancers, malignant melanoma appears to develop as a result of occasional severe sunburn, rather than by prolonged,

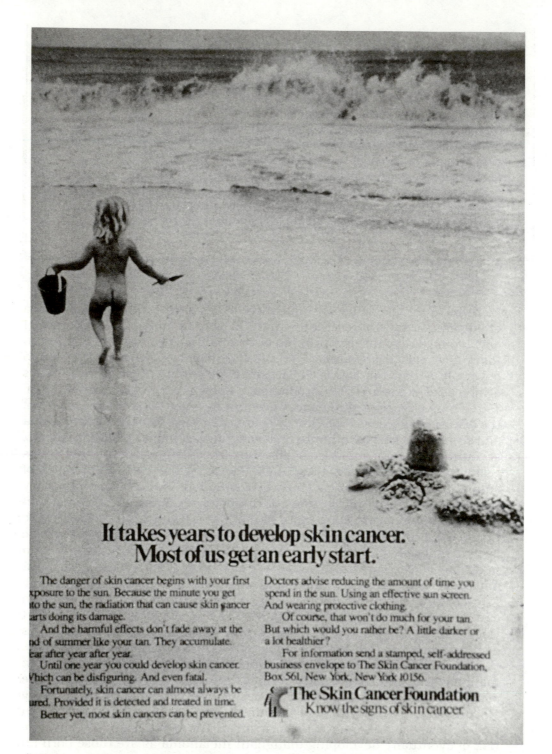

It takes years to develop skin cancer. Most of us get an early start.

The danger of skin cancer begins with your first exposure to the sun. Because the minute you get into the sun, the radiation that can cause skin cancer starts doing its damage.

And the harmful effects don't fade away at the end of summer like your tan. They accumulate. Year after year after year.

Until one year you could develop skin cancer. Which can be disfiguring. And even fatal.

Fortunately, skin cancer can almost always be cured. Provided it is detected and treated in time.

Better yet, most skin cancers can be prevented.

Doctors advise reducing the amount of time you spend in the sun. Using an effective sun screen. And wearing protective clothing.

Of course, that won't do much for your tan. But which would you rather be? A little darker or a lot healthier?

For information send a stamped, self-addressed business envelope to The Skin Cancer Foundation, Box 561, New York, New York 10156.

The Skin Cancer Foundation
Know the signs of skin cancer.

Health education efforts such as this poster from the Skin Cancer Foundation attempt to alert parents to the dangers of excessive childhood sun exposure. [Courtesy of The Skin Cancer Foundation, New York, N.Y.]

low-dose exposure to sunlight. A blistering sunburn experienced during childhood or adolescence seems to double or triple the risk of subsequently developing malignant melanoma. Interestingly, while basal cell and squamous cell carcinomas develop only on sun-exposed portions of the body, malignant melanomas frequently occur on areas normally covered. They also tend to occur at a younger age than do the other two forms of skin cancer, the highest percentage of malignant melanomas occurring in victims under age 50. Because of the suspected link between childhood sunburn and melanoma, groups such as The Skin Cancer Foundation are urging parents to be particularly careful in protecting youngsters from excessive sun exposure.

Ill effects of UV-light exposure are not limited to cancer and sunburn. Premature wrinkling, drying, and mottling of the skin are among the less desirable consequences of UV exposure. In recent years the growing popularity of tanning parlors has been accompanied by claims from the owners of such establishments that they provide a safe alternative to sunbathing because they utilize UVA radiation rather than UVB and hence cannot result in burning. Nevertheless, tanning parlor patrons are exposing themselves to several other serious risks. While the link between UVA and skin cancer is still somewhat controversial, the ability of UVA to cause premature aging of skin and to induce cataracts is indisputable. UVA also enhances the effect of sunlight: individuals who sunbathe outdoors shortly after a stint in a tanning parlor frequently suffer extremely severe sunburns. Photosensitive reactions to either tanning parlors or outdoor sunbathing can occur when unwary sun-worshippers expose themselves to UV light while taking antibiotics (especially tetracycline), antihistamines, birth control pills, even certain cosmetics. Such a toxic reaction is generally manifested as an unusually severe sunburn immediately following exposure to UV light. Exposure to even moderate amounts of ultraviolet radiation can be dangerous for individuals suffering from *lupus erythematosus*, an autoimmune ailment. Between 40–60% of lupus patients experience aggravation of skin disease or systemic symptoms when exposed to either UVA or UVB light. Many researchers contend that the threat of UV damage to the body's immune system should be regarded just as seriously as its ability to induce skin cancer. Studies have shown that ultraviolet radiation from both natural and artificial sources can alter the proportions of various types of white blood cells and depress the activity of natural killer-T cells in the bloodstream. Immune system dysfunction caused by UV exposure is not related to the amount of pigmentation in a person's skin, as is the case with skin cancer. Individuals with black or brown skin are just as likely to suffer immune system damage if they spend too much time in the sun as are fair-skinned people. Unfortunately, most sunscreens do *not* appear to be effective in preventing the type of immune system damage provoked by UVB exposure (Sontheimer, 1992; "Sunscreens," 1992). Weighing serious long-term health risks against short-term fashion benefits, dermatologists are unanimous in their recommendation that all UV exposure, whether on the beach or at a tanning salon, be avoided to the greatest extent possible.

Figure 10-3 Hazards of UV Radiation

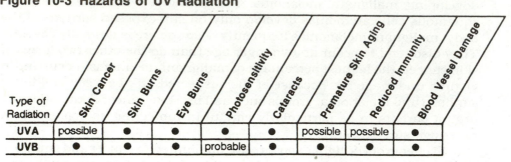

Type of Radiation	Skin Cancer	Skin Burns	Eye Burns	Photosensitivity	Cataracts	Premature Skin Aging	Reduced Immunity	Blood Vessel Damage
UVA	possible	●	●	●	●	possible	possible	●
UVB	●	●	●	probable	●	●	●	●

Source: Food and Drug Administration, U.S. Department of Health and Human Services/Public Health Service.

Ultraviolet light has some beneficial as well as harmful effects. A certain amount of skin exposure is necessary to promote the bodily synthesis of vitamin D, a deficiency of which can result in the development of rickets, a bone deformity. The germicidal properties of UV light have recommended its use in operating rooms to reduce the danger of bacterial or viral infections. Ultraviolet light applications have also been successfully employed to treat such bacterial skin diseases as acne and boils (Schreiber, 1986).

Microwaves

Electromagnetic radiation comprising wavelengths ranging from approximately one millimeter to one meter (intermediate between infrared and short-wave radio wavelengths) is termed microwave radiation. Since microwave energies are so low, such radiations are typically characterized by their frequencies which, in the case of microwaves of biological interest, generally fall between 100 and 30,000 megahertz (MHZ).

Humans today are continuously bombarded with microwaves from such diverse sources as military radar installations, radio and television transmitters, communications and surveillance satellites, radar and radio-frequency transmitters at airports and on planes and ships, microwave ovens, telephone and TV-signal relay towers, walkie-talkies, video display terminals, automatic garage door openers, and so on. Whether or not microwave radiation, particularly at lower levels of exposure, presents a public health threat remains a matter of controversy among researchers. Unlike X-rays, microwaves are nonionizing; instead, when absorbed they cause an increased rate of vibration in the molecules of the absorbing material, resulting in the production of heat. Depending on frequency, microwaves are differentially absorbed by bodily tissues. Those of very low energy (below 150 MHZ) simply pass through the body without being

BOX 10-8
Electromagnetic Fields (EMF): Cause for Concern?

Residents of Meadow Street in Guilford, Connecticut, were frightened. Five people in that small neighborhood had developed tumors or malignancies and people were convinced that a nearby electrical substation was somehow to blame. This wasn't the first time that electromagnetic fields had been incriminated in localized "cancer clusters." In 1979 researchers at the University of Colorado Medical Center in Denver reported that children who are exposed to stronger than average magnetic fields, such as those living in the vicinity of large power transmission lines, have a 2–3 times greater risk of developing leukemia than do children living at a distance from such sources. While the Denver study was subsequently discredited as methodologically flawed, several other researchers reported similar linkages between EMFs and childhood cancers. In Sweden scientists compared leukemia rates among children living within 1000 feet of power lines with national averages and found that those exposed to the strongest magnetic fields experienced a cancer incidence three times higher than what would normally be expected.

Such findings sent power company physicists scurrying to their laboratories to try to determine whether such reports were valid and, if so, what could be done to mitigate the problem—a major dilemma in the present-day U.S. where per capita electricity use has increased more than 300-fold since 1900. From the beginning, many scientists were skeptical of any cancer-EMF association, simply because the amounts of radiation emanating from power lines and appliances are so minute in comparison with the earth's own magnetic field. The fact that per capita residential use of electricity has increased 20-fold during the past half century would suggest that if EMFs *did* have carcinogenic potential,

childhood cancer rates should have soared during the past 50 years—but they haven't. Nor does the doubling or tripling of leukemia rates cited by the University of Colorado researchers translate into a large number of additional cancer cases. Even if results of the 1979 study are valid (and many scientists claim they are not), a doubling of risk would increase the rate of childhood leukemia from 1 case per 20,000 children per year to 2 cases. Numerous research efforts to verify a possible EMF-cancer association have been carried out since the early 1980s with inconclusive results. While some epidemiologic studies, such as those previously cited, showed a slight risk of cancer with EMF exposure, others found no such association; significantly, experiments using animal models failed to demonstrate any correlation between laboratory exposure to low frequency radiation and the induction or promotion of cancer. In 1992, two major reports concluded that scientific evidence supporting claims of EMF-provoked health damage simply doesn't exist. Summing up the general consensus within the scientific community, a study sponsored by the Oak Ridge Associated Universities (a group representing 65 universities in the southeastern U.S.) concluded that "Epidemiologic findings of an association between electric and magnetic fields and childhood leukemia or other childhood or adult cancers are inconsistent and inconclusive."

While activist groups remain convinced that EMF is a very real problem which shouldn't be allowed to fade from public consciousness, the lack of any conclusive proof of health damage has prompted second thoughts among those who just a few years ago regarded EMF as a potentially significant environmental health issue. In June 1992, the Connecticut Academy of Science and Engineering concluded that the power company's substation had nothing to do with the Guilford cancer cases; the following year, in the first lawsuit of its kind to go to trial, a jury in San Diego rejected the plaintiffs' claim that their 5-year-old daughter's kidney cancer had been caused by the transmission lines above their home. The lack of solid scientific information on EMF health effects has prompted a proposal by EPA to eliminate its fledgling EMF program. Stressing that it doesn't want to see the issue disappear, the agency, nevertheless, will recommend the program be temporarily phased out because data on EMF health effects are insufficient for standard-setting purposes. Predicting that the program will be revived in a few years after ongoing studies provide more definitive answers, an EPA official commented, "It's not like the agency is out of it. The program will just wind down for a while and then wind back up."

References

Illinois Department of Public Health. 1992. *EMF Facts* (Jan.).

Taubes, Gary. 1993. "Electrical Emissions: Dangerous or Not?" *New York Times*, June 22.

absorbed; those of intermediate frequency (150–1200 MHZ) are absorbed by the deeper tissues without any noticeable heating of the skin. This poses a danger of serious bodily harm, since internal organs can receive highly damaging doses of microwave radiation without the victim realizing that anything is wrong. As microwave frequency increases, tissue penetration decreases and at 3500 MHZ warming of the skin can be felt; above 10,000 MHZ only the surface of the skin is heated and no penetration of the body occurs.

Differential absorption of microwave energy by bodily tissues is to a large degree a function of their water content. Moist tissues such as skin, muscle, and the intestines absorb more microwaves than do bones and fatty tissues. Sensitivity of specific organs to microwaves depends not only on how readily such radiation is absorbed, but also on how effectively blood circulating through the organ can dissipate the excess heat. Experiments have shown that body parts with poor circulation—the eyes, gastrointestinal tract, testes, urinary bladder, and gall bladder—are the areas most susceptible to injury from microwaves (Dalrymple, 1973).

Excessive heating of internal organs is the best understood type of microwave-induced injury. One extreme case involved a 42-year-old radar repairman who stood in the beam of a radar transmitter while working within 10 feet of the antenna. He felt a sensation of heat in his abdomen which became intolerably painful in less than a minute. He quickly moved aside, but within 30 minutes he began to experience acute abdominal pains and vomiting and soon lapsed into shock. Despite prompt hospitalization and subsequent surgery, he died 11 days later from tissue destruction caused by absorption of microwave energy, his doctor reporting that his small intestine appeared to be "cooked" (Brodeur, 1977).

That high levels of microwave absorption can cause serious biological damage is not disputed. Much more controversial is the question of microwave radiation damage from prolonged low levels of exposure. The federal government has set 10 milliwatts/cm² of body area as the maximum permissible level for continuous exposure to microwaves, but a number of researchers claim to have evidence showing that much lower levels of exposure can cause a wide variety of ill effects, including cataracts, cancer, chromosomal abnormalities, birth defects, heart attacks, and a tendency among irradiated men to father only girl babies. Unfortunately there has been little support in this country for research into the long-term health effects of microwave exposure. It is interesting, however, that the Russians and East Europeans who have been studying the biological effects of microwaves for many years have set a level of permissible exposure 1000 times lower than current U.S. regulations permit ∎

References

Basso-Ricci, S. 1985. "Cancer Following Medical Irradiation: The Validity of Gray's Hypothesis." *Panminerva Medica* 27.

Beasley, Conger, Jr. 1994. "The Dirty History of Nuclear Power." *E Magazine*, Jan./Feb.

Brodeur, Paul. 1977. *The Zapping of America*. W. W. Norton.

Browne, Malcolm W. 1992. "Russia Will Continue Operating Its Notorious Types of Reactors." *New York Times*, Nov. 8.

Carter, L. J. 1978. "Uranium Mill Tailings: Congress Addresses a Long-Neglected Problem." *Science* 202, 191.

_____. 1977. "More Burning of Coal Offsets Gains in Air Pollution Control." *Science* 198.

Cooper, George, Jr. 1973. "The Development of Radiation Science," In *Medical Radiation Biology*, edited by Glenn V. Dalrymple, M. E. Gaulden, G. M. Kollmorgen, and H. H. Vogel, Jr. W. B. Saunders.

Cushman, John H. 1993. "U.S. Drops Test Plan at Bomb Waste Site." *New York Times*, Oct. 22.

Dalrymple, Glenn V. 1973. "Microwaves." In *Medical Radiation Biology*. Edited by Glenn V. Dalrymple et al. W. B. Saunders.

DeLeo, Vincent, M.D. 1992. Testimony before the Senate Committee on Governmental Affairs, June 5.

Eisenbud, M. 1973. *Environmental Radioactivity*. Academic Press.

Environmental Defense Fund and Robert H. Boyle. 1979. *Malignant Neglect*. Vintage Books.

Hall, E. J. 1976. *Radiation and Life*. Pergamon Press.

Hawkes, Nigel, Geoffrey Lean, David Leigh, Robin McVie, Peter Pringle, and Andrew Wilson. 1987. *Chernobyl: The End of the Nuclear Dream*. Vintage Books.

Health Implications of Nuclear Power Production. 1977. World Health Organization.

International Atomic Energy Agency (IAEA) and OECD Nuclear Energy Agency. 1983. *Uranium Extraction Technology*.

"Ionizing Radiation Exposure of the Population of the United States." 1987. National Council on Radiation Protection and Measurements, Report No. 93, September 1.

Kahn, Patricia. 1993. "A Grisly Archive of Key Cancer Data." *Science* 259 (Jan. 22).

Kneale, George W., and Alice M. Stewart. 1993. "Reanalysis of Hanford Data: 1944–1986 Deaths." *American Journal of Industrial Medicine* 23 (March).

League of Women Voters Education Fund. 1993. *The Nuclear Waste Primer*. Lyons & Burford.

Macklis, Roger M. 1993. "The Great Radium Scandal." *Scientific American* (Aug.).

Maxfield, W. S., G. E. Hanks, D. J. Pizzarello, and L. H. Blackwell. 1973. "Acute Radiation Syndrome." In *Medical Radiation Biology*, edited by Dalrymple et al. W. B. Saunders.

"Mescaleros Prepare Business Plan for Private MRS Facility." 1994. *Nuclear Waste News* 14, no. 14 (April 7).

"New Study Suggests Recommended Radiation Dose Limit Is Too High." 1992. *Environmental Health Letter*, Feb. 11.

Norwood, Christopher. 1980. *At Highest Risk*. Penguin Books.

Perera, Judith. 1993. "New Radiation Standards Urged for British Workers." *Environmental Health Letter*, June 11.

Schreiber, Michael M. 1986. "Exposure to Sunlight: Effects on the Skin." *Comprehensive Therapy* 12, no. 5.

Simons, Marlise. 1993. "West Is Warned of the High Cost of Fixing Risky Soviet A-Plants." *New York Times*, June 22.

Sontheimer, Richard D., M.D. 1992. "Photosensitivity in Lupus Erythematosus." *Lupus News* 12, no. 2.

Spiers, F. W. 1957. "Radioactivity in Man and His Environment." *Nature of Radioactive Fallout and Its Effects on Man*. U.S. Atomic Energy Commission, U.S. Government Printing Office.

Sternglass, E. J. 1972. *Low Level Radiation*. Ballantine.

"Sunscreens May Not Afford Protection." 1992. *Environmental Health Letter*, June 12.

Upton, Arthur C. 1973. "Radiation Carcinogenesis." *Medical Radiation Biology*, edited by Glenn Dalrymple et al. W. B. Saunders.

Wald, Matthew L. 1993. "Energy Chief Vows Moral Obligation of U.S. to Take Atom Waste." *New York Times*, Dec. 3.

————. 1993. "Nuclear Storage Divides Apaches and Neighbors." *New York Times*, Nov. 11.

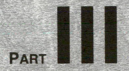

PART **III**

Environmental Degradation
How We Foul Our Own Nest

The fouling of the nest which has been typical of man's activity in the past on a local scale now seems to be extending to the whole system.
—Kenneth Boulding

Air pollution, water pollution, excessive levels of noise, and the accumulation of disease-breeding refuse are not phenomena unique to the latter half of the 20th century. Wherever humans have congregated in appreciable numbers, the burning of fuel, the thoughtless disposal of excreta and material wastes, and the din arising from a multitude of human activities have created conditions which adversely affected the health and well-being of the very people responsible for those conditions. For most of human history, environmental degradation was primarily local in scope, concentrated in the relatively few places where humans established urban centers. The extent of pollution in these cities, however, often far exceeded the levels of filth plaguing our environmentally conscious society of today. Streets and gutters clogged with human body wastes, animal excrement, and garbage were a result of both overcrowding and a transference to the city of more casual rural practices. By the time of the Industrial Revolution in the late 18th and early 19th centuries, belching smokestacks from thousands of factories and the noise of machinery and transport vehicles further degraded the quality of urban life. Indeed, back in the "good old days" health and sanitary conditions due to air and water pollution and to inadequate (or nonexistent) refuse collection and disposal were far worse than anything with which we are familiar in the 1990s. When repeated epidemic outbreaks of waterborne disease killed thousands of citizens or when smog-laden air caused millions to wheeze, cough, and occasionally die, the more enlightened civic leaders began to question society's shortsightedness in fouling its own nest. Many of the most important reforms in civic life which occurred late in the last century involved implementation of public health measures to deal with water pollution, refuse collection, and smoke abatement. However, throughout this period when urban pollution levels were rising, the countryside remained relatively uncontaminated, except for those areas where a local industry—perhaps a metal smelter or pulp mill—created noxious conditions within its own sphere of influence.

The changes which transformed local pollution problems into national ones have occurred largely in the years since the end of the Second World War. Reverse migration from urban centers into sprawling suburbia was made possible by a quantum increase in the number of automobiles ("infernal combustion engines") whose exhaust fumes guaranteed that air pollution would no longer be restricted to areas of smoke-generating heavy industry. The escalating energy demands of a growing, affluent population were accompanied by construction of massive new power plants, most of them coal-burning and many located in regions of the country previously noted for pristinely clean air. Perhaps most significant was the vast outpouring of new, synthetic chemical products, many of them toxic compounds, which do not break down readily and can be transported immense distances by air currents, water, or in the tissues of living organisms to wreak their havoc far from their place of origin. In spite of the warnings of a few farsighted individuals, several decades of experience were required before society as a whole became aware of the insidious nature and now-massive scope of environmental degradation.

During the decade of the 1970s, a national awakening regarding issues of ecology and environmental health produced a flood of federal and state legislation aimed at pollution abatement. The battle has been joined and some successes have already been achieved, but it has become increasingly evident that the problem of environmental pollution is far more complex than originally perceived. Issues not even considered until fairly recently— issues such as acid precipitation, carbon dioxide accumulation, ozone layer depletion, contamination of groundwater with toxic organic chemicals, and the fearsome dilemma of what to do about abandoned chemical waste dumps—present policymakers, scientists, and citizens with thorny technical and political problems. Solutions to older questions pertaining to community waste disposal practices, air pollution abatement measures, or stormwater runoff control are well understood but often fail to be implemented due to fiscal constraints.

The concluding chapters of this book attempt to delineate the nature of the pollution problems confronting society as we approach the 21st century. They also describe the legislative tools with which we are now attempting to combat the contamination of our nation's air and water resources in order to prevent future generations from perpetuating the "fouling of the nest" which so endangers our health and well-being■

The Atmosphere

When I look at thy heavens, the work of thy fingers, the moon and the stars which thou hast established; what is man that thou art mindful of him . . . ?

—Psalms 8:3–4

The airy canopy above Earth which so inspires poets and painters is a physical characteristic of our planet unique in the solar system. Its existence makes possible the rich diversity of life forms found on Earth, making this globe a veritable oasis in space.

Questions regarding the origin of Earth's atmosphere have intrigued scientists for decades. It is generally assumed that the Earth formed almost five billion years ago when particles in a gigantic whirling cloud of dust and gases were pulled together into an aggregate body by enormous gravitational forces. This infant planet had an atmosphere consisting primarily of light gases such as hydrogen and helium, very similar to the present-day atmosphere on the larger planets of Jupiter and Saturn. However, due to Earth's smaller size, gravitational forces were insufficient to retain these elements and they subsequently dissipated into space. This original atmosphere was gradually replaced by a secondary atmosphere produced through the outgassing of volatile materials from the interior of the Earth as the once-molten orb began to cool. Modern phenomena such as volcanic eruptions provide vivid evidence that such outgassing continues right up to the present day.

While there is widespread agreement among scientists that the primitive Earth's atmosphere was significantly different in chemical composition from that of the present, opinions vary as to precisely which compounds were the major constituents of the early atmosphere. For many years it was widely accepted that a mixture of hydrogen, methane, ammonia, and water vapor would have provided the most congenial environment for the origin of life; these must have been the predominant gases in prebiotic times. Recently, however, this assumption has been challenged by observations that gases ejected by volcanoes consist largely of carbon dioxide and water vapor, leading to the conclusion that, unless volcanoes operated very differently in the past than they do today, the main component of Earth's early atmosphere was carbon dioxide, just as it is today on our neighboring planets of Mars and Venus. This concept of a carbon dioxide-rich primitive atmosphere, with mere traces of ammonia and notably devoid of free oxygen, constitutes the prevailing view at present. The origin of our modern oxygen-rich atmosphere is traced to the evolution of green plants, about two billion years ago, whose photosynthetic activities resulted in the uptake of considerable quantities of atmospheric carbon dioxide and the subsequent release of free oxygen—a necessary precursor for the evolution of higher forms of life (Budyko, 1986; Gribbin, 1982).

Although the chemical constituents of the atmosphere have existed in roughly their present proportions for at least several hundred million years, these constituents are in a constant state of flux, reacting with the continents and oceans to form our weather patterns, constantly being removed and recycled (see chapter 1 on "Geochemical Cycles") as a part of great natural processes. The intimate interrelationships between the atmosphere and land, water, and living things make it relevant to refer to such interactions as the **earth-atmosphere system**. This system is essentially a closed one—every material that goes into the air, though it may circulate and change in form, nevertheless remains within the earth-atmosphere system. This fact has disquieting implications for humans who have always viewed the skies as a convenient garbage dump for their volatile wastes—unfortunately the concept of a pollutant or any other substance "vanishing into thin air" is an impossibility.

Composition of the Atmosphere

The modern atmosphere consists of a mixture of gases so perfectly and consistently diffused among each other that pure dry air exhibits as distinct a set of physical properties as is possessed by any single gas. By volume, the composition of dry air can be broken down as follows:

> 78% Nitrogen (N_2)
> 21% Oxygen (O_2)
> 0.9% Argon (Ar)
> 0.03% Carbon Dioxide (CO_2)
> trace amounts—neon, helium, krypton, xenon, hydrogen, methane, and nitrous oxide

Of the four major atmospheric components, only two, oxygen and carbon dioxide, directly enter into biological processes. Oxygen is required by most living organisms for the production of energy, a process known as aerobic respiration; carbon dioxide constitutes the carbon source for photosynthesis—a series of photochemical reactions whereby chlorophyll molecules in green plants absorb sunlight and use its energy to synthesize simple sugars from carbon dioxide and water. Atmospheric nitrogen, on the other hand, can be utilized only by a few species of nitrogen-fixing bacteria and cyanobacteria, while argon is chemically and biologically inert and thus plays no significant role in the biosphere.

Regions of the Atmosphere

Although the composition of its component gases is uniform throughout the atmosphere from sea level to an altitude approximately 50 miles (80 km) above the earth's surface, scientists subdivide this extent into three distinct regions based on temperature zones.

Troposphere.   Extending from sea level to an altitude about 8–9 miles above the earth (slightly less above the poles, more above the equator) is the region known as the troposphere. Virtually all life activities occur within this region and most weather and climatic phenomena occur here.

Figure 11-1 Regions of the Atmosphere

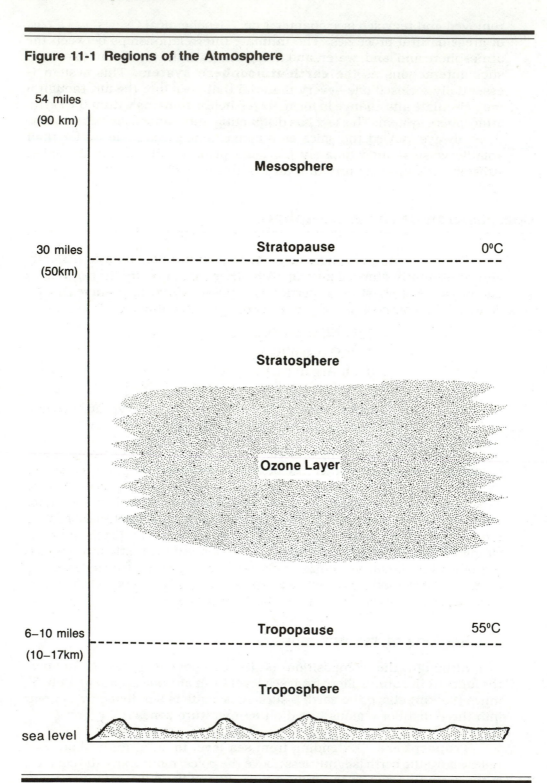

54 miles
(90 km)

Mesosphere

30 miles   Stratopause   0ºC
(50km)

Stratosphere

Ozone Layer

6–10 miles   Tropopause   55ºC
(10–17km)

Troposphere

sea level

In addition to the usual gases, the troposphere also contains varying amounts of water vapor and dust particles. Within the troposphere temperature steadily falls with increasing altitude, a decrease of 5.4 °F per 1000 feet (10 °C/km). The upper limit of the troposphere is known as the **tropopause**.

Stratosphere.   Above the troposphere lies the stratosphere, a region distinguished by a temperature gradient reversal. Here the temperature slowly rises with increasing altitude until it reaches 32 °F (0 °C) at a height of about 30 miles (50 km), the upper boundary of the stratosphere known as the **stratopause**. Unlike the troposphere, the stratosphere contains almost no water vapor or dust. It is the site, however, of the **ozone layer**, a region characterized by higher-than-usual concentrations of the rare gas ozone (O_3), an isotope of oxygen (O_2). The ozone layer extends from about 10–30 miles above the earth's surface, being most concentrated between 11–15 miles. Amounts of ozone vary depending on location and season of the year. Ozone concentrations are lowest above the equator, increasing toward the poles; they also increase markedly between autumn and spring.

Mesosphere.   Above the stratopause is the region known as the mesosphere, where temperature once again begins to fall with increasing altitude. Since the air becomes progressively more diffuse as the altitude above the earth increases, it is difficult to say precisely where the atmosphere ends. In terms of mass, 99% of our atmosphere lies within 18 miles of the earth's surface—an astonishingly thin blanket nurturing beneath it all the life known to exist in the universe (Strahler and Strahler, 1973).

Radiation Balance

In addition to providing the major source of certain chemical elements necessary for life, the atmosphere performs a vital role in controlling the earth's surface environment by regulating both the quality and quantity of solar radiation that enters and leaves the biosphere.

The source of all energy on earth, of course, is the sun, but solar energy can be subdivided into several categories, depending on wavelength of the various forms of radiation involved:

Type of Radiation	% of Total Energy	Wavelength (in micrometers)
Ultraviolet rays	9	0.1–0.4
Visible light rays	41	0.4–0.7
Infrared rays (heat)	50	0.7–3000

These forms of electromagnetic radiation travel outward from the sun at a rate of 186,000 miles (300,000 km) per second, taking slightly over nine minutes to reach the earth. Although none of the sun's energy is lost as it travels through space, once it begins to penetrate earth's atmosphere both a depletion and diversion of solar radiation begin to occur.

Most of the ultraviolet radiation present in sunlight is absorbed by the ozone layer as it passes through the stratosphere, though some of the UV wavelengths longer than 0.3 micrometers (the so-called UV-B region) manage to penetrate to the earth's surface where they can produce sunburn and skin cancers. The ozone layer itself is actually created by ultraviolet light, since UV radiant energy causes ordinary oxygen molecules to break apart, releasing single atoms of oxygen which then react with intact oxygen molecules to form ozone. Since, as was explained in chapter 10, ultraviolet radiation can have serious adverse effects on living organisms, the existence of the ozone layer is of great biological significance (Panofsky, 1978).

Visible light rays and infrared radiation penetrate through the upper stratosphere unaffected by the ozone layer. However, as the atmospheric gas molecules increase in density closer to the earth, these molecules cause a random scattering of the incoming visible light waves (infrared waves are not so affected and for the most part continue to stream directly toward the earth). Entering the troposphere, additional scattering and diffuse reflection of visible light waves occur due to contact with dust particles and clouds (a clear sky appears blue because the shorter blue wavelengths are scattered to a greater extent than are the longer red wavelengths and thus reach our eyes from all parts of the sky). Additional amounts of incoming solar radiation are lost by reflection from the upper surfaces of clouds, oceans, or from the land (particularly when covered with snow or ice). Energy losses also occur when carbon dioxide and water vapor absorb infrared radiation (heat waves) as sunlight enters the lower atmosphere. This heat absorption results in an increase in air temperature. Although the carbon dioxide content of the air is constant everywhere, the amount of water vapor varies considerably and is the main factor accounting for differences in the amount of infrared absorption in various climatic regions (e.g. arid regions experience greater temperature extremes during a 24-hour period than do more humid areas at the same latitude because the low water vapor content of desert air minimizes the absorption of the infrared waves). Altogether, scattering, reflection, and absorption of sunlight can result in the loss of as little as 20% of incoming solar radiation when skies are clear to nearly 100% under conditions of heavy cloud cover. On a global yearly average it is estimated that the earth-atmosphere system absorbs about 68% of the total incoming solar radiation, 32% being lost due to the factors just mentioned.

In order to maintain a global radiation balance, energy absorbed by the earth from incoming sunlight must be equalled by outward radiation of energy from the earth's surface. This so-called "ground radiation" occurs in the form of infrared waves longer than 3 or 4 micrometers (referred to as "long wave radiation"), which are continually being radiated back into the atmosphere, even at night when no solar radiation is being received. Some of the infrared waves leaving the earth (those in the 5–8 and 12–20 micrometer range) are absorbed by water vapor and carbon dioxide in the

Figure 11-2 Reflection and Absorption of Solar Radiation

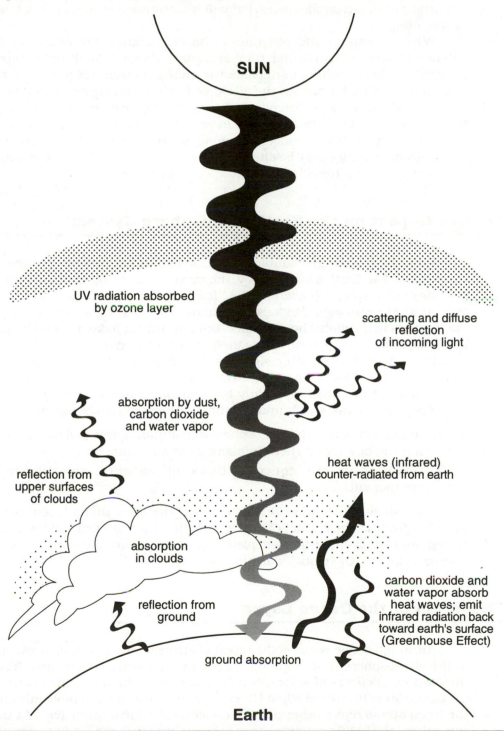

SUN

UV radiation absorbed
by ozone layer

scattering and diffuse
reflection
of incoming light

absorption by dust,
carbon dioxide
and water vapor

heat waves (infrared)
counter-radiated from earth

reflection from
upper surfaces
of clouds

absorption
in clouds

carbon dioxide and
water vapor absorb
heat waves; emit
infrared radiation back
toward earth's surface
(Greenhouse Effect)

reflection from
ground

ground absorption

Earth

atmosphere, a portion of which are reradiated back to the earth's surface, thereby keeping the earth's climate warmer than it would otherwise be. This phenomenon, known as the greenhouse effect, has extremely important climatic implications that will be discussed in more detail later in this chapter.

While incoming and outgoing units of radiation are often not in balance at any one particular time and place (indeed, such imbalances provide the forces behind our constantly changing weather patterns), an equilibrium of such units for the world as a whole during any given year exists, resulting in the maintenance of annual average global temperatures which fluctuate very little from year to year (Strahler and Strahler, 1973). One of the most pressing concerns among atmospheric scientists today is that human activities may be altering the global radiation balance in ways which may have far-reaching climatic consequences.

Human Impact on the Earth-Atmosphere System

Geologic records give ample indication of drastic climatic changes at various times in Earth's long history, the most recent being four successive periods of widespread glaciation (the "Ice Ages"), the last of which ended only 10,000 years ago. Obviously humans had nothing to do with past fluctuations in the global heat balance, but our impact today may no longer be so negligible. Temperature measurements compiled over many decades clearly indicate that possibly significant changes in climate are already underway; the extent to which human activities are provoking or enhancing such trends is presently the topic of heated academic debate.

The major causes of human-induced atmospheric change are:

1. introduction into the atmosphere of pollutant gases and particles not usually found there in significant amounts, and
2. changes in the concentrations of natural atmospheric components.

The following sections illustrate two of the most difficult issues we must confront as the impact of human activities on the earth-atmosphere system inexorably intensifies—depletion of the ozone layer and rising levels of atmospheric CO_2 (global warming).

Depletion of the Ozone Layer

Although ozone is one of the rarest of atmospheric gases, its presence in the stratosphere is of vital importance in protecting life on earth from the damaging effects of solar ultraviolet radiation. As mentioned earlier, the ozone layer is created when UV energy splits the oxygen molecule and the freed atoms rejoin other oxygen molecules to form ozone (O_3). At the same time, the highly reactive ozone is being broken down again to normal

Figure 11-3 Formation of Ozone in the Stratosphere

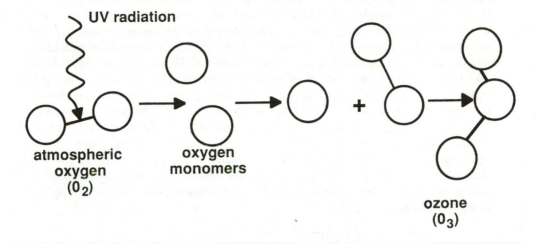

oxygen (O_2); thus the ozone layer is maintained in a state of dynamic equilibrium, daytime increases being balanced by nighttime decreases.

Since the early 1970s, fears have been growing that certain pollutant emissions into the atmosphere are beginning to disrupt this equilibrium, threatening the long-term integrity of the ozone layer. Initially attention focused on the damage potential of nitrous oxides emitted with jet airplane exhausts (particularly from supersonic transports such as the Anglo-French Concorde) and the use of nitrogen fertilizers. It gradually became apparent, however, that a far more serious threat to the ozone layer is posed by the widespread use of a group of synthetic chemicals called chlorofluorocarbons (CFCs), one of the best known of which is the refrigerant Freon. Used in a number of industrial processes, as solvents and refrigerants, in making plastic foams, and as spray can aerosol propellants until their use for this purpose was banned in 1978, CFCs are particularly troublesome because they are such stable chemicals; when released into the environment through vaporization or leakage from enclosed systems or by direct spraying into the air, as in the case of aerosol containers, CFCs do not break down but instead drift upward through the troposphere into the stratosphere where the molecules are finally broken down by solar radiation, releasing atoms of chlorine that react with and destroy ozone. The chlorine-ozone reaction is a catalytic one, meaning that the same chlorine atom can repeat the reaction with tens of thousands of ozone molecules. This, plus the fact that the chlorine atoms will remain in the atmosphere for 100 years or more, explains why CFCs' destructive impact on the ozone layer will be much greater than emission levels might suggest.

Depletion of the ozone layer is worrisome from a human health perspective because of stratospheric ozone's role in absorbing biologically damaging ultraviolet radiation. It is now well-established that for each 1% decrease in atmospheric ozone, penetration of UV radiation to the earth's surface will increase by 2%. Since more than 90% of nonmelanoma skin cancers are associated with exposure to UV radiation in sunlight, any increase in ultraviolet exposure is expected to result in a rising incidence of skin malignancies. A National Academy of Sciences report in 1982 estimated that for every 1% decrease in the concentration of atmospheric ozone, there will be a 2–5% increase in cases of basal cell carcinomas and a 4–10% increase in squamous cell carcinomas. The impact of rising UV exposure on the incidence of more dangerous malignant melanomas is unclear (Maugh, 1982). An EPA analysis concluded that between now and 2075, increasing levels of UV exposure due to ozone layer depletion could result in as many as 200 million additional cases of skin cancer among Americans, as well as damage to the body's immune system. In 1992, estimates released by the United Nations Environment Program forecast a 26% worldwide increase in nonmelanoma skin cancers if stratospheric ozone levels fall by 10%.

The "Hole in the Sky"

During the early 1980s, both government and many scientists downplayed the ozone depletion threat, asserting that earlier forecasts of ozone loss had been exaggerated and assuring skeptics that CFC production had leveled off and thus presented little cause for concern. This sense of complacency was suddenly shattered in 1985 when members of the British Antarctic Survey announced the existence of a large hole in the ozone layer over the South Pole. Although the gap was temporary, opening in early September (Antarctic spring) and closing by mid-October as the southern atmosphere grew warmer, it had been increasing in size each year since the British researchers first noticed it in 1981; by the time of their startling revelation, the "hole" represented a 40% decline in ozone concentrations. Subsequent confirmation by NASA that the ozone hole was real led to intensified research efforts to learn what was going wrong in the polar skies. United States scientists sent to McMurdo Bay in the years following discovery of the "hole in the sky" revealed that the springtime depletion of ozone was steadily getting larger, appearing earlier, and lasting longer. In 1987, ozone losses totalled 50%; by 1991 they reached 70% over an area four times the size of the United States and measurements of UV radiation reaching the ground were the highest ever recorded in Antarctica up to that time. In 1992 and 1993 the "ozone hole" grew even larger; the area of severe depletion extended over 9.4 million square miles above Antarctica in 1992—the most extensive depletion yet observed—while springtime in 1993 brought the lowest recorded ozone levels ever, with total destruction of ozone over Antarctica between altitudes of 8.4 and 11.8 miles. Conflicting theories regarding the cause of this depletion—chemical pollution, cyclical solar flares, and natural atmospheric variation were the main contenders for chief villain—were vigorously debated by researchers. Within a few years the weight of evidence tilted toward the chemical pollution theory with the discovery that concentrations of ozone-destroying chlorine molecules were 400–500 times higher within the ozone hole than outside. The presence of chlorine was widely regarded as a "smoking gun"— evidence establishing a direct cause-and-effect link between CFC emissions and ozone layer destruction.

Since the late 1980s, evidence has continued to mount that the pace of ozone loss is accelerating, not only over the South Pole but also above the more populous regions of the Northern Hemisphere. Since 1979 the U.S. government has been collecting data on atmospheric ozone from ground-based survey stations and the Nimbus-7 satellite. By 1993 NASA scientists were reporting record low concentrations of stratospheric ozone above the middle latitudes of North America and Eurasia—down by as much as 20% from their normal levels. While this dramatic drop in ozone may be blamed, at least in part, on debris hurled into the upper atmosphere by the massive 1991 eruption of the Philippine volcano, Mt. Pinatubo, researchers point out that even prior to this event about 3% of the ozone layer above the United States, Europe, Russia, Japan, and China had been lost. Moreover, when the ozone dipped by 3% over the United States, it dropped by 4% over Australia and New Zealand, and 6% in Scandinavia. More ominously, this loss was occurring in the spring and summer when human exposure to sunlight is at peak levels (Science, 1993; World Resources Institute, 1992). Until recently, a major weakness in the claim that observed declines in stratospheric ozone levels represent a serious environmental health threat was the scarcity of data documenting an actual increase in ultraviolet light penetration anywhere except in Antarctica— where the number of exposed humans is negligible. That data gap was essentially closed in November 1993, with the publication of a five-year study conducted in Toronto by two scientists working with Environment Canada (Canadian equivalent of EPA). From 1989 to 1993, the researchers took ground-level measurements of UV radiation every hour from sunrise to sunset during winter and summer (seasons when UV levels are at their highest and lowest, respectively). They found that at wavelengths around 300 nanometers (the portion of the UV spectrum most strongly absorbed by stratospheric ozone), ultraviolet radiation increased by 35% per year in winter, 6–7% per year in summer. Since measurements of stratospheric ozone concentrations above Toronto had documented a 4% annual decrease in winter and a 2% summer decline each year during the study period, skeptics' arguments that air pollution or cloud cover will counteract the effect of ozone loss have been proven wrong (Kerr and McElroy, 1993).

Policy Response—the Montreal Protocol

After years of controversy among scientists, the chemical industry, and government policymakers as to the extent of ozone depletion, the identity of the main culprits, and the most effective approach for halting—or at least slowing down—the process, consensus is gradually emerging that ozone depletion is real, that it presents a major threat to life on this planet, and that global cooperation is required to combat a phenomenon that threatens us all. A major step forward to meet this challenge was taken in September 1987, when diplomats from 29 nations, meeting in Montreal, Canada, signed an international accord aimed at controlling the chemicals most responsible for ozone layer depletion. As originally ratified, the Montreal Protocol called for the freezing of CFC consumption at 1986 levels by 1990, to be followed by a 50% reduction in the production of these chemicals by the end of the century. The treaty went into effect in January 1989, after ratification by nations representing more than two-thirds of the world's CFC production. A year later, spurred by scientific evidence that ozone was disappearing at a much faster rate than had previously been anticipated, the Montreal Protocol was substantially strengthened by an agreement to halt use of most CFCs entirely by the end of 1999, to eliminate halons (potent ozone-destroying chemicals used in fire extinguishers) as well, and to establish new controls for several other ozone-depleters such as carbon tetrachloride and methyl chloroform. This time representatives of more than 80 countries, meeting in London, signed the agreement, making the treaty a truly international accord. By November 1992, reports of a large, unexpected decline in stratospheric ozone over northern Europe and North America during the winter of 1991–1992 prompted yet another revision in the terms of the Montreal Protocol. This time delegates from more than 100 nations gathered in Copenhagen, Denmark, and agreed to advance the timetable for a CFC phaseout to January 1, 1996, and to effect a 75% reduction in these chemicals (relative to 1986 levels) by January 1, 1994. Halon production was to cease entirely by the 1994 date. While a few exceptions to the ban will be permitted on a case-by-case basis in situations where no practical substitutes for CFCs yet exist (e.g. as propellants in anti-asthma inhalers), production of these chemicals is already declining rapidly (Rowlands, 1993).

Unfortunately, even full implementation of the treaty's requirements will not prevent further losses of ozone. Millions of pounds of CFCs already released are gradually drifting up toward the ozone layer and will remain in the atmosphere for many decades. Nevertheless, the cutbacks in CFC production called for in the Montreal Protocol are already having an impact. In August 1993, atmospheric physicists working for the National Oceanic and Atmospheric Administration (NOAA) announced that the unexpectedly rapid drop in industrial production of CFCs even prior to the implementation deadlines set by the treaty had resulted in a substantial slowdown in the rate at which ozone-depleting chemicals were accumulating in the atmosphere. Consequently, it is expected that if this trend continues, the peak period of ozone layer destruction will occur around the turn of the century, after which declining CFC concentrations will permit a gradual regeneration of stratospheric ozone over a period of 50–100 years. The good news was hailed by Dr. James Elkins, leader of the NOAA team, as "a beautiful case study of science and public policy working well" (Stevens, 1993). As such, the international efforts to protect the ozone layer exemplified by the Montreal Protocol are extremely significant in that they represent the first time in history that the nations of the world have agreed to work together to prevent a disaster of global proportions before it's too

BOX 11-1

Ozone Enemy #1

The early phaseout of chlorofluorocarbons (CFCs) mandated by the Montreal Protocol will be neither easy nor cheap. For many years CFCs were regarded as near-perfect chemicals and were used in hundreds of products that typified our modern way of life. The chilling agent in refrigerators, freezers, and air conditioners; the blowing agents used to inject the bubbles that gave buoyancy and lightness to styrofoam, carpet pads, and foam cushions; the propellants in aerosol cans—all were chlorofluorocarbons. So how has such a universally acclaimed product of modern industry suddenly found itself at the top of environmentalists' "hit list" of pollutants posing a threat to the global ecosystem? Why are CFCs the target of an international effort to phase out their production by 1996?

The answer lies in one of the properties of CFCs that makes them so useful to industry—their extreme chemical stability. When released, CFCs don't break down; instead they persist in the environment for as long as 150 years. They eventually migrate into the upper atmosphere where, upon contact with solar UV radiation, they break apart, releasing highly active chlorine atoms that catalyze the breakdown of ozone. As if this weren't bad enough, they also act as "greenhouse gases," trapping outgoing heat waves and contributing to global warming.

As evidence of large-scale, pollutant-induced atmospheric changes continued to accumulate during the late 1970s and early 1980s, calls for banning CFC production and consumption became more vocal. In 1978 Congress responded by prohibiting the use of CFCs as propellants in aerosol containers; Canada and the Scandinavian countries followed the U.S. example, but elsewhere in the world use of the chemicals continued without restriction. Indeed, the large chemical companies manufacturing the product took the position that CFCs, like citizens in a free country, should be considered innocent until proven guilty, and they continued to insist that conclusive evidence linking CFC use with ozone layer depletion was lacking. They stressed the profound economic consequences of phasing out CFC production. By 1987, when concerns about ozone layer depletion prompted signing of the Montreal Protocol, the value of goods and services related in some way to CFC use totalled about $28 billion annually in the United States alone and approximately 715,000 American workers were employed in jobs directly dependent on the availability of chlorofluorocarbons.

Nevertheless, by 1988 the weight of evidence incriminating CFCs as the prime cause of ozone layer destruction could no longer be denied. E.I. du Pont de Nemours & Co., the corporate giant that invented CFCs and remained the world's largest manufacturer of these chemicals, announced its intention to try to eliminate production of CFC-11 and CFC-12 (the most heavily used CFCs and the ones considered most damaging to ozone) by the year 2000. Two other U.S. producers, Pennwalt Corp. and Allied Signal, Inc., indicated they, too, saw the handwriting on the wall and intended to get out of the CFC business at some unspecified time. (Taking its cue from the giants, McDonald's fast-food chain also declared its intention to phase out the use of CFC-related packaging materials in its U.S. establishments.) Accordingly, a scramble to find ozone-safe alternatives to CFCs has been underway since the late 1980s, an effort that has been given added urgency by recent revisions of the Montreal Protocol which pushed forward the date for halting CFC production from 2000 to 1996—and added methyl chloroform and carbon tetrachloride to the roster of ozone-depleters which were to be eliminated by that date. Production of another group of chemicals used in fire-extinguishers, halons, was halted even earlier, in January 1994. It also appears likely that EPA will extend the ban to include methyl bromide, hydro-bromofluorocarbons (HBFCs), and, by early in the next century, a number of hydrochlorofluorocarbons (HCFCs)—chemicals that until recently were viewed as likely CFC substitutes. EPA insists that most of the soon-to-be-banned chemicals can be replaced without undue hardship. Presenting perhaps the greatest challenge is CFC-12 (Freon), the refrigerant found in automotive air conditioners and household refrigerators. Several substitutes for use in industrial refrigerators ("chillers")—HCFC-22 and HCFC-123—have already been introduced onto the market and car manufacturers in 1993 began replacing Freon with HFC-134a; by the end of 1995 no CFCs will be used in the production of American automobile air conditioners. Nevertheless, the overall decline in

the use of CFCs for refrigerants will be slower than their phaseout in other categories of use. The solvent cleaner, CFC-113, has already largely been replaced by the adoption of CFC-free technologies, such as the use of aqueous or semi-aqueous cleaners. Methyl chloroform, also used as a solvent cleaner and in a variety of other products, will be more difficult to replace, but efforts to find alternatives are moving forward.

CFCs won't suddenly vanish on New Year's Day, 1996. The ban that takes effect on that day specifically pertains to those who produce, export, or import CFCs. Thus the thousands of companies that still use the targeted ozone-depleters for a wide variety of purposes can continue to do so. However, replacement supplies will dwindle rapidly, their cost will soar, and eventually CFCs will be unavailable at any price. Far-sighted users of CFCs have already begun evaluating alternative options, realizing that replacements for CFCs, once they're found, will also be expensive—and may not perform as well. Drastic steps to save the ozone layer are justified—but they won't be painless.

References
"The Ozone Layer." 1987. *Chemecology* 16, no. 8 (Oct.).
"The Unforgiven: Faster Pace for Banning Ozone Depleters." 1993. *The Environmental Manager's Compliance Advisor,* no. 349 (April 19).

late. Initial indications of the success of this approach offer hope for similar cooperation in tackling even more difficult environmental challenges—such as global climate change.

Rising Levels of Atmospheric CO_2— Moving Toward a Warmer World?

The inhabitants of Planet Earth are quietly conducting a gigantic environmental experiment. So vast and so sweeping will be the impacts of this experiment that, were it brought before any responsible council for approval, it would be firmly rejected as having potentially dangerous consequences. Yet, the experiment goes on with no significant interference from any jurisdiction or nation. The experiment in question is the release of carbon dioxide and other so-called greenhouse gases to the atmosphere.

—Wallace S. Broecker, geochemist, Columbia University (Mintzer, 1987)

As mentioned earlier in this chapter, the relative concentrations of the four major atmospheric gases—nitrogen, oxygen, argon, and carbon dioxide—have remained constant for at least several hundred million years. Within recent decades, however, scientists have been expressing concern that a decrease in oxygen levels and an increase in the amount of atmospheric carbon dioxide might be occurring due to the sharp rise in fossil fuel combustion (a process that consumes O_2 and releases CO_2), the worldwide destruction of forest cover, and the poisoning of oceanic photoplankton by pollution of the seas. (Plants are the source of atmospheric oxygen and also capture and store huge amounts of CO_2, thereby removing it from the atmosphere.) Fortunately, recent studies of the oxygen balance have shown that no oxygen depletion has yet occurred and forces operating at the present time are deemed far too insignificant to constitute a real threat so far as oxygen supply is concerned (Broecker, 1970).

The fears regarding carbon dioxide increase, on the other hand, have proven to be well founded and the prospect of a long-term global warming due to CO_2-induced enhancement of the greenhouse effect promises to be one of the biggest environmental issues of the late 20th century. Levels of atmospheric CO_2 have been gradually rising ever since the dawn of the Industrial Revolution as a result of the ever-increasing use of coal, oil, and gas to power the world's factories and vehicles. When fossil fuels are burned, one of the primary combustion products is carbon dioxide; the combustion of one ton of coal, for example, releases three tons of CO_2. In past ages, excess carbon dioxide released through volcanic outgassing was gradually absorbed into the oceans and eventually incorporated into carbonate rock or was photosynthetically "fixed" by green plants. These natural processes, however, are now being overwhelmed by the sheer volume of excess carbon dioxide being released. While fossil fuel combustion has received most of the attention—and blame—in relation to rising CO_2 concentrations, the widescale destruction of natural vegetation, particularly deforestation in the tropics, contributes nearly one-fourth (23%) of all global CO_2 emissions. Both forests and the organic matter in soil humus hold immense quantities of carbon which are oxidized and released as carbon dioxide when vegetation is destroyed. Recently space satellite monitors have revealed that the impact of forest destruction on CO_2 release may be even greater than previously realized. Data collected over the Amazon basin indicate that the thousands of fires deliberately set every year by settlers and ranchers clearing the Brazilian rain forest are generating such enormous quantities of gases and particles that they alone may account for at least one-tenth of the carbon dioxide released by human

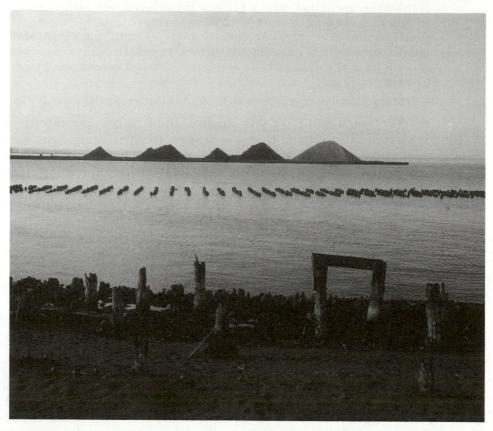

Piles of coal tower above Escanaba Harbor, Michigan. The widespread combustion of coal and other fossil fuels to power the world's factories and cars has significantly increased carbon dioxide emissions. [Thomas A. Schneider]

activities each year (Watson et al, 1990). The equilibrium that has prevailed for millennia has been disrupted, with the result that atmospheric CO_2 levels are now sharply increasing. Measured at 355 ppm in 1990 and currently rising by 1.5 ppm each year (a 0.5% annual rate of increase), the concentration of atmospheric carbon dioxide has grown by 25% since the beginning of the Industrial Revolution, a full 12% of this increase occurring since 1960. Scientists predict that a continuation of existing trends will result in a doubling of CO_2 from preindustrial levels by about 2075—with further increases in succeeding decades. Even if coal use were to be curtailed, EPA officials assert that a doubling of carbon dioxide concentrations would only be postponed for a few decades.

The sense of alarm felt by those monitoring this situation relates not to any adverse effect that CO_2 might exert on human health—the gas is not a toxic pollutant but a natural and necessary constituent of the biosphere—but rather is due to the impact increasing levels of carbon dioxide will have on global climate. As mentioned earlier in this chapter, atmospheric CO_2 plays a vital role in moderating the earth's temperature, a phenomenon known as the **greenhouse effect**. Just as the glass in a greenhouse permits light to enter but prevents the escape of heat, thereby warming the air within, so the absorption of infrared ground radiation by carbon dioxide and its subsequent re-radiation back toward the earth helps to maintain an average global temperature of 59 °F. Without CO_2 in the atmosphere, the earth's average surface temperature would fall to about 0 °F, making the existence of life as we know it impossible. By way of comparison, the planet Venus, with a dense, CO_2-rich atmosphere, has a surface temperature of 890 °F—hot enough to melt lead—while Mars, whose atmosphere consists primarily of CO_2 but is very diffuse and contains but a trace of water vapor, is colder than Antarctica, with an average temperature of -53 °F (Revkin, 1992; Houghton, Jenkins, and Ephraums, 1990). However, as carbon dioxide levels increase, more infrared radiation will be absorbed and over time average global temperatures will correspondingly rise.

Suggesting that perhaps global warming has already begun, results obtained independently in 1988 by researchers at NASA's Goddard Institute for Space Studies and by a team of British scientists showed that global mean temperature is now almost 1 °F (0.5 °C) higher than it was a century ago; the gradual retreat of most mountain glaciers around the world during the 20th century also gives evidence that a sustained climatic warming may be occurring (another piece of anecdotal evidence was advanced recently by scientists in Antarctica who reported that penguins on that icy continent are now observably fatter than they were a few years ago—a fact they postulate could be due to the birds' overindulging on fish which are now more plentiful in polar waters due to CO_2-induced warming of the oceans!). Scientists' efforts to demonstrate a direct cause-and-effect relationship between rising levels of CO_2 and climatic warming have been bolstered by the recent findings of a team of French and Russian researchers working in Antarctica. Drilling deep into a glacier on that frigid continent, they have extracted mile-long cores of ice that provide a frozen record of annual snow layers extending back to 160,000 years ago. Chemical analyses of the air found in tiny bubbles trapped in consecutive layers of ice have yielded information on fluctuations in the content of atmospheric CO_2 over long periods of geologic time. Using the same ice samples, measurements were also made of the ratio between several isotopes of oxygen found in water molecules, thereby giving an indication of climatic warming and cooling (heavier isotopes of oxygen tend to predominate when temperatures are high, while the lighter isotopes are proportionally more abundant during cool periods). A comparison of these two sets of analyses reveals a near-perfect correlation between rising levels of carbon dioxide in the air and rising global temperatures. Although it is not yet possible to discern from ice core evidence whether increasing levels of CO_2 caused climatic warming or whether warming somehow provoked a rise in CO_2 emissions, it is now quite clear that the two changes occur in tandem. After a comprehensive review of the experimental evidence to date, the International Panel on Climate Change (IPCC), a group of several hundred eminent scientists working under the sponsorship of the United Nations, concluded that the reality of global warming can no longer be

Figure 11-4 Greenhouse Index Ranking and Percent Share of Global Emissions, 1991

Rank	Country	Percent	Rank	Country	Percent
1.	United States	19.14	26.	Czechoslovakia	0.70
2.	Former Soviet Union	13.63	27.	Malaysia	0.61
3.	China	9.92	28.	Colombia	0.61
4.	Japan	5.05	29.	Netherlands	0.59
5.	Brazil	4.33	30.	Philippines	0.59
6.	Germany*	3.75	31.	Myanmar	0.55
7.	India	3.68	32.	Argentina	0.54
8.	United Kingdom	2.37	33.	Turkey	0.53
9.	Indonesia	1.89	34.	Romania	0.52
10.	Italy	1.72	35.	Bulgaria	0.51
11.	Iraq	1.71	36.	Bolivia	0.48
12.	France	1.63	37.	Pakistan	0.46
13.	Canada	1.62	38.	Belgium	0.40
14.	Mexico	1.43	39.	Peru	0.39
15.	Poland	1.16	40.	Yugoslavia	0.36
16.	Australia	1.13	41.	Nigeria	0.35
17.	South Africa	1.12	42.	Egypt	0.34
18.	Spain	1.01	43.	Viet Nam	0.32
19.	Venezuela	1.01	44.	Greece	0.31
20.	Republic of Korea	0.98	45.	Ecuador	0.30
21.	Zaire	0.93	46.	Bangladesh	0.29
22.	Thailand	0.88	47.	Hungary	0.26
23.	Korea, Democratic		48.	Austria	0.25
	People's Republic	0.84	49.	Denmark	0.24
24.	Islamic Rep of Iran	0.82	50.	Algeria	0.23
25.	Saudi Arabia	0.78			

*Data for Germany include both the former Federal Republic of Germany and the former German Democratic Republic.

Source: World Resources Institute, *World Resources 1994–1995*.

denied. In a 1990 report the IPCC warned that the projected doubling of atmospheric carbon dioxide will result in an average global temperature increase of 3–8 °F (1.5–4.5 °C) within the next one hundred years—an unprecedentedly short time for a change that would represent conditions warmer than any the earth has experienced during recorded history.

Turning up the Heat: Other Greenhouse Gases

As if humanity doesn't have enough to worry about with the seemingly inexorable rise in carbon dioxide levels, climatologists now warn that increasing atmospheric concentrations of several other gases—

specifically, methane, nitrous oxide, and chlorofluorocarbons (CFCs)—are further enhancing the greenhouse effect by capturing wavelengths of infrared radiation not readily absorbed by CO_2. Although present in concentrations far below that of carbon dioxide, these trace gases are much more efficient than CO_2 in absorbing outgoing heat waves. A molecule of methane, for example, can trap 20–30 times more infrared radiation than does a molecule of CO_2. Equally worrisome is the fact that emissions of trace gases are increasing at a substantially faster rate than CO_2 and originate from sources that may be even more difficult to control. A brief look at the situation regarding the other "greenhouse gases" reveals the following picture:

Methane (CH_4).   Although current atmospheric concentrations of this gas are less than 2 ppm, as opposed to CO_2 levels of 355 ppm, methane is far more potent as a greenhouse gas and is increasing at a 1% annual rate. Curtailing methane emissions will not be easy, since over half originate from rice cultivation (due to the respiration of anaerobic bacteria in waterlogged paddy fields) and from microbial activity in the intestines of cattle and termites (it is estimated that a cow belches methane approximately twice a minute!). Other significant sources more amenable to controls include emissions from gas and coal production, flares on oil rigs, landfills, and tropical deforestation (when vegetation is burned during clearing activities).

Nitrous Oxide (N_2O).   Up by 8% since the beginning of the 20th century and increasing at a rate of 0.25% annually, the so-called "laughing gas" sometimes used as a painkiller by dentists is a more efficient greenhouse gas than CO_2 but because its total atmospheric concentrations are in the parts per billion range, its overall contribution to global warming is still fairly limited. Nitrous oxide is a natural by-product of the metabolism of certain soil microbes, but the generation of this gas has been boosted significantly by the increased worldwide use of nitrogen fertilizers. Combustion of fossil fuels, increased land cultivation, burning of biomass, and the decomposition of agricultural wastes and sewage are presumed to be additional sources of N_2O.

Chlorofluorocarbons (CFCs).   The prime villains in ozone layer destruction, CFCs are also potent greenhouse gases, each molecule of which has a direct warming effect 12,000–20,000 times greater than that of a CO_2 molecule. While atmospheric concentrations of CFCs are considerably lower than those of other greenhouse gases, they are rising much more rapidly—approximately 5% per year.

It should be noted that water vapor is another important greenhouse gas, but because human activities have negligible impact on its atmospheric concentrations and because the amount of water in the air varies widely from place to place and day to day, levels of this atmospheric constituent are not taken into consideration when discussing global warming scenarios.

While the lion's share of public attention regarding climate change has thus far focused on carbon dioxide emissions, it is now agreed that the cumulative effect of the other greenhouse gases will be nearly equivalent to that of CO_2. An estimate of the relative contribution of the various greenhouse gases to global warming can be seen in Figure 11-5.

Figure 11-5 Relative Contribution of Various Greenhouse Gases to Global Warming

CO_2—55%

CFC-11 & CFC-12—17%

other CFCs— 7%

CH_4—15%

N_2O— 6%

Source: Data from 1990 IPCC report.

Thanks to the additional heat-capturing potential of methane, nitrous oxides, and CFCs, the timetable for the onset of noticeable climate change has markedly accelerated. Whereas atmospheric scientists project a doubling of CO_2 concentrations over pre-industrial levels to be reached somewhere around 2075, the anticipated 3–8°F temperature increase associated with such a doubling may occur as early as 2030 due to the added impact of these other greenhouse gases (World Resource Institute, 1990; Stern, Young, and Druckman, 1992; Revkin, 1992).

Impacts of Global Warming

To many people, the prospect of temperatures a few degrees higher than they are at present seems little cause for dismay—particularly when they happen to be contemplating such a scenario during a January blizzard. The major impact of a global warming trend, however, would not be felt in terms of human physical discomfort but rather in a possibly drastic alteration of worldwide rainfall and temperature patterns.

While climatologists are unable to make accurate detailed predictions regarding CO_2-induced climatic changes in specific areas of the globe, their computer modeling studies support widespread agreement that while temperatures everywhere are rising to some extent, the global warming trend is not evenly distributed. The high latitude regions of the Northern Hemisphere are expected to experience the greatest temperature increases (perhaps twice as high as the world average), particularly during the winter months. In mid-latitude regions also (including the continental United States) greenhouse warming will exceed the global average, with winter temperatures increasing more than summer temperatures. Regional

BOX 11-2

Freeze or Fry? Greenhouse Uncertainties

Convincing a skeptical public that drastic—and expensive—steps should be taken immediately to ward off a hypothetical future threat is a difficult business, particularly when the experts themselves disagree on the nature, direction, and extent of potential climate change. Those who have followed the debate over the past two decades may be understandably bewildered as some scientists warn of a future hothouse world while others predict a return to Ice Age conditions. In recent years the preponderance of scientific opinion has shifted in support of the general theory of human-induced global warming, as opposed to cooling, but numerous remaining uncertainties make it impossible as yet to say exactly when, where, and how much temperatures are likely to rise in the years ahead.

The greenhouse warming scenarios described in this chapter have been derived from computer-generated global climate models which, while valuable for depicting the broad outlines of what is likely to happen, are at present incapable of detailed predictions on the timing, extent, and exact mechanism of warming—and of its consequences in any given locality. Such models are not yet sophisticated enough to account adequately for the highly complex interactions which characterize the earth-atmosphere system and routinely influence climate. To understand the nature of the current debate over global warming—that is, those points on which there is still considerable controversy in spite of general agreement on the main thesis—it is helpful to examine the areas of uncertainty that are currently the subjects of intense scientific investigation.

1. **Role of the Oceans.** Covering approximately three-fourths of the surface of the planet, the world's oceans constitute perhaps the single greatest confounding influence for computer models because so little is currently known about ocean dynamics or the ways in which the oceans and atmosphere interact. By absorbing huge amounts of excess heat to warm the enormous volume of water they contain, oceans may even now be slowing the rate of atmospheric warming; this thermal inertia of sea water may explain why the 0.5°C rise in average world temperature observed during the 20th century is only about half of that predicted by climate models, based on the level of greenhouse gas emissions. Existing climate models ignore the complexities of the mixing of ocean waters and the manner in which deep currents transport heat from one part of the globe to another, yet such factors play an extremely important role in determining world climate. Similarly, the part played by oceans in absorbing excess carbon dioxide is imperfectly understood. About half the CO_2 released to the atmosphere by fossil fuel combustion or deforestation is taken up by various components in the world's carbon cycle (see chapter 1), much of it by the oceans. Gas exchange at the sea surface results in enormous amounts of carbon dioxide cycling in and out of the oceans each year. While it is believed that oceans currently absorb much more CO_2 than they release, some researchers worry that even minor changes in the temperature, chemistry, or circulation of ocean currents could provoke unpredictable changes in the way oceans absorb or release carbon dioxide. Obviously, much more understanding of ocean

dynamics is necessary in order to improve the accuracy of global warming predictions.

2. **Influence of Clouds.** The clouds that drift above 60% of the earth's surface at any given time constitute another important variable in climate change predictions. Greenhouse warming might generate more cloud cover than currently exists if the anticipated rise in ocean temperatures results in higher evaporation rates. Although clouds both reflect and absorb heat, at present they exert a net cooling effect which some observers conclude will more than offset the amount of warming that a doubling of greenhouse gas concentrations would produce. According to this line of thinking, a self-regulating mechanism is thus built into the system, precluding realization of the more extreme greenhouse scenarios. However, other researchers warn that matters are not so simple and current realities (i.e. the net cooling effect of cloud cover) may not apply to future conditions. The degree to which clouds reflect or retain heat depends on their altitude and water content. High altitude cirrus clouds, for example, tend to trap heat while lower to mid-level cumulus and stratus clouds reflect it. Thus if global warming causes an increase in the proportion of cirrus clouds, the greenhouse effect would be further intensified; if cumulus and stratus clouds predominate, they may counteract temperature increases. Unfortunately, while observers agree that cloud dynamics will have a major impact on future climate, computer models are not yet able to predict the direction of such change.

3. **Biofeedback Mechanisms.** As atmospheric CO_2 content and temperatures rise, the metabolic processes of living organisms may respond in ways that could either intensify or diminish the amount of warming that actually occurs. Just as the oceans serve as an important "sink" for CO_2, ecosystems on land play an integral role in the biogeochemical cycling of carbon. Each year plants take up about 100 billion metric tons of carbon through their photosynthetic activities and give off approximately the same amount as they respire or decay. Since the total amount of carbon involved represents close to one-third of all the carbon in the atmosphere, any change in the equilibrium between photosynthesis and respiration could have a rapid and dramatic impact on the overall level of atmospheric CO_2. Some observers have suggested that the photosynthetic rate of green plants will be accelerated as the carbon dioxide content of the atmosphere rises (a phenomenon referred to as "CO_2 fertilization"), thereby effecting a net increase in the amount of carbon bound up in plant tissues and acting as a negative feedback mechanism preventing further CO_2 buildup in the atmosphere. Proponents of this theory point to laboratory experiments which show that some, though not all, plant species exhibit a 30% increase in growth rate when CO_2 content of the surrounding air is doubled. However, outside the laboratory real-world conditions cast doubt on this rosy scenario. Insufficient amounts of mineral nutrients or water are more often the main limitation to plant growth than is the level of CO_2—and rising temperatures are likely to have an adverse impact on availability of the latter in many parts of the world. Additionally, as temperatures rise, the rate of respiration also increases. Many researchers believe that temperature-induced increases in the rate of CO_2-releasing respiration will equal the CO_2-consuming rise in photosynthetic rates, thus resulting in no net change in the biosphere's carbon-storage capacity. Some observers take this scenario a step further, arguing that just as respiration rates will increase as the climate becomes warmer, decay

rates also will accelerate. Peat deposits in the tundra regions of the far north constitute an enormous reservoir of carbon, the decay of which has thus far been retarded by the cold temperatures that characterize this biome. However, as climate warms, microbial action in the wet, oxygen-deficient tundra soils could release huge amounts of methane gas—a much more potent greenhouse gas than CO_2—and thus serve as a powerful positive feedback mechanism, further boosting the extent of global warming.

While much remains to be learned about the variables mentioned above—as well as about the possible role of sunspot activity, volcanic eruptions, reflectivity of the planet, and the influence of soil chemistry on the carbon cycle—current climate models are reliable and consistent enough to dispel notions that the threat of climate change needn't be taken seriously. Detailed predictions of where, when, and how much may be years in coming, but existing information provides a sound basis to begin formulating long-range policies to confront the daunting challenges that changing climate will pose.

References

Revkin, Andrew. 1992. *Global Warming.* Abbeville Press.

World Resources Institute. 1990. *World Resources 1990–91.* Oxford University Press.

changes in rainfall patterns are even more difficult to predict, but computer models suggest that our grandchildren's generation may witness heavier precipitation in the already-wet equatorial regions, more winter precipitation in the polar regions, much drier summers in the midwestern United States, and drier winters in California. Along with such widespread regional climatic alteration, more localized weather changes such as the frequency and intensity of storms and hurricanes will also be pronounced. More frequent "January thaws" during winter and more unusually hot days during the summer may become commonplace. Whereas Washington, D.C. now averages only one day each year when the mercury tops 100°F, a doubling of CO_2 levels could result in two sweltering weeks of triple-digit temperatures in our nation's capital; residents of Dallas, who currently suffer through 100°F heat approximately 19 days each year, can look forward to 78 such days in the warmer world projected by climatologists.

Scientists and policymakers alike are now striving to determine what changes are likely to occur as temperatures climb and to formulate strategies to ameliorate detrimental effects as much as possible. The more significant potential impacts of global warming are discussed in the following sections.

Diminishing Crop Yields

The hotter, drier weather forecast for some of the world's most productive agricultural lands is bad news at a time when global food demand is steadily increasing. For farmers, major climatic change could bring benefits to some regions, severe hardship to others. Climate models predict that greenhouse warming would result in shifting rainfall patterns that could bring substantially heavier monsoon rains to India but 30–60% less summer precipitation to the American Midwest. Higher temperatures could force a northward shift of agricultural zones, perhaps boosting crop yields in Canada and Russia while turning the American "Breadbasket" into a dustbowl. Although some observers have suggested that rising concentrations of CO_2 might actually enhance food production by increasing photosynthetic rates, the combined impact of excessive heat and drought could counteract this effect. Similarly, soils in the northern latitudes that may benefit from increasing temperatures are generally too acidic and not fertile enough to support intensive grain production.

Global warming could have other less obvious impacts on agricultural productivity. Livestock production will suffer due to heat-induced declines in animal fertility; pastures and rangelands can be expected to sustain heat damage. As temperatures rise, the range of plant pathogens and crop-destroying insects expand considerably; pests currently confined to southern latitudes may spread northward, causing serious agricultural losses. A shift in the balance between pest and predator species, prompted by changing environmental conditions, could also have adverse repercussions for farming by favoring the survival of more resilient pest species over that of their natural enemies. These increased pest infestations may prompt farmers to increase applications of chemical pesticides, raising the probability of more surface and groundwater pollution problems. Crop losses are likely to be further compounded by increasing levels of tropospheric ozone, a pollutant gas that forms most readily on hot, sunny days. Conflicts over access to irrigation water is bound to increase, pitting farmers against city dwellers within nations and heightening international tensions where disputed water supplies cross national borders.

The extent to which greenhouse warming will affect agricultural production will depend in large measure on the rate at which these climatic changes occur. Most of the world's major food crops are already adapted to a wide range of environmental conditions and if climatic change is gradual, agricultural scientists will have time to develop new, even more tolerant varieties. However, if changes occur rapidly, the prospect for world harvests is far less comforting. Since world agriculture is now so highly adapted to existing conditions, any change at all is bound to be disruptive, at least in the short term. At a time when world food reserves are marginal and world food demand is rising, any threat to sustained high crop yields is a cause for serious concern.

Loss of Biodiversity

Climate change will impose even greater stresses on natural ecosystems than on domesticated plants and animals, since many nonagricultural species have gradually become adapted to life in a specific habitat and have a rather narrow range of tolerance to changing environmental conditions. Plants and animals, particularly those living in temperate regions, will be forced to move hundreds of miles toward the poles (or thousands of feet up mountainsides) in order to maintain the temperature conditions to which they have become adapted. For many species such migration will be virtually impossible. Plants, for example, can shift location only as far as their seeds are dispersed. A gradual poleward migration might be conceivable if the rate of climate change is very slow, but if warming is so rapid that the present habitat becomes unsuitable before a new area can be colonized, then the species will die out.

One might assume that animals, capable of moving under their own power, would find migration to more congenial climes relatively easy. In today's world, however, barriers to migration in the form of cities, highways, dams, and so on make large-scale movements of many species highly problematic (visualize the challenges faced by a group of alligators heading north out of Okefenokee Swamp as they attempt to traverse Atlanta!). While some animal species migrate easily, others are genetically programmed to be highly territorial and wouldn't even try to move as their environment became uninhabitable; others might be capable of migrating, but if the plant species on which they feed don't move also, they would perish of starvation. Biodiversity, already suffering severely from pressures imposed by overhunting, pollution, and habitat destruction, may find greenhouse warming the most devastating blow of all.

Rising Sea Levels

The most dramatic consequence of global warming will be a worldwide rise in sea level due to both the thermal expansion of water as temperatures in the ocean rise and to the melting of the Greenland and Antarctic ice sheets. Although this development could be a boon to navigation in the Arctic (the fabled "Northwest Passage" might become a practical alternative to the Panama Canal!), its impact on densely populated coastal regions worldwide will be devastating. A sea level rise of just six feet (and most estimates predict significantly greater increases than this) would totally obliterate many low-lying coral islands. Entire populations in the Marshall Islands, Maldives, and parts of the Caribbean face the prospect of their homelands disappearing beneath the waves within the foreseeable future. Along the edges of continents, towns and cities built on barrier islands, river deltas, or low-lying shorelines can anticipate a similar scenario unless they soon embark on multi-billion dollar coastal defense construction projects. In many desperately poor, densely populated regions of the world, such expenditures are obviously impossible. It is anticipated that Egypt may lose 15% of its arable land to encroaching seas by the mid-21st century; in Bangladesh even a three-foot rise in sea level would inundate one-sixth of the country's land area. When one pauses to consider the number of major world cities now located at or near sea level, the impact of such a rise on human settlement patterns becomes clear. Although sea level will advance gradually (no one foresees the likelihood of Boston or Galveston or Miami being submerged overnight!), even a slight increase can have significant consequences. Some experts feel that a six-inch rise during the present century has been responsible for much of the coastal erosion that has occurred. As water levels rise, the coastal wetlands so important to commercial fisheries and to many bird populations will be inundated and cease to exist. Wildlife biologist Norman Myers laments that "all in all, the demise of coastal wetlands could prove to be the greatest wildlife-related impact of the Greenhouse Effect in the U.S."

Human Illness

Although global warming is primarily an environmental problem rather than a human health issue, the increasing frequency of heat waves will have an impact on morbidity and mortality rates. Extreme heat will result in some excess deaths, mainly due to heart attacks and strokes. Certain vectorborne diseases currently confined to the tropics may spread into regions where they are currently unknown, and the elevated levels of tropospheric ozone common when temperatures are high can be expected to aggravate human respiratory ailments (Lyman et al., 1990).

Rate of Global Warming

As mentioned earlier, the *rate* at which global temperatures rise will be extremely important in determining how serious the impacts of climate change will be. Humanity may be able to adjust reasonably well to a very gradual warming trend, whereas a more rapid change could be catastrophic. Which of these two scenarios is more likely? Several years ago Columbia University geochemist Wallace Broecker, in testimony submitted to a congressional hearing, remarked that:

> Earth's climate does not respond in a smooth and gradual way; rather it responds in sharp jumps. If this reading of the natural record is correct, then we must consider the possibility that the major responses of the system to our greenhouse provocation will come in jumps whose timing and magnitude are unpredictable. Coping with this type of change is clearly a far more serious matter than coping with a gradual warming.

In this context, recent reports from scientists working in Greenland provide considerable cause for alarm. Analysis of oxygen in layers of ice from cores drilled 10,000 feet deep through the island's massive ice cap has provided a record of temperature change extending back 250,000 years. To the surprise of project members, the evidence revealed that climate change in the past occurred much more rapidly and more frequently than had previously been realized. During at least one inter-glacial period, average global temperature changed by 18°F in just a few decades. Indeed, an examination of the ice core record suggests that the relatively stable climate of the past 8000–10,000 years (the period during which human civilizations have developed) is a climatologic anomaly—an exception to the rule of frequent and sudden change throughout much of geologic time. These important new findings prompted Dr. J. W. C. White, a researcher at the University of Colorado's Institute of Arctic and Alpine Research, to warn that "adaptation—the peaceful shifting of food-growing areas, coastal populations, and so on—seemed possible, if difficult, when abrupt change meant a few degrees in a century. It now seems a much more formidable task, requiring global cooperation with swift recognition and response" (Sullivan, 1993).

The Greenhouse Policy Debate

Since the early 1970s, climatologists have been raising increasingly strident warnings about the impending greenhouse warming, urging policymakers to take action to forestall this so-called "Doomsday Issue." While the general public until recently tended either to ignore such predictions or to regard them as plot material for a science fiction novel, there has been a steadily growing chorus of experts who claim that global climate change has already begun. Testifying before a Senate subcommittee during the torrid summer of 1988, James Hansen of the NASA Goddard Institute for Space Studies told the assembled lawmakers that "the greenhouse effect has been detected and is changing our climate now." Hansen cited the fact that the four hottest years then on record had all occurred in the 1980s (since then, the world has experienced several more years of record-breaking heat, with 1990 enjoying the distinction of being the warmest yet documented). Such statements add a sense of urgency to demands that governments shake off their inertia and launch efforts to reduce the continued emission of greenhouse gases. As Howard Ferguson, a meteorologist with the Canadian Atmospheric Environmental Service, remarked: "All the greenhouse scenarios are consistent. These numbers are real. We have to start behaving as if this is going to happen. Those who advocate a program consisting only of additional research are missing the boat."

Calling for action is easier than implementing such changes, however. At the Earth Summit in Rio de Janeiro in 1992 (see Part I: Introduction), signing of the Convention on Climate Change was the first substantive action taken by delegates. This document, signed by representatives from a dozen countries, commits the signatories to stabilize concentrations of greenhouse gases at 1990 levels; at the insistence of the Bush Administration, no timetable for achieving the agreed-upon objective was established, much to the dismay of several European nations (Austria, Switzerland, and the Netherlands) who wanted a legally binding stabilization deadline of 2000 for carbon dioxide emissions and who threatened to take stronger action on their own. Ironically, more than a year after the Rio pact was approved, the United States had done more to comply with the terms of the agreement than had its European critics. In October 1992, the U.S. Senate ratified the treaty and the following April President Clinton pledged the United States would stabilize greenhouse gas emissions at 1990 levels. By contrast, as of mid-1994, the European Community had neither ratified the treaty nor taken any group actions to meet its objectives. There are also serious concerns regarding rising levels of greenhouse gas emissions in Third World nations, as efforts to bolster national development gain momentum. Already the People's Republic of China is the world's third largest producer of CO_2, with a rate of increase faster than anywhere else in the world. As China strives to promote rapid industrialization and electrification for its still-growing population, the need to exploit its vast coal reserves to fuel development goals will doubtless take precedence over international commitments to cap greenhouse gas emissions. And if the populations of demographic giants such as China and India achieve levels of affluence even remotely resembling those of more industrialized countries, the impact of emissions from millions of additional cars, refrigerators, and so on would be far higher than those currently generated in the West.

Unfortunately, even if all signatory nations were to move immediately and wholeheartedly to fulfill treaty commitments, capping emissions at or near their present levels will not be sufficient to forestall global warming. This is because current rates of CO_2 emissions, stable or not, are so much higher than those of the pre-industrial period that natural processes of absorption or destruction—which formerly maintained a rough equilibrium—cannot keep pace and the atmospheric reservoir of CO_2 continues to increase. Only if emissions were slashed by more than 60% of their 1990 levels (a drastic step no government is contemplating at present) would there be a realistic prospect of halting a continued rise in the atmospheric concentration of carbon dioxide—and a further increase in average global temperature (EPA, 1990; Houghton, Jenkins, and Ephraums, 1990).

Policy Options

A number of approaches for reducing greenhouse gas emissions have been proposed and need to be pursued simultaneously if the world is to have any hope of achieving climate stability. Several of the most important initiatives are outlined in the following sections.

Improving Energy Efficiency. The United States is only half as energy efficient as western Europe (though considerably more efficient than China, India, or the nations of eastern Europe). Policy actions such as mandated efficiency standards for automobiles, electrical appliances, and lighting or tax credits for manufacturers who invest in new, more efficient plants are examples of ways government could boost energy conservation by encouraging innovations that produce more work out of energy. In this context, President Clinton's announcement in the fall of 1993 of a joint undertaking with the auto industry to develop a car capable of achieving 80 miles per gallon fuel efficiency is a promising development. Even if the fuel efficiency of the average American car were raised to just 45 mpg, per vehicle CO_2 emissions would drop by 40%.

Replacing Fossil Fuels with "Soft Energy Path" Technologies. Switching to solar, wind, or wave power to heat homes and generate electricity could provide an infinitely renewable source of energy with zero emissions of carbon dioxide. But greatly increased funding for research and

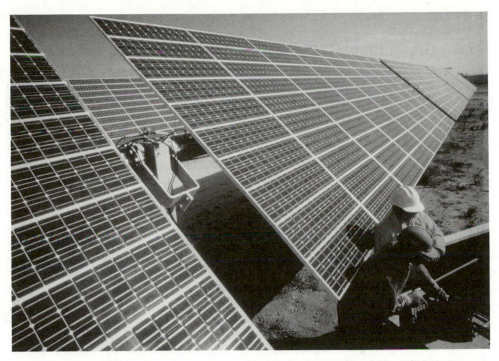

Solar energy panels are one of several alternative energy sources that produce no carbon dioxide emissions. [Courtesy of Siemens Solar Industries]

development is urgently needed to facilitate rapid development of these promising energy alternatives. Although nuclear power generation also avoids the CO_2 emissions problem, scientists do not generally regard the rapid expansion of nuclear capacity as a viable response to thwart global warming. According to a 1990 Greenpeace report, replacing fossil fuel-burning power plants with nuclear facilities would require building one new plant somewhere in the world every 2½ days from now until the year 2025 at a cost of $144 billion annually, nearly half of which would need to be spent by Third World nations. Aside from the fact that the nuclear power industry still confronts some serious unresolved problems, the economic obstacles to a massive program to build nuclear power plants appear insurmountable at present.

Reversing Forest Loss.   Since forests act as carbon "sinks," removing CO_2 from the air during photosynthesis, the worldwide destruction of forests has had a significant contributory impact on rising levels of atmospheric CO_2. Reversing the ongoing loss of tree cover through massive reforestation efforts has been a widely discussed option, though skeptics claim that it would be necessary to replant an area larger than the continent of Australia simply to offset the CO_2 emitted over the next four to five decades, assuming that annual emission rates during those years remain at current levels. Attempting to prove the naysayers wrong, a Connecticut-based utility, Applied Energy Services, recently launched

BOX 11-3
Green Lights—Combating Global Warming

Improving the efficiency of energy use is arguably the single most important action societies must undertake to reduce carbon emissions. The potential is enormous: experts estimate that energy needs could be reduced by amounts ranging from 30–90% by making buildings, appliances, automobiles, motors, etc., more energy-efficient. One small but promising step in this direction was taken a few years ago when the U.S. Environmental Protection Agency launched its **Green Lights** program to transform electrical lighting systems in American industries and institutions. A voluntary program of cooperation between government, utilities, lighting manufacturers, and corporate consumers of electricity, Green Lights attempts to reduce U.S. electric consumption—and the pollution associated with fossil fuel power production—by encouraging the replacement of standard incandescent and fluorescent lighting with new, energy-saving compact fluorescent lamp (CFL) systems.

Of all the electricity generated in the United States each year, 20–25% is consumed by lighting, and among lighting users, office buildings, warehouses, and manufacturing facilities account for the lion's share—between 80–90%. Thus it was logical for EPA to target these large industrial consumers in an effort to make a substantial dent in the high level of carbon dioxide emissions.

Green Lights has enjoyed considerable success in recruiting corporate "Partners" who pledge to upgrade lighting efficiency and quality over a five-year period. In return, EPA promises to facilitate the process by providing information and computer software for evaluation and selection of the most appropriate lighting. Financial assistance for the changeover is also provided through a utility and financing data base. Program-related information (contact lists, pollution prevention statistics, available computer programs, etc.) is available through a Green Lights electronic bulletin board and Green Lights public service announcements tout the successes of participant companies while promoting program objectives. EPA has also enlisted "Allies"—primarily utility companies, lighting manufacturers, and lighting management companies—to assist Green Lights Partners with technical and financial matters. Utilities cooperate by informing corporate customers about the benefits of energy-efficient lighting and by documenting achieved savings due to lighting improvements within their service area. Some utilities offer rebates or financial incentives to companies that agree to retrofit existing systems, figuring that reductions in power demand will help the utility improve generating systems and postpone the need to build expensive new power plants. Lighting manufacturers share their expertise with Green Lights by conducting customer workshops on the various lighting options available and providing warranties on the new technologies being marketed. Lighting management firms assist Green Lights by providing lighting audits, recommending products, and helping EPA to develop training and certification guidelines. Green Lights' success has also been enhanced by numerous "Endorsers"—organizations that promote the program's goals to their members via informational materials or presentations.

Although still relatively young, the Green Lights program has expanded rapidly since its inception in 1991. Less than three years after the program was launched Green Lights could claim over 1100 participants (555 Partners, 450 Allies, and 117 Endorsers) and prospects for future growth appear bright. For the Partners who have pledged their cooperation, participation in Green Lights signals not only corporate environmental responsibility but also good business sense, since pollution prevention translates into profitability. Those companies that have installed energy-efficient lighting save, on average, 52% on electrical bills for lighting, spend less on lighting maintenance (compact fluorescent lamp bulbs last approximately 10 times longer than regular bulbs), and enjoy better lighting quality in the bargain. Thus even though the initial cost of each CFL bulb at present is significantly higher than that of a conventional bulb, over its lifetime the CFL version is actually cheaper. According to EPA, participating companies average a 25% rate of return on their investment in energy-efficient lighting.

While bottom-line considerations may be the prime inducement for Partners to sign on with Green Lights, a reduction in pollutant emissions is EPA's ultimate program goal. The Agency estimates that if electricity consumers would install energy-efficient lighting everywhere such a change is profitable, U.S. electrical demand would drop by more than 10%. This decline in power use, in turn, would reduce CO_2 emissions by 202 million metric tons annually—4% of all U.S. carbon emissions—and would constitute an important first step toward forestalling a greenhouse future.

References

Environmental Protection Agency.
Melody, Mary. 1993. "Green Lights Program Casts New Light on Industry." *Hazmat World* 6, no. 3 (March).

For information on the Green Lights program or workshops, call the Green Lights Hotline at (202)775-6650.

a "carbon offset" project in Guatemala where, with the help of the Guatemalan forestry department, Peace Corps volunteers, CARE, and the U.S. Agency for International Development, the company donated $2 million for the planting of 52 million trees. Project sponsors are hopeful that the amount of carbon dioxide removed from the atmosphere by this enormous woodlot will exceed that emitted by a new fossil fuel plant the company is building in Connecticut.

Reducing CFC Emissions and Other Greenhouse Gases. Full implementation of the terms of the Montreal Protocol should result in an eventual decline in atmospheric CFC concentrations, though the longevity of these chemicals guarantees that they will continue to exert an influence for nearly a century after emissions cease. However, not all scientists agree that the phaseout of CFCs currently underway will slow global warming. Evidence has been mounting that loss of stratospheric ozone exerts a cooling effect on lower levels of the atmosphere great enough to offset the warming caused by the heat-absorptive properties of CFCs (this may explain why observed temperature increases thus far haven't been as large as those predicted by climate models). If this cooling effect of ozone loss really is counteracting global warming as theorized, then ending the use of CFCs won't have any impact on reversing the greenhouse problem. Strategies for reducing emissions of methane and nitrous oxide, two other potent heat-trapping gases, are less well-defined. Developing rice varieties that don't require flooding could help to eliminate the methane-generating anaerobic microbes that currently make rice cultivation the single largest source of this greenhouse gas. Certain additives to livestock fodder could reduce belching of methane by modifying fermentation in the rumen of cattle. Capping manure piles to capture methane (which can then be converted to fuel in biogas plants) and repairing leaks in natural gas pipelines could further reduce emissions of methane to the atmosphere. Lowering nitrous oxide emissions would require cutting back on the use of nitrogen fertilizers.

Taxing the Use of Fossil Fuels.   In his best-selling book, *Earth in the Balance*, Vice-President Gore advocated imposition of a so-called "carbon tax," in which production of gasoline, heating oil, coal, natural gas, and electricity generated from fossil fuels would be taxed incrementally according to their carbon content. Such a tax scheme recognizes that not all fossil fuels pollute equally: coal burning emits twice as much CO_2 as does natural gas, 1.5 times more than oil. A differential tax would provide financial motivation for energy purchasers to choose less-polluting fuels and would incorporate the environmental costs of energy use into energy prices.

Obstacles to Success

Action to implement these long-term strategies must begin immediately on a global scale if the changes already underway are to be minimized. The obstacles to success are great, since the basic problem stems from the energy use decisions of billions of individuals in every nation of the world. Some observers conclude that it is already too late; the degree of worldwide cooperation and coordination necessary to achieve any meaningful reduction in CO_2 releases would, in their view, be impossible to attain in a world "hooked" on fossil fuels. Instead of a crash fuel-switching effort, such voices call for accelerating research on CO_2 and its effects and for a policy to improve society's ability to adapt to changing circumstances, preparing the economy for the consequences of global warming. Perhaps the best summation of the differing assessments of what society's response to greenhouse warming ought to be is that given at a 1988 climate change conference by Harvard planetary scientist Michael McElroy:

> If we choose to take on this challenge, it appears we can slow the rate of change substantially, giving us time to develop mechanisms so that the cost to society and the damage to ecosystems can be minimized. We could alternatively close our eyes, hope for the best, and pay the cost when the bill comes due (Lyman et al., 1990; Revkin, 1992; EPA, 1992)■

References

Broecker, Wallace S. 1970. "Man's Oxygen Reserves." *Science* 168 (June 26).

Budyko, M. I. 1986. *The Evolution of the Biosphere.* D. Reidel Publishing Company.

Environmental Protection Agency. 1992. *Climate Change Discussion Series: Agriculture.* Office of Policy Planning and Evaluation, May.

Environmental Protection Agency. 1990. *Policy Options for Stabilizing Global Climate: Report to Congress.* Washington, D.C.

Gribbin, John. 1982. "Carbon Dioxide, Ammonia—and Life." *New Scientist* 94(1305), 413–416, May 13.

Houghton, J. T., G. J. Jenkins, and J. J. Ephraums, eds. 1990. *Climate Change: the IPCC Scientific Assessment.* Cambridge University Press.

Kerr, J. B. and C. T. McElroy. 1993. "Evidence for Large Upward Trends of Ultraviolet-B Radiation Linked to Ozone Depletion." *Science* 262 (Nov.).

Lyman, Francesca, with Irving Mintzer, Kathleen Courrier, and James J. MacKenzie. 1990. *The Greenhouse Trap: What We're Doing to the Atmosphere and How We Can Stop Global Warming.* World Resources Institute.

Maugh, Thomas H. 1982. "New Link Between Ozone and Cancer." *Science* 216 (April 23).

Mintzer, Irving M. 1987. "A Matter of Degrees: the Potential for Controlling the Greenhouse Effect." World Resources Institute, Research Report 5, April.

"Ozone Takes a Nose Dive After the Eruption of Mt. Pinatubo." *Science* 260 (April 23, 1993).

Panofsky, Hans A. 1978. "Earth's Endangered Ozone." *Environment* 20, no. 3 (April).

Revkin, Andrew. 1992. *Global Warming: Understanding the Forecast.* Abbeville Press.

Rowlands, Ian H. 1993. "The Fourth Meeting of the Parties to the Montreal Protocol: Report and Reflection." *Environment* 35, no. 6 (July/Aug.).

Stern, Paul C., Oran R. Young, and Daniel Druckman, eds. 1992. *Global Environmental Change: Understanding the Human Dimensions.* National Academy Press.

Stevens, William K. 1993. "Scientists Report an Easing in Ozone-Killing Chemicals." *New York Times*, Aug. 26.

Strahler, Arthur N., and Alan H. Strahler. 1973. *Environmental Geoscience.* Hamilton Publishing Company.

Sullivan, Walter. 1993. "Study of Greenland Ice Finds Rapid Change in Past Climate." *New York Times*, July 15.

Watson, R. T., H. Rohde, H. Oeschger, and U. Siegenthaler. 1990. "Greenhouse Gases and Aerosols." In *Climate Change: the IPCC Scientific Assessment*, edited by J. T. Houghton, G. J. Jenkins, and J. J. Ephraums. Cambridge University Press.

World Resources Institute. 1992. *World Resources 1992–93.* Oxford University Press.

World Resource Institute. 1990. *World Resources 1990–91.* Oxford University Press.

CHAPTER 12

Air Pollution

> *If you visit American city, You will find it very pretty: just two things of which you must beware: don't drink the water and don't breathe the air!*
>
> —Tom Lehrer, lyrics from ''Pollution''
>
> *Every American expects and deserves to breathe clean air.*
>
> —President George Bush

Humans have undoubtedly been coping with a certain amount of polluted air ever since primitive *Homo sapiens* sat crouched by the warmth of a smoky fire in their Paleolithic caves. An inevitable consequence of fuel combustion, air pollution mounted as a source of human discomfort as soon as people began to live in towns and cities. It has become an extremely serious problem on a worldwide basis during the past century for two primary reasons: 1) there has been an enormous increase in world population, particularly in urban areas, and 2) since the early 1800s the rapid growth of energy-intensive industries and rising levels of affluence in the developed countries have led to record levels of fossil fuel combustion.

Prior to the 20th century problems related to air pollution were primarily associated, in the public mind at least, with the city of London. As early as the 13th century small amounts of coal from Newcastle were being shipped into London for fuel. As the population and manufacturing enterprises grew, wood supplies diminished and coal burning increased, in spite of the protestations of a long series of both monarchs and private citizens who objected to the odor of coal smoke. One petitioner to King Charles II in 1661 complained that due to the greed of manufacturers, inhabitants of London were forced to "breathe nothing but an impure and thick Mist, accompanied by a fuliginous (sooty) and filthy vapour, which renders them obnoxious to a thousand inconveniences, the Lungs, and disordering the entire habit of their Bodies. . . ." (Evelyn, 1661).

In spite of such railings, English coal consumption increased even faster than the rate of population growth and by the 19th century London's thick, "pea-soup" fogs had become a notorious trademark of the city. Numerous well-meaning attempts at smoke abatement were largely ignored during the heyday of laissez-faire capitalism, epitomized by the industrialists' slogan, "Where there's muck, there's money."

The same conditions that had made London the air pollution capital of the world began to prevail in the United States as well during the 19th and early 20th centuries. St. Louis, plagued by smoky conditions, passed an ordinance as early as 1867 mandating that smokestacks be at least 20 feet higher than adjacent buildings. The Chicago City Council in 1881 passed the nation's first smoke abatement ordinance. Pittsburgh, once one of the smokiest cities in the United States, was the site of pioneer work at the Mellon Institute on the harmful impact of smoke both on property and human health. In spite of gradually increasing public awareness of the problem, levels of air pollution and the geographical extent of the areas affected continued to increase. Although by the late 1950s and 1960s large-scale fuel-switching from coal to natural gas and oil had significantly reduced smoky conditions in many American cities, other newer pollutants—products of the now-ubiquitous automobile—had assumed worrisome levels. Today foul air has become a problem of global proportions; no longer does one have to travel to London or Pittsburgh or Los Angeles to experience the respiratory irritation or the aesthetic distress which a hazy, contaminated atmosphere can provoke. As the 20th century draws to a close, virtually every metropolitan area in the world—New York, Moscow, Athens, New Delhi, Bankok, Beijing, Mexico City—capitalists and socialists, industrialized and developing nations alike, all are grappling with the problem of how to halt further deterioration of air quality without impeding industrial productivity and industrial development.

Sources of Air Pollution

Where is all this dirty air coming from? Not surprisingly, the sources of air pollution are quite diverse and vary in importance from one region to another. Some air contaminants are of natural origin; volcanic eruptions, forest fires, and dust storms periodically contribute large quantities of pollutant gases and particles to the atmosphere. In June 1991, immense quantities of volcanic ash and an estimated 18 million metric tons of sulfur dioxide (roughly equivalent to U.S. emissions of this pollutant gas during an entire year) were spewed into the atmosphere during a single massive eruption of Mt. Pinatubo in the Philippines. Earlier that same year, in a vengeful act of environmental terrorism during the Persian Gulf War, Iraqi dictator Saddam Hussein ordered the systematic firing of Kuwaiti oil fields in a fruitless attempt to hamper the advance of United Nations forces toward Kuwait City. Before Iraqi troops were pushed back across their own borders, they had damaged or destroyed almost 85% of Kuwait's 950 oil wells, thereby generating a pall of pollution from oil fires that extended eastward as far as Afghanistan and northern India. Less dramatic but worthy of note, considerable amounts of methane gas are released into the air when organic matter decays in the absence of oxygen, and some plant species produce volatile hydrocarbons that are thought to be responsible for the blue haze observed in the Smoky Mountains and other forest regions. However, most of the pollutants befouling our air today come from emission sources that have proliferated with the development of industries and transportation networks.

At present in the United States the largest sources of air pollution, in order of importance, are 1) transportation, primarily automobiles and trucks; 2) electric power plants that burn coal or oil; and 3) industry, the major offenders being steel mills, metal smelters, oil refineries, and pulp and paper mills. Of less importance now than in past decades is the contribution made from heating homes and buildings and burning refuse. The general trend toward heating with oil, gas, or electricity instead of with coal greatly reduced pollution from space heating. At the same time, increasingly common municipal bans on home refuse burning, along with the utilization of sanitary landfills or incinerators equipped with pollution control devices for community solid waste disposal, have accounted for a marked decline in emissions from trash combustion. Within any one region or community, of course, the relative importance of various emission

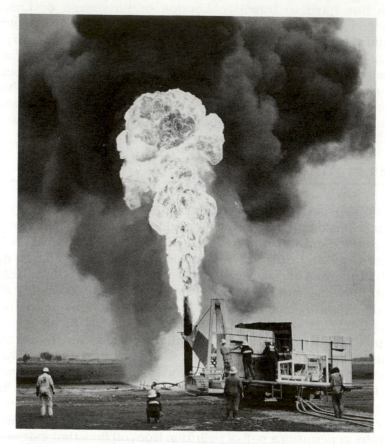

A burning oil well in Kuwait discharges thick, black smoke into the air. Hundreds of oil wells were set ablaze by the retreating Iraqi army during the Persian Gulf War. [Reuters/Bettmann]

sources may differ from the overall national rankings noted here. In most metropolitan areas, automobiles contribute by far the largest amount of air pollutants; in small towns, by contrast, significant levels of contamination may be caused by just one polluting factory.

Criteria Air Pollutants

Air pollution, of course, is no single entity; thousands of gaseous, liquid, and solid compounds contribute to the atmospheric mess. The nature of some of these substances is well known while others are only now being studied and their threat to human health assessed. The most common and widespread air pollutants include six that the federal government has designated **criteria pollutants**, requiring the Environmental Protection Agency to gather scientific and medical information on their environmental and human health effects. These are the pollutants for which **National Ambient Air Quality Standards (NAAQS—**familiarly referred to as ''nax'') have been set, specifying the maximum levels of concentration of these pollutants allowable in the outdoor air. The six criteria air pollutants are discussed in the following sections (it should be noted that most industrialized countries, and some developing nations as well, now have regulations controlling these same air contaminants).

Particulate Matter (PM_{10}). All airborne pollutants that occur in either liquid or solid form, including pollen, dust, soot, smoke, acid condensates, and sulfate and nitrate particles are referred to as particulate matter. Particulates range in size from pieces of fly ash as large as a thumbnail to tiny aerosols less than 1 micrometer in diameter—so small that they remain suspended in the air and are transported on wind currents as easily as are gases. To many people, particulate matter and "air pollution" are synonymous, since easily visible dark plumes of smoke and soot or clouds of dust are the only forms of air pollution of which they are aware. Marked reductions in particulate levels in a number of urban areas in recent years have led many citizens to conclude erroneously that air quality is no longer a problem, since most other air pollutants are invisible.

Particulate matter is generated by a wide variety of activities—fuel combustion, road traffic, agricultural activities, certain industrial processes, and natural abrasion. The most visible damage caused by particulate matter is the layer of grime deposited on buildings, streets, clothing, and so on. Prior to pollution-control efforts launched during the 1970s, it was estimated that in the most polluted areas of big cities as much as 50–100 tons of particulate matter per square mile fell each month (Air Pollution Primer, 1969). Particulate matter can obscure visibility and corrode metals; most important is the fact that when inhaled, particulates irritate the respiratory tract. Most dangerous in this regard are the tiny aerosols that, because of their very small size, can evade the body's natural defense mechanisms and penetrate deeply into the lungs (in most cities, these very small particles comprise 50–60% of suspended particulates). In recognition of this fact, the EPA in 1987 replaced the original standard for total particulates with a revised standard that applies to those particles with a diameter of 10 micrometers or less (PM_{10}) that are small enough to penetrate to the highly sensitive alveolar region of the lungs.

Sulfur Dioxide (SO_2). The major source of this colorless pollutant gas is fuel combustion, inasmuch as sulfur is present to a greater or lesser degree as an impurity in coal and fuel oil. When these sulfur-containing fuels are burned, the sulfur is oxidized to form SO_2. By itself sulfur dioxide is not particularly harmful, but it readily reacts with water vapor in the atmosphere to form other sulfur compounds such as sulfuric acid, sulfates, and sulfites which irritate the respiratory system, corrode metals and statuary, harm textiles, impair visibility, and kill or stunt the growth of plants. Sulfur dioxide is also one of the main precursors of acid precipitation, recognized now as an environmental threat of major proportions and a subject which will be dealt with in greater detail later in this chapter.

Carbon Monoxide (CO). No other pollutant gas is found at such high concentrations in the urban atmosphere as is the extremely toxic, odorless,

Figure 12-1 Criteria Pollutants

Pollutant	Form	Major Source	Effects
PM_{10}	solid or liquid	Combustion, industrial processes	1. grime deposits 2. obscures visibility 3. corrodes metals
SULFUR DIOXIDE (SO_2)	gas	Coal-burning power plants, metal smelters, industrial boilers, oil refineries	1. respiratory irritant 2. corrodes metal & stone 3. damages textiles 4. toxic to plants 5. precursor of acid rain
CARBON MONOXIDE (CO)	gas	Motor vehicles	1. aggravates cardiovascular disease 2. impairs perception and mental processes 3. fatal at high concentrations
NITROGEN DIOXIDE (NO_2)	gas	Motor vehicles, power plants	1. respiratory irritant 2. toxic to plants 3. reduces visibility 4. precursor of ozone 5. precursor of acid rain
OZONE (O_3)	gas	Motor vehicles (indirectly)	1. respiratory irritant 2. toxic to plants 3. corrodes rubber, paint
LEAD (Pb)	metal aerosol	Motor vehicles	1. damage to nervous system, blood, kidneys

and colorless carbon monoxide. Any type of incomplete combustion produces CO, but the most significant source in terms of urban air pollution is automobile emissions (in indoor situations, cigarette smoking is a major source of carbon monoxide). When inhaled, CO binds to hemoglobin in the blood, displacing oxygen and thereby reducing the amount of oxygen carried in the bloodstream to the various body tissues. For this reason, carbon monoxide is the air pollutant that provokes the most severe reactions among heart patients. Studies have shown that more deaths among heart attack victims occur during periods of high CO concentrations than at other times. Patients suffering from angina pectoris, a coronary disease in which there is an insufficient supply of oxygen to the heart during exercise, experience a much more rapid onset of pain during periods of increased carbon monoxide pollution. Depending on the concentration of CO in the air and the length of exposure, inhalation of carbon monoxide can result in adverse health effects ranging from mild headaches or dizziness at relatively low levels of exposure to death at high levels. Fortunately, the health effects of short-term carbon monoxide exposure are reversible, but people who work for many hours in areas of heavy traffic (e.g. police officers, toll collectors, parking garage attendants) are obviously receiving substantial doses. Some evidence indicates that blood absorption of CO slows down mental processes and reaction time, raising the suspicion that many rush-hour traffic accidents can be at least partially attributed to low-level carbon monoxide poisoning.

Nitrogen Oxides (NO$_x$). Consisting primarily of nitrous oxide (NO) and nitrogen dioxide (NO$_2$), oxides of nitrogen are formed when combustion occurs at very high temperatures. Nitrogen oxides enter the atmosphere in approximately equal amounts from auto emissions and power plants (in urban areas, cars are generally the predominant source of NO$_x$ emissions). Nitrogen dioxide is the only criteria pollutant gas that is colored. The yellow brown "smoggy" appearance typical of southern California on bad days is due to the high concentrations of NO$_2$ in the air. At high levels of pollution, nitrogen dioxide has a pungent, sweetish odor. At commonly encountered ambient levels, NO$_2$ causes lung irritation and can increase susceptibility to acute respiratory ailments such as pneumonia and influenza. Nitrogen dioxide stunts plant growth and visibly damages leaves. It reduces visibility and, like sulfur dioxide, contributes to the formation of acid rain.

Ozone (O$_3$). The main constituent of a group of chemical compounds known as **photochemical oxidants**, ozone and such fellow travelers as peroxyacetylnitrate (PAN) and various aldehydes are considered to be auto-associated pollutants even though they are not emitted directly from the tailpipe into the atmosphere. Instead, these substances form in a complex series of chemical reactions when nitrogen dioxide and **volatile organic compounds (VOCs)**, especially certain hydrocarbons from both auto exhausts and a variety of stationary sources, react with oxygen and sunlight to produce a witch's brew of chemicals dubbed **photochemical smog**. First observed in the Los Angeles area in the 1940s (the bright sunlight, warm temperatures, frequent atmospheric inversions, and heavy traffic make southern California particularly well-suited for photochemical smog formation), photochemical smog is now often observed in other cities as well, especially on bright summer days ("ozone season" is considered to extend from May 1 through September 30). Ozone, an early and continuing product of the photochemical smog reaction, is the chemical whose presence is used to measure the oxidant level of the atmosphere at any given time. This pungent, colorless gas irritates the mucous membranes of the respiratory system, causing coughing, choking, and reduced lung capacity. Heart patients, asthmatics, and those suffering from bronchitis or emphysema are at special risk during periods of high

O_3 levels. Ozone also cracks rubber, deteriorates fabrics, and causes paint to fade. The eye irritation and watery eyes frequently experienced during smog episodes is caused both by ozone and by PAN, another member of the photochemical oxidant family. Photochemical smog has caused extensive plant damage, killing or injuring plants directly or increasing their vulnerability to attack by insects. A classic example of photochemical oxidant damage to plants can be seen in the ailing ponderosa pine forests of the San Bernardino Mountains, about 70 miles downwind from Los Angeles. The profound impact of photochemical oxidants on agricultural yields was highlighted in a report issued by the World Resources Institute which documented crop damage due to air pollution, primarily ozone, as costing U.S. farmers up to $5 billion a year. Crops most seriously affected included soybeans, cotton, winter wheat, kidney beans, and peanuts.

Lead (Pb).   The adverse impact of this toxic metal on the intellectual development of children (see chapter 7) caused it to be added to the list of criteria pollutants when the Clean Air Act was reauthorized in 1977. Since most airborne lead can be traced to automobile emissions, the major control strategy for this pollutant is to phase out the use of leaded gasoline.

Hazardous Air Pollutants (HAPs)

In addition to the criteria air pollutants, a large number of less common, but much more hazardous, chemicals are released into the atmosphere from a wide range of industries and manufacturing processes. Although the sources of these emissions are more localized than are those of the criteria pollutants, the fact that many of them are either toxic or carcinogenic suggests that they deserve special attention. In 1970 Congress directed the EPA to develop a list of industrial air pollutants that can cause serious health damage even at relatively low concentrations and to establish protective emission standards for those so listed. No deadline date for listing substances as hazardous was mandated, however, and implementation of the congressional directive was exceedingly slow.

By 1990, twenty years after the original congressional mandate, only eight toxic air pollutants had been listed—**asbestos, mercury, beryllium, benzene, vinyl chloride, arsenic, radionuclides, and coke oven emissions**—and standards had been set only for the first seven (a standard for coke oven emissions was finally promulgated in 1993). Frustrated with this snail's pace, environmentalists for years had prodded EPA to speed up the evaluation process, urging the agency to list and set standards for additional toxic air pollutants which pose a special hazard to public health. In 1986, congressional passage of the Emergency Planning and Community Right-to-Know Act (SARA Title III), prompted by the tragic chemical accident in Bhopal, India two years earlier, led to heightened public awareness of the toxic threats lurking in hundreds of communities across the nation. By requiring that manufacturers disclose information on the kinds and amounts of toxic pollutants they discharge into the local environment each year, this law prompted demands from community activists and the media for tighter controls on health-threatening emissions.

In turn, the necessity of revealing data that might alarm previously complacent local residents prompted voluntary emissions reductions by a number of firms eager to maintain a positive corporate image. In 1990 Congress responded to the mounting pressure to "do something" about air toxics by identifying 189 chemicals that it ordered EPA to regulate as hazardous air pollutants and by establishing comprehensive, technology-based controls for dealing with this widely acknowledged yet largely ignored public health threat. The new regulatory approach to controlling air toxics will be discussed in greater detail later in this chapter.

Impact of Air Pollution on Human Health

If dirty skyscrapers or sick ponderosa pines were the only consequence of polluted air, concern about the phenomenon would undoubtedly be considerably less than it is today. The unfortunate fact is, however, that over the years there has been a steadily growing mass of evidence indicating that the quality of the air we breathe has a measurable impact on human health.

Some of the ill effects of air pollution have, of course, been known for a long time: Los Angelenos knowingly curse the smog as they wipe tears from their burning eyes; motorists hopefully roll up their car windows in heavy traffic, trying to avert a carbon monoxide-induced headache; and asthmatics resignedly brace for an attack when the weather forecaster proclaims an ozone alert. For many years discomforts such as these were shrugged off as necessary consequences of economic growth, since smoke-belching factories were acknowledged symbols of prosperity and progress. Only after several air pollution "disasters" made world headlines did the general public begin to realize the extent of the threat to human health posed by dirty air. The great London smog of 1952 (see Box 12-1) involved the largest number of casualties, but it wasn't the first such episode. Eighteen years earlier a very similar scenario unfolded in the heavily industrialized Meuse River Valley of Belgium. During a three-day inversion, 60 people died of the foul air, while thousands of others became seriously ill, coughing and gasping for breath. In the fall of 1948, the small (pop. 14,000) Pennsylvania town of Donora, near Pittsburgh, fell victim to a five-day inversion. Situated in a heavily industrialized valley, Donora was enveloped in a cold, damp blanket of smoggy air, permeated with the smell of sulfur. During this time, fully 42% of the town's population suffered eye, nose, and throat irritation; chest pains; coughing; difficulty in breathing; headaches; nausea; and vomiting. When the inversion finally lifted, it was found that 20 people had died during the period (Waldbott, 1978).

The dramatic examples of pollution-induced death and disease described above were all associated with levels of air contamination considerably worse than those experienced by most urban residents today, even those living in visibly smoggy cities. For many years researchers have been trying to determine whether air pollution at levels typically encountered in metropolitan areas can, by itself, increase mortality and

Box 12-1

Atmospheric Inversions

Shortly before Christmas of 1952, the city of London experienced a killer smog that even in that notoriously polluted metropolis was exceptionally severe. For a period of five days the cold, moist air hung over the city like a heavy wet blanket, with scarcely a trace of breeze to carry away the thickening cloud of smoke and fumes from millions of coal-burning fireplaces, factories, and motor vehicles. Even in the middle of the day, the pervading gloom was so thick that car-train collisions were common and a steam ferry ran into an anchored ship along the Thames River. When the fog finally lifted, health officials revealed the grim human toll of this episode—nearly 3000 excess deaths, most of them due to respiratory or heart disease, had occurred during the week of foul air. The London situation was not solely a result of pollutants being dumped into an overburdened atmosphere. The volume of emissions during the time period in question was not substantially different than at many other times during the year. Though London, like most other metropolitan areas, suffered regularly from unhealthy levels of contaminated air, pollution was seldom bad enough to cause acute respiratory distress as it did during this event. The chief villain in this situation, and in virtually every other air pollution "disaster" on record, was an atmospheric anomaly known as an **inversion**.

Under normal conditions air is in a constant state of flux. As the air near the earth's surface is warmed it expands and rises, carrying with it pollutant particles and gases. Cooler, cleaner air moves in to replace it, setting up convection currents. These forces, combined with the earth's rotation, generate winds that further aid in dispersing pollutants.

The vertical extent to which warm air rises until it cools to the same temperature as the air above is referred to as the **mixing depth**—an expanse that corresponds with the upper boundary for pollution dispersal. The amount of mixing depth varies depending on the time of day and the season of the year, being greater during daytime and in summer than it is at night and during winter.

In contrast to this usual situation, a reversal of the normal pattern can occur in which the air closest to the surface of the ground is cooler than the layer above it. In such a situation the cool air, being heavier than warm air, is unable to rise and mix and remains atypically stable. This state of affairs is known as an **atmospheric inversion**—a condition where a layer of cool surface air is trapped by an overlying layer of warmer air. In such a case, the mixing depth will be minimal and pollutant emissions, if any, within the affected area can accumulate to levels that may threaten human health.

The two most important types of inversions are:

a) *radiation inversion*—This normal nocturnal situation often occurs on clear nights when absorbed daytime heat is radiated quickly out into space and the temperature of surface air drops below that of the air above it. Generally a radiation inversion presents little health threat because it breaks up as soon as the morning sun warms the earth, reestablishing normal convection currents. In most cases a radiation inversion simply doesn't persist long enough to permit build-up of dangerously high concentrations of pollutants.

b) *subsidence inversion*—More troublesome than radiation inversions are subsidence inversions, caused when a layer of air within a high-pressure mass settles down over a region, being compressed and thereby heated by the high pressure area above. At ground level the air temperature remains unchanged and hence is relatively cooler than the air layer directly above. Subsidence inversions are particularly worrisome because they may remain in place for days, the surface air becoming increasingly foul as time passes. While inversions can occur at any time (southern California experiences inversions as often as 340 days of the year), they are more frequent and last longer during the fall and winter months. They are particularly common in valleys, since at night cool air flows down the hillsides and is trapped at the bottom. Not until the sun is directly overhead will the surface air be sufficiently warmed to break up the inversion layer, and in winter such an inversion may persist all day.

It should be pointed out that an atmospheric inversion per se is a perfectly natural occurrence and presents no threat to human health—if there are few sources of pollutant emissions within the affected region. Inversions become major problems only when they occur in industrialized or densely settled areas where noxious pollutants can steadily accumulate to dangerous concentrations.

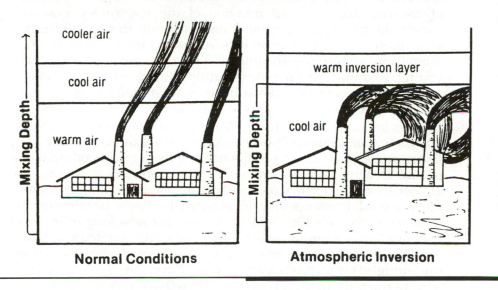

Normal Conditions   **Atmospheric Inversion**

morbidity rates and, if so, which specific pollutants pose the greatest hazard. Results obtained from a number of studies within the past few years confirm fears long suspected—air pollution kills, and at levels of pollutant concentration well within the legally allowable limits established by the NAAQS.

The Air Pollution-Health Connection

Investigations aimed at determining precise cause-and-effect relationships linking given levels of pollution with specific health responses have encountered numerous difficulties. One such problem relates to scientific ethics: it simply isn't acceptable to expose the most vulnerable members of society—children, the elderly, asthmatics, etc.—to high levels of air pollution and then watch to see what happens to them. In addition, because urban air contains so many different pollutants, determining with certainty *which* pollutant at *what level* is causing an observed health effect has been problematic. The likelihood that synergistic effects play a role in determining the response to polluted air is a further complicating factor, as is the possibility of contributory occupational exposure. Particularly troublesome to researchers striving to elucidate the air pollution-health connection has been the overwhelming influence of cigarette smoking—i.e. how much is due to the pollutants in city air and how much is due to self-inflicted tobacco pollutants? In spite of these challenges, a substantial body of evidence regarding the health effects of air pollutants has been assembled from three basic sources.

1. *Animal studies*—Using experimental animals to test the pathological effects of varying doses of a single air pollutant is common procedure for determining dose-response curves. Such studies provide a valid method of assessing cause-and-effect relationships and provide a way of determining precisely how a given pollutant affects the structure and function of the respiratory system—something that would be much more difficult to do with human subjects since in most cases it involves sacrificing the experimental animal and performing an autopsy. The major weakness of animal testing, of course, lies in extrapolating the quantitative results of such tests to human exposure levels, since animals may be either more or less sensitive to a given pollutant than are humans.

2. *Studies on human volunteers*—When conducted under controlled laboratory conditions, exposure studies on volunteers can be used to determine at precisely what concentration a given pollutant can induce an acute (short-term) health effect. Since such studies are almost always performed on healthy adults and are limited to short-term, reversible effects they are of limited value in predicting how more sensitive individuals might respond or how long-term exposure might affect public health. Such tests with isolated pollutants also ignore the synergistic effects to be expected when numerous intermingled air pollutants are inhaled. Nevertheless, such tests do help to quantify human responses to individual pollutants.

3. *Epidemiologic studies*—By investigating the distribution of suspected air pollution-related ailments within a relatively large population, researchers can study the effects of real-life exposures in various subgroups. Such studies are more realistic than controlled laboratory experiments in terms of actual exposure experienced by the general public, but they are frequently difficult to interpret because of the impossibility of controlling variables. In epidemiologic studies it is seldom possible to attribute an observed health effect to any one specific pollutant, and differences among members of the community in such terms as age, health status, socioeconomic level, and smoking habits compound the difficulties faced by epidemiologic investigators.

In spite of the inherent shortcomings of each method, results of all three lines of research today are converging to provide evidence that strongly supports the need for government regulation of air pollution in order to protect human health.

Major Health Effects

Not surprisingly, air pollution's major impact on health is the result of irritants acting on the respiratory tract. Not all air pollutants are equally harmful, however. Research indicates that the most serious health effects associated with polluted air can be attributed to elevated levels of PM_{10}, especially to the fine particulates with an aerodynamic diameter of 2.5 micrometers or less and to sulfate particles. These pollutants have been more directly associated with heightened risk of death and disease than have any other contaminants in the ambient air; the fatalities that occurred during the air pollution disasters previously described have all been attributed to this group of pollutants. These tiny aerosols, generated primarily by the combustion of fossil fuels, present a particularly serious threat to human health because they tend to be more toxic than larger particles and can be inhaled deeply into the lungs where they lodge in sensitive pulmonary tissue and constitute a chronic source of irritation. Epidemiologic studies conducted from 1975–1988 in six U.S. cities have convincingly demonstrated the link between high levels of particulate air pollution and death due to lung cancer, respiratory disease, and heart ailments—even after controlling for individual risk factors such as smoking, occupational exposure, excessive weight gain, and so on. The correlation was most dramatically evident in Steubenville, Ohio, the most polluted city in the survey group, where adjusted mortality rates were 26% higher than in Portage, Wisconsin, the least polluted of the six communities studied. Interestingly, the link between pollution levels and increased risk of premature death was statistically significant only in relation to concentrations of fine, inhalable particles; varying levels of total suspended particulates, NO_x, SO_2, or ozone appeared to have no measurable impact on death rates—an indication that fine particulates constitute the most dangerous form of air pollution in terms of human health impact (Dockery, 1993).

When polluted air is inhaled, both the structure and the functioning of the respiratory tract can be altered. Although much remains to be learned about the precise physiologic mechanisms by which exposure to air pollution can kill, some of the ways in which air pollutants can induce illness include the following.

Inhibit or Inactivate Natural Body Defenses. The human respiratory system is well constructed to restrict entry of foreign particles and to rid the body of such intruders if they succeed in penetrating the first lines of defense. As a result, the approximately 10,000–20,000 liters of germ- and particle-laden air inhaled by a person each day are effectively cleansed by the time they reach the lungs. Particles are removed both by

Figure 12-2

Human Respiratory System

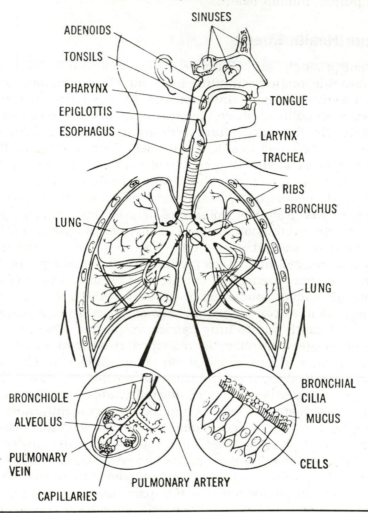

SINUSES

ADENOIDS

TONSILS

PHARYNX

EPIGLOTTIS

ESOPHAGUS

TONGUE

LARYNX

TRACHEA

RIBS

BRONCHUS

LUNG

LUNG

BRONCHIOLE

ALVEOLUS

PULMONARY VEIN

CAPILLARIES

PULMONARY ARTERY

BRONCHIAL CILIA

MUCUS

CELLS

Chronic Airway Resistance

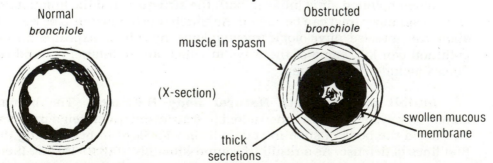

Normal
bronchiole

Obstructed
bronchiole

muscle in spasm

(X-section)

swollen mucous membrane

thick secretions

Source: American Lung Association, *Air Pollution Primer*, 1969.

deposition and by clearance, the precise site at which this occurs depending on particle size. Large particles may be trapped by nasal hairs or are deposited on the walls of the nose or throat, while smaller particulates generally escape these defenses and travel deeper into the respiratory tract where the slower air movement causes all but the smallest to settle out on the surface of the trachea or bronchi (the conducting airways). Upon settling, the invading particles are trapped by mucus produced by cells lining the airways. They are then swept upward by the constant beating movement of millions of tiny **cilia**, hair-like projections of epithelial cells lining the respiratory tract. This mucociliary action transports dirt and pathogens to the upper respiratory passages from whence they are expelled by nose-blowing, coughing, sneezing, or swallowing. The tiniest aerosol particulates that evade removal in this manner and are deposited on the lining of the **alveoli** (terminal air sacs) may be attacked and devoured by specialized scavenger cells called **macrophages**, thus removing them from the lungs. Although not always successful, these defense mechanisms are extremely important in shielding the respiratory system from assault. Research has shown that exposure to certain air pollutants can induce health problems due to the effect of these contaminants on the body's natural defenses. When pollutant gases, especially ozone, NO_2, or SO_2 are inhaled, the action of the cilia lining the airways may be slowed down or halted altogether. At high pollutant concentrations, patches of ciliated cells may be killed and slough off; function of the macrophage cells in the alveoli also may be inhibited. Any of these effects greatly reduces the body's ability to withstand invasion from pathogenic organisms such as bacteria or viruses. Thus a common health consequence of breathing polluted air is increased susceptibility to infectious airborne diseases such as pneumonia or acute bronchitis.

Cause Constriction of the Airways ("chronic airway resistance"). Exposure to gases such as O_3 or SO_2 may result in a swelling of the membrane lining the airways, thereby reducing the diameter of the opening and resulting in more labored breathing.

Induce Fibrosis and Thickening of Alveolar Walls. Ozone is particularly effective in altering the wall structure of the delicate terminal air sacs. When ozone comes into contact with sensitive alveolar cells, tiny lesions are formed. The breaks subsequently heal, but in the process scar tissue is formed. Lung tissue becomes thicker and stiffer, making it more difficult for air to penetrate and thereby reducing functional lung capacity ("Health Effects," 1978).

Fortunately, in most of the industrial democracies, the public has recognized the serious health hazards posed by air pollution and have demanded air quality controls that have significantly reduced the high levels of contamination commonly encountered in urban air in former years. Although air quality continues to worsen in many developing nations and in parts of the former Soviet empire, today in most parts of the United States, Japan, and western Europe it is very unlikely that another air

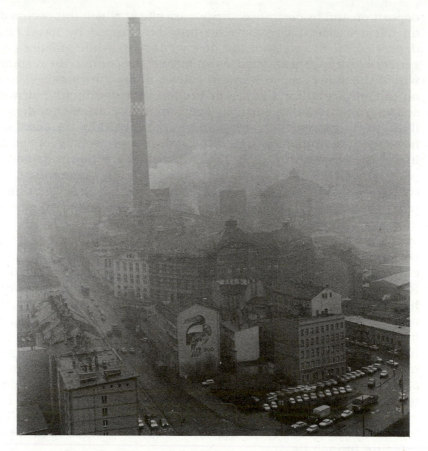

Heavy smog settles on downtown Leipzig, Germany. Decades of authoritarian government and central planning have resulted in severe pollution problems throughout the former Soviet Union and the former communist states of eastern and central Europe. [Reuters/Bettmann]

pollution disaster such as that of Donora in 1948 or London in 1952 could occur again. For this we can thank the persistent efforts of a dedicated coalition of citizens and scientists who wouldn't allow the public to ignore the air pollution-health connection and the legislators, both state and federal, who had the political courage to impose mandatory controls on polluters.

Pollution Control Efforts—The Clean Air Act

As air quality in the United States steadily deteriorated during the 1950s and 1960s, it became increasingly evident that a broad-based, concerted effort was needed to deal with what was increasingly perceived as a problem of national scope. Until 1955 any attempts to regulate pollutant emissions were based solely at the local or state level; in that year

BOX 12-2

Lenin's Environmental Legacy

There is no worse ecological situation on the planet than ours in the USSR. Pyoth Chadayev said 150 years ago that it was Russia's fate to serve as an example to the world of how not to live. I would say that we have become both an environmental testing ground for the whole world and an ecological threat to the entire planet.

—Dr. Grigory M. Barenboim, environmental analyst
comments during 1990 interview in Moscow

From the grimy industrial centers of Russia and Ukraine to the soot-laden cities of Poland, Slovakia, and the Czech Republic, a pall of pollution hangs like a shroud, darkening skies, depressing spirits, and undermining the health of millions of citizens throughout the former Soviet empire. For those who once thought of air pollution as a peculiarly capitalist problem, the belated recognition that Communists could be equally adept at environmental despoliation came as a shock; yet in retrospect, Leninist ideology and socialist economic policies deserve much of the blame for current ecological problems. The fierce determination of Lenin, following the 1917 Bolshevik Revolution, to abandon all tradition and constraints in order to build a socialist state led to wholesale exploitation of natural resources and the subordination of human welfare to utopian goals. Both Lenin and his successor Stalin ruled with an iron hand, indifferent to pollution and the health of the populace so long as industrial production continued to expand. Public opinion had no influence on decision makers and a centrally planned economy made no adjustments based on local needs or preferences. Communities adversely affected by a polluting enterprise had no right to protest or to receive compensation for the harm they suffered. Production goals, set by Moscow, were measured solely by gross output; unrealistically low prices for energy and natural resources encouraged overconsumption and waste. Although the Soviet government had enacted strict antipollution laws decades before similar legislation was passed in the West, such mandates were almost never enforced. Since all manufacturing enterprises belonged to the State, local government officials who might have been expected to insist on compliance with pollution abatement laws typically supported factory managers whose pollutant emissions were regarded as the price of progress.

That price has been heavy indeed. Because of questionable monitoring and data-collection procedures in Russia and the former East-bloc nations of central Europe, air quality statistics for the region are of somewhat doubtful accuracy. The fact that it was not uncommon for inspectors to warn factory managers of an impending visit, providing time to cap especially dirty equipment, leads some observers to conclude that published figures of pollutant concentrations are likely to be decidedly conservative estimates. Even so, the picture such statistics paint is a bleak one. In the former Soviet republics, 103 urban areas, home to more than 50 million people, experience levels of air pollution regularly exceeding government standards. Nowhere is the problem worse than in the Siberian city of Norilsk, 300 miles above the Arctic Circle, where in 1990 more than two million tons of industrial emissions poisoned the air. Smokestacks throughout the city belch sulfur dioxide, which on calm days regularly reaches concentrations more than 70 times the legally allowable limits. Carbon disulfide, phenol, and hydrogen fluoride, all well above maximum permissible concentrations, further contribute to the toxic miasma in a city reputed to have the highest male lung cancer rate in the world. Norilsk may top the pollution charts, but scores of other urban centers in Russia are smog-shrouded as well.

Pollution is blamed for fully one-fifth of all illnesses in Moscow, a city of nine million people. Only 8% of Muscovites live in areas considered "ecologically acceptable," thanks to industrial emissions (only 30% of stationary sources in the capital have installed pollution control equipment) and to exhausts from close to a million motor vehicles burning leaded gasoline, most unequipped with catalytic converters. By the late 1980s, due at least in part to dangerously high levels of air pollution, the incidence of bronchial asthma among children in Moscow was seven times higher than it had been 30 years earlier. Among residents living along the "Garden Ring"—the heavily-traveled inner beltway circling central Moscow—cardiovascular and nervous system disorders are 2½ times as common as they are elsewhere in the Moscow region. In the most polluted neighborhoods of the capital city, rates of physical retardation among children are 1½ times more prevalent than in cleaner areas; in one exclusive maternity clinic, fully eight out of ten babies born during a six-month period in the early 1990s entered the world prematurely or with birth defects. Elsewhere throughout the Russian republic, the story sounds depressingly similar. High concentrations of air toxics contribute to an elevated incidence of pneumonia and other respiratory diseases, birth defects, cancerous tumors, digestive tract infections, and kidney ailments.

Several hundred miles to the west a comparable situation confronts inhabitants of the former Communist states of central and eastern Europe, where 40 years of authoritarian government and central planning resulted in environmental degradation as bad as that in the Soviet republics. Here, too, air pollution is an overwhelming problem, exacerbated by massive dependence on brown coal (lignite) as the region's primary fuel. Eastern Europe's brown coal deposits are high in sulfur and have only half the heat value of hard coal. Consequently, much larger amounts must be burned to meet the required energy demand than would be the case with higher BTU fuel. Since few of the coal-fired plants in the region are equipped with any kind of pollution controls, emissions from these facilities exact a heavy environmental toll. Ambient levels of sulfur dioxide in eastern Europe are among the highest in the world; particularly hard-hit are the industrial areas of eastern Germany, northern Bohemia (Czech Republic), and Silesia (Poland) where SO_2 concentrations average well in excess of limits established by the World Health Organization. Nitrogen oxide levels are also high, particularly in the Czech Republic and Poland; particulates, another group of pollutants associated with coal combustion, are prevalent as well, especially in eastern Germany. Perhaps the most visually dramatic example of the devastation caused by dirty air can be seen in the village of Copsa Mica in Romania. Thanks to a nearby factory that produces a black powder used in the manufacture of rubber, the entire town and all its inhabitants are covered with a film of black soot; the spectacle of pollution presented by Copsa Mica caused a visiting *New York Times* reporter to remark that everything in the entire valley looks as though it had been "dipped in ink." As in the former Soviet Union, industrial emissions are now augmented by the noxious fumes of a steadily-expanding fleet of private automobiles. Although the total number of cars in eastern Europe is still low by Western standards, each vehicle on the road produces substantial amounts of pollution. In Hungary, almost half the carbon monoxide and NO_x, one-third of the hydrocarbons, and most of the airborne lead can be traced to auto emissions. As a result, Budapest, Hungary's capital, is already experiencing unacceptable levels of photochemical smog. Similar problems are reported from Poland where the number of passenger cars (five million in 1992) is expected to double within 20 years.

Failure of national governments to protect air quality has had a devastating impact on both the environment and human health in eastern Europe. Forest damage, caused by acid deposition, is worse here than anywhere else in the world. Dead or dying trees are a common sight throughout the once-verdant woodlands of southern Poland, southeastern Germany, and northern regions of the Czech Republic. A 1989 survey by the U.N.'s Economic Commission for Europe tallied the following percentage of forests showing some signs of damage within the countries of eastern Europe: Poland, 82%; Bulgaria, 78%; Czechoslovakia, 73%; East Germany, 57%; and Hungary, 36%. Crop losses, too, are presumed to be significant. In the most polluted regions of Poland, yields of potatoes, beans, and barley have been falling in recent years. Czechs complain that their alfalfa, cereals, and lettuce have been adversely affected by air pollution.

In eastern Europe as in Russia, however, the most insidious impact of dirty air is on the health and well-being of the region's people. While many factors (e.g. high percentage of smokers, high-fat diets, occupational safety hazards, stress, etc.) undoubtedly account for the rather bleak health prospects among eastern Europeans, air pollution is believed to be an important contributing influence. In the most contaminated areas of the Czech Republic, life expectancy is five years less than in cleaner parts of the country. In Poland's industrial region of Silesia, inhabitants suffer 30% more cancer, 47% more respiratory disease, and 55% more cardiovascular illness than in other parts of the country. This may explain why average life expectancy there is three or four years less than elsewhere in Poland. The incidence of mental retardation in Silesia, attributed to high concentrations of lead in air, water, and food, has been described by Polish researchers as "appalling." In the Czech Republic, high SO_2 levels appear to be responsible for a five-fold increase in respiratory ailments among preschoolers in comparison to the rest of the country. A long-suppressed report recently released in Bulgaria documented a shocking litany of health problems experienced by people living in the vicinity of industrial complexes in that nation: asthma, ulcers, skin disease, rickets, liver ailments, hypertension, nervous system disorders—all at significantly higher rates of incidence than elsewhere in Bulgaria.

Responding to the enormity of the environmental and public health catastrophe brought about by decades of exploitation and neglect indigenous "green movements" have proliferated throughout Russia and eastern Europe in recent years. Antipollution laws have been enacted, and governments in the region declare their strong commitment to environmental cleanup. Nevertheless, at a time of unprecedented uncertainty and upheaval throughout the former Soviet bloc, the outlook for a rapid reversal of environmental ills is not encouraging. Public demand for closing industrial polluters has given way to fears of massive layoffs and shortages of essential goods if enterprises are closed—"better a dirty factory than no factory" seems to be the prevailing attitude. Scarcity of hard currency to purchase needed pollution control equipment, the lack of any feasible alternative to coal as an energy source, and simple preoccupation with day-to-day survival make it unlikely that environmental restoration will be a high government priority in the years immediately ahead. Nevertheless, the people of eastern Europe have at last recognized the dimensions and consequences of the eco-catastrophe that confronts them. Well-wishers can only hope that this new environmental consciousness will lead—sooner rather than later—to the difficult but essential actions that must be implemented if these ravaged lands are to avoid ecological collapse.

References

Feshbach, Murray, and Alfred Friendly, Jr. 1992. *Ecocide in the USSR: Health and Nature Under Siege*. Basic Books.

French, Hilary F. 1990. Green Revolutions: Environmental Reconstruction in Eastern Europe and the Soviet Union." *Worldwatch Paper* 99, Worldwatch Institute (November).

the first federal law dealing exclusively with air pollution offered research and technical support to states and municipalities, thereby initiating a policy of federal-state-local partnership in the pollution control effort. By 1963, worsening levels of air pollution generated pressure for more effective action and led to passage of the first Clean Air Act, which gave the federal government a modest degree of authority to attack interstate air pollution problems and which further increased the flow of federal dollars to state and local pollution control agencies. By 1965 recognition of the automobile's contribution to air quality problems precipitated the first emission standards for automobiles (these standards, set for carbon monoxide and hydrocarbon emissions, took effect with 1968 model year cars). In 1967 the comprehensive Air Quality Act established a regional approach for establishing and enforcing air quality standards, though the main responsibility for control of emission sources (except for automobiles) remained at the state and local levels of government. This gradual transition from total reliance on state and local authorities to an increasing federal involvement grew out of general recognition that the problems of air pollution were so immense, diverse, and complex that environmental improvement could be achieved only through intergovernmental cooperation at all levels.

Although such laws were well intentioned, they relied on voluntary compliance by states, many of which were reluctant to adopt strict controls for fear of driving away industry, thereby forfeiting jobs and tax revenues. As a result, pollutant levels continued to rise and public outcry mounted. By 1970, spurred by a grassroots demand that something be done about the environmental crisis facing the nation (a public outcry that culminated in the national observance of "Earth Day" on April 22, 1970), an historic turning point was reached with congressional passage of the Clean Air Act Amendments of 1970 (henceforth referred to here simply as the Clean Air Act). This landmark piece of environmental legislation provided the first comprehensive program for attacking air pollution on an effective nationwide basis.

The 1970 Clean Air Act established a number of legal precedents that form the basis of U.S. air quality control regulations in effect today—and, coincidentally, served as a model subsequently adopted by many other nations struggling with dirty air problems of their own. Some minor modifications to the law, primarily in the form of deadline extensions for meeting stringent new auto emission requirements, were made in 1977. However, by the early 1980s, continuing problems with high levels of certain auto-related pollutants, complaints that portions of the act had not been implemented with sufficient vigor, and the emergence of acid rain as a troublesome new issue not even addressed by the 1970 mandate, gave rise to vociferous demands from the environmental community for changes that would make the Clean Air Act both stronger and more comprehensive. At the same time, the new Reagan Administration viewed its mission as one of dismantling many of the environmental programs enacted during the 1970s. Although Congress refused to approve most of the changes proposed, decisions by the Reagan EPA to waive implementation of certain regulations deemed burdensome to industry resulted in a gradual reversal of air quality improvements that had been on the upswing during the decade of the 1970s. On the most contentious issue of all—what to do about acid rain—the Reagan White House adamantly opposed any new initiatives other than further study, remaining steadfastly unconvinced that the phenomenon posed any real problems.

As a result of this impasse, efforts to reauthorize the Clean Air Act as required by law languished throughout the 1980s, in spite of continued public support for improving air quality. The legislative logjam remained unbroken until 1988 when newly elected President George Bush, citing his desire to be remembered as the "Environmental President," threw his active support behind efforts to resolve the clean air controversy. Within Congress the clash among regional interests and competing ideologies frequently threatened to derail negotiations, but eventually, after months of heated debate, the differences were resolved. Passage of the Clean Air Act Amendments of 1990, signed into law by President Bush in November of that year, marked a significant strengthening of U.S. air quality legislation. The amendments expanded the scope of regulatory requirements, addressed new issues ignored by the 1970 act, and made the law more consistent with other environmental mandates. Although these amendments won't be fully implemented until 2010, assuming all deadlines are met on time (three years after passage of the law, half of all states had missed the deadline for filing smog-reduction plans), they should result in major measurable improvements in U.S. air quality. Some of the most significant provisions of the Clean Air Act are discussed in the following paragraphs.

National Ambient Air Quality Standards (NAAQS)

In setting NAAQS standards for the six criteria air pollutants, the EPA reviews the existing medical and scientific literature to establish **primary standards** at levels intended to safeguard human health, allowing a margin of safety to protect more vulnerable segments of the population such as young children, asthmatics, and the elderly. These standards are subject to periodic revision as new data become available. Currently the EPA is debating whether the NAAQS for particulate matter should be lowered to reflect recent findings of elevated mortality rates in cities where PM_{10} levels are well below the current standard of 150 $\mu g/m^3$ of air. These primary standards are to be set without regard for pollution control costs

Figure 12-3 National Ambient Air Quality Primary Standards

Pollutant	Averaging Time	Maximum Concentration (approximate equivalent)
Particulate matter (PM$_{10}$)	Annual arithmetic mean 24-hour	50 $\mu g/m^3$ 150 $\mu g/m^3$
Sulfur dioxide (SO$_2$)	Annual arithmetic mean 24-hour	80 $\mu g/m^3$ (0.03 ppm) 365 $\mu g/m^3$ (0.14 ppm)
Carbon monoxide (CO)	8-hour 1-hour	10 mg/m^3 (9 ppm) 40 mg/m^3 (35 ppm)
Nitrogen dioxide (NO$_2$)	Annual arithmetic mean	100 $\mu g/m^3$ (0.053 ppm)
Ozone (O$_3$)	Maximum daily 1-hour average	235 $\mu g/m^3$ (0.12 ppm)
Lead (Pb)	Maximum quarterly average	1.5 $\mu g/m^3$

and were originally mandated to be attained by 1975, with penalties (e.g. bans on the construction of new sources of pollution, cut-off of federal highway construction funds, etc.) to be imposed on those **non-attainment areas** which failed to bring their pollution levels into conformance with the NAAQS. Twenty years after passage of the original legislation, numerous urban areas were still in violation of the primary standard for ozone, historically the most difficult-to-control pollutant, and many cities also exceeded the standard for carbon monoxide as well. Therefore, with the enactment of the 1990 amendments, Congress revised its approach for dealing with non-attainment areas. Under the current program, regions still in violation of any of the air quality standards are classified according to the seriousness of their pollution problems (categories range from

Figure 12-4 Classification of Non-Attainment Areas

Pollutant	Class	Level-PPM	Attainment Date
Ozone	Marginal	.121 to .138	3 years
	Moderate	.138 to .160	6 years
	Serious	.160 to .180	9 years
	Severe 1	.180 to .190	15 years
	Severe 2	.190 to .280	17 years
	Extreme	.280 and above	20 years
Carbon Monoxide	Moderate	9.1 to 16.4	12/31/95
	Serious	16.5 and up	12/31/00
PM_{10}	Moderate	N/A	12/31/94 6 years for future areas
	Serious	N/A	12/31/01 10 years for future areas

For Ozone and CO: Adjustment possible based on 5% rule; EPA may grant two one-year extensions of attainment date

Possible extension of attainment date up to five years for serious areas

"marginal" to "extreme"), and are given varying amounts of time—anywhere from 3–20 years, depending on the severity of non-attainment—to come into compliance with the standards. The higher the pollution levels, the more regulatory steps states must take in dealing with the problem. Lest affected areas postpone action until deadlines are imminent, the 1990 amendments require specified annual emission reduction goals to ensure steady progress toward the ultimate objective of full compliance with NAAQS primary standards.

In addition to the primary standards, EPA was told to set more stringent **secondary standards** that would promote human welfare by protecting agricultural crops, livestock, property, and the environment in general. No timetable for compliance with secondary standards has been set. However, since the secondary standards set by the EPA are, in most cases, identical to the primary standards, the lack of a deadline date is largely irrelevant.

It is difficult to over-emphasize the importance of national as opposed to state or local air quality standards. As experience prior to 1970 amply demonstrated, drifting air pollutants pay little heed to political boundaries, a fact that largely nullified feeble state attempts at improving air quality within their own borders. States or cities that tried to impose emission controls on polluters within their jurisdictions found that air quality gains were minimal due to airborne pollutants arriving from less concerned—or less courageous—states upwind. Threats by polluting industries to leave a particular state and relocate in a more lenient regulatory environment made many state legislatures extremely reluctant to get tough with polluters. Thus, establishing uniform nationwide standards has been a key element in improving air quality since 1970.

Emission Limitations for New Stationary Sources of Pollution

The intent in establishing **new source performance standards (NSPS)** for factories and power plants is to reduce pollutants at their point of origin by ensuring that pollution controls are built in when factories and plants are newly constructed or substantially modified. Note that this requirement is not retroactive; that is, polluting power plants or factories already in operation at the time the Clean Air Act was passed are not affected by the NSPS guidelines. The new source performance standards are set on an industry-by-industry basis, taking into account such factors as economic costs, energy requirements, and total environmental impacts such as waste generation and water quality considerations. The 1990 amendments strengthened this provision by adding a requirement for all stationary sources to obtain operating permits from the state regulatory agency, specifying allowable levels of pollutant emissions, as well as required control measures. By consolidating all the requirements pertaining to a particular facility into one document, this new permit program should facilitate the enforcement of air quality provisions.

Strict Emission Standards for Automobiles

Emission standards for automobiles and other mobile sources form an integral part of Clean Air Act requirements, inasmuch as four of the six criteria air pollutants originate chiefly from motor vehicle exhausts. Detroit eventually settled upon modified engine design plus installation of catalytic converters as the chief means by which American car manufacturers would reduce emissions. Claiming financial difficulties and the impossibility of meeting the deadline imposed by Congress, the auto industry won several deadline extensions and a relaxed standard for NO_x emissions. In spite of much foot-dragging on the part of industry, new model automobiles can now meet federal standards and average emission levels are steadily dropping. Further declines will occur in the years ahead as stricter emission standards for new motor vehicles, mandated by the 1990 amendments, take effect. By 1996 tailpipe emissions of hydrocarbons and nitrogen oxides, both precursors of ozone formation, must be reduced by 35% and 60%, respectively, in all new cars, with a further 50% reduction in the year 2003 if conditions at that time warrant such action. Acknowledging the limitations of a strategy focused exclusively on reducing tailpipe emissions, Congress also included amendments requiring

BOX 12-3
Fighting Smog: The I/M Approach

Much of the documented improvement in urban air quality since passage of the 1970 Clean Air Act has been achieved through strict pollution controls on motor vehicles—a prime source of carbon monoxide, nitrogen oxides, ozone, volatile hydrocarbons, and lead. The device chosen by auto manufacturers to limit such emissions was the catalytic converter, installed in all non-diesel American cars since 1975. Within the catalytic converter carbon monoxide, hydrocarbons, and nitrogen oxides are burned at temperatures between 2000–3000°F and thereby converted to non-polluting water vapor and carbon dioxide. Improvements in catalytic converters over the years since they were first introduced have made these devices highly efficient; according to the Motor Vehicle Manufacturers Association, the emission control systems on late model cars have decreased CO and HC emissions by 96% and NO_x by 76% below the levels emitted by vehicles without emission controls.

Unfortunately, the theoretical air quality gains achievable if all vehicles were equipped with properly functioning catalytic converters have not been fully realized. Poor auto maintenance and illegal tampering with pollution control devices (due to the mistaken belief that catalytic converters reduce gasoline mileage and engine efficiency) has impaired the effectiveness of catalytic converters to the extent that air quality gains in many metropolitan regions are being seriously jeopardized (age also has an impact on the functioning of auto emission controls; most catalytic converters are designed to capture pollutants efficiently for only 50,000 miles—half the lifetime mileage for the average

U.S. car—and because only the newer-model catalytic converters achieve the pollution reduction efficiencies mandated by the EPA, older cars, regardless of vehicle miles traveled, emit more pollutants than newer models). Because of excessive auto emission levels, a number of metropolitan areas consistently violate the NAAQS for ozone and carbon monoxide, resulting in the threat of federal sanctions. Recognizing that just 15% of cars in the United States are responsible for 75% of troublesome emissions and that further reductions in auto-related pollutants in congested urban areas are unlikely to be achieved without strict transportation controls, Washington has pushed states to implement auto **inspection and maintenance (I/M)** programs within non-attainment areas. Such programs require motorists to bring their cars to an approved testing station where a computer-linked probe inserted into the exhaust pipe measures pollutant emissions. Many I/M programs also include a tamper inspection and require that any missing or tampered pollution control devices be replaced before a car is certified as passing the test.

Beginning in 1974 when New Jersey became the first state to institute an I/M program, the concept has spread nationwide. The 1990 Clean Air Act Amendments made what had been a strongly recommended effort mandatory by requiring all of the approximately 110 non-attainment areas in the country to begin emissions inspection programs. As a result, 55 urban areas which in 1990 had not yet instituted a testing program were ordered to do so by July of 1993. Not only did the

1990 amendments expand the geographic extent of I/M efforts, they also required that existing tests become much more stringent in those areas where the degree of ozone non-attainment is categorized as "serious," "severe," or "extreme" (as opposed to merely "moderate" or "marginal"). In the 84 metropolitan areas currently so designated, test stations will be required to install expensive new treadmills with highly sensitive computer-assisted diagnostic equipment. Such devices, to be phased in over several years beginning in July 1994, will be capable of detecting emissions violations from millions of poorly maintained cars which could slip by the less rigorous tests used formerly. EPA asserts that when the new program is operational, smog levels in many cities will be reduced by 30% and carbon monoxide by 50% or more. The cost for these anticipated air quality improvements will be borne largely by motorists whose cars fail to pass inspection; the government estimates out-of-pocket expenses to drivers for repairing a vehicle with excessive emissions could be as low as $25 (sometimes a simple engine tune-up is all that's needed) or as high as $450. If a vehicle still fails to pass inspection after the owner has spent $450 or more on repair costs, emission requirements will automatically be waived.

In spite of the fact that expanded, tougher I/M programs are likely to result in longer waits at testing stations, slightly higher fees for testing, and more costly repairs to correct violations, public reaction to the revised rules has been generally positive. Acknowledging the need to take some sort of action to deal with an obvious problem, an official with the Automobile Club of New York views tighter I/M controls as the least objectionable and most effective option. "Everybody is for cleaner air," he remarked; "this is a way for motorists to do their bit."

References

McFadden, Robert D. 1992. "Changes Seen in Urban Auto Emissions Tests." *New York Times*, Nov. 8.

Schneider, Keith. 1992. "EPA Is Proposing Strict New Testing of Auto Emissions," *New York Times*, July 14.

the use of reformulated gasoline and less-polluting alternative fuels such as ethanol, methanol, and natural gas to achieve emissions reductions (in December 1993, the Clinton Administration pleased the nation's corn producers by stipulating that at least 30% of clean-burning gasoline must be made from renewable resources, thereby giving a major boost to ethanol as opposed to petroleum-based methanol). This program was initiated in CO non-attainment areas such as Denver in 1992 and will be expanded in 1995 to include the nine cities with the most serious ozone problems (i.e. Los Angeles, San Diego, Houston, Chicago, Milwaukee, Baltimore, Philadelphia, New York, and Hartford). In addition, service stations in areas plagued by high ozone levels must install vapor recovery systems on gasoline pumps to capture hydrocarbons that would otherwise be released during refueling. The law also established a pilot program in California requiring car manufacturers to produce 150,000 clean fuel cars (presumably electric) for sale in that state by 1996; by 1999 the number

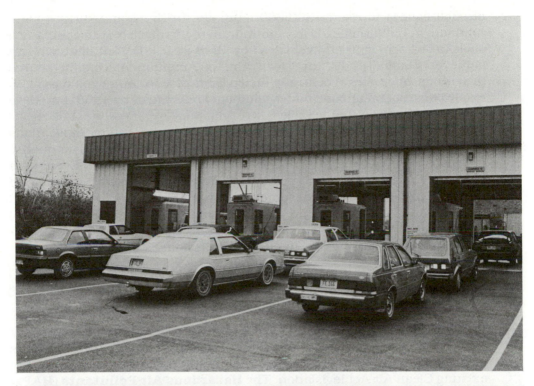

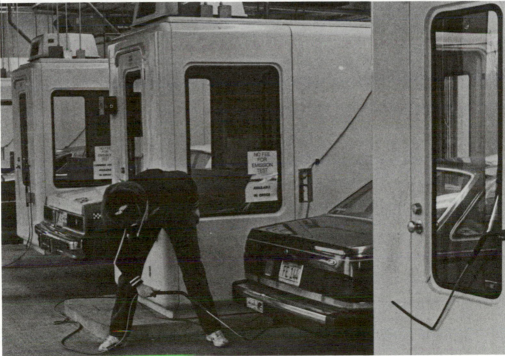

Inspection/Maintenance program: (top) vehicles await their turn for emissions testing in Chicago; (bottom) a monitor inserted into the tailpipe of an automobile measures emissions of carbon monoxide and hydrocarbons. [Illinois Environmental Protection Agency]

of such cars is to rise to 300,000 annually (in the same spirit, a state mandate in California calls for a minimum of 2% of each auto company's sales to be "zero emission vehicles" by 1998—a feat Detroit doubts it can achieve). Finally, under the Clean Air Act Amendments mobile source provisions, operators of centrally fueled fleets of 10 or more vehicles in 26 ozone or carbon monoxide non-attainment areas must, by 1998, purchase and use only clean fuel vehicles.

The success or failure of these initiatives holds important implications for the future because there is little hope of solving auto-related air quality problems solely through reliance on catalytic converters. Even with extremely strict standards for tailpipe emissions, the sheer increase in numbers of cars on the road (some experts predict this figure will exceed 600 million worldwide by the year 2000 and reach one billion by 2030) guarantees a reversal of air quality gains in the years ahead unless a radically different approach to curbing emissions is adopted.

Regulation of Hazardous Air Pollutants Through Technology-Based Controls

The requirement included in the 1990 amendments that EPA identify and set emission limitations for all major sources of any of the 189 air toxics targeted by Congress for such controls marked a major change in the existing Clean Air Act legislation. The **Hazardous Air Pollutants (HAPs)** mandate will impact thousands of manufacturing facilities and small businesses never previously affected by requirements for operating permits or emission controls. After issuing standards for HAP source categories, a task due for completion in 2000 (and already behind schedule), EPA is required to promulgate health-based standards for those chemicals believed to present a cancer risk of 1:1,000,000 exposed persons or greater. Emission reductions are to commence by 1995 and by 2003 the level of airborne toxics should be down by as much as 90% from pre-control levels. A requirement that EPA subsequently reevaluate health threats that may persist (i.e. "residual risk") after controls have been established means that publication of final emission standards may not be truly final—a further tightening of restrictions on HAP emissions may be ordered if conditions call for such action. Finally, the 1990 air toxics regulations also created an independent Chemical Safety Board, charged with investigating the cause of chemical accidents.

Acid Deposition Controls

Perhaps the most bitterly debated issue during the Clean Air Act reauthorization process was acid rain controls. Such controls became a part of federal clean air legislation only after passage of the 1990 amendments. The main focus of the new program was a mandate to cut sulfur dioxide emissions in half—a 10 million ton annual reduction from 1980 levels by the year 2000, with an interim SO_2 reduction target of 5 million tons by January 1, 1995. Nitrogen oxides, another major contributor to acid rain

BOX 12-4

Quest For Clean Air: New Approaches to an Old Problem

For the past 25 years, efforts to improve urban air quality by reducing pollutant emissions from motor vehicles have focused on increasing the efficiency of tailpipe controls (i.e. catalytic converters) and producing cleaner fuels. The degree to which these efforts have been successful is reflected in data showing that between 1981 and 1992 highway emissions of volatile organic hydrocarbons dropped by 46%, carbon monoxide by 45%, and NO_x by 25%—all at a time when the number of vehicle miles traveled (VMT) grew by more than one-third. In the years immediately ahead, technological improvements mandated by the 1990 Clean Air Act Amendments should result in even more impressive gains. Nevertheless, the continued steady increase in vehicle miles traveled, projected to grow by 2% annually for at least the next 15 years, spell trouble ahead. More vehicles on the road driving more miles translates into more pollution, even when tailpipe emissions per car are lower than ever before. EPA projects that by 2005 pollution due to motor vehicles will once again be on the upswing.

For years the standard approach to reducing pollution while simultaneously easing traffic congestion has been the promotion of alternatives to single-occupant vehicle (SOV) trips. By encouraging drivers to carpool or to use mass transit, so the argument goes, fewer cars would clog the highways and air quality would improve. Unfortunately, such efforts have met with minimal success in a society long-accustomed to the convenience and freedom of travel afforded by private autos, especially when fuel has been relatively cheap, parking inexpensive, and road use essentially free. One of the most touted alternatives, public transit, is extremely costly to build, relies heavily on subsidies for operating expenses, yet nationwide accounts for a mere 2.1% of all person-trips. Similarly, carpooling—encouraged by the provision of high-occupancy vehicle lanes and parking spaces—has met with a lukewarm response.

One factor hindering acceptance of these conventional travel alternatives is their focus on home-to-work travel at a time when non-work trips or "chained" trips from home to daycare to work to shopping areas, etc., are the fastest-growing category of travel. In addition, the movement of jobs out of the central city areas to scattered suburban locations makes it difficult for commuters to be well-served by alternatives to the single-occupant car. With statistics showing that over 20% of all U.S. households today have three or more cars, it is clear that automobiles continue to dominate American transportation decisions.

Seeking a radically different approach to achieving air quality improvements and reducing traffic congestion, some observers propose a number of innovative strategies to **manage transportation demand**, utilizing pricing incentives or disincentives rather than, or in addition to, regulation as a means of influencing driving decisions. Advocates of this approach point out that pricing, unlike regulation, applies uniformly to all categories of drivers and trips, giving all drivers, not just workday commuters, incentive to change travel behavior. Pricing strategies leave decision-making as to the value of a given trip up to the individual driver—people who would be inconvenienced by forgoing use of a car need not do so if they are prepared to pay the additional cost their decision entails. Among the proposals receiving serious consideration are the following:

1. **feebates**—Intended to affect new car purchasing decisions, feebates could be applied as either a credit or a surcharge on the sales tax or vehicle registration fee at the time a vehicle is bought. The size of the credit or surcharge would depend on such parameters as the amount of criteria pollutant emissions, greenhouse gas emissions (CO_2), or fuel economy of the car in question. The feebate approach would generate consumer demands that manufacturers produce cleaner, more fuel-efficient automobiles.

2. **scrappage**—Based on evidence that older cars are responsible for a disproportionate share of pollutant emissions, programs such as the "Cash for Clunkers" effort promoted recently by the Illinois EPA offer monetary incentives to get aging, high-emitting vehicles off the road. Proponents have argued that companies confronted with regulatory requirements to reduce overall emissions might find it more cost-effective to provide employees with new, catalytic converter-equipped cars while scrapping their old vehicles, rather than invest in multi-million dollar smokestack controls. In the short term, scrappage programs may bring some air quality benefits, but analyses suggest the gains may be shortlived, since most of the scrapped cars would have been off the road soon regardless, due to inevitable fleet turnover.

3. **VMT tax**—Based on odometer readings taken during annual registration or I/M checks, a tax on vehicle miles traveled could be a strong incentive for drivers to eliminate unnecessary trips. If combined with the results of I/M emissions testing, the tax per mile could be adjusted up or down, depending on the vehicle's emissions profile, thus providing a double incentive to drive less and minimize pollutant emissions.

4. **congestion pricing**—Just as electric utilities, telephone companies, and airlines charge higher rates for using their services during peak hours, so could differential fees be assessed for highway use during peak and off-peak hours. Already new technologies are making it possible to collect such fees effectively and inexpensively. An example of one such method is currently being used on the Oklahoma Turnpike where cars and trucks equipped with a small transponder can choose to pay tolls electronically. In 1993 the nation's first "smart card" system, which automatically charges the driver's account as he/she passes a tolling area, was installed by AT&T in Orange County, California. Such schemes can encourage motorists to defer trips to off-peak hours, or to use mass transit or other alternatives.

5. **cash-out tax subsidies for employer-paid parking**—Free parking provided by employers for their work force is a powerful disincentive to the use of public transit or other travel options. Income tax laws treat free parking as a fringe benefit, excluding its value (which may be as high as $155 per month) from employees' taxable income. Some authorities have proposed changing the tax codes to require that employers offer their employees a choice between continuing to receive free parking or the market value of that parking as cash-in-hand. The assumption is that many, if not most, employees would choose the cash payment and would find alternative, less polluting ways of traveling to work.

While few of the options just described have yet been implemented, they have prompted considerable discussion among policymakers at the state and federal level. As a market-based approach to tackling environmental problems continues to gain favor, the use of pricing strategies to influence driving decisions becomes increasingly likely.

Reference

Kessler, Jon, and William Schroeer. 1993. *Meeting Mobility and Air Quality Goals: Strategies that Work*. USEPA, Office of Policy Analysis (Oct. 13).

formation, are targeted for emission reductions of 2 million tons annually, based on 1980 emission levels. A novel feature of the acid deposition regulations that is attracting widespread interest and attention is a market-oriented system of emissions allowances that utilities can buy, sell, or trade to help finance the costs of pollution controls (see Box 12-5).

The provisions described here represent only the highlights of this extremely complex piece of legislation. Responsibility for implementing and enforcing the federal mandate falls primarily on the environmental agencies of state government, which must develop **State Implementation Plans (SIPs)**, detailing strategies for compliance with Clean Air Act requirements. SIPs must list all the pollution sources within the state, estimating the quantities of each pollutant emitted annually, including both mobile and stationary sources. They must issue operating permits for stationary sources, as well as timetables for compliance, and must include some kind of transportation control strategy for dealing with auto-related pollutants in areas of heavy traffic. States must have their SIPs approved by the federal EPA or be working with the Agency to improve a conditionally approved plan before they can issue a construction permit for any new polluting facility.

Enforcement provisions under the Clean Air Act, and the civil and criminal penalties for violation of the law, were significantly strengthened under the 1990 amendments. EPA can levy large financial penalties against facilities in violation of air quality requirements—penalties sufficiently stiff to cancel any economic benefits a firm might derive from delaying compliance. Criminal liability, which may be imposed on persons *knowingly* violating the law, can result in fines, imprisonment, or both. The Clean Air Act gives citizens the right to file suit against polluters if the EPA fails to take action. To encourage "whistle-blowing" by persons aware of Clean Air Act violations, Congress has authorized EPA to pay informants up to $10,000 for information leading to a civil penalty or criminal conviction (Bryner, 1993; "Easy Guide," 1993; *Environmental Law Handbook, 1993*).

Global Air Quality Trends

Deadline dates have come and gone, hot summers are punctuated with ozone alerts, and a haze of smog still hovers over many of our cities. Nevertheless, nearly a quarter century after the Clean Air Act ushered in a "get tough" approach regarding air pollution control, overall trends in American skies are favorable. Elsewhere in the world, progress in cleaning up dirty air varies considerably from one country to another.

A comprehensive assessment of international air quality trends is complicated by the fact that scarcely any routine monitoring of air quality has been conducted in the developing nations that comprise the bulk of world population. Anecdotal information suggests that pollution levels in Third World cities are far higher than in most industrialized countries—

and getting steadily worse. Problems appear especially serious in terms of particulate pollution, known to have the most serious adverse health impact of all air contaminants. A report issued by the World Health Organization (WHO) estimates that 70% of the entire world population, primarily residents of developing nations, breathe air that contains health-threatening levels of particulates. Concentrations of sulfur dioxide, another pollutant known as a respiratory irritant and a precursor of acid rain, are increasing dramatically in a number of developing nations, as well as in Russia and eastern Europe, as plentiful supplies of sulfur-laden coal are burned without pollution controls. Reports from China indicated a steady rise in SO_2 levels throughout the 1980s; in cities such as Beijing, Xian, and Guangzhou, SO_2 readings all exceeded WHO guidelines; residents of other Third World metropoli such as Manila, São Paulo, and Tehran similarly suffer unhealthy levels of exposure to SO_2. Acid rain, a consequence of SO_2 and NO_x pollution, is no longer confined to western Europe and North America where the phenomenon was first described; China is experiencing serious problems of acid deposition downwind of its manufacturing centers, while in remote areas of Africa, investigators are reporting levels of acid rain and smog equivalent to those in the industrial wastelands of central Europe, possibly owing to regular burning of vast areas of the savanna by herders and farmers.

Auto-related pollutants are also mounting rapidly in Third World cities as car ownership becomes synonymous with "the good life." Few developing nations require that vehicles be equipped with emission controls and the vast majority continue to sell leaded gasoline. A similar situation prevails in eastern Europe and the former Soviet Union. The fact that many of the vehicles on the road are old and poorly maintained—and frequently fueled with adulterated gasoline—ensures choking levels of pollutant emissions that can scarcely be imagined by motorists in Los Angeles or London.

In contrast with the downward trends in air quality evident in many developing countries, in parts of the industrialized world emission levels from both stationary sources and motor vehicles have been drastically cut in recent years. While the United States was the pace-setter in air pollution control initiatives until the early 1980s, more recently several European nations and Japan have equalled or surpassed the American record. Since the 1970s, levels of SO_2 have fallen by more than 60% in Sweden, Switzerland, Austria, and Germany. Japan requires state-of-the-art controls on automobiles, incinerators, power plants, and steel mills and is the only country in the world that compensates victims of air pollution—deriving monies for those so injured from a tax on SO_2 emissions. The Canadian province of Ontario has an ambient air standard for SO_2 considerably more stringent than that of the United States. Germany, jolted out of complacency in the early 1980s by reports of widespread forest damage due to acid rain, since 1983 has implemented one of the world's most vigorous air quality control programs. Unlike the situation in the United States, where power plants in operation prior to promulgation of New Source Performance Standards were exempted from the requirement for the best available technological controls, Germany has mandated the

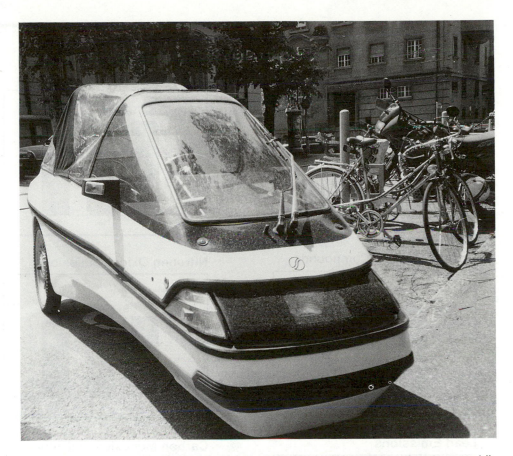

The "mini-el" is an electric car currently being used in Switzerland, where automobile emissions levels have been drastically reduced in recent years. [Markus Schefer]

retrofitting of all its medium and large-size power plants, regardless of age, with state-of-the-art pollution control devices. The Swiss and Austrians, similarly concerned about dying forests, have adopted what may be the most stringent air quality regulations in the world, setting emission standards even for motorcycles!

The trend toward tighter controls on mobile sources has been relatively recent outside the United States. In 1980 Japan was the only other country with strict requirements for automobiles. Within a decade, however, all major industrialized nations, with the exception of Russia and the eastern European countries, were regulating tailpipe emissions, many of them with standards equivalent to those in America. Several developing nations—Mexico, Brazil, Taiwan, and South Korea—also have adopted U.S. emission standards (World Resources Institute, 1990).

In the United States, air quality in most parts of the country has improved significantly since passage of the Clean Air Act. In spite of population growth, increased traffic volume, and continued industrial development, emissions of most pollutants have declined and the number of days rated as "unhealthy" has dropped dramatically since the 1970s.

Figure 12-5 U.S. Air Pollution Trends, 1970–90

Total Particulates

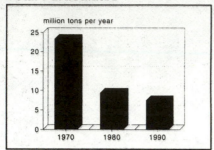

Sulfur Dioxide Emissions

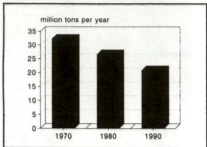

Volatile Organic Compounds

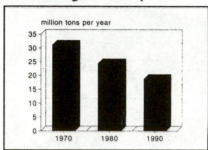

Nitrogen Oxides Emissions

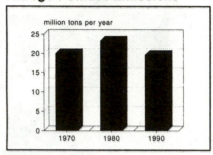

Lead Emissions

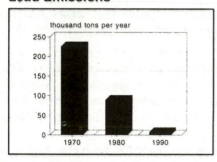

Carbon Monoxide Emissions

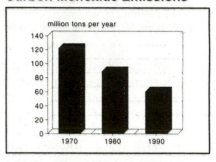

Source: U.S. Environmental Protection Agency, *National Air Quality and Emissions Trends Report*, 1990.

Progress in cleaning up the nation's air has not been uniform—concentrations of some pollutants have declined more than others and some regions of the country have experienced air quality trends better or worse than national averages would indicate. Of the criteria air pollutants, since 1970 ambient levels of lead have dropped by a precipitous 97%, but nitrogen oxides have actually risen slightly due to increased fossil fuel combustion. Emissions of particulates, SO_2, CO, and the volatile organic compounds that contribute to ozone formation have all declined measurably since passage of the Clean Air Act. An indirect indication of progress in reducing CO emissions, due primarily to improvements in automobile control systems, is the sharp drop in accidental carbon monoxide fatalities, over 80% of which are caused by inhalation of car exhausts. Since the number of people, the number of cars, and the amount of fuel consumed are all increasing, it would be logical to expect the number of auto-associated CO poisonings to increase as well. However, the reverse has been the case. In 1979, accidental CO-related fatalities in the United States totalled 1,513—a number that dropped steadily to 878 in 1988. Researchers attribute this welcome news to the fact that catalytic converters have achieved CO emission reductions of more than 90% over levels prevailing prior to imposition of pollution controls (CO in the ambient air fell by 28% during this period, in spite of a 39% increase in vehicle miles traveled). As a consequence, it now takes much longer for CO emissions from a car left idling in an enclosed space to reach life-threatening concentrations (Cobb and Etzel, 1991).

However, levels of the criteria pollutants in a number of urban areas still remain high enough to endanger the health of their residents. In 1990 the EPA reported that at least 74 million Americans lived in areas that regularly exceed the NAAQS for at least one criteria pollutant and as many as 140 million—more than half the U.S. population—were resident in areas where ozone (i.e. smog) levels had violated national standards at least once during that year. The latter figure emphasizes the fact that ozone, and, to a lesser extent, carbon monoxide, remains our most troublesome pollutant in terms of numbers of people affected. In fact, a 1991 report issued by the National Academy of Sciences suggests that tropospheric ozone concentrations have actually been increasing over extensive regions of the United States (unfortunately, for those who question why we don't solve the ozone layer depletion problem by pumping excess ground-level ozone up into the stratosphere, it can't be done!). It is likely that in the years immediately ahead there will be much more aggressive efforts to tighten controls for nitrogen oxides, whose emissions appear to be more important contributors to ozone formation than previously realized, while continuing to expand controls over a wide range of formerly unregulated sources of VOCs such as dry cleaning establishments, furniture refinishers, auto body shops—and possibly even consumer items such as charcoal lighter fuel, spray starch, and power lawn mowers! Of all regions of the United States, the Los Angeles area will be most heavily impacted by stricter air quality regulations. A non-attainment area for four of the six criteria pollutants, southern California is in violation of the NAAQS more frequently than New York, Houston, Chicago, Denver, and Pittsburgh (other non-attainment areas) combined. Although present ozone levels in Los Angeles are only one-quarter of the choking, eye-watering levels prevailing in the mid-1950s, they still must be cut by half to comply with existing standards. As a result, California has adopted the toughest, most aggressive air quality regulations in the nation—some of which are now being copied by several northeastern states grappling with smog problems of their own.

In spite of these remaining challenges, air quality trends in the United States are generally encouraging. While declining levels of pollutant emissions are due in some measure to energy conservation, fuel-switching, and the demise of many smokestack industries, a large share of the credit must be given to the regulatory programs that have mandated significant investment in pollution control technologies. Although the battle to control air pollution is by no means over, progress to date proves that the Clean Air Act is working.

Acid Deposition

An air quality problem virtually unrecognized and unmentioned at the time the 1970 Clean Air Act was passed, the issue of acid deposition (commonly referred to in popular jargon as "acid rain," though the phenomenon includes not only rain but also snow, fog, dry SO_2 and NO_2 gas, and sulfate and nitrate aerosols) became political dynamite during the 1980s, pitting region against region, nation against nation. Although the domestic policy battles generated by the debate over acid rain controls were largely resolved by key provisions of the 1990 Clean Air Act Amendments, the problem itself persists and the damage toll continues to climb. Nor are all the facts concerning acid deposition completely understood even today. To comprehend what the fuss is all about requires a brief look at the nature of acid deposition, how it is formed, and the types of damage it causes.

What Is Acid Deposition?

Rainfall by nature is slightly acidic due to its tendency to react chemically with atmospheric CO_2, thereby forming a weak solution of carbonic acid. Thus while distilled water has a pH value of 7.0, a pH of 5.6 is considered normal for natural, unpolluted rain. Thus, by definition, any precipitation measuring less than 5.6 on the pH scale is considered acid deposition (some researchers who have been measuring pH levels in remote areas far from sources of industrial emissions suggest that the pH of unpolluted rain is closer to 5.0 than 5.6 and advocate a downward revision of what level of rainfall acidity should be considered "normal"). Since the pH scale is logarithmic, rainfall with a pH of 4.0 is ten times more acid than precipitation with a pH of 5.0 and 100 times more acid than that of pH 6. The below-2.0 reading recorded during a three-day drizzle in the fall of 1978 at Wheeling, West Virginia, represented a level 10,000 times more acid than unpolluted rainfall.

Extent of the Problem

Acid precipitation has been observed as a local phenomenon in the vicinity of coal-burning facilities for more than a century. In fact, the term "acid rain" was first coined by an English chemist, Robert Angus Smith, to describe the corrosive brew falling on industrial Manchester more than 100 years ago. Only recently, however, has acid rain emerged as a regional problem, affecting areas far from the source of pollutant emissions. The alarm was first raised in 1972 by Swedish delegates attending the U.N.

Conference on the Human Environment in Stockholm. After initial disbelief by many national governments, Swedish views about the extent and seriousness of this newly recognized environmental threat have become widely accepted. On the basis of measurements taken during the past few decades, scientists believe that the pH of rainfall has been gradually dropping throughout large areas of both North America and Europe. Not only is rainfall becoming more acid in the affected areas, but the geographical extent of the problem is widening also. Early measurements of rainfall pH indicated that in the years 1955–1956 only 12 northeastern states were experiencing acid precipitation. By 1972–1973 the number of states experiencing average rainfall acidity below pH 5.6 extended over the entire eastern portion of North America, except for the southern tip of Florida and the far northern regions of Canada. In addition, acid rain was detected in several of the major urban areas of California and in the Rocky Mountain region of Colorado.

Today the pH of rainfall averages 5.0 or less throughout the United States east of the Mississippi River, with substantially lower readings being obtained during some individual storm episodes. However, encouraging news was reported recently by scientists working for the U.S. Geological Survey who documented a steady drop in the concentrations of acid-forming sulfates in precipitation from 1980–1991, with a corresponding rise in the pH or rainfall during that time period. Such field data are hailed as evidence that pollution control technologies aimed at curbing SO_2 emissions are having the intended impact. Unfortunately, USGS monitoring stations have not seen an equivalent decline in rainfall nitrate concentrations, nor has a nearly 35-year trend toward increasing acidification of waterways been reversed. Indeed, in the streams being monitored, pH levels have continued to fall year after year (Hilchey, 1993).

Beyond North America, acid deposition today also affects most countries of Europe and has recently been identified as a serious environmental concern in the rapidly industrializing southern provinces of China; Japan also has reported problems of acid rain. Indeed, although extensive monitoring has not been done outside North America and Europe, it is assumed that acid rain is a problem everywhere that coal and oil are intensively used (Rodhe, 1989; "Evidence of Acid Fog," 1989).

Mystery of the Dying Lakes

During the 1960s and 1970s anglers, campers, and resort owners raised the first alarms concerning what was to become a major environmental tragedy. From the sparkling lakes of the remote Adirondacks, to the popular vacationlands of Ontario and Quebec, to the waterways of Scandinavia, reports of the mysterious disappearance of once-abundant fish, amphibians, and aquatic insects began to generate public concern. The fact that such lakes and streams were far from any of the usual sources of water pollution which have traditionally been associated with fish kills only increased the bewilderment. To a casual observer the water remained blue and clear, uncontaminated by chemical spills or sewage overflows;

beneath the surface, however, the affected lakes had become watery deserts, devoid of life. Today in the Adirondacks alone, 280 lakes once renowned for their trout fishing are devoid of fish; 2600 lakes in Minnesota's Boundary Waters Canoe Area are on the brink of suffering the same fate; in Canada 140 Ontario lakes are now fishless and the expectation is that within 20 years another 48,500 will be dead; 10,000 Scandinavian lakes no longer contain any fish and another 10,000 are threatened. Such lakes are acid dead, poisoned by pollutants falling from the sky in the form of sulfuric and nitric acid.

Formation of Acid Rain

Acid precipitation forms when its major precursors, sulfur dioxide and nitrogen dioxide, are chemically converted through a complex series of reactions involving certain reactive hydrocarbons and oxidizing agents such as ozone to become sulfuric or nitric acid. The reactions involved can take place either within clouds or rain droplets, in the gas phase, on the surface of fine particulates in the air, or on soil or water surfaces after deposition (Rhodes and Middleton, 1983).

Sulfur dioxide, one of the two pollutants primarily responsible for acid rain formation, is discharged into the atmosphere in amounts averaging 30 million tons annually in the United States. Of this amount, approximately two-thirds originates from coal- and oil-burning power plants; the remainder is primarily from smelters and industrial boilers. A certain amount of SO_2 enters the atmosphere from natural sources such as volcanoes or mud flats, but such emissions contribute relatively little to the problem of acid rain; it is estimated that in the northeastern U.S. 90% of the sulfur in the air comes from human sources of pollution.

Nitrogen oxides, of which about 20 million tons per year are currently emitted in the United States, come predominantly from auto emissions, power plants, and industry. NO_x emissions have declined by only about 6% since 1978, considerably less than reductions achieved for SO_2. Some observers worry that soon after the turn of the century, NO_x levels will once again begin to climb as the automobile fleet continues to grow and as new factories and power plants come on line. Until recently, SO_2 emissions have widely been perceived as posing a more serious problem that NO_x in terms of acid rain formation; however, as technological controls are increasingly successful at reducing levels of airborne sulfur compounds, the role of nitrogen oxides as acid rain precursors will grow in importance (Hilchey, 1993).

Long-Distance Transport

The aspect of acid rainfall that makes it such a politically charged issue is the fact that the pollutant emissions that are the precursors of acid rain formation may be produced hundreds of miles from the regions suffering the effects of acid deposition. Because some pollutants can remain in the air for a relatively long period of time, they can be carried on the prevailing winds across geographical and political boundaries far from their place of origin—a phenomenon known as long-distance transport. There are documented examples of acid rain-forming pollutants being carried more than 600 miles before being deposited on the earth's surface.

Ironically, pollution control technologies adopted early in the 1970s to reduce *local* levels of ambient air pollution had the unintended effect of increasing the long-distance transport problem. The approach adopted most often by utilities striving to lower SO_2 concentrations in the vicinity of their plants was to pursue a **tall stack strategy**; that is, to build extremely tall "superstacks" that discharged pollutant gases into the persistent air currents more than 500 feet above the ground. This approach was indeed effective in reducing local pollution levels, but it promoted long-distance transport and thereby increased the range and severity of acid deposition in regions downwind. Until the 1990 Clean Air Act Amendments committed the United States to aggressive acid rain control efforts, relations between Canada and the United States were seriously strained because half of the corrosive rain falling over southeastern Canada originates in the heavily industrialized Ohio River Valley and upper Midwest. New York and the New England states harbored a similar grudge against Illinois, Indiana, and Ohio—the source of fully one-fourth of all U.S. sulfur emissions. In the same way, the acid rain currently wreaking havoc on lakes and forests in Norway and Sweden is produced primarily in central Europe and Great Britain. Such circumstances make the formulation of acid rain control policies politically difficult because those bearing the cost of pollution abatement strategies and those reaping the benefits are not one and the

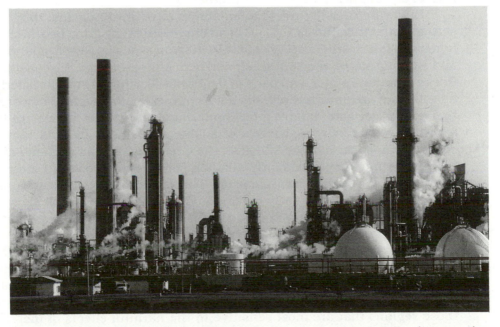

Tall smokestacks are effective in reducing local levels of pollutant gases, however they contribute to the long-distance transport problem. [Thomas A. Schneider]

same. Effective action toward resolving this dilemma was taken first in Europe where 35 countries in 1979 signed the **Convention on Long-Range Transboundary Air Pollution**, an agreement requiring the signatory nations to achieve a 30% reduction in SO_2 emissions from 1980 levels by 1993. Targets have subsequently been set for reducing NO_x and VOC emissions as well. In the United States, the acid rain debate raged in Congress for years. Legislators from the Midwest were nearly unanimous in their opposition to proposed federal rules that would impose more stringent sulfur emission controls on coal-burning power plants in their region. Citing the financial burden that would be passed along to electric consumers and the inherent threat controls would pose to coal-mining interests in states like Illinois and West Virginia, Midwestern representatives were acutely aware that the environmental gains achieved by tougher regulations would be enjoyed by citizens outside their own constituencies. Conversely, legislators from such states as New Hampshire and Maine, areas that had few large sources of emissions yet were suffering severe economic and ecological damage due to acid rain, were among the most vocal in demanding regulatory action.

Regional Vulnerability to Acid Rain

Although the entire eastern United States is now experiencing acid rainfall, not all areas are suffering adverse ecological effects. An ecosystem's sensitivity to acid precipitation is determined primarily by the chemical composition of the soil and bedrock—an attribute referred to as the **buffering capacity** of that environment.

Buffering capacity refers to an ability to neutralize acids, the buffer acting to maintain the natural pH of an environment by tying up the excess hydrogen ions introduced by acid rain. Regions such as New England, the Mid-Atlantic states, the Southeast, northern Minnesota and Wisconsin, the Rocky Mountain states, and parts of the Pacific Northwest are characterized by soils that are naturally already acidic or underlain by granitic bedrock; these areas are said to have a low buffering capacity and hence are very sensitive to the increased levels of acidity introduced by acid rain. By contrast, most parts of the Midwest, the Great Plains, and portions of the Southwest have predominantly alkaline soils and bedrock of limestone, giving them a high buffering capacity. This fact explains why a state such as Illinois, which is currently experiencing rainfall almost as acid as that falling in New York or New England is not suffering comparable ecological damage. Nevertheless, such apparent invulnerability is not guaranteed to last forever. Over time, a given soil's buffering capacity can be overwhelmed by continual acid inputs, a phenomenon that seems to be occurring already in parts of the upper Midwest. It seems a cruel twist of fate that prevailing wind currents are transporting acid rain-forming pollutants to precisely those regions that are most sensitive to the harmful effects of increased acidification.

Figure 12-6 Areas Sensitive to Acid Deposition

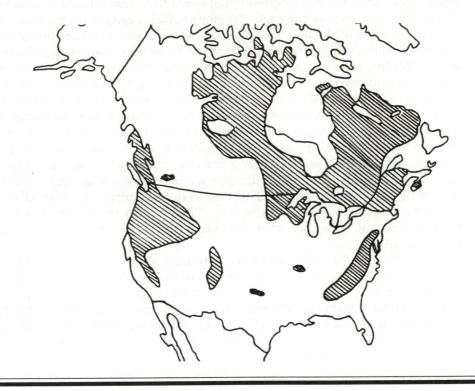

Environmental Effects of Acid Rain

Acid precipitation can cause a number of adverse environmental changes, the best-understood of which include the following.

Damage to Aquatic Ecosystems.   That acid rain can decimate the biotic communities inhabiting lakes, ponds, and streams in those regions where natural buffering capacity is low has been well documented in numerous studies. Most freshwater organisms do best in waters that are slightly alkaline—about pH 8. As lakes gradually become acidified due to steady inputs of acid rain, one aquatic species after another disappears. The first affected are the tiny invertebrates that constitute a vital link in aquatic food chains; at pH 6.0 the freshwater shrimp are eliminated; at pH 5.5 the bacterial decomposers at the lake bottom begin to die off, as do the phytoplankton, the producer organisms in aquatic ecosystems. Fish populations, the subject of most human attention, are somewhat more tolerant to increasing acidity; little change in their numbers is noticed until the pH drops below 5.5. Under pH 4.5 all fish species disappear, as do most frogs, salamanders, and aquatic insects ("Acid Rain," 1982).

Interestingly, falling pH levels seldom kill adult fish directly. The primary cause of fish de-population is acid-induced reproductive failure; pH values below 5.5 can prevent female fish from laying their eggs, and those eggs which are laid frequently fail to hatch or result in the production of deformed fry (just as the early developmental stages of humans are the most vulnerable to the adverse influence of environmental contaminants, the same holds true for the larval stages of lower organisms). Interference with hatching is accentuated by the fact that the most critical developmental period usually coincides with the time of the annual snow melt when several months' accumulation of acid suddenly inundates the spawning areas in one massive dose, a situation known as **shock loading**. This large-scale reproductive failure leads to a situation in some lakes where the older fish grow larger and larger, thanks to decreased competition for food, and anglers boast of their excellent catches until, with further increases in acidity, all the fish disappear. As a professor at the University of Toronto succinctly states: "There is no muss, there is no fuss, there is no smell. The fish quietly go extinct . . . They simply fail to reproduce and become less and less abundant, and older and older, until they die out" (Weller, 1980).

At one time it was assumed that acid rain's impact on aquatic environments was limited to freshwater ecosystems. In 1988, however, this assumption was shattered by a report published by the Environmental Defense Fund, a nonprofit environmental organization, documenting acid rain-induced eutrophication of Chesapeake Bay. EDF cited evidence showing that nitrates entering the bay through acid precipitation were as important as farmland fertilizer runoff in stimulating the algal blooms which are degrading water quality in that important saltwater estuary.

Mobilization of Toxic Metals.   Contact with acidified water can cause tightly bound toxic metals such as aluminum, manganese, lead, zinc, mercury, and cadmium to dissolve out of bottom sediments or soils and leach into the aquatic environment. Such metals, especially aluminum, can kill fish by damaging their gills, thereby causing asphyxiation. Acid-induced release of aluminum, even at concentrations as low as 0.2 mg/L, has resulted in fish kills at water pH levels which wouldn't have been lethal in the absence of the toxic metal. Toxic metals in the water also can bioaccumulate in fish tissues, making them dangerous for humans to eat.

Mobilization of poisonous metals also presents a direct threat to human health if the acidified lakes are a source of drinking water supplies. A resort owner from the Adirondacks testified before a congressional committee that, in response to his children's complaints about the taste of water piped to their lodge, he had the water tested and found it contained 5 times the safe level for lead and 10 times that for copper. In other communities, acidified water that was originally free of toxic metals became contaminated upon passing through lead or copper plumbing systems—the low pH of the water caused corrosion of the pipes, resulting in leaching of toxic metals into the water. Homeowners who obtain their drinking water from roof catchments in areas affected by acid rain are also at special risk (Boyle and Boyle, 1983).

Deterioration of Buildings, Statuary, and Metals.   While it is extremely difficult to assign a precise monetary value to the impact of acid rain on materials, it is nevertheless acknowledged that the scope of the damage is large indeed. Most pronounced are the effects of acid deposition on stone and metal buildings and statues, on textiles, leather, and paint, and to some extent on paper and glass. Many monuments of great historic and cultural significance are today slowly disintegrating under the impact of airborne pollutants, of which various sulfur compounds are by far the most important. Corroding surfaces of the Statue of Liberty, the Washington Monument, the Capitol Building in Washington, D.C., Canada's Parliament buildings in Ottawa, and the Field Museum in Chicago all give evidence of the ravages produced by acid rain (Scholle, 1983).

Reduction of Crop Yields.   The extent of acid rain damage to field crops is less clear-cut than with other types of acid-induced environmental damage, partly because few studies were conducted prior to 1979 and research on this topic is still considered somewhat ambiguous. Preliminary results indicate a wide range of responses, depending on the particular crop variety in question. Yields of some species appear to be diminished by acid rain, some are stimulated, while others show no change as pH levels of rainfall drop (Cohen, Grothaus, and Perrigan, 1982). Since even slight reductions in yield can have a profound impact on farm economics, more research on acid rain and crop yields is urgently needed.

Damage to Forest Productivity.   From the wooded slopes of the Adirondacks to the forests of central Europe and Scandinavia, acid-laden rain and fog are contributing to death and reduced growth rates among an ever-increasing number of important tree species. Most affected are conifer forests at high elevations, frequently shrouded in acid fog or mist. At many sites above 850 meters in the White Mountains of New Hampshire or the Green Mountains of Vermont, over half the red spruce have died since the early 1960s. In Germany, the rate at which wide areas of forest have been similarly affected just since the early 1980s has been so dramatic that distraught German scientists have coined a word for the phenomenon—*waldsterben* ("forest death"). By 1989 German scientists were estimating that more than half the trees in the country were suffering some degree of defoliation. Fortunately, in the last few years the rate of forest decline in Germany appears to be slackening, possibly in response to the aggressive pollution control policies enacted specifically for that purpose in 1983. The situation looks less hopeful for Germany's central European neighbors, whose forests are dying at an alarming rate. In the Czech Republic and Poland over a third of all forests are moderately or severely affected (75% of Polish trees show some signs of damage); more than 60% of the conifers in Lithuania are ailing—and the situation is worsening annually. One analysis published in 1990 calculated that three-fourths of European commercial forests were experiencing damage caused by sulfur deposition and 60% were receiving more nitrogen than they could assimilate without harm; this pollution-induced damage was estimated to cost the European

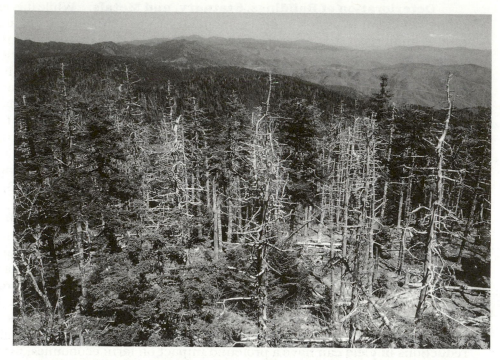

Hundreds of balsam fir trees have been killed or damaged by acid deposition on this mountain ridge in the Great Smoky Mountains National Park. [Thomas A. Schneider]

forest industry approximately $30 billion each year (World Resources Institute, 1992).

The extent to which acid rain can be blamed for the decline of forests on two continents is currently a subject of intensive investigation by scientists in Europe and North America. In some cases acid rain causes direct damage to leaves, resulting in nutrients being lost from foliage faster than they can be replaced by root absorption. This phenomenon is particularly associated with the acid fog which commonly occurs on ridgetops and it is further enhanced by the presence of ozone. With a pH as low as 2.2, acid fog and clouds with high ozone content are blamed for much of the damage apparent in the red spruce forests at higher elevations. For the most part, however, it appears that acid rain's role in the forest decline drama is less direct. The increasing acidity of soils due to years of acid deposition has led to more rapid leaching of essential plant nutrients—calcium, potassium, magnesium—and has also increased the solubility and migration of aluminum which acts as a poison to the fine root hairs most directly responsible for nutrient uptake. Excess deposition of nitrogen (some European forests are now receiving four to eight times more than they need) is over-stimulating plant growth and worsening nutrient deficiencies. The additional impact of ozone, which in areas such as the mixed broadleaf forests of the Appalachian Mountain region may occur at concentrations three times higher than the estimated tolerance level, may be the final environmental insult leading to premature forest death. It is theorized that the interaction of all these factors has undermined the natural resistance to disease and insect attack that formerly ensured the health and sustained viability of these biotic communities. Whatever the final verdict on the cause of the problem, the extent and severity of forest damage now so apparent has increased environmentalists' conviction that we must act now to control acid rain while there are still trees left to save (Flynn, 1994).

Acid Rain Controls

Throughout the 1980s a growing awareness of the extent and severity of the acid rain problem has led to increasingly vociferous public demands to "Stop Acid Rain!" through regulatory action, primarily in the form of laws requiring stringent pollution controls on coal-burning power plants. Passage of the 1990 Clean Air Act Amendments, containing the strong acid rain control provisions previously discussed, ended nearly a decade of vituperative debate. The innovative market mechanism devised to make the requirements more financially feasible for the affected utilities (see Box 12–5), permits polluters to choose among numerous technological options for meeting mandated emission limits.

BOX 12-5

Marketing Pollution

No longer are the commodities being bought and sold amidst the pandemonium at the Chicago Board of Trade restricted to such mundane items as soybean futures or pork bellies. Thanks to the revolutionary new concept known as **allowance trading** created by the 1990 Clean Air Act Amendments, utility companies can now broker government-assigned allowances for SO_2 emissions in an innovative attempt to make acid rain controls more effective and affordable. First proposed by the Environmental Defense Fund, the idea of allowance trading was welcomed by legislators as a means of breaking congressional gridlock over who should pay for rescuing acid-threatened lakes and forests. Now in the early stages of implementation, this novel market-based approach to environmental cleanup is being followed with intense interest by government regulators here and abroad; if successful, the use of marketplace incentives to finance pollution cleanup is likely to expand far beyond its current focus on acid rain.

Under the strategy devised by Clean Air Act negotiators, EPA will shelve its traditional regulatory approach that requires polluters to install controls on each piece of equipment. Instead, the agency has been directed to set enforceable limits on the amount of sulfur dioxide that power plants can emit each year and to assign these plants a designated number of emission "allowances." For each allowance granted, the recipient is permitted to discharge one ton of SO_2 annually (the number of allowances assigned to each facility is determined by a complex formula and is specified in the plant's operating permit). The emission limits imposed on individual plants must collectively correspond with the congressionally-mandated 10 million ton annual reduction in SO_2 emissions nationwide required by the Clean Air Act to be achieved by the year 2000. Utilities can subsequently adopt any pollution reduction strategy they wish in order to achieve the mandated reductions. A plant's annual emissions cannot exceed the allowances allocated to it for that calendar year— *unless the utility purchases surplus allowances at market rates from another plant whose emissions were below the designated limit.*

The beauty of allowance trading is that it encourages polluting facilities not merely to reduce emissions to the legal limit, but to cut them as low as possible, thereby accumulating unused emissions allowances which can then be sold, at a profit, to another power plant. Thus utilities which choose to install newer, cleaner technologies and make efforts to find the most cost-efficient means of reducing pollutant emissions can help cover the cost of their investment by selling surplus allowances to those facilities—usually older, dirtier plants—for which the cost of installing new equipment substantially exceeds that of purchasing another company's pollution credits. Since the value of one allowance is expected to range between $500–$700, while the EPA-imposed penalty for exceeding allowance allocations is $2000/ton, it is obviously cheaper for utilities to purchase extra allowances than to pollute the air.

Proponents of emissions trading are convinced this market approach will significantly reduce the cost of complying with the Clean Air Act's acid rain provisions because some facilities are inherently cheaper to clean up than others. While some critics complain that emissions trading is promoting the "right to pollute," on a nationwide basis the same amount of SO_2 will be removed from the air, thus achieving Clean Air Act goals but at a substan-

tially lower dollar cost than would be possible under the old "command-and-control" regimen.

While the federal program is just now getting underway (Phase I, targeting 110 of the dirtiest power plants, all in the eastern half of the U.S., requires compliance with specified emissions reductions by January 1995), Los Angeles has seized the emissions trading concept and carried it beyond the acid rain arena, applying the strategy to a broad-based smog control effort. Early in 1994 the South Coast Air Quality Management District (AQMD) launched its RECLAIM program (Regional Clean Air Incentive Market), focusing on 390 of the Los Angeles area's biggest polluters—companies that emit in excess of four tons of smog-generating NO_x or SO_2 each year. AQMD will set annual emission limits on the amounts of these pollutants for each company, limits that will be reduced 5–8% annually through the year 2003. As in the federal program, buying and selling of pollution credits will be a key feature of RECLAIM, with anticipated pollution control savings of $58 million.

Three thousand miles to the east, in the first such interstate agreement, New Jersey and Connecticut agreed early in 1994 to experiment with pollution credits in a deal whereby a New Jersey utility, Public Service Electric and Gas, will cut its emissions of nitrogen dioxide by 2,400 tons more than required under the Clean Air Act over the next five years and sell its pollution rights to Northeast Utilities, a Connecticut-based company which would find it much more costly to comply with federal clean air mandates if installing new equipment were the only compliance option. In a slightly different twist from the rules governing SO_2 allowance trading, the market-based approach to reducing nitrogen dioxide emissions requires that such deals be "directionally correct," meaning that the buyers of pollution credits must be downwind from the sellers. In this instance, for example, prevailing air currents travel from west to east; so any additional pollutants generated by the Connecticut utility are expected to blow out to sea and dissipate before they can harm anyone. In neighboring New York State, officials are delighted by the agreement since each year of its five-year duration it will spare their state exposure to the 500 tons of NO_2 which the New Jersey utility otherwise would have emitted. As an additional benefit of the arrangement, the broker who will handle the trade has announced his company's intention to retire 10 percent of the credits, so that over five years total NO_2 emissions will decrease by 140 tons—a win-win situation for everyone involved.

By expanding emissions trading beyond a narrow SO_2/acid rain focus, advocates are wagering that a "smog market" approach to environmental regulation is the wave of the future and represents the only way of achieving air quality at a price the public is willing to pay.

References
Armstrong, Scott. 1993. "Market Plan Set to Clean Up L.A. Smog." *The Christian Science Monitor* (Nov. 12).
Fulton, William. 1992. "The Air Pollution Trading Game." *Governing* (March).
Wald, Matthew L. 1994. "Unusual Interstate Tradeoff: Clean Air for Dirty." *New York Times*, March 16.

Fuel Switching.   Burning natural gas or low-sulfur coal or oil instead of high-sulfur coal constitutes perhaps the simplest way of reducing SO_2 emissions (low-sulfur coal has a significantly lower BTU value than high-sulfur coal, however). Natural gas in particular is likely to play an important role in the effort to combat acid deposition since it has a minimal sulfur content and emits far less NO_x when burned than do either coal or oil.

Coal Washing.   Though only partially effective, this simplest of clean-coal technologies can remove 20–50% of the sulfur content of coal at a moderate cost; coal washing might be an effective pollution control strategy in developing countries such as China and India, determined to exploit their sizeable coal reserves yet unable to afford more efficient, but costly, emission control technologies.

Flue Gas Desulfurization (stack gas "scrubbers").   The most common "technological fix," scrubbers are quite expensive, particularly when older facilities must be retrofitted, but they can achieve impressively high levels of emission reduction. By chemically precipitating out pollutant gases as they pass through the smokestack, scrubbers can remove up to 95% of the SO_2 and 70–90% of NO_x. In the process, however, large amounts of waste sludge are generated, constituting a disposal dilemma.

Fluidized Bed Combustion or Integrated Gasification/Combined Cycle.   These constitute two relatively new—and expensive—advanced combustion technologies. These also exhibit high pollutant removal efficiencies for both SO_2 and NO_x.

It is quite possible that the facilities targeted for acid rain controls may need to employ a combination of these methods in order to reach their reduction goals, especially as emissions limitations become more stringent in the years ahead. Nevertheless, it is encouraging that a variety of proven options exist and that the resolve to employ them has now been codified by federal mandate (World Resources Institute, 1992).

Indoor Air Pollution

While the attention of scientists, citizens, and government regulators has until recently been focused almost exclusively on problems of ambient air pollution, recent studies suggest that more serious air quality threats lurk much closer to home. It is now apparent that contaminants within private dwellings may pose a greater risk to human health than do outdoor air pollutants. In fact, levels of several health-threatening air contaminants are often significantly higher indoors than out, prompting the EPA to rank indoor air pollution at the top of a list of 18 leading cancer risks. This is particularly worrisome because the majority of people spend more of their time indoors than outside; thus their exposure to indoor air pollutants is nearly continuous. Such pollutants pose a special threat to the very young, the ill, and the elderly—the groups most susceptible to pollution's adverse health effects and also the ones most likely to spend long periods of time inside.

In recent years justifiable concerns about energy conservation may have worsened the indoor air pollution problem because thick insulation, triple-glazed windows, and magnetically sealed doors greatly reduce air exchange with the outside, effectively retaining and accumulating contaminants inside the home.

While most people tend to equate the risk of harm they might suffer from toxic pollutants to the total amount and toxicity of such substances, in fact the main determinant of danger is the dose actually received by the individual. Thus in reality large amounts of toxic pollutants such as benzene, formaldehyde, or carbon monoxide, for example, when emitted from a factory smokestack or the tailpipe of a car, pose minimal risk to the average citizen because they break down or are diluted in concentration before he/she is directly exposed to them. By contrast, much smaller amounts of the same chemicals, released in close proximity to individuals inside the confined environs of their homes or offices, have a quick, direct route into the body and hence pose a much greater overall risk of health damage. Studies carried out to date demonstrate that personal exposures and concentrations of indoor air pollutants exceed those occurring outdoors for all of the 15 most prevalent chemicals studied (Wallace, 1987). In addition, peak pollutant concentrations, as well as overall averages, are generally higher indoors than in the ambient air.

Some of the more common air pollutants known to be present in the home environment include the following.

Radon Gas

When Stanley Watras started radiation-detection alarms ringing at the Limerick nuclear power plant near Philadelphia one December morning in 1984, he didn't realize that he was about to become a national celebrity, alerting Americans to a hitherto unsuspected menace within their own homes. The radioactive contamination that was detected by Watras when he arrived for work that fateful winter morning had obviously come from outside the nuclear facility, so Watras requested Philadelphia Electric, the utility company that owned the plant, to check his home in Colebrookdale Township. To everyone's amazement, tests revealed that the Watras home had levels of radon gas approximately 1000 times higher than normal. Investigators estimated that Watras, his wife, and two young sons were receiving radiation exposure equivalent to 455,000 chest X-rays a year simply by living in their house. As officials of Pennsylvania's Division of Environmental Radiation hastened to determine the extent of the indoor radon threat, it quickly became apparent that the Watras family was not alone in its predicament. Throughout sections of eastern Pennsylvania, New Jersey, and New York, underlain by a uranium-rich geological formation known as the Reading Prong, thousands of homes exhibit elevated levels of radon. Nor is the problem limited to a few mid-Atlantic states. In the autumn of 1988 the EPA announced that their data indicate radon contamination problems span the country and urged that most homes be tested for the presence of radon. While some scientists feel EPA figures overstate the number of homes affected, there is general agreement that indoor radon exposure represents a serious health hazard.

Radon originates from the natural radioactive decay of uranium. It is present in high concentrations in certain types of soil and rocks (e.g. granite, shale, phosphate, pitchblende), but most soils contain amounts high enough to pose a potential health hazard. Radon dilutes to harmless concentrations in the open air, but when it enters the confined space inside a structure it can accumulate to potentially hazardous levels. Since radon is a gas, it readily moves upward through the soil; small differences in air pressure between indoors and outdoors (very slight negative air pressure inside a heated building results from the "stack effect," created by air's tendency to rise whenever it is warmer than the surrounding atmosphere) cause the gas to seep into homes through dirt floors or crawl spaces, through cracks in cement floors and walls, through floor drains, sump holes, joints, or pores in cinder-block walls. Occasionally, radon gets into wellwater supplies and enters homes when water is used, particularly for showers or baths. Radon is dangerous because it is radioactive, undergoing decay to produce a series of "radon daughters," the most troublesome of which are alpha-emitters polonium-218 and 214. These can be inhaled and deposited in the lungs where they constitute an internal source of alpha radiation exposure, increasing the risk of lung cancer. Radon's contribution to overall human exposure to ionizing radiation is considerable. The National Council on Radiation Protection and Measurement estimates that the average individual receives fully 55% of his or her yearly dose of ionizing radiation from radon inside homes. The health consequences of

Figure 12-7

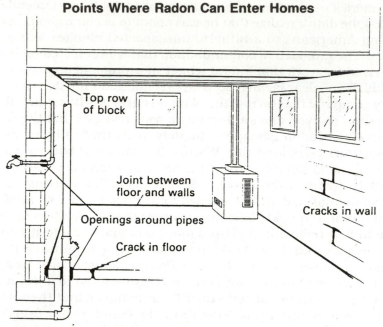

Points Where Radon Can Enter Homes

Top row
of block

Joint between
floor and walls

Openings around pipes

Crack in floor

Cracks in wall

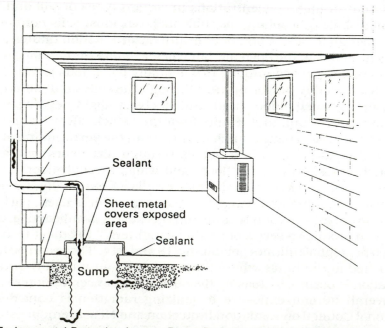

Radon Reduction Methods

Outside fan
draws radon
away from house

Sealant

Sheet metal
covers exposed
area

Sealant

Sump

Source: U.S. Environmental Protection Agency, *Radon Reduction Methods*, August 1986.

such exposure, according to EPA estimates, are between 7,000–30,000 lung cancer deaths annually—a number which would make radon the second-leading cause of lung cancer deaths in the United States, behind cigarette smoking. In some parts of the country where radon levels are unusually high, hundreds of thousands of Americans are receiving as much radiation exposure from radon in their homes as that received by the Ukrainian citizens who lived near Chernobyl at the time of the nuclear accident there in 1986. The extent of an individual's chances of developing radon-induced lung cancer depends on radon concentrations inside the home and on the length of time one is exposed. It is thought that long-term exposure to slightly elevated levels of radon poses a greater cancer threat than does short-term exposure to much higher levels. Cigarette smoking has a synergistic effect in enhancing the radon/lung cancer risk by a factor of 10.

Until recently radon was regarded as a health hazard only to uranium miners, so estimates of risk to residents of radon-contaminated homes have simply been extrapolated from standards set for occupational exposure in the mines. Indoor radon concentrations are measured as the number of picocuries of radiation per liter of air (pCi/L). Outdoors, radon concentrations in the ambient air typically measure about 0.4 pCi/L, while the average indoor level approximates 1.3 pCi/L. Acknowledging that *any* amount of exposure to ionizing radiation entails *some* degree of risk, for practical reasons EPA regards 4 pCi/L as the **action level**—the point at or above which homeowners are advised to take some kind of remedial action (although Congress has established a long-term goal of lowering indoor radon concentrations in every home to a level equivalent to that prevailing outdoors, such a goal is not yet technologically achievable; nevertheless, the EPA believes that reducing elevated radon levels to around 2 pCi/L should be possible almost everywhere). Readings above 20 pCi/L are considered cause for serious concern and may require significant abatement measures (as a basis for comparison, radon levels in the Watras home measured 2700 pCi/L!)

Results from an EPA-sponsored survey of residential radon levels in nine million homes nationwide revealed that an estimated one out of every 15 homes in the U.S. has average indoor radon levels in excess of 4 pCi/L. Nor is the problem limited to private residences. Another study carried out under the auspices of the 1988 Indoor Radon Abatement Act found that out of 927 public school buildings surveyed throughout the country, 19% had at least one ground floor room where radon concentrations were above EPA's action level. Such findings have prompted a strong EPA recommendation that all homes and schools in the nation should be tested for the presence of radon.

Since it is impossible to predict with certainty which structures are likely to have elevated radon levels (some homes in the Watras neighborhood were essentially radon-free), the need for radon reduction measures can only be determined by actual measurements, which often can be done by the homeowner with relatively inexpensive devices (see Box 12–6). If test results indicate the need for some sort of radon remediation efforts, a variety of options are available. Most require the services of a professional

Figure 12-8 Indoor Radon Survey Results

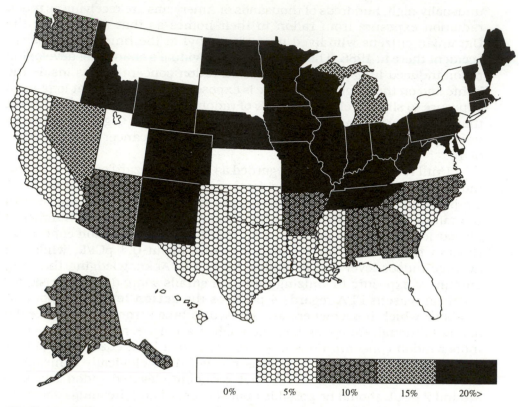

Estimated Percent of Homes with Screening Levels Greater than 4pCi/L

Source: U.S. Environmental Protection Agency, *Securing Our Legacy: An EPA Progress Report 1989–1991*, 1992.

contractor, though some can be as simple as covering sump holes or improving ventilation. More extensive—and expensive—possibilities include installing fans or air-to-air heat exchangers to replace radon-contaminated indoor air with outdoor air; covering any exposed earth inside homes with concrete, gas-proof liner, or sheet metal; sealing all cracks and openings with mortar, polyurethane sealants, or other impermeable materials; installing a drain tile suction system around the outer foundation walls of a house; or by installing a series of exhaust pipes inside hollow-block basement walls or baseboard to draw radon out of the voids within such walls before it can enter the living space. In structures with significantly elevated levels of radon, it may be necessary to utilize several methods to achieve sufficient reductions.

BOX 12-6
A Hidden Menace in Your Home?

Radon detection businesses have been proliferating rapidly following EPA's announcement advising that homes nationwide be tested for the presence of this apparently ubiquitous indoor air pollutant. Concerned home-owners, deterred by the hefty fee charged by many entrepreneurs offering radon monitoring services, should be heartened to learn that they can purchase relatively inexpensive devices that will give a reasonably accurate indication of the extent of radon problems in the user's home.

The two most popular do-it-yourself home radon detectors are charcoal canisters—small containers of activated charcoal that should be opened and left in place for three to seven days, then sealed and returned to the manufacturer for analysis—and alpha track detectors that are left in place for several weeks to as long as one year. Since radon levels can fluctuate considerably from day to day and season to season, alpha track detectors are good for determining yearly averages; charcoal canisters are useful for short-term screening tests, but since their results are indicative only of radon levels during the few days when the test was performed, they may over- or under-represent the actual extent of hazard. Both devices, how-ever, can be effectively used by nonprofessionals to give a rough approximation of radon pollution. If laboratory analysis reveals that radon levels are high, consultation with a radon abatement specialist would be advisable, but if the screening test indicates negligible amounts of the gas, the homeowner is saved the expense of contracting for a radon survey which might cost several hundred dollars.

Those interested in doing their own radon monitoring can improve the accuracy and relevance of the results by understanding a few basic concepts about radon. Because radon infiltrates into homes through the ground, basements are likely to exhibit the highest radon levels. For this reason, if residents want to know the peak concentrations to which they may be exposed, a monitoring device should be located in the basement (or lowest level of the dwelling), placed about 3–6 feet above the floor and away from walls, doors, or windows. However, if occupants spend little time in the basement and want a measurement more representative of the exposure they are receiving, monitors can be placed in living areas of the next highest floor. Another likely spot for monitor placement is near suspected sources of radon entry, such as sump holes or crawl spaces (however, don't use charcoal canisters in humid environments such as bathrooms and kitchens; the charcoal absorbs moisture and test results will not be accurate). Since monitoring devices are relatively inexpensive, it may be advisable to use two or three simultan-eously in different areas of the house. Radon concentrations in most states tend to be highest in winter, so this is the best time for using short-term monitoring devices.

Home radon detectors are available for purchase at hardware stores or supermarkets; information regarding companies offering mail-order services for radon monitoring devices can be obtained from local health departments or by placing a toll-free call to one of the State Radon Contacts listed in Figure 12-9. Although there are as yet no mandatory standards which radon monitoring equipment or testing laboratories are required to meet; manufacturers may voluntarily submit their products or facilities for EPA evaluation. Therefore, it's a good idea for those considering purchase of a radon detection device to check whether the company is listed as "EPA-approved." Similarly, EPA publishes regularly updated lists of radon measurement and abatement firms which meet the agency's voluntary proficiency standards and recommends that anyone planning to hire a contractor for radon-related work first check that person's professional qualifications as determined by the agency's proficiency programs.

Products of Combustion

Carbon monoxide, nitrogen oxides, and particulates can reach very high levels inside homes where gas stoves or other gas appliances are used, where kerosene heaters or wood-burning stoves are operating, where auto emissions from a garage can enter the house, or where there are cigarette smokers. In homes with gas ranges, for example, nitrogen oxide levels are frequently twice as high as those outdoors. Carbon monoxide emissions from wood, coal, or gas stoves often exceed Clean Air Act standards for outside air. The growing popularity of woodburning stoves is a particular cause for concern, since wood is a much dirtier fuel than either oil or gas. Wood smoke contains approximately 100 different chemicals, at least 14 of which are the same carcinogens found in cigarette smoke. In many developing nations, where burning of wood, charcoal, or other biomass fuels is an everyday event, exposure to combustion products emitted by poorly vented household stoves constitutes the leading indoor air quality problem. One study carried out in Kenya by the World Health Organization revealed that average particulate levels were more than 20 times higher than WHO guidelines in homes where wood or plant residues were burned as fuel.

Cigarette smoking (the by-product of which is now referred to technically as **ETS**—"Environmental Tobacco Smoke") may constitute the most significant source of indoor air pollution in many homes; particulate levels may go as high as 700 micrograms/m^3, far above the primary ambient air quality standard of 50, when there are smokers in a house. A study conducted by researchers at Harvard University found that household tobacco smoke is the main source of exposure to particulate pollutants for most children. It also demonstrated that whereas typical particulate levels in a home without smokers is 10–20 micrograms/m^3, each smoker contributes an additional 25–30 micrograms/m^3, more than doubling the base level amount (Ware et al., 1984). Particulate matter and carbon monoxide are not the only indoor air pollutants generated by smokers—cigarette smoking represents the major source of human exposure to benzene, a known carcinogen and a listed toxic air pollutant. Nonsmokers living or working in the same room with a smoker are exposed to at least five times the amount of benzene as those who work in the

Figure 12-9 State Radon Contacts

Alabama 800/582-1866	Montana 406/444-3671
Alaska 800/478-4845	Nebraska 800/334-9491
Arizona 602/255-4845	Nevada 702/687-5394
Arkansas 501/661-2301	New Hampshire 800/852-3345
California 800/745-7236	New Jersey 800/648-0394
Colorado 800/846-3986	New Mexico 505/827-4300
Connecticut 203/566-3122	New York 800/458-1158
Delaware 800/554-4636	North Carolina 919/571-4141
District of Columbia 202/727-5728	North Dakota 701/221-5188
Florida 800/543-8279	Ohio 800/523-4439
Georgia 800/745-0037	Oklahoma 405/271-5221
Hawaii 808/586-4700	Oregon 503/731-4014
Idaho 800/445-8647	Pennsylvania 800/237-2366
Illinois 800/325-1245	Puerto Rico 809/767-3563
Indiana 800/272-9723	Rhode Island 401/277-2438
Iowa 800/383-5992	South Carolina 800/768-0362
Kansas 913/296-1560	South Dakota 605/773-3351
Kentucky 502/564-3700	Tennessee 800/232-1139
Louisiana 800/256-2494	Texas 512/834-6688
Maine 800/232-0842	Utah 801/538-6734
Maryland 800/872-3666	Vermont 800/640-0601
Massachusetts 413/586-7525	Virginia 800/468-0138
Michigan 517/335-8190	Washington 800/323-9727
Minnesota 800/798-9050	West Virginia 800/922-1255
Mississippi 800/626-7739	Wisconsin 608/267-4795
Missouri 800/669-7236	Wyoming 800/458-5847

vicinity of coke ovens, the single largest industrial source (Smith, 1988). In the past few years, growing militancy on the part of the nonsmoking public, aroused by data such as that just cited, has led to some highly publicized lawsuits against facilities that continue to allow patrons or employees to smoke. In the spring of 1993, four Connecticut residents suffering from diseases (e.g. asthma and lupus) which rendered them especially sensitive to ETS, made news by filing lawsuits against McDonald's Corporation, Wendy's, and Burger King. Using the Americans With Disabilities Act as the basis for legal action, the four claimed that because of their medical condition the restaurants cited were inaccessible to them because the presence of ETS, even within designated no-smoking sections, caused such severe breathing difficulties that they were, in effect,

This Is A "Non-Smoking" Restaurant.

Thank You.
318A

Signs such as this are increasingly being seen in shopping malls, restaurants, and other public places where environmental tobacco smoke has become an unwelcome indoor air pollutant. [Nora Byrne]

disabled. The plaintiffs sought no monetary compensation—instead they asked the court to impose a total smoking ban on all Connecticut restaurants belonging to these fast food chains. Stressing that his clients were being discriminated against, the lawyer for the plaintiffs argued that "the intent of the Americans With Disabilities Act is that disabled people should be able to participate. Just as ramps allow access to people in wheelchairs, so do smoking bans open up doors to those with respiratory ailments" (Taylor, 1993). A subsequent request by a group of more than a dozen state attorneys general that fast food restaurants voluntarily phase out smoking on their premises and a lawsuit filed against five large fast food chains by the Texas attorney general finally prompted a 1994 agreement by McDonald's to ban smoking in all of its 1400 company-owned restaurants and to urge that its franchise owners enforce a similar prohibition (several other fast-food chains have also implemented total smoking bans, including Dairy Queen, Arby's, and Taco Bell). In the United States, even in the absence of enforceable federal standards, ETS is rapidly becoming a socially unacceptable indoor air pollutant.

Formaldehyde

Known to cause skin and respiratory irritation, formaldehyde is now suspected of being carcinogenic as well. A wide variety of household products contain formaldehyde, most notably urea formaldehyde foam insulation, particleboard, plywood, and some floor coverings and textiles. Levels of formaldehyde are particularly likely to be high in mobile homes where residents frequently complain of rashes, respiratory irritation, nausea, headaches, dizziness, lethargy, or aggravation of bronchial asthma. Within the same home, formaldehyde levels can fluctuate dramatically, depending on environmental conditions. A 15 °F increase in temperature can result in a doubling of formaldehyde levels, while the lowest formaldehyde concentrations have been recorded on cold winter days; similarly, increases in relative humidity cause a corresponding rise in formaldehyde emissions. In terms of its effect as an irritant, there does not appear to be a threshold level for formaldehyde exposure. The National Academy of Sciences estimates that as many as 10–20% of the population experiences some form of irritation due to formaldehyde exposure even at very low levels of concentration. The Consumer Product Safety Commission has advised consumers against using urea formaldehyde foam insulation, citing complaints from 5,700 persons who blame the product for causing various respiratory and health problems. A former commission-imposed ban on such insulation was overturned in 1983.

Chemical Fumes and Particles

Numerous household products (including furniture polish, hair sprays, air fresheners, over-cleaners, paints, carpeting, pesticides, disinfectants, solvents, etc.), release chemical fumes and particles that can reach very high levels indoors. While relatively little research has been done on the health impact of inhaling these substances on a regular basis, it is known that several commonly used household chemicals cause cancer in laboratory animals. Paradichlorobenzene, the active ingredient in moth crystals and many air fresheners and room deodorants, as well as limonene, another odorant, present perhaps the highest cancer risk among indoor organic chemicals. Tetrachloroethylene, a solvent used in dry cleaning, is another carcinogen to which household residents may receive significant exposure when wearing freshly dry-cleaned garments or by breathing emissions from closets in which such articles were stored (Smith, 1988).

When used in accordance with instructions, most household chemicals are not known to provoke acute health effects. However, use of pesticides inside homes has occasionally resulted in a wide range of health complaints, including headaches, nausea, vertigo, skin rashes, and emotional disorders. Chlordane, which for almost 40 years was the most widely used insecticide for controlling termites, was taken off the market in 1988 in response to hundreds of complaints about alleged chlordane-induced illnesses among residents following pesticidal applications in homes.

Biological Pollutants

A diverse group of living organisms, most of them too small to be seen with the naked eye, can also pose serious air quality problems inside homes and public buildings. Bacteria and fungal spores can enter structures via air handling systems and occasionally cause disease outbreaks (the

Figure 12-10 A Day in the Life of . . . One Person's Exposure to Respirable Particles

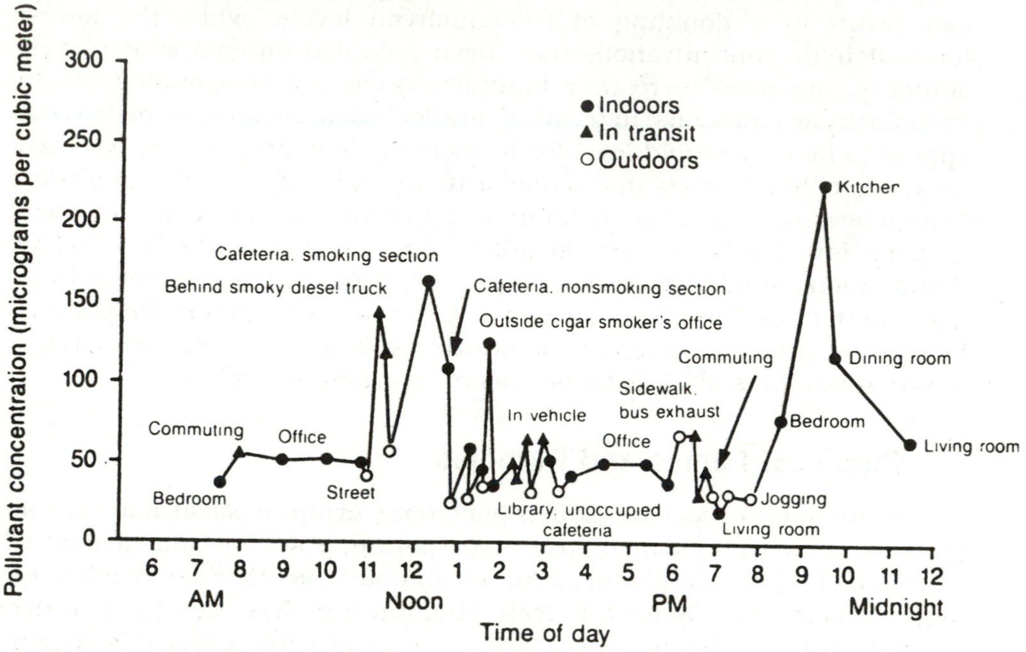

Source: U.S. Environmental Protection Agency.

Legionnaires' Disease episode in Philadelphia in 1976 is the classic example of this sort of occurrence). Many allergies are associated with exposure to household dust which may contain fungal spores, bacteria, animal dander, and feces of roaches or mites. Perhaps most significant in stimulating allergic reactions are live dust mites, tiny arthropods less than 1 millimeter in size that are found in enormous numbers on bedsheets and blankets where they feed on sloughed-off scales of skin. Humid conditions or the presence of stagnant water seem to favor buildup of large populations of these unwanted guests and their dissemination has sometimes been associated with the use of humidifiers or vaporizers which harbored fungal or bacterial growth.

Sick Building Syndrome

Some indoor air pollutants can provoke complaints among building occupants of problems such as chest tightness, muscle aches, cough, fever, and chills. These symptoms of what is now termed **building related illness (BRI)** may persist for an extended time period after affected persons leave the building, but they have clearly identifiable causes and can be clinically diagnosed. By contrast, a somewhat more mysterious malady

BOX 12-7
Multiple Chemical Sensitivity: Fact or Fantasy?

An emerging new public health problem occasionally referred to in such apocalyptic terms as "20th Century Disease" is being reported with increasing frequency across the nation, its symptoms provoking angry debate among health care providers and toxicologists who have not yet reached consensus on whether the ailment reported by thousands of sufferers is real or simply "in their heads."

Multiple chemical sensitivity (MCS) represents a condition in which some people claim to develop a wide range of potentially debilitating symptoms from exposure to an ever-expanding range of chemical substances at lower and lower levels. While the nature and extent of MCS remains poorly understood, a National Academy of Sciences internal document suggests that close to 15% of the U.S. population may experience some degree of chemical sensitivity. Those reporting such problems tend to fall into one of four groups: 1) industrial workers exposed on the job; 2) occupants of poorly ventilated buildings; 3) people living in areas with high levels of air or water pollution; and 4) individuals who have experienced unique exposures to chemicals in pesticides, consumer products, and so forth. A common thread that binds these disparate groups together is that all of them experience a number of different symptoms involving several body organs. The symptoms develop within a relatively short time after a change of some sort in that person's environment. Exposure to vapors from a newly installed carpet, moving into a recently constructed office building, being accidentally sprayed with a pesticide—all are examples of typical events triggering the subsequent development of MCS. In some cases sufferers are unable to recall any single, obvious high-dose exposure leading to the onset of symptoms, causing some researchers to conclude that repeated, cumulative exposure to low levels of certain chemicals may also give rise to MCS symptoms. Clinical ecologists, a group of physicians involved in MCS research and treatment, hypothesize a two-step process in the development of sensitivity:

1. high level and/or chronic low-level exposure to a chemical which *induces susceptibility* to future exposures;

2. a "*triggering*" of symptoms by low-level exposure either to the same chemical which caused induction or to a variety of other chemicals; these triggering substances can provoke symptoms in sensitized individuals at concentrations far below those known to cause toxicological damage.

As time passes, MCS sufferers experience problems with a steadily widening spectrum of chemicals (detergents, deodorants, perfumes, plastics, synthetic fabrics, petroleum products, etc.) and develop an increasingly broad range of symptoms which can render them partially to totally disabled. Many victims find they can no longer engage in such commonplace activities as shopping, working in conventional office or industrial settings, dining in restaurants—even living in a typically furnished home. One young woman afflicted with MCS felt compelled to move out of her house to live year-round in a tent due to the multiple chemical exposures indoors which rendered her constantly ill.

Beyond the despair and sense of isolation experienced by those afflicted with MCS is the psychological distress caused by the insensitivity of family, friends, physicians and employers who frequently assume the illness is a figment of the sufferer's overactive imagination—a result of stress, depression, or some other psychosocial condition. Indeed, many serious researchers are highly skeptical, if not downright disbelieving, of the existence of MCS as a true physiological disease. Their resistance is based on the fact that MCS violates all the fundamental tenets of toxicological science. Such critics are troubled by the fact that MCS produces no objective evidence of disease which can be tested and observed in the clinical setting; the major symptoms are subjective ones—headache, fatigue, stomach pains, difficulty in concentrating, emotional disturbances, "woozy head"—which can't be independently verified. The ailment is not associated with any specific chemical nor with any specific effect; in fact, descriptions of MCS include accounts of how symptoms spread from one organ to another over time for no apparent reason. The dose-response relationships so basic to toxicological theory appear foreign to MCS—severity of symptoms appears to be entirely independent of the amount of exposure. Finally, there is no proven mechanism of illness, no generally accepted physiological data to explain how trace amounts of chemicals could produce the adverse health effects being reported. And MCS sufferers generally *look* reasonably healthy, even when they *feel* miserable!

Nevertheless, even though skeptics are still in the majority, a growing number of researchers are coming to the conclusion that MCS is a real illness, pointing to the fact that those afflicted generally can identify a specific exposure to environmental chemicals which caused or seriously aggravated the symptoms they are experiencing. The legal system, too, is taking MCS seriously. Hundreds of personal injury lawsuits involving MCS have been filed, alleging harm from a wide variety of consumer products. Thousands more worker compensation claims have been filed and the number continues to grow. Many of these cases are settled out of court or dismissed. When cases *do* come to trial, lack of credible expert witnesses make causation difficult to prove. This situation is expected to change, however, as new findings enhance understanding of the condition.

Certainly the need for more research on chemical sensitivity is sorely needed, particularly in light of its severe social, financial, and emotional repercussions. Perhaps additional studies will merely confirm the contention of mainstream physicians that MCS is a mental ailment, not a physical one. On the other hand, it is also conceivable that just as many disbelievers 25 years ago scoffed at the existence of "sick building syndrome," only later to be confronted with the reality of Legionnaires' Disease, so in the years ahead, today's MCS sufferers may be regarded as those "miners' canaries," warning us of the dangers of an increasingly toxic environment.

References

Ashford. Nicholas A., and Claudia S. Miller. 1993. "Multiple Chemical Sensitivity: Fact or Fiction." *Health & Environment Digest* 6, no. 11 (March).

Castlemen, Michael. 1993. "This Place Makes Me Sick," *Sierra*, (Sept./Oct.).

Davis, Earon S., and Mary Lamielle. 1991. "Toxic Reaction: Legal Responses Vary To Chemical Illness." *Indoor Pollution* 5, no. 7 (Dec).

reported with increased frequency since the mid-1970s is a condition described as **sick building syndrome (SBS)**. SBS refers to situations where building occupants experience various forms of acute discomfort—eye irritation, scratchiness in the throat, dry cough, headache, itchy skin, fatigue, difficulty in concentrating, nausea and dizziness—but no causative agent of such symptoms can be found. Furthermore, these symptoms generally vanish soon after sufferers leave the building (sometimes the complaints are associated with only one part of the building or even with a single room). This situation has become so widespread in recent years that a committee of the World Health Organization has suggested that as many as 30% of the world's new and remodeled buildings may be generating complaints. While some of the symptoms reported may, in fact, be caused by illnesses contracted somewhere else, by preexisting allergies, or by job-related stress, in many cases poor indoor air quality is the major culprit. Although some of the reported outbreaks of sick building syndrome are eventually traced to specific pollutants—e.g. microorganisms spread through ventilation systems, vehicle exhausts entering intake vents, ozone emissions from photocopying machines, VOCs outgassing from new carpeting—in most cases these contaminants aren't present in concentrations high enough to provoke the reported symptoms. Synthetic mineral fibers released into the air from acoustical ceiling tile and insulating material have recently been identified by researchers at Cornell University as the prime cause of many SBS situations. Most often, however, SBS has been traced to inadequate ventilation and its rise in frequency parallels efforts since the 1973 Arab oil embargo to incorporate energy conservation features into building design.

Unlike the situation in homes, most new nonresidential structures are equipped with mechanical heating, ventilation, and air conditioning (HVAC) systems and feature windows tightly sealed to restrict air infiltration from outside. These HVAC systems recirculate air throughout the building, with a significant portion of the air being reused several times prior to being exhausted, the purpose of such reuse being to lessen energy costs for heating or cooling incoming fresh air. Building codes require that a specified minimum amount of outside air be provided in order to establish an acceptable balance between oxygen and CO_2 indoors, to dilute odors, and to remove contaminants generated within the structure. Prior to 1973 that specified minimum was approximately 15 cubic feet per minute (cfm) per building occupant; after 1973 the standard was reduced to just 5 cfm, an amount which, in a number of situations, proved inadequate for maintaining healthy, comfortable conditions. In some situations HVAC systems were improperly installed, had defective equipment, or functioned poorly because of improper vent placement. When errors such as these occur, an insufficient amount of ventilation air will be supplied. Once such problems are identified, they can generally be corrected by repairing or adjusting the air handling system to provide additional outside air; in some cases, however, building design itself may be at fault, requiring much more extensive renovations (Turiel, 1985; EPA, 1991; Beek, 1994).

In general, the public has been slow to demand action on this problem because access to information about indoor air pollutants has been very limited and possibly because people don't want to believe that pollution problems have invaded the home. Nevertheless, an increasing awareness of the threat posed by indoor air pollutants has stimulated thinking on new ways of dealing with this recently recognized problem. Monitoring and enforcing air quality standards inside 80 million American homes is obviously impossible. However, standards could be set to control pollutant emissions by modifying product design or manufacture. For example, the United States has set standards regulating emissions of formaldehyde from plywood and is considering regulating emissions from unvented fossil-fuel heating appliances; there have even been proposals to require catalytic converters on wood stoves! In the future, updated building codes which incorporate design features and materials which minimize release and retention of indoor air pollutants could ensure that most new structures have acceptable air quality. In the meantime, efforts must be made to educate homeowners and occupants on the impact personal behavior and consumer choices can have on the quality of the indoor environment. Decisions as to which products we buy, how we use certain appliances, our consideration for the health of others as reflected in personal smoking habits—all have a profound impact on indoor air quality and will ultimately determine the success or failure of any government effort to minimize indoor air pollution (Nero, 1988).

References

Acid Rain: What It Is. 1982. National Wildlife Federation.

Air Pollution Primer. 1969. National Tuberculosis and Respiratory Disease Association.

Beek, Jim. 1994. "Man-Made Minerals Could Be Key to SBS." *Indoor Air Review* 3, no. 11 (Jan.).

Boyle, Robert, and R. Alexander Boyle. 1983. *Acid Rain.* Schocken Books/Nick Lyons Books.

Bryner, Gary C. 1993. *Blue Skies, Green Politics: The Clean Air Act of 1990.* CQ Press.

Cobb, Nathaniel, and Ruth A. Etzel. 1991. "Unintentional Carbon Monoxide-Related Deaths in the United States, 1979 through 1988." *Journal of the American Medical Association* 266, no. 5 (Aug.).

Cohen, C. J., L. C. Grothaus, and S. C. Perrigan. 1982. "Effects of Simulated Sulfuric and Sulfuric-Nitric Acid Rain on Crop Plants: Results of 1980 Crop Survey." *Special Report* 670, Agricultural Experiment Station, Oregon State University, Corvallis.

Dockery, Douglas W., et al. 1993. "An Association Between Air Pollution and Mortality in Six U.S. Cities." *The New England Journal of Medicine* 329, no. 24 (Dec. 9).

"Easy Guide to the Air Toxics Law." 1993. *The Environmental Manager's Compliance Advisor,* no. 344 (Feb. 1).

Environmental Law Handbook, 12th ed. 1993. Government Institutes, Inc.

Environmental Protection Agency. 1991. *Indoor Air Facts* No. 4 (revised), *Sick Building Syndrome.* (ANR-455-W), April.

Evelyn, John. (1661). *Fumifugium.* London National Society for Clean Air, 1969.

"Evidence of Acid Fog Found on Mount Ohiyama." 1989. *Japan Times,* Sept. 13.

Flynn, John. 1994. "The Falling Forest." *Amicus Journal* 15, no.4 (Winter).

Health Effects of Air Pollution. 1978. American Thoracic Society.

Hilchey, Tim. 1993. "Government Survey Finds Decline in a Building Block of Acid Rain." *New York Times*, Sept. 7.

Nero, Anthony V., Jr. 1988. "Controlling Indoor Air Pollution." *Scientific American* 258, no. 5 (May).

Rhodes, S. L., and P. Middleton. 1983. "The Complex Challenge of Controlling Acid Rain." *Environment* 22, no. 4 (May).

Rodhe, Henning. 1989. "Acidification in a Global Perspective." *Ambio* 18, no. 3.

Scholle, Stephen R. 1983. "Acid Deposition and the Materials Damage Question." *Environment* 25, no. 8 (Oct.).

Smith, Kirk R. 1988. "Air Pollution: Assessing Total Exposure in the United States." *Environment* 30, no. 8 (Oct.).

Taylor, Steven T. 1993. "McSuit: American Fast food Icon Hit with Litigation over ETS." *Indoor Air Review* 3, no. 4 (June).

Turiel, Isaac. 1985. *Indoor Air Quality and Human Health.* Stanford University Press.

Waldbott, George L. 1978. *Health Effects of Environmental Pollutants.* C. V. Mosby.

Wallace, L. A. 1987. *Total Exposure Assessment Methodology* (TEAM Study: Summary and Analysis), vol. 1, Environmental Protection Agency.

Ware, J. H., et al. 1984. "Passive Smoking, Gas Cooking, and Respiratory Health of Children Living in Six Cities." *American Review of Respiratory Disease* 129:366–74.

Weller, Phil. 1980. *Acid Rain: The Silent Crisis.* Between the Lines & the Waterloo Public Interest Research Group.

World Resources Institute. 1992. *World Resources 1992–1993.* Oxford University Press.

World Resources Institute. 1990. *World Resources 1990–1991.* Oxford University Press.

CHAPTER 13

Noise Pollution

> *. . . I've shot my hearing; it hurts and it's painful, and it's frustrating when little children talk to you and you can't hear them.*
> —Pete Townshend, 1989 press conference
>
> *Pete Townshend has good hearing compared with me. My left ear is there just to balance my face, because it doesn't work at all.*
> —Ted Nugent

Confessions by Pete Townshend and Ted Nugent that careers as rock musicians had irreversibly damaged their hearing may not have dampened their fans' enthusiasm for ear-splitting concerts, but it did serve as a warning to the general public that "feeling the beat" may produce longer-lasting results than the temporary high elicited by good vibrations. As the sounds of modern life become steadily more raucous, Townshend and Nugent join the ranks of an estimated 10 million Americans who have suffered full or partial hearing loss due to excessive noise exposure. Unfortunately, public and policymakers alike tend to regard noise as an inevitable by-product of modern life, sometimes unpleasant but largely unavoidable. At the same time, polls taken among urban residents in both the United States and Europe reveal that most city dwellers certainly are bothered by noise. Typically, those questioned rank excessive noise among the top environmental issues of greatest concern to them and as one of the major considerations that might cause them to move to another part of town.

Sources of Noise

Most concerns about noise as a pollutant have focused on the occupational environment where high levels of noise associated with machinery, equipment, and general work practices have long been recognized as a serious threat to both the physical and psychological health of workers. However, the sources of noise that torment the general public are far more diverse than those which constitute an occupational hazard. Around the world, rapidly growing numbers of cars, trucks, and motorcycles have been boosting noise levels on crowded streets and highways, while the not-so-friendly skies above metropolitan neighborhoods are regularly deafened by the roar of jets taking off or landing at urban airports. Even once-quiet residential areas are losing their tranquility as noise-generating home appliances and motorized yard tools are increasingly regarded as essential components of the good life. While most people perceive community noise as a general din, originating from a multiplicity of sources, vehicular noise—particularly that from motorcycles and large trucks—seems to be regarded as the most annoying by community residents. Unfortunately, overall noise levels are growing steadily worse, in part because modern life-styles and transportation habits are changing in ways that inevitably result in more noise generation. We are also carrying noise with us to places that formerly were havens of peace and quiet. The advent of snowmobiles, trail bikes, and powerful motorboats have brought noise pollution to once-silent wilderness areas; amplified music now jars city parks when partying crowds forget that not everyone finds loud rock

Figure 13-1 Examples of Outdoor Day-Night Average Sound Levels in dB Measured at Various Locations

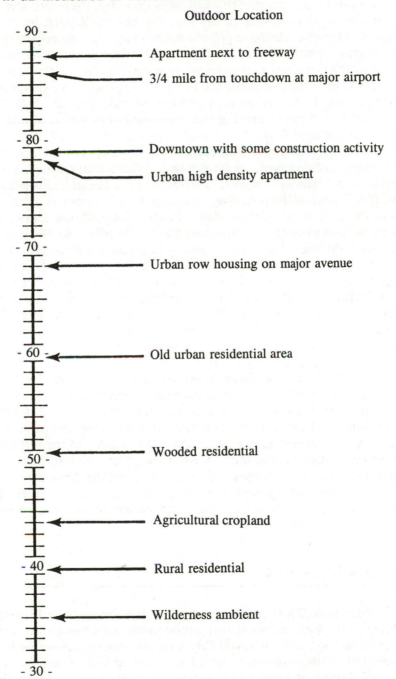

Outdoor Location

- 90 -

Apartment next to freeway

3/4 mile from touchdown at major airport

- 80 -

Downtown with some construction activity

Urban high density apartment

- 70 -

Urban row housing on major avenue

- 60 -

Old urban residential area

Wooded residential

- 50 -

Agricultural cropland

- 40 -

Rural residential

Wilderness ambient

- 30 -

Source: U.S. Environmental Protection Agency, *Protective Noise Levels*, EPA 550/9–79–100, Nov., 1978.

bands pleasurable and the desert air occasionally reverberates to a similar beat, thanks to "boom car" sound-offs where enthusiasts compete to see whose car stereos are the most ear splitting.

Beyond the technological and life-style changes that have made contemporary life noisier than in days gone by, there are simply more of us on the planet, adding to the din. For the most part, levels of outdoor noise are directly related to population density—the more populous the city, the noisier conditions are likely to be. Predicted trends in noise levels to the year 2000 are not particularly encouraging. One of the most important sources of excessive community noise, urban traffic, is expected to increase considerably in the years immediately ahead, with the U.S. Department of Transportation estimating that the number of automobiles on the road will increase by 0.6–0.7% annually through the end of the century. Overseas, a recent study on noise control strategies revealed that efforts taken to reduce traffic noise in several western European countries (e.g. screens along main highways) helped to offset the increase in traffic noise but didn't result in an overall lowering of noise exposure—simply because of the rapid increase in size of the car fleet. In the Netherlands alone, private car ownership is projected to increase from 4.6 million in 1985 to 7.9 million by 2010, during which time passenger traffic on that nation's highways will grow by 70%; truck traffic is expected to increase by an even larger percentage. Europeans have been experimenting with rerouting traffic, prohibiting vehicles entirely in certain areas, and constructing noise screens, a combination of which has resulted in some lowering of noise levels in central cities. However, the spread of residential suburbs into rural areas is resulting in a steady expansion of noise exposure into areas formerly undisturbed by such problems (OECD, 1991). Air traffic noise, on the other hand, has been declining slightly in both the United States and abroad, thanks to the introduction of the quieter planes required by stricter certification standards of the International Civil Aviation Organization. However, the substantial increase in air traffic witnessed in recent years threatens to reverse the gains achieved through engineering advancements and regulations. After the year 2000, it is anticipated that the land area and numbers of people exposed to unacceptable levels of aircraft noise will again increase, particularly since efforts to prohibit residential development or commercial construction on land near airports have proven largely futile.

Noise As a Nuisance

More than 2000 years ago, the Roman Emperor Julius Caesar grappled with the issue of noise as a public nuisance when he attempted to ban chariot racing on the Eternal City's cobblestone streets due to the racket it created. History doesn't record whether or not he was successful, but as the clamor of urban life continued to increase during the ensuing centuries, the irritant value of noise grew apace and has occasionally caused frayed tempers to snap. Several years ago a Japanese newspaper

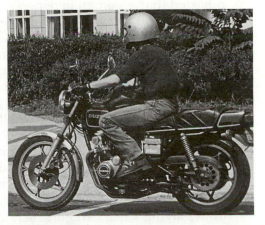

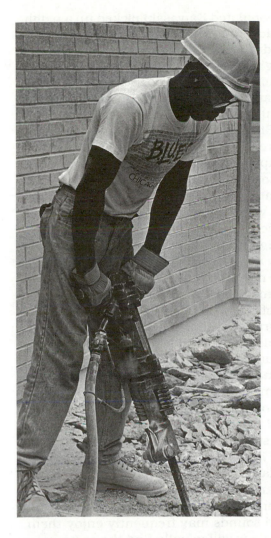

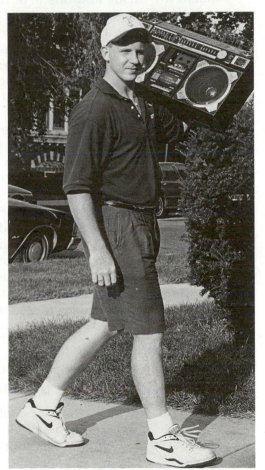

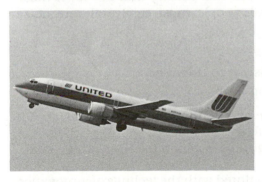

Millions of Americans are daily being exposed to levels of noise that could permanently damage their ability to hear. [Photos by Nora Byrne]

reported that a woman in densely populated Kawasaki picked up a neighbor's dog and threw it out the window of her apartment, exclaiming that the animal's constant barking was driving her to distraction. The enraged neighbor then retaliated by stabbing the woman to death! Perhaps to avoid just such altercations, more and more Japanese city dwellers are having their canine pets' vocal cords cut or are fitting them with antibarking shock collars to make sure they remain quiet all day in the tiny, yardless living quarters typical of modern Japan (Shapiro, 1989). Noise also was causing friction recently in New Orleans' French Quarter, where priests and worshippers at St. Louis Cathedral complained they couldn't hear themselves pray, thanks to the spirited outdoor jazz band performances held in adjacent Jackson Square. Fortunately, in this case an amicable compromise was eventually worked out, with the musicians agreeing to abstain from playing when cathedral services were being held (Suro, 1991). Even outside the hustle and bustle of big city life, noise can provoke bizarre behavior. A few years ago an elderly man in rural Los Angeles County was arrested for using a four-foot square mirror to reflect sunlight into the eyes of pilots landing and taking off at a small regional airport. When questioned as to his motives for engaging in actions with potentially disastrous consequences, he attested to holding a grudge against the private planes whose drone prevented him from hearing his small portable radio! (Rotella, 1989). In a more humorous vein, international tennis star Monica Seles was frequently the target of caustic remarks from distracted opponents who complained that her lusty grunts, measured as high as 98 decibels, constituted a noise pollution problem on the courts (Finn, 1992).

Just as beauty is in the eye of the beholder, the perception of a sound as "noise" (arbitrarily defined by some writers as "unwanted sound") depends on the point of view of the individual listener. Unfortunately for those attempting to set up standards regulating noise exposure, the loudness of a noise and the annoyance it causes are not always directly correlated. As any college student partying near a residential neighborhood well knows, people *generating* loud sounds may frequently enjoy them, while those forced to listen against their will usually find the same noise profoundly objectionable. In general, people most easily tolerate noise when:

1. they are causing it;
2. they feel it is necessary or useful to them; or
3. they know where it is coming from.

To the extent that other people exposed to the same sounds do not experience equivalent benefits from the noise, conflict between participating and nonparticipating groups is generated (Bugliarello et al., 1976).

While most people are well acquainted with the feelings of annoyance and irritation that unwanted sounds can arouse, noise is frequently shrugged off as an inescapable part of modern life about which little can be done. It is becoming increasingly evident, however, that noise levels commonly encountered in thousands of cities, factories, places of recreation, and even inside homes represent far more than a simple nuisance. Noise today has become a public health hazard; more insidious than easily-recognized air and water pollution, noise is invisibly undermining the physical and psychological well-being of millions of people around the world. The remainder of this chapter will describe the ways in which noise affects human health, but first it is necessary to take a brief look at the physical nature of sound and at how noise levels are measured.

Nature of Sound

Sound is produced by the compression and expansion of air created when an object vibrates. The positive and negative pressure waves thus formed travel outward longitudinally from the vibrating source. Two basic characteristics of sound, **frequency** (or **pitch**) and **amplitude**, are related to how loud and annoying a sound will be perceived.

Frequency describes the rate of vibration—how fast the object is moving back and forth. The more rapid the movement, the higher the frequency of the sound pressure waves created. The standard unit used today for measuring frequency is the **hertz (Hz)**, equivalent to one wave per second passing a given point. Most people can hear sounds within a frequency range of 20-20,000 Hz, though there exists a great deal of individual variation in ability to perceive very low or very high frequency sounds.

Amplitude refers to the intensity of sound—how much energy is behind the sound wave. Sound waves of the same frequency can be heard as very loud or very soft, depending on the force with which they strike the ear. In technical terms, amplitude measures the maximum displacement of a sound wave from its resting, or equilibrium, position, but it is perceived psychologically as **loudness**. The unit for measuring intensity, or amplitude, of sound is the **decibel (dB)**; the decibel scale ranges from 0, which is regarded as the threshold of hearing for normal, healthy ears, to 194, regarded as the threshold for pure tones. Because any increase of 10 dB will result in a doubling of perceived loudness, even a small rise in decibel values can make a significant difference in noise intensity.

A listener's perception of a sound as loud, however, does not depend entirely on its amplitude, being affected to some extent by its frequency as well. Although hearing ability ranges from 20–20,000 Hz, not all of these frequencies sound equally loud to the human ear. Maximum sensitivity to sound occurs in the 1000–5000 Hz range. For reference, normal human speech frequencies can vary from 500–2000 Hz. However, sounds at the very low or very high ends of the full audible range (20–20,000 Hz) seem much fainter to our ears than do those in the middle frequencies. Thus, for example, an extremely low-pitched sound must have an amplitude many times greater than a sound of medium pitch in order for both to be heard as equally loud. For this reason, decibel values are sometimes weighted to take into account the frequency response of the human ear. When this is done, the unit measurement designation may be written as dB(A). Figure 13-2 indicates approximate decibel values for a number of commonly encountered sounds.

Figure 13-2 Sound Levels and Human Reponse

Common Sounds	Noise Level (dB)	Effect
Air raid siren	140	Painfully loud
Jet takeoff	130	
Discotheque	120	Maximum vocal effort
Pile driver	110	
Garbage truck	100	
City traffic	90	Very annoying, hearing damage
Alarm clock	80	Annoying
Freeway traffic	70	Phone use difficult
Air conditioning	60	Intrusive
Light auto traffic	50	Quiet
Living room	40	
Library	30	Very quiet
Broadcasting studio	20	
	10	Just audible
	0	Hearing begins

Source: U.S. Environmental Protection Agency

Noise and Hearing Loss

Almost everyone has experienced irritation due to noise, but many people are unaware that the sounds which annoy them also may be affecting their hearing. The EPA estimates that at least 20 million Americans are daily being exposed to levels of noise that are permanently damaging their ability to hear.

Most people are familiar with the temporary deafness and ringing in the ears that occurs after sudden exposure to a very loud noise such as a cap gun or firecracker exploding close to one's head. This type of partial hearing loss generally lasts a few hours at the most and is referred to as **temporary threshold shift (TTS)**. In addition to the obvious impact of sudden, high-intensity sounds, noise research has found that TTS can also result from longer-term exposure (16–48 hours) to noise and that recovery to normal hearing may take as long as two days, depending on both the intensity and duration of noise exposure (Melrick, 1991). The type of short-term hearing loss typified by TTS is an accepted fact of life among workers in noisy occupations, performers and patrons at rock concerts, wildly-cheering spectators at sporting events, and many others. However, most people don't realize that regular, prolonged exposure to noise, even at levels commonly encountered in everyday life, can eventually result in

BOX 13-1
Warning Signs of Hearing Impairment

Perhaps the most difficult aspect of persuading people that the noise levels to which they are exposed present a real threat to their hearing is the fact that such a loss usually is gradual and because the inner ear has no mechanism for registering pain. Nevertheless, certain warning signs can indicate that noise levels are high enough to cause hearing impairment. If heeded, such warnings as the following can help to forestall serious damage:

1. when conversation is difficult or impossible because of high-level background noise (e.g. such as that at a rock concert or noisy sporting event)

2. when ears ring or buzz after leaving a noisy environment

3. when temporary threshold shift is experienced after exposure to very loud noise

4. when pain due to over-stressing of the eardrum occurs after exposure to extremely high-intensity noise

5. when noise exposure results in sensations of unsteadiness, dizziness, or nausea

6. when prolonged noise leaves one highly tense and irritable

permanent hearing impairment. Because damage to the ear is usually painless and seldom visible, few people recognize the injury they are incurring until it is too late. The Occupational Safety and Health Administration (OSHA) has determined that exposure to daily noise levels averaging just 85 decibels (approximately the loudness of an electric shaver or a food processor) over an eight-hour period will result in a slight irreversible loss in hearing; for particularly sensitive individuals, average sound levels as low as 70 dB may be dangerous. The noise of city traffic, subways, power lawnmowers, motorcycles, certain household appliances, babies screaming, and even people shouting all exceed the decibel level considered "safe." Above 85 dB, progressively higher levels of noise exposure exert ever-increasing risk of damage—and the louder the noise, the shorter the exposure time required to wreak lasting harm. With each additional five decibels of loudness, the time required to cause permanent injury is cut in half (Jaret, 1990). For revelers rocking with the beat at a nightclub, where the intensity of sound may hit 120 dB, the damage is done in less than 30 minutes.

Mechanism of Hearing Loss

Noise results in hearing loss through its destructive effect on the delicate hair cells in the Organ of Corti within the cochlea of the inner ear.

These hair cells convert fluid vibrations in the inner ear into impulses which are carried by the auditory nerve to the brain, resulting in the sensation of sound. The outer hair cells at the base of the cochlea, primarily associated with high-frequency sounds, are the first to be affected, but continued exposure to loud noise will eventually result in damage to hair cells in other areas of the cochlea. Over a period of time, prolonged exposure to excessive noise levels may result in the complete collapse of individual hair cells, thus affecting the transmission of nerve impulses. The average individual is born with approximately 16,000 sensory receptors within the Organ of Corti; while 30–50% of these hair cells can be destroyed before any measurable degree of hearing loss is detectable, losses above this level result inevitably in an impairment of hearing ability. Unfortunately, there is no method at present by which a doctor can diagnose the beginning stages of noise-induced hearing loss. The earliest warning signs—inability to hear high-frequency sounds—are unlikely to be noticed unless the affected individual has his or her hearing tested for some other reason. By the time enough hair cells have been lost to affect perception of lower-frequency sounds, a process that may require many years of excessive noise exposure, the damage has been done.

Figure 13-3 How We Hear

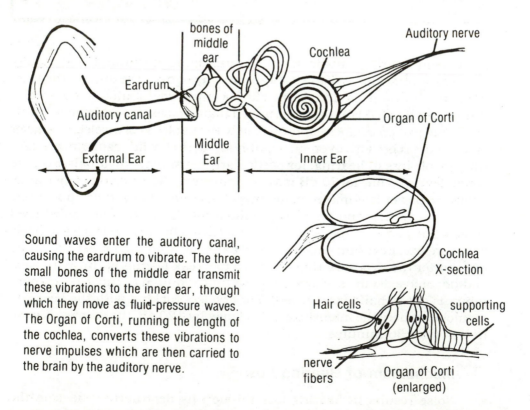

Sound waves enter the auditory canal, causing the eardrum to vibrate. The three small bones of the middle ear transmit these vibrations to the inner ear, through which they move as fluid-pressure waves. The Organ of Corti, running the length of the cochlea, converts these vibrations to nerve impulses which are then carried to the brain by the auditory nerve.

This type of hearing loss, categorized as **sensorineural**, is irreversible and cannot be restored by the use of a hearing aid since both the auditory nerve and cochlear structures have been affected. By contrast, hearing loss resulting from infections (e.g. "swimmer's ear," mumps, measles, etc.) or by trauma (e.g. a blow to the head that ruptures the eardrum or puncturing the eardrum with a cotton-tipped swab or toothpick) is referred to as **conductive** hearing loss and can often be corrected by surgery or medication (Thurston and Roberts, 1991). To a limited extent the ear can protect itself against loud continuous noise by a tightening of the membrane at the entrance to the inner ear, thereby dampening sound. However, in situations where noise volume increases very rapidly or instantaneously, as when a military jet makes a low-altitude flyover or someone fires a rifle close to the ear, adaptation processes and reflex protective mechanisms don't have time to function effectively. In such cases damage risk to the inner ear is greater than it would be if the volume of noise were increasing more slowly (Ising et al., 1990).

Many people take it for granted that a gradual loss of hearing is one of the inevitable consequences of growing older, a belief bolstered by statistics which report that by the age of 65, one out of four Americans is experiencing hearing loss significant enough to interfere with communication; by the time they reach their nineties, nine out of ten seniors are so afflicted. Many researchers are convinced, however, that the extent of the problem is considerably greater than it need be. Some years ago, an audiologist traveled to a remote African village near the Sudan-Ethiopian border to test the hearing of tribe members who had never heard the blare of amplified music or the din of urban traffic. He found that 70+-year-old Africans, unlike their American peers, could easily hear sounds as soft as a murmur from as far as 300 feet away (Jaret, 1990). While some degree of age-related hearing loss (clinically described as **presbycusis**) may be inevitable, the Sudanese experience provides a meaningful lesson—one of the best ways to preserve lifelong sharpness of hearing is to limit as much as possible one's exposure to a noisy environment.

Effects of Hearing Loss

Hearing disability caused by noise can range in severity from difficulty in comprehending normal conversation to total deafness. In general, the ability to hear high-frequency sounds is the first thing to be affected by noise exposure; for this reason, tests for early detection of hearing loss should pay special attention to hearing ability in the 4000 Hz range. People affected often have difficulty hearing such sounds as a clock ticking or telephone ringing and cannot distinguish certain consonants, particularly s, sh, ch, p, m, t, f, and th. Individuals suffering hearing loss not only have trouble with the volume of speech, but also with its clarity. They frequently accuse people with whom they are speaking of mumbling, particularly when talking on the telephone or when background noises interfere with conversation; listening to the radio or television may become impossible.

BOX 13-2

Just Turn It Down!

They seem to be the height of fashion in headgear these days, adorning joggers panting along the roadside, accompanying children walking to school, soothing rush-hour commuters on trains and subways, staving off boredom for those engaged in yard chores, providing background music for college studies. Everyone is wearing them, especially young people who find in these Walkman-type portable stereos and headphones a way to carry their music with them wherever they go. The proliferation of these devices and their enormous popularity worldwide has sparked intense debate among noise experts as to the extent to which use of personal stereos has contributed to the documented hearing loss among teenagers and young adults. The question is given urgency by the fact that in the United States alone, more than 20 million personal stereos with headsets have been sold annually in recent years.

While the amount of noise exposure received by a listener obviously varies, depending on the volume setting chosen, most brands are capable of reaching decibel levels of 105 to 126—considerably higher than the 85dB volume at which damage to hearing begins. Loudness alone, of course, is not the sole determinant of how damaging to the ears personal stereos can be; equally important are the frequency and duration of their use. While the majority of researchers agree that most users select volume settings lower than 90 dB and hence are at minimal risk of long-term hearing damage, a sizable minority turn up the sound levels to more than 100 dB and listen for extended periods of time. Many who misuse their personal stereos in this way report experiencing tinnitus or a sensation of fullness in the ears, indicative of a temporary hearing loss. Unfortunately, incremental hearing loss can't be felt at the time it is occurring unless decibel levels are in excess of 140, the "threshold of pain." To assist listeners in determining when the volume of their Walkman is high enough to present a hearing threat, some noise experts urge that manufacturers provide some sort of warning device on stereo units, such as an indicator that lights up when sound intensity exceeds 90 dB or a volume control logo painted red for settings that exceed this noise level. In the absence of such aids, Walkman aficionados wishing to safeguard their hearing should keep in mind two simple rules-of-thumb: on a scale of 1–10, any setting above 4 is potentially ear-damaging; and if music from one's headphones is loud enough to be heard by passers-by, it's loud enough to be causing noise-induced hearing loss.

Overall, personal stereos present a minimal auditory hazard, particularly when compared to target-shooting or playing in a rock band. Nevertheless, such devices do have the potential for harm if misused and efforts to educate the public on the importance of protecting their hearing not only from personal stereos but from all sources of excessive environmental noise is sorely needed.

The psychological impact of such difficulties—the fear of being laughed at for misunderstanding questions or comments, the frustration of not being able to follow a conversation, the feeling of isolation or alienation experienced as friends unconsciously avoid trying to converse—are frequently as severe as the physical disability. Individuals experiencing hearing loss tend to become suspicious, irritable, and depressed; their careers suffer and their social life becomes severely restricted, sometimes to the point of complete withdrawal (Perham, 1979). Some researchers even suspect that the confusion and unresponsiveness blamed on Alzheimer's disease may actually, in some cases, be due to hearing loss.

In addition to these problems, a person with partial hearing loss may suffer sharp pain in the ears when exposed to very loud noise and may experience repeated bouts of **tinnitus**—a ringing or buzzing sound in the head that can drive the victim to distraction, interfering with sleep, conversation, and normal daily activities. Probably the single most common side effect of noise-induced hearing loss, tinnitus can become a permanent condition, though it is usually only a temporary nuisance. To sufferers, the intensity of the noise in their heads can be maddening, likened by one victim to "holding a vacuum cleaner to your ear" (Murphy, 1989). The pitch of the ringing characterizing tinnitus can sound like a high scream and volume levels as high as 70 dB have been measured. Among those afflicted with permanent tinnitus, certain medications, diet, or relaxation therapies may ease the symptoms, but the condition at this stage is essentially irreversible (Cohen, 1990).

Other Effects of Noise

Hearing loss is the most obvious health threat posed by noise pollution, but it is by no means the only one. Noise can adversely affect our physical and psychological well-being in a host of other ways.

Stress and Related Health Effects

Exposure to unwanted noise involuntarily induces stress, and stress can lead to a variety of physical ailments including an increase in heart rate, high blood pressure, elevated levels of blood cholesterol, ulcers, headaches, and colitis.

Stressful reaction to loud or sudden noise undoubtedly represents an evolutionary adaptation to warnings signalling approaching danger. Bodily responses to the snarl of a predatory beast or the rumble of a boulder crashing down a mountainside cause a surge of adrenalin, an increase in heart and breathing rates, and the tensing of muscles—all physiological preparations for fight or flight that have important survival value. However, these same metabolic responses are today being triggered repeatedly by the innumerable noises of modern society. As a result, our bodies are subjected to a constant state of stress which, far from being advantageous, is literally making millions of people sick—even though they may not

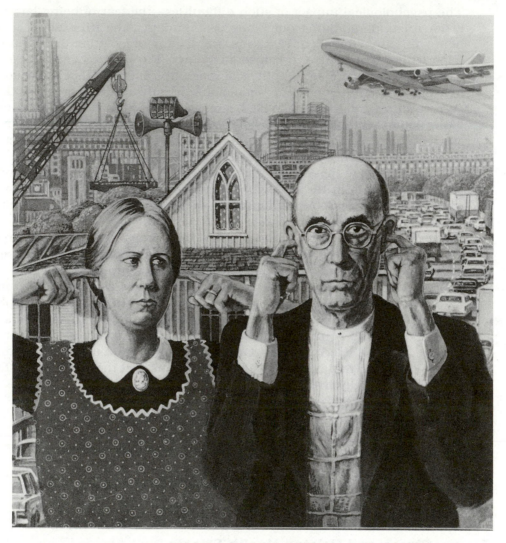

Contemporary American life is much noisier than in days gone by due in part to advanced technology, life-style changes, transportation habits, and population density. [EPA Journal]

attribute their problems to noise. While many individuals insist that they have "gotten used to noise" and are no longer bothered by it, the truth is that no one can prevent the automatic biological changes which noise provokes. Research into the association between noise exposure and stress-related disease has produced findings such as the following:

> Workers exposed to high levels of occupational noise were found to exhibit up to five times as many cases of ulcers as would normally be expected among people in quieter surroundings.

> A five-year study of factory workers revealed that employees assigned to noisy areas of the plant had a higher frequency of diagnosed medical problems, including respiratory ailments, than did workers in quieter sections of the same plant.

Exposure of a laboratory population of rhesus monkeys to noise levels typically experienced on a daily basis by factory workers resulted in a 30% elevation of the monkeys' blood pressure—a level which persisted for a long period after the experiment ended.

Such findings indicate that adverse noise-induced health effects cannot be reversed quickly simply by removing the noise source (Terry, 1979).

Teratogenic Effects of Noise

The human uterus is not an inner sanctum of peace and quiet. Research has shown that fetal development proceeds amidst constant internal noise generated by the throbbing of maternal arteries and rumbling of bowels. Background noise levels within the pregnant uterus have been variously estimated as ranging anywhere from 56 to 95 dB (as compared with, for example, a typical office environment where decibel levels average about 50). Although the mother's body tissues to some extent attenuate penetration of external noise into the womb, both experimental and anecdotal evidence indicate that outside noise can provoke a physical response in the developing unborn child.

For over half a century, one method used by physicians for determining fetal viability has been to place a sound source near the mother's abdomen and expose the fetus to noise of 120 Hz frequency. Since a fetus' hearing ability is well-developed by the 28th week of pregnancy, such noise exposure causes a noticeable increase in heart rate and kicking among third-trimester fetuses. Less scientific but equally persuasive testimony comes from pregnant women who have reported that they felt considerably more fetal movement while listening to music in a concert hall, the kicking reaching a peak when the audience began to applaud!

While the fact that noise exposure begins well before birth is undisputable, it is less clear whether such exposure presents any risk of hearing impairment to the unborn child. The question is of some concern because approximately 45% of the U.S. work force is now female and many of these women will experience one or more pregnancies during their working years. Since occupational noise pollution control frequently is focused on providing ear protection to workers, the question of possible noise-induced hearing damage to the fetuses of pregnant employees is of more than academic interest. While a few epidemiologic studies have reported some degree of hearing impairment among children whose mothers received occupational noise exposures up to 100 dB during pregnancy, most of the limited research done to date indicates that hearing loss induced in a fetus by external noise is highly unlikely. The insulating effect of maternal tissues which limits the amount of outside sound penetrating the uterine environment renders noise an unlikely teratogenic agent (Thurston and Roberts, 1991).

Much more research is needed to define the extent of the relationship, if any, between noise and birth defects, as well as to establish how high noise levels must be to cause developmental problems. Lacking definitive information, some doctors recommend that pregnant women try to avoid noise exposure to the greatest extent possible, one such expert offering the tongue-in-cheek advice that "any expectant mother should get out of New York."

Effects of Noise on Learning Ability and Work Performance

Noisy surroundings at home and school can adversely affect children's language development and their ability to read. High noise levels interfere with a youngster's capacity to distinguish certain sounds such as "b" and "v," for example, and can foster a tendency to drop the endings of words, thereby distorting speech. Research has shown that reading skills are seriously impaired when the student's surroundings are noisy. One study focused on children living in a noisy apartment complex found that the longer they had resided in that environment, the poorer was their reading development. The investigators conducting the study concluded that a noisy home environment has more of an impact on reading skills than do such factors as parents' educational level, number of children in the family, or the child's grade level. Another study that examined the effect of classroom exposure to noise revealed that in one school located adjacent to an elevated railway, students whose classrooms faced the track scored significantly lower on reading tests than did those whose rooms were on the opposite side of the school.

Figure 13-4 Noise around our Homes

Noise Source	Sound Level for Operator (in dBA)
Refrigerator	40
Floor Fan	38 to 70
Clothes Dryer	55
Washing Machine	47 to 78
Dishwasher	54 to 85
Hair Dryer	59 to 80
Vacuum Cleaner	62 to 85
Sewing Machine	64 to 74
Electric Shaver	75
Food Disposal (Grinder)	67 to 93
Electric Lawn Edger	81
Home Shop Tools	85
Gasoline Power Mower	87 to 92
Gasoline Riding Mower	90 to 95
Chain Saw	100
Stereo	Up to 120

A comparable situation relating to decreased efficiency on the job faces millions of American workers. Several years ago the National Institute for Occupational Safety and Health conservatively estimated that more than 2.5 million U.S. industrial workers were exposed to harmful levels of noise. Aside from the health aspects of this exposure, noise hinders the performance of tasks requiring high levels of accuracy (total *quantity of work*, as opposed to quality, does not appear to suffer appreciably). Very loud or sporadic noises seem to be the most disruptive, distorting time perception, increasing the variability in work performance, disturbing concentration, and making it more difficult to remain alert. The effects of working all day in a noisy environment frequently carry over into domestic life, making the worker more prone to aggravation and frustration when he or she comes home. Pent-up stress from daytime noise exposure may prevent relaxation in the evening, and if the home environment is noisy also, the worker may remain tense and irritable (EPA, 1979).

Safety Aspects of Noise

Safety, as well as health, can be in jeopardy when noise levels are high. Some years ago a worker in an auto glass manufacturing plant caught his hand in a piece of equipment; he frantically screamed for help, but no one came to his aid because noise levels in the factory were so high that he couldn't be heard. On another occasion, two people in Elizabeth, New Jersey, were struck and killed by a locomotive while watching Senator Robert Kennedy's funeral train pass through the city; they hadn't heard the warning whistle because of the noise from the Secret Service and news media helicopters. In an auto pressroom in Ohio, two workers were permanently disabled when noisy working conditions prevented their hearing warning shouts about approaching panel racks (Stansbury, 1979). Many traffic accidents are thought to be caused by drivers' inability to hear emergency sirens. Both by interfering with shouts for help or by masking warning signals, high levels of background noise pose a very real threat to public safety.

Figure 13-5 Permissible Noise Exposures Established By OSHA

Duration per day (hours)	Sound level (dB)
8	90
6	92
4	95
3	97
2	100
1½	102
1	105
½	110
¼ or less	115

Source: OSHA

Sleep Disruption

Sleep is a biological necessity. We need sleep to repair the wearing out of bodily tissues and to rejuvenate them; deprivation or disruption of sleep can thus directly threaten both physical health and mental well-being.

BOX 13-3

Play Can Be Deafening!

The association between high noise levels and hearing loss in the occupational environment has been recognized—and regulated—for years. The Occupational Safety and Health Administration (OSHA) has set an eight-hour time-weighted average of 90 dB(A) as the maximum permissible noise exposure for the American worker. In recent years, however, it has become increasingly clear that dangerous levels of noise are found not only in factories but also in the home and in association with a wide range of recreational activities. The same individual whose hearing is protected by regulations while on the job may, during off-work hours, incur irreparable damage by engaging in noisy activities where sound levels are totally unregulated and where those exposed seldom wear ear protection.

Perhaps most at risk of nonoccupational noise-induced hearing loss are millions of children and young adults whose ideas of fun are often inseparable from noise: listening to amplified music, playing electronic arcade games, participating in noisy sports events, playing in the school band. Researchers have been surprised to discover that noise-induced hearing loss can begin at 10–20 years of age, much earlier than they previously had thought possible. In 1990 a group of British researchers reported unexpected frustration in their efforts to study hearing damage among youths aged 15–23. Their project was stymied because they couldn't assemble a sufficient number of young people to serve as "controls"—virtually all the candidates had already been exposed to loud music!

Hearing impairment among rock musicians is legendary, as testimony by such notables as Pete Townshend, Ted Nugent, Joey Kramer, and others bears witness. The impact on those whose exposure is limited to *attending* rock concerts or noisy nightclubs is probably less dramatic. Attendees are typically exposed to noise levels of 100 dB or higher (OSHA standards permit no more than 2 hours exposure to noise of this intensity in the workplace). They frequently experience temporary threshold shift (TTS) but generally recover within a few hours to a few days after exposure (Clark, 1991).

The roar of the crowd at athletic events may be endangering fans' hearing, particularly if the event in question happens to be a Minnesota Twins game at the Metrodome. Perhaps because its dome is smaller than average, with a roof configuration that returns noise to the field, the Metrodome may reverberate with noise levels exceeding 100 dB when the stands are full and the home team is winning. As in the situation with rock concerts, spectators who spend a limited amount of time in these raucous surroundings are at minor risk of long-term harm, but Twins players and the concessionaires who spend most of the season amidst the cheering throngs are at serious risk of permanent hearing impairment (Gauthier, 1988).

Many household appliances expose persons of all ages to noise levels that frequently exceed the 85 dB "safe" level; fortunately the duration of exposure to such noises as the whir of a food processor or the drone of a vacuum cleaner is generally quite brief. On the other hand, certain power tools such as chainsaws or leaf blowers could present a risk if used for prolonged periods without hearing protection. Similarly, farm equipment such as tractors can be a significant cause of hearing impairment for rural youngsters. A study conducted in Wisconsin revealed that more than half the children involved in farm work experienced some degree of noise-induced hearing loss, double the rate of children *not* working on farms.

Of all the dangerous forms of recreational noise exposure, however, the greatest toll on young ears (and older ears as well!) is wrought by hunting and target shooting, activities regularly enjoyed by an estimated 13% of the U.S. population. With decibel levels frequently exceeding the threshold of pain, the crack of gunfire, or even cap pistols, can instantly destroy receptor cells in the inner ear and irreversibly damage hearing ability. Among a study group of 94 children or teenagers who were victims of noise-induced hearing loss, an analysis of the noise sources revealed that fully 46% suffered because of guns or fireworks; only 12% had been damaged by exposure to live or amplified music, 8% by power tools, and 4% by recreational vehicles.

Since noise-induced hearing loss is cumulative, growing slowly but steadily worse with continued exposure to a wide variety of high-decibel activities,

people of all ages, but especially children, need to become more aware of how to protect themselves. For those young people who shrug off the importance of ear protection, down-playing the impact hearing loss could have on their lives, an analogy by Congressman Richard Durbin of Illinois, a member of the House Committee conducting hearings on noise pollution, seems particularly apt: "If you are color blind you can visit an art museum, but you miss a lot. People who have lost their hearing are missing so much. They hear *something*, but they are missing a lot in the process" (U.S. Congress, 1991).

References

Clark, William W. 1991. "Noise Exposure from Leisure Activities: A Review." *Journal of the Acoustical Society of America* 90, no.1 (July).

Gauthier, Michele M. 1988. "Clamorous Metrodome Hard on Ears and Foes." *The Physician and Sports Medicine* 16, no. 3 (March).

U.S. Congress. House. 1991. *Turn It Down: Effects of Noise on Hearing Loss in Children and Youth.* Hearing before the Select Committee on Children, Youth, and Families, July 22. Washington, D.C.: U.S. Government Printing Office.

Noise can prevent people from going to sleep, can waken them prematurely, or can cause shifts from deeper to lighter stages of sleep. While individual response to noise in relation to its impact on sleep varies widely, in general adults are wakened by noise more easily than are children; the elderly are more sensitive than the middle-aged; sick persons are more affected than healthy ones; and women are more easily disturbed than men (Bugliarello, 1976).

Noise Control Efforts

Historically, noise abatement efforts have consisted primarily of local ordinances directed at specific community nuisances. One of the earliest of such laws was a London ordinance that went into effect in 1829

(Lipscomb, 1974), allowing stagecoach horses to be confiscated if they disrupted church services! Over the years since then, cities have adopted a wide variety of local restrictions on noise sources. A brief sampling of such regulations include: requirements for mufflers on cars; prohibitions against construction activity, garbage collection, or lawn mowing during early morning or evening hours; bans on roosters or other noisy animals within city limits; restrictions on auto horn-blowing; bans on truck traffic through residential neighborhoods; and prohibitions on "boom cars" or other forms of amplified music outdoors.

The federal government entered the noise control arena in 1972 with passage of the Noise Control Act—the first national law aimed at relieving over-stimulated American ears by regulating certain commercial products considered to be major noise sources. The law called for noise emission limits to be set for products such as medium- and heavy-weight trucks, buses, motorcycles, power lawnmowers, jackhammers, and rock drills. In addition, the EPA was to draft noise labeling requirements for noisy products as well as conduct studies on the health impact of noise in order to provide an objective basis for the numerical noise standards yet to be promulgated.

In 1978 the Noise Control Act was amended by the Quiet Communities Act which authorized EPA to work in partnership with state and local governments, helping them to develop anti-noise programs appropriate to their own special needs and abilities. Federal funding provided aid in the form of grants, seminars, and training programs to assist lower levels of

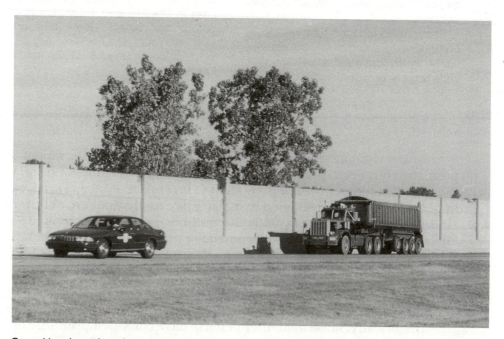

Sound barriers along busy highways help protect nearby residents from the incessant rumble of heavy traffic. [Thomas A. Schneider]

government. With the EPA serving as a coordinating agency and providing seed money for local initiatives, hundreds of community noise abatement programs were launched during the 1970s. Noise control efforts suffered a serious setback in the 1980s, however, with the advent of a Reagan Administration committed to an anti-regulatory agenda on environmental issues. In 1982, to the dismay of noise experts, EPA's Office of Noise Abatement and Control (ONAC) was disbanded and has yet to be restored. With the EPA leadership terminated and its technical assistance and funding eliminated, research on the impact of noise on health and hearing has declined sharply since the early 1980s. Most information on noise pollution appearing in current textbooks is still based on studies conducted during the 1970s. The promising proliferation of municipal noise abatement efforts which characterized the late 1970s has suffered a similar reversal. Of the more than 1100 state and local noise control programs that

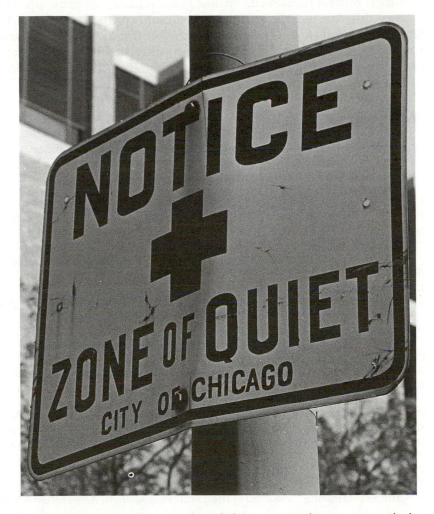

In most urban areas noise-control regulations are nonexistent or are routinely ignored. [Nora Byrne]

existed 20 years ago, only about 15 are still functioning. Although the Noise Control Act mandates are still theoretically in effect, they are not being enforced. Regulations that were about to be promulgated at the time ONAC closed were never completed and those that had been finalized have been ignored. Of the wide range of equipment targeted by the Noise Control Act, the only products for which noise emission standards have yet been promulgated are air compressors, motorcycles, trucks, and waste compactors. In 1991 hearing experts testified before a Congressional Committee, urging restoration of EPA leadership in national noise abatement efforts and calling for renewed noise emission information and warning labels on dangerously noisy equipment (U.S. Congress, 1991). Whether a more environmentally friendly Clinton Administration will heed their appeal remains to be seen. Undoubtedly the most serious obstacle to implementing effective programs is the difficulty of convincing both policymakers and the public that noise pollution is really important. As one EPA official remarked, "Noise is something we grow up with, and it is very difficult to believe that such a common pollutant could be doing anything serious to our health or the environment." Until an aroused public insists that excessive noise is a community health hazard that must be controlled, it is unlikely that elected officials will give noise abatement efforts the attention they deserve.

References

Bugliarello, George, Ariel Alexandre, John Barnes, and Charles Wakstein. 1976. *The Impact of Noise Pollution.* Pergamon Press.

Cohen, Peter. 1990. "Drumming: How Risky Is It To Your Hearing?" *Modern Drummer* (October).

Environmental Protection Agency. 1979. *EPA Journal* 5, no. 9 (Oct.).

Finn, Robin. 1992. "No Stereo Necessary In a Graf-Seles Final." *New York Times*, July 3.

Ising, Hartmut, Ekkehard Rebentisch, Fritz Poustka, and Immo Curio. 1990. "Annoyance and Health Risk Caused by Military Low-altitude Flight Noise." *International Archives of Occupational and Environmental Health* 62:357–363.

Jaret, Peter. 1990. "The Rock & Roll Syndrome." *In Health* (July/Aug.).

Lipscomb, David M. 1974. *Noise: The Unwanted Sounds.* Nelson-Hall.

Melrick, William. 1991. "Human Temporary Threshold Shift (TTS) and Damage Risk." *Journal of the Acoustical Society of America* 90, no. 1 (July).

Murphy, Elliott. 1989. "Townshend, Tinnitus and Rock & Roll." *Rolling Stone*, July 13–27.

OECD. 1991. *Fighting Noise in the 1990s.* Paris: OECD.

Perham, Chris. 1979. "The Sound of Silence." *EPA Journal* 5, no. 9 (Oct.).

Rotella, Sebastian. 1989. "Man Accused of Using Mirror to Harass Pilots." *New York Times*, Dec. 30.

Shapiro, Margaret. 1989. "Crowds are Made in Japan Too." *Washington Post*, Feb. 13.

Stansbury, Jeff. 1979. "Noise in the Workplace." *EPA Journal* 5, no. 9 (Oct.).

Suro, Roberto. "In the Birthplace of Jazz, It's Just a Little Too Loud." *New York Times*, Sept. 3.

Terry, Luther L., M.D. "Health and Noise." *EPA Journal* 5, no. 9 (Oct.).

Thurston, Floyd E., M.D., and Stanley L. Roberts, PA-C, M.P.H. "Environmental Noise and Fetal Hearing." *Journal of the Tennessee Medical Association* 84, no. 1 (Jan.)

CHAPTER 14

Water Resources

All the rivers run into the sea, yet the sea is not full; to the place from whence the rivers come, thither they return again.
—Ecclesiastes 1:7

Although the ancient writer of Ecclesiastes expressed his scientific observations in poetic form, his statements relating to the cycling of water through the hydrosphere are basically correct, albeit overly simplified. Water moves in what is essentially a closed system, circulating from one part of the earth to another, changing in form from liquid to solid or gas and back to liquid again, yet remaining relatively constant in total amount. Water occurs as vapor in the atmosphere, as rain or snow falling on the earth or oceans, as ice locked in massive glaciers or ice caps, and as rivers, streams, lakes, seas, and subterranean groundwater. The manner by which water moves from place to place, changing from one form to another, is called the **hydrologic cycle**.

Hydrologic Cycle

The hydrologic cycle, like virtually all other processes on earth, is powered by energy from the sun that causes water to evaporate from the surface of the oceans, rivers, lakes, and from the soil. The movement of this water vapor in the atmosphere is an important factor in the redistribution of heat around the earth. Because heat is absorbed when water evaporates, the atmosphere becomes a reservoir of heat energy. This heat energy then drives the hydrologic cycle which gives rise to the atmospheric forces involved in weather and climate.

The principal processes involved in the hydrologic cycle are:

1. Evaporation of water from surface waters and from the soil.
2. Transportation of water by plants; because both evaporation and transpiration produce the same result (i.e. the addition of water vapor to the atmosphere), the two processes are often collectively called evapotranspiration.
3. Transport of atmospheric water from one place to another either as water vapor or as liquid water droplets and ice crystals in clouds.
4. Precipitation when atmospheric water vapor condenses and falls as rain, hail, sleet, or snow.
5. Runoff, whereby water that has fallen on land finds its way back to the oceans, flowing either on or under the surface of the continents.

The amount of time required for the completion of the cycle can vary widely from place to place and from one part of the cycle to another. On the average, a water molecule spends nine days in the atmosphere from the time it evaporates until it falls again as rain or snow (Ehrlich, Ehrlich,

Figure 14-1 Hydrologic Cycle

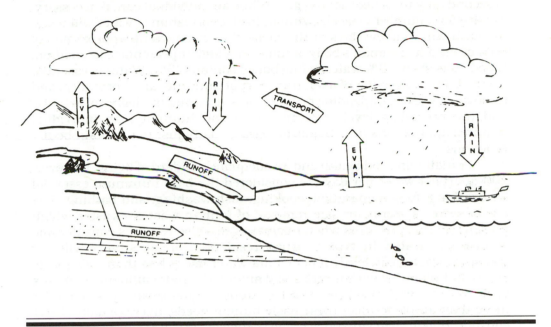

and Holdren, 1977). However, if it happens to fall as a snowflake on the Antarctic ice sheet, it may remain there for thousands of years before it breaks off as part of an iceberg and melts into the ocean; conversely, if it falls during a desert thunderstorm, it might evaporate in an hour or two.

Approximately 71% of the earth's surface is covered with water, a resource amounting to almost 1.5 billion km^3 in total volume. Of this amount, however, only a very small percentage is readily available for human use. Most of the water on the planet, about 97.4%, is found in the world's seas and oceans—enormously abundant but too salty for drinking or agricultural use; 2% is fresh water locked up in glaciers and polar ice caps; the remainder, less than 1% of the total, consists of fresh water in rivers, lakes, groundwater, and water vapor in the atmosphere (World Resources Institute, 1992; Maurits la Riviere, 1989). Obviously, for humans this is the portion of greatest significance, since it constitutes the water we drink, bathe in, and use for irrigation and industrial purposes. Of this small percentage of water on which human life depends, only a minuscule portion is found in the rivers, streams, and lakes of the world. Likewise, at any given moment only a tiny amount of the world's water occurs as atmospheric water vapor. By far the greatest amount of all available fresh water, approximately 96.5% of the total, is found beneath the surface of the soil in the form of groundwater.

Water Quantity and Health

The human body's absolute dependence on regular intake of water is second only to its need for oxygen. While an individual can, if necessary, survive for a number of weeks without food, deprivation of water will result in death within a few days at the most. Water makes up approximately 65% of the adult human's body, a somewhat higher percentage in children. Blood consists of 83% water, while bones contain 25%. Water is essential for the body's digestion of food, transport of nutrients and hormones, and removal of wastes. Depending on a person's size, weight, degree of activity, and the prevailing level of temperature and humidity, an individual requires approximately 1–3 quarts of water daily just to maintain bodily functions.

To maintain good health and an adequate standard of living, however, 100 quarts of water per day are considered the bare minimum essential for drinking, food preparation, cooking, dish washing, and bathing. The use of sewer systems for safe removal of human wastes—wastes which present serious problems when mismanaged—also requires considerable amounts of water. In typical urban residential areas, sewers will not transport wastes efficiently if per capita water use is less than 100 quarts a day. In industrialized countries and among the more affluent segments of the urban population in developing nations, water quantity is generally more than ample to meet these basic human needs; average daily water consumption in such situations ranges between 200–400 quarts per person per day. However, in developing countries more than a billion people still lack access to adequate supplies of safe water, in spite of impressive gains made during the United Nations-sponsored 1981–1990 International Drinking Water Supply and Sanitation Decade (World Bank, 1992). In many rural areas the problem is not the lack of water per se, but rather that the source of such water is far from the point of use. In some countries, women may spend several hours each day hauling water from a distant river, well, or standpipe to their homes, leaving little time for more economically productive tasks such as gardening or trading in the marketplace. The sheer physical effort involved in carrying water long distances also exerts a toll on the health of rural women who, not infrequently, may be malnourished and overworked. In most urban areas of the Third World, water supply systems are in place, but frequently they are in poor condition or are unreliable, functioning perhaps only a few hours each day. While walking distances for the urban poor are less than for their country cousins, such people nevertheless spend hours waiting in long lines for their turn at the standpipe. Among many poor urban residents in the Third World, water is obtained by purchasing it from vendors at a cost many times higher than the cost per unit of a piped-in municipal supply. The necessity of buying water imposes a heavy financial burden on family incomes; in Port-au-Prince, Haiti, 20% of a typical slum-dweller's household budget is spent on water.

In situations such as these, where safe water is in short supply, difficult or time-consuming to obtain, or exorbitantly expensive, important aspects of personal hygiene and basic sanitation such as washing hands and eating

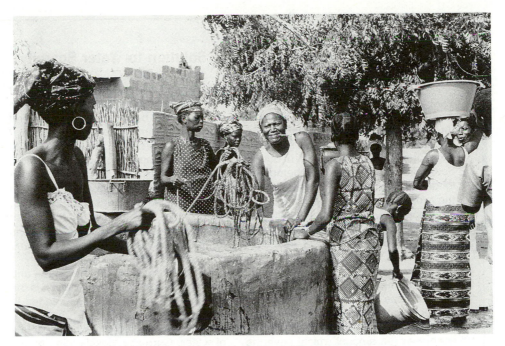

Women in Senegal gather at the community well. [© Beryl Goldberg]

utensils is frequently neglected. In addition, there is a strong temptation to utilize polluted sources of water if higher-quality supplies are not easily accessible. A recent study published by the World Health Organization demonstrated that improved access to water reduced the incidence of diarrheal cases by 25%, while improvements in both water quality and access reduced such illnesses by fully 37%. Perhaps the most essential prerequisite for improving the health and living standards among the Third World poor is an increase in the quantity of readily available safe water supplies (Briscoe, 1993).

Water Supply: Our Next Crisis?

While water is indeed a renewable resource, the *rate* at which it is renewed within the global hydrologic cycle is both fixed and slow. Water is also a finite resource—although human technologies can devise means for utilizing the existing supply more efficiently, science cannot create additional water nor alter the rate at which water is circulated through the biosphere. Faced with these realities, many water resource experts view current water use trends with alarm, warning that the approaching "water crisis" which they foresee could be the first resource constraint to impose serious limits on further world economic growth. Such fears are based on the fact that over the past 300 years worldwide withdrawals from fresh-water resources have increased more than 35-fold and continue to grow

BOX 14-1

Water from the Sea: The Ultimate Solution to Water Scarcity?

"Water, water everywhere, but not a drop to drink." The lament of Coleridge's Ancient Mariner has reverberated through the centuries as inhabitants of arid coastal regions wistfully dreamed of transforming sea water into a potable beverage. Today such schemes no longer seem unrealistic, as pressures on the world's freshwater resources spur developments that make desalination projects both technologically feasible and increasingly common in water-short areas of the world. Currently there are more than 7500 desalination plants in operation in 120 countries around the globe. Of various sizes and types, these facilities produce, collectively, nearly 5 billion cubic meters of fresh water from the sea each year (an amount which, nevertheless, represents only 0.1% of total water use). The leading producer of desalted seawater is the oil-rich desert kingdom of Saudi Arabia which boasts 29 desalination plants that annually yield fully 27% of total world capacity of desalted water. A distant runner-up for second place, at 12%, is the United States, with more than 100 small plants in southern Florida and several others in California, including the nation's largest desalination facility at Santa Barbara, completed early in 1992. The Persian Gulf nations of Kuwait and the United Arab Emirates rank just below the United States in desalination capacity, while numerous other facilities are scattered around the Caribbean, in Australia, Spain, and elsewhere.

The technologies for desalting seawater are straightforward and relatively simple. Large plants, such as the 1 million m^3/day facility at Jubail, Saudi Arabia, and the plant at Key West, Florida, typically employ a multistage flash distillation process, in which water is heated under pressure and then injected into a low pressure chamber where it instantly "flashes" into steam which is captured and condensed into pure water. The fact that pressurized hot water from a single source can be flashed into several chambers simultaneously makes it possible to produce large amounts of water quite dependably by this method. Smaller plants more commonly rely on reverse osmosis, a process by which seawater is forced, under high pressure, through a membrane that permits passage of water molecules but screens out the slightly larger ions of sodium and chlorine.

The problem with both methods—and the main factor limiting their use—is the enormous amount of energy needed to power both processes, a requirement which translates into a high price per unit of water. Currently, desalination of sea water is three to four times more expensive than obtaining the same amount from conventional freshwater sources. Brackish water, with its lower salt content, costs less than half as much to treat as does seawater, but even so, desalination remains one of our most costly water supply options, well beyond the reach of many poor countries. It is conceivable that eventually, as technology is refined and as the price of water from other sources continues to increase, desalinated water may become more cost-competitive than it is at present. For the foreseeable future, however, it is unlikely that desalination offers a realistic option for satisfying more than a small fraction of the world's water needs.

References

Ashworth, William. 1982. *Nor Any Drop to Drink*. Summit Books.

Postel, Sandra. 1992. *Last Oasis: Facing Water Scarcity*. W. W. Norton & Co.

World Resources Institute. 1992. *World Resources 1992–93*. Oxford University Press.

at a 2–3% annual rate, down slightly from a 4–8% yearly increase in the decades prior to the 1990s (World Resources Institute, 1992). Recent water emergencies, precipitated by drought or water mismanagement, in such diverse areas as California, eastern Africa, southeastern India, and Uzbekistan are, these experts insist, but harbingers of more difficult times to come. At first glance, such gloomy predictions seem at variance with the facts. Although the amount of fresh water readily available for human use constitutes less than 0.01% of all the water on earth, it still represents an abundant supply—theoretically sufficient to satisfy the needs of 20 billion people if equally divided (Maurits la Riviere, 1989). Obviously, however, neither the planet's water resources nor its human population are evenly distributed. Depending on local patterns of annual precipitation and evaporative demand (i.e. the maximum amount of moisture the atmosphere is capable of absorbing), water availability varies widely from one region to another. In the United States, for example, average annual rainfall is approximately 30 inches. This amount is distributed quite unevenly, however; whereas the Pacific Northwest receives about 80 inches of precipitation annually and the states east of the Mississippi River average 40–45 inches, the Great Plains and the Southwest are chronically water-short. The driest state, Nevada, receives only 9 inches of rainfall in an average year (Pringle, 1982). Viewing the world as a whole, nations lying between 20–30 degrees of latitude both north and south of the equator (the transition zone between temperate and tropical regions) tend to have the lowest annual rates of precipitation and are also most subject to recurrent droughts. Perhaps not by coincidence, these lands also are home to some of the world's poorest countries and experience some of the highest population growth rates. Even within regions where water supplies are usually adequate, periodic dry spells and increasing industrial and municipal demands may result in localized shortages. Compounding the problem of regional disparities in water supply is the fact that everywhere—both in water-rich and water-poor areas of the world—pollution is rendering much of the available supply unusable without extensive (and expensive) treatment.

Impact of Population Growth on Water Demand

To some extent, water demand within a society is determined by that society's level of affluence and technological development. On a per capita basis, today's largest water consumers are the rich nations of the industrialized world. The average American currently consumes, directly or indirectly, more than 70 times as much water each year as the average Ghanaian (Maurits la Riviere, 1989). However, in the years ahead the major factor accounting for increased water demand, especially in urban areas, will be the explosive growth of human populations. Within any region, the amount of available water, determined primarily by precipitation, is finite. Thus the amount available per capita is directly proportional to population size. While more efficient water management can help to ensure more equitable distribution and prevent wastage, unchecked population growth will inevitably result in chronic water shortages. The problem is most acute today for the countries of the Middle East (see Box 14–2), a naturally arid, drought-prone region with some of the world's highest birth rates. In Gaza, Jordan, Syria, and Iraq, populations will double in less than 20 years, yet water availability will remain unchanged. In Africa and southern Asia also, rapid population growth is increasing the stress on water supplies; by 2025 it is expected that more than a billion people throughout this area will be plagued by a scarcity of water (Falkenmark and Widstrand, 1992).

The impact of burgeoning population on water supplies promises to be most sorely felt in Third World cities. Even in countries where national averages indicate adequate water resources, runaway rates of urbanization and industrialization are seriously endangering both the quantity and quality of water supplies within many metropolitan areas. In the Chinese capital, Beijing, for example, excessive pumping of groundwater to slake the city's thirst has caused one-third of the wells to go dry and is lowering the water table by as much as 6 feet each year (Linden, 1990). Bodily wastes generated by soaring numbers of urban poor lacking the most basic sanitation facilities have so polluted many urban water supplies with microbial pathogens that cities from Shanghai to Lima have been forced to divert millions of dollars from other urgently needed projects to finance increased levels of wastewater treatment. Such problems will become even more severe in the years ahead if current population growth trends persist. Projections indicate that global water use by the end of this decade will be twice as high as it was in 1980, thanks to expanding development efforts and increasing human numbers (McCaffrey, 1992).

Groundwater

Mention "water resources" and most people immediately think of rivers, lakes, and constructed reservoirs—surface water sources that are visible, accessible, and useful not only for direct consumption but for transportation and recreation as well. However, as pointed out earlier, over 96% of all available fresh water supplies occur in the form of groundwater, a resource whose immense importance is often overlooked and little understood by the general public. Approximately half of all Americans and more than 95% of farm families depend on groundwater for their drinking water supplies; in addition, 40% of all water used for irrigation in the United States is drawn from groundwater reserves (Council of Environmental Quality, 1981; Miller, 1991). This vast unseen reservoir flows very slowly toward the sea and is a major source of replenishment for most surface water supplies. Estimates indicate that most rivers receive as much of their flow from groundwater seepage as from surface runoff.

Groundwater supplies constitute an invaluable natural resource—one that has long been regarded as having certain inherent advantages over surface water supplies. Groundwater is usually cleaner and purer than most surface water sources. This is true because the soil through which it percolates filters out most of the bacteria, suspended materials, and other

BOX 14-2

Water Wars in the Middle East

The only matter that could take Egypt to war again is water.
　　　　　　　　—Anwar Sadat, 1979

This candid declaration by the former Egyptian president soon after signing the historic peace treaty with Israel reflects basic Middle Eastern realities which are assuming more menacing proportions today than at the time they were uttered. Growing competition, both within and between nations, for the increasingly scarce water resources of that geopolitically strategic area of the world, threatens regional security and convinces many observers that the next Middle East war will be waged over water, not oil. Within this volatile region, all major rivers are shared by two or more countries which to date have exhibited scant willingness to cooperate in solving the looming water supply crisis. In addition, several countries of the Middle East draw groundwater from common aquifers that are being overpumped and, to an increasing extent, polluted. Indeed, when U.S. intelligence services listed the ten places in the world where war was most likely to erupt over dwindling shared water supplies, most of the candidates were in the Middle East. Throughout the region, the nature of each country's water woes is remarkably similar: a naturally arid to semiarid climate, rapidly falling water tables due to overpumping, and—at the crux of the problem—exploding population growth.

The potential for trouble appeared particularly ominous during the brief Persian Gulf War in 1991. Since all the countries of the Gulf rely heavily on desalination plants for their drinking water, Iraqi sabotage of such facilities loomed as a major concern. Although international law prohibits the poisoning or contamination of an enemy's water supply, Iraqi forces nevertheless destroyed or disabled most Kuwaiti desalination plants. Worries that the major Saudi facility at Jubail might be damaged by massive oil slicks in the Gulf proved unfounded, but given the minimal security precautions taken to protect such vital facilities throughout the region, their safety during any future conflict cannot be taken for granted.

Egypt presents a classic example of a country almost entirely dependent on water supply sources beyond its own frontiers. Sadat's comments following the 1979 peace accord with Israel, quoted above, were not directed at the Zionist state but rather at Ethiopia, in whose highlands originate the headwaters of the Blue Nile. To Egyptians, unhindered access to Nile waters is a life-or-death matter and a top national security issue. Their densely crowded population of 59 million (1994) is growing by an additional one million every 10 months and is projected to reach 75 million by the year 2000. With fully 86% of all the water they use coming from the Nile—and with the magnitude of water needs mounting with every additional birth—Egyptians can't afford any reduction in current withdrawal rates. Nevertheless, Egypt has little influence over the decisions of governments upstream; population growth and development ambitions in Sudan and the nations bordering Lake Victoria are increasing water demands on the Nile long before its waters flow across the Egyptian border. Political antagonism between the regimes in Cairo and Khartoum has made the water issue even more volatile. During the Gulf conflict, rumors that Iraq had missiles in Sudan, aimed at the Aswan High Dam on the Nile, prompted a stern warning by Egypt that any attack on the dam would be regarded as an act of war. Adding to the pressure on water resources, more than a decade of drought in East Africa has reduced the level of the Nile to its lowest point in the past one hundred years. Looking at regional supply and demand trends, Egyptian officials foresee severe water deficits in both their country and the Sudan by 2010.

Hundreds of miles to the northeast, in the Tigris-Euphrates watershed, two other nations with rapidly growing populations—Syria and Iraq—nervously speculate on the water-grabbing intentions of an upstream neighbor. Turkey, one of the few Middle Eastern countries with an adequate supply of water within its borders, has embarked on a major water development project in the arid southeastern region of Anatolia. Consisting of a series of irrigation and hydroelectric dams on the Tigris and Euphrates Rivers, including the massive Ataturk Dam on the Euphrates, the project when complete will supply nearly half of Turkey's current energy demand and bring irrigation water to millions of acres of Anatolian cropland. Turkey's downstream neighbors, not surprisingly, are less sanguine about the project's potential benefits. Unless water-sharing agreements can be negotiated among the three countries, something which Turkey as yet has been unwilling to commit itself, Syria could eventually lose 40% of its Euphrates water; even further downstream, Iraq could experience flows down as much as 90%. Tensions reached a high point in January 1990, when Turkey cut off the flow of the Euphrates for one month to begin filling the reservoir behind the Ataturk Dam. Syria and Iraq both complained loudly about the temporary diversion in spite of Turkey's efforts to compensate for the inconvenience by increasing down-stream flow 50 days prior to the closure. The furor over the Ataturk Dam was not the first time countries in the region came close to blows over water: in 1975 Syrian diversions of Euphrates water to fill its Ath-Thawrah Dam nearly resulted in armed conflict with Iraq. Reports of an alleged Syrian plot to blow up the Ataturk Dam and a Turkish threat to limit the flow of Euphrates water into Syria in retaliation for Syrian support of Kurdish terrorists operating in Turkey have further soured relations among these countries.

Nowhere in the Middle East is the potential for war over water greater than in the Jordan Valley, where Israelis, Jordanians, and Palestinians compete for dwindling water supplies which, even if shared, are not sufficient to meet current demand. In Israel, renewable water supplies are being overdrawn by 15–20% annually, a figure that experts predict will rise to 30% by the end of the decade. Citing mounting pressures generated by a rapidly growing population (thanks to extremely high birth rates among the Arab population and unprecedented levels of Jewish immigration from the former Soviet Union) and the limitations imposed by a naturally arid environment, a researcher at Haifa University recently warned government officials that "Israel is on the threshold of a catastrophe." Certainly the current water situation is complicating efforts to conclude a lasting peace agreement with Israel's Arab neighbors, who feel Israel is taking more than its fair share of the region's inadequate water resources. Jordanians protest Israeli diversions from the Sea of Galilee into an aqueduct serving Tel Aviv, thereby diminishing the flow of the Jordan River and rendering it too saline for irrigation. Jordanian attempts to stave off impending water shortages by drilling deeper wells and improving the efficiency of irrigation constitute little more than stop-gap solutions to the challenge of supplying the water needs of a nation whose population will double in just 19 years. Palestinians in the occupied West Bank chafe under military orders that cut off their access to irrigation water from the Jordan while simultaneously setting limits on the amount of water they can withdraw from existing wells and prohibiting the digging of new ones. In the meantime, Palestinians charge, Israeli settlers pumping from the same aquifer are under no such restrictions and have withdrawn so much water from recently drilled wells that many Arab wells have gone dry. In the occupied Gaza Strip, whose current population growth (5%) is among the highest in the world, the water situation is even more critical. Completely dependent at present on a single heavily polluted aquifer, Gazans are pumping water out of the ground at more than twice the rate of natural recharge. As a consequence, the water table is falling rapidly and saltwater intrusion into the coastal aquifer, added to the chemical and biological contamination, will render Gaza's groundwater reserves undrinkable within the next few years.

As pressures on water resources throughout the region steadily increase, logic would suggest that Middle Eastern leaders set aside the fear, mistrust, and hostility that have poisoned their relations in recent decades and seek common ground in forging cooperative water management agreements. Unfortunately, there are few indications as yet that either regional leaders or the world community as a whole are giving the issue the priority it deserves. By the time they do, it may be too late to prevent disaster.

References

Cowell, Alan. 1991. "More Precious Than Oil, and Maybe as Volatile." *New York Times*, March 17.
Moffett, George D., III. 1990. "If Jordan Valley Wells Run Dry." *Christian Science Monitor*, March 14.
Starr, Joyce R. 1991. "Water Wars." *Foreign Policy*, no. 82 (Spring).

contaminants that find easy access to rivers and lakes. In addition, because evaporation is virtually nil and seasonal fluctuations in supply are small, groundwater supplies are dependable year-round. In terms of cost, groundwater has advantages also. The expense of digging a well is generally less than that of piping surface water to its place of use and because of its greater purity it is less expensive to treat prior to consumption.

Until recently, communities relying on groundwater for their municipal supplies tended to take this resource largely for granted, assuming that adequate quantities of high-quality water would always be available. Today, however, a sense of alarm is spreading with the realization that the twin evils of pollution and over-use are threatening the integrity of groundwater supplies. To understand how this situation has come about, it is necessary to take a brief look at the physical characteristics of our groundwater resource.

Nature of Groundwater

When rain falls upon the earth, that which is not taken up by plant roots or lost as surface runoff percolates downward through the soil until it reaches the water table. Contrary to what some people think, the water table is not a vast underground lake or river, but the upper limit of what

Figure 14-2 Nature of Groundwater

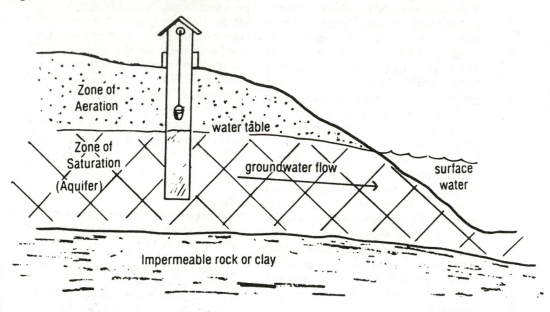

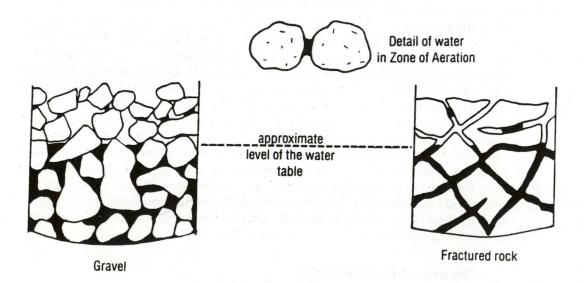

How Water Occurs in the Rock

Source: U.S. Geological Survey, *A Primer on Ground Water*

hydrologists call the **zone of saturation**—an area where the spaces between rock particles are completely filled with water. Such moisture-laden strata are called **aquifers** (Latin for "water carriers"). Above the zone of saturation lies the **zone of aeration**, where some soil moisture may be found as capillary water—useful for plants but incapable of being pumped out by humans. The zone of saturation extends downward until it is limited by an impermeable layer of rock. Sometimes there are successive layers of groundwater separated by impermeable rock layers. Aquifers may range from a few feet to several hundreds of feet in thickness and they may underlie a couple of acres or many square miles. They may occur just below the soil surface or thousands of feet below the earth, though seldom deeper than two miles.

The amount of water that any given aquifer can hold depends on its **porosity**—the ratio of the spaces between the rock particles to the total volume of rock. Sand and gravel aquifers are examples of rocks with high porosity. Additionally, if water is going to move through an aquifer, its pores must be interconnected. To qualify as a good aquifer, a rock layer must contain many pores, cracks, or both. The rate of water movement through an aquifer varies, not surprisingly, with the type of rock: through gravel it may travel tens or hundreds of feet per day; in fine sand only a few inches or less per day. When hydrologists measure the flow of surface streams, they do so in terms of feet per second; when measuring groundwater flow, figures in feet *per year* are the rule.

Groundwater Pollution

The inherent superiority of groundwater over surface water due to its supposed freedom from contamination can no longer be taken for granted. Since the early 1980s, more than 225 different chemical, biological, and radiological pollutants have been identified in groundwater deposits throughout the United States. Estimates by the National Research Council suggest that the extent of groundwater pollution is still quite limited—just 0.5–2% of total reserves. However, such cases tend to occur in populated areas where the aquifer in question may be the principal or only source of local drinking water. Such findings have raised legitimate concerns among the public regarding both acute and chronic health effects and have resulted in the closure of hundreds of wells, affecting the water supplies of millions of Americans. In numerous cases involving synthetic organic chemicals, levels of contamination have been many times higher than those found in the most heavily polluted surface waters. Within affected communities the discovery that wells are contaminated frequently has come as an unwelcome surprise since, contrary to the situation in lakes and rivers, groundwater pollution is in a sense hidden, out of sight and difficult to detect without sophisticated chemical analyses. Since many pollutants in groundwater are colorless, odorless, and tasteless, many citizens unknowingly consume health-threatening poisons for years. Because routine tests performed to ensure drinking water safety have only recently been expanded to include monitoring for toxic chemicals, well

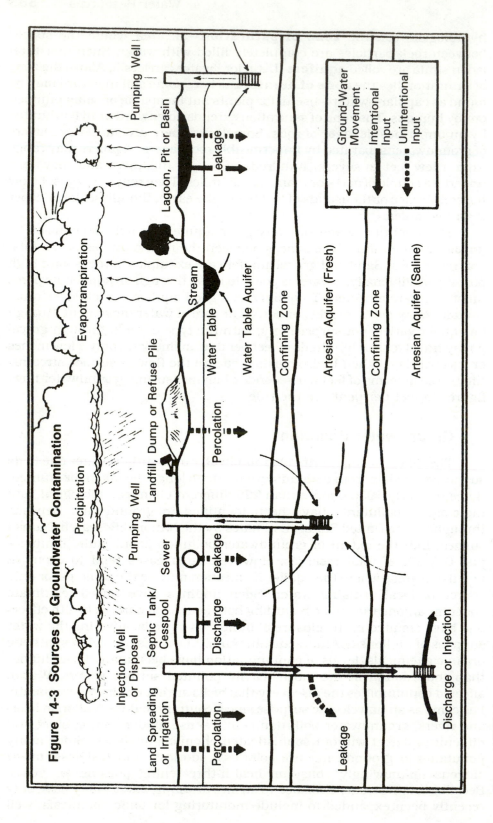

Figure 14-3 Sources of Groundwater Contamination

Source: U.S. Environmental Protection Agency.

water pollution in the past was often detected only when noticeable numbers of people began to fall ill. Amendments to the Safe Drinking Water Act in 1986 significantly expanded the number of contaminants for which public water systems must monitor in both surface and groundwaters. However, these regulations do *not* cover the approximately 10.5 million private wells, mostly in rural areas, which frequently are shallower and thus even more vulnerable to pollution than municipal wells (Sanford and Oosterhaut, 1991).

Degradation of groundwater supplies by human-generated pollutants occurs largely due to faulty waste disposal practices or poor land management. The most significant sources of contamination include:

Septic Systems and Injection Wells. Here liquid wastes are deliberately discharged directly into the ground. If such facilities are properly sited, waste discharges pose little hazard, but if located adjacent to or uphill from an aquifer or well, a potential for pollution exists. Contamination from septic systems, which serve approximately 30% of U.S. households, can be either microbial or chemical. A number of outbreaks of waterborne diarrheal diseases such as salmonellosis, hepatitis A, and typhoid fever have been traced to well water contaminated by sewage from septic tanks. Similarly injection wells, which dispose of an estimated 60% of the nation's liquid hazardous wastes into supposedly confined geological formations deep underground, have, on occasion, been responsible for polluting nearby aquifers.

Waste Storage, Treatment, or Disposal Facilities. Unplanned seepage from open dumps, landfills, waste ponds, underground storage tanks, tailings piles—even graveyards!—constitute a well-recognized and severe groundwater pollution threat if such facilities are improperly sited. A large percentage of all federal Superfund sites involve groundwater contamination originating from sources such as these. Design requirements for the development of new land disposal facilities emphasize incorporation of barriers to prevent leachate migration, thereby protecting groundwater quality.

Pipes, Materials Transport, Transfer Operations. Unintentional leakage from sewers or oil pipelines or accidental spills during transport or transfer of hazardous substances can be another source of groundwater pollution. Studies of well water contamination with agricultural chemicals conducted by the Illinois EPA revealed that the majority of problems— and all those involving high concentrations of pollutants—could be traced to locations where pesticidal formulations were routinely prepared (and routinely spilled on the ground!) prior to field application.

Nonpoint Sources of Pollution. Many instances of groundwater contamination can be traced to substances discharged as a result of other activities: irrigation practices, mine drainage, field application of farm chemicals or manures, de-icing of highways, and urban street runoff, among the most notable examples. Sources such as these are responsible for a host of water quality problems, among them the elevated nitrate levels found in numerous private wells in farming areas and the high chloride content in wells in some northern states where large quantities of road salts are applied during the winter months.

The most disturbing aspect of groundwater pollution is the fact that by the time the problem is discovered, it is generally too late to do anything about it. Because of the very slow rate of groundwater flow, chemical pollutants will not be flushed out of an aquifer for many years after the source of contamination is cut off (conversely, and for the same reason, contamination of one part of an aquifer does not necessarily affect the use of other parts). Unlike the situation in surface waters, where naturally occurring microbes gradually break down organic pollutants, groundwater is largely devoid of the oxygen needed by the bacteria and other decomposer organisms that endow streams and lakes with their capacity for self-purification. Cleanup of a polluted aquifer, while theoretically possible, is so expensive and time-consuming that it is usually not feasible. The process generally involves drilling numerous wells, pumping out enormous quantities of water, treating the water to remove the contaminants, and then reinjecting the water into the aquifer (Rail, 1989). For all practical purposes, a community that finds its groundwater seriously contaminated has little choice but to close the affected wells and seek a new water supply. Groundwater protection strategies, therefore, logically focus on preventing pollution in the first place rather than on efforts to clean up an aquifer after the damage is done.

Groundwater Depletion

With water demand and per capita water consumption increasing steadily in recent decades, many groundwater-dependent regions of the world have experienced an alarming decline in the water table, a direct result of overpumping. Periodic fluctuations in the level of the water table are normal, with levels rising during wet periods and falling during dry spells (generally the water table is highest in the late spring, sinks in summer, rises somewhat during the fall, and reaches its lowest point just before the spring thaw). However, when the water table lowers persistently it means that more water is being taken out of the groundwater reservoir than is being returned to it through precipitation or stream flow. Such a situation is akin to mining an aquifer, and if continued over an extended time period it can permanently deplete the groundwater supply or render it uneconomical to exploit due to excessive pumping costs. Groundwater depletion problems have assumed major proportions in parts of the Middle East, North Africa, India, China, Thailand, Mexico, and the western United States (Postel, 1992).

Instances of groundwater "mining" can occur even in well-watered areas when demand generated by rapid population growth, along with residential and commercial development, result in a sharp decline in groundwater reserves. In the United States, however, depletion is most acute in arid regions such as the Great Plains and Southwest where the insatiable demand for irrigation water and the water needs of homes and industries in the booming cities of the Sunbelt have resulted in serious groundwater overdrafts.

A classic case of groundwater depletion in the American West is exemplified by the exploitation of the Ogallala Aquifer, the world's largest underground water reserve. Underlying portions of six states in the High Plains, the Ogallala supplies almost one-third of all the groundwater used for irrigation in the United States. This enormous sand and gravel formation was deposited millions of years ago as the eastern front of the Rocky Mountains eroded. The plentiful rains of Pleistocene times saturated the formation with water, but due to subsequent changes in the geology and climate of the region, replenishment of the aquifer by natural recharge ceased long ago. Consequently, the Ogallala in a very real sense represents **"fossil" water**—a nonrenewable resource much like coal or oil which, once gone, is gone forever. Thus the heavy rates of groundwater withdrawal which, beginning in the early 1940s, transformed 11 million acres of shortgrass prairie into lush expanses of corn, cotton, and alfalfa raised serious concerns about the region's long-term economic viability as the water table plummeted. Overpumping has been most pronounced in the Texas Panhandle where, by 1990, 24% of that state's portion of the aquifer had been depleted. Rates of extraction during the peak years of the early 1970s led some experts to project that the Ogallala's reserves would last only 40 more years and predicted that production of corn, the crop with the highest water demand, would cease entirely within a few years. Recently, however, cutbacks in the acreage irrigated and implementation of more efficient irrigation techniques have reduced water use in the Texas High Plains by 43% and groundwater depletion rates have slowed. Nevertheless, the fact that the water reserves of the Ogallala remain a finite resource calls into question the wisdom of consuming fossil waters to cultivate crops that can be grown at far less environmental cost on rain-watered land further east (U.S. Water Resources Council, 1978; Postel, 1992).

The impact of groundwater overdrafts extends well beyond constraints on irrigated agriculture. In arid western states, aquifer depletion can precipitate serious environmental problems, the most visible of which is the drying up of many surface streams (recall that many rivers, particularly in dry climates, receive the bulk of their flow from underground sources with which they are in hydrologic contact). In coastal areas around the world, excessive pumping of groundwater to meet the demands of growing urban populations has resulted in migration of seawater into depleted aquifers, contaminating existing freshwater supplies. Saltwater intrusion is now a serious problem in such far-flung cities as Dakar, Senegal; Jakarta, Indonesia; and Lima, Peru. Along Israel's Mediterranean shoreline, 20% of the important coastal aquifer is now polluted and officials fear that one out of five coastal wells may have to be abandoned within the next few years. In the United States, saltwater intrusion is endangering water supplies in southern California, south Florida, and in portions of Long Island and New Jersey (World Resources Institute, 1992; Postel, 1992; Ashworth, 1982). In addition, as groundwater reserves are depleted, land

BOX 14-3

Here Today, Gone Tomorrow: Mining Fossil Water

Pursuing the mirage of food self-sufficiency in an arid environment, the governments of Saudi Arabia and Libya have embarked on short-sighted efforts to irrigate desert fields with prodigious amounts of nonrenewable groundwater. Ignoring the lessons to be learned from depletion of the Ogallala Aquifer in the United States, Saudi and Libyan planners press forward with initiatives that guarantee a similar fate for their countries' groundwater resources.

Fully 90% of the water used for agricultural purposes (and 75% of all water consumption) in Saudi Arabia is fossil groundwater, pumped from reserves that accumulated thousands of years ago. Natural recharge of the aquifer has long since ceased, making Saudi groundwater—like Saudi oil—a finite resource which, once gone, is gone forever. In spite of the hydrologic realities, in the late 1970s Saudi officials launched a major effort to diversify their economy, redistribute oil revenues, and decrease the country's reliance on food imports by encouraging large-scale wheat production in the desert. By heavily subsidizing agricultural inputs—land, equipment, and water—the government has obtained impressive increases in crop production. By the end of the 1980s, land under cultivation had reached nearly 7.5 million acres (3 million hectares), approximately 20 times the amount cropped in 1975, and in 1991 Saudi farmers reaped a record wheat harvest of 4 million metric tons, up from just 3000 tons only 15 years earlier. With domestic consumption at less than a million tons, the kingdom has now become one of the world's leading wheat exporters, selling or giving away its bountiful surplus.

The price of such success has been considerable, however. Subsidizing wheat production to the tune of approximately $500/metric ton, the Saudi government has been paying farmers more than 8 times what it would have cost to purchase wheat abroad. More significant in the long term than Saudi agriculture's drain on the royal treasury is its impact on the kingdom's water reserves. It is estimated that groundwater depletion has been averaging over 5 billion cubic meters annually in recent years, a rate that is expected to increase substantially throughout the 1990s. United States government analysts estimate that if depletion trends persist, Saudi reserves of fossil groundwater will be exhausted by 2007.

In Libya a similar scenario is unfolding as that nation's mercurial leader, Muammar Qaddafi, lavishes petrodollars on promotion of his "Great Man-Made River Project"—a massive $25 billion effort to pipe fossil groundwater from an aquifer under the Sahara Desert to irrigate cereal crops and pasturelands in more fertile regions near Libya's Mediterranean coast. If completed as planned, the project will double the country's water supply—temporarily. As in Saudi Arabia, the reserves that Qaddafi is tapping are nonrenewable; engineering estimates suggest that within 40–60 years, the much-heralded Great Man-Made River will run dry. Future generations of Libyans, like their Saudi counterparts, may well question the wisdom of national leaders whose nonsustainable development goals led them to squander an irreplaceable resource, leaving their successors diminished options for ensuring national water security in the years ahead.

References

Al-Ibrahim, Abdulla Ali. 1991. "Excessive Use of Groundwater Resources in Saudi Arabia: Impacts and Policy Options." *Ambio*, 20, no. 1.

Pearce, Fred. 1991. "Will Qaddafi's Great River Run Dry?" *New Scientist*, Sept. 7.

World Resource Institute. 1990. *World Resources 1990–91*. Oxford University Press.

Figure 14-4 Groundwater Withdrawals

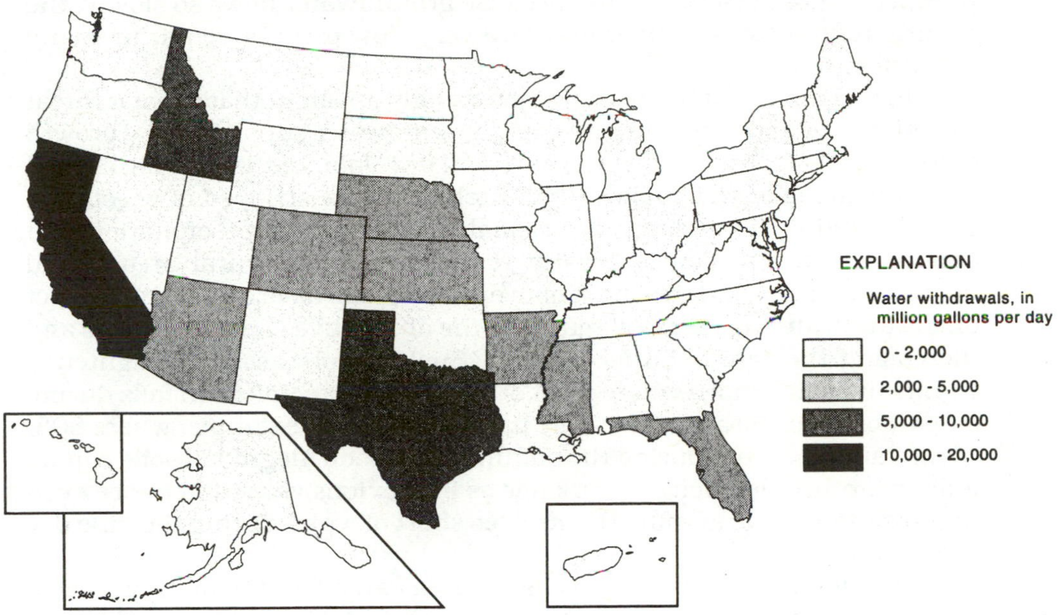

EXPLANATION

Water withdrawals, in million gallons per day

0 - 2,000

2,000 - 5,000

5,000 - 10,000

10,000 - 20,000

Source: U.S. Geological Survey, Department of the Interior.

subsidence is occurring, accompanied by the formation of fissures and faults that disrupt irrigation canals and highways, as well as endangering buildings. In Mexico City, where the pumping of groundwater to supply the needs of 18 million people greatly exceeds the rate of natural recharge, the 16th century Metropolitan Cathedral dominating the city's historic plaza is one of many structures now sagging precariously, a victim of land subsidence. Around Orlando, Florida, overexploitation of groundwater reserves has created huge sinkholes that virtually overnight swallow up chunks of roads, yards, and, occasionally, homes. Falling water tables are also resulting in the abandonment of hundreds of thousands of acres of irrigated lands, as energy costs render pumping too expensive to make such farming economically feasible. These abandoned fields thereupon become subject to excessive rates of erosion and desertification. Native vegetation as well as crop plants suffer as water tables drop below the level of the deepest root systems. In the American West, an area equivalent to 10% of all U.S. lands is experiencing severe desertification and an additional 10% is seriously threatened (Ashworth, 1982).

Natural Recharge

Under natural conditions aquifers are recharged by moisture filtering downward from the surface or by seepage from a lake or stream. The area of land which, because of its permeable soils, is the main source of the groundwater inflow is called the **recharge area** of the aquifer. This recharge zone may be many miles from the point at which the water is pumped out of the ground; and because groundwater flows so slowly, the natural refilling of an aquifer may be a very slow process, requiring many centuries in some cases.

In recent years it has become increasingly apparent that a major threat to both the quality and quantity of our groundwater supplies is the growth of industrial, commercial, and residential development within the critical recharge areas of an aquifer. When such areas are stripped of vegetation and covered with buildings and asphalt the amount of precipitation that can penetrate the soil is greatly reduced. Even in rural areas, land degradation due to deforestation or overgrazing can have an adverse impact on groundwater recharge by reducing the absorptive capacity of soils and increasing the rate of surface runoff. Such factors assume heightened significance in regions where most of the annual precipitation falls during a distinct "rainy season." In some parts of India, for example, where 80% of the rainfall occurs during the summer monsoon, degraded soils can no longer capture as much of the deluge as in previous years and hence even high-rainfall areas now find themselves short of water during the nine dry months of the year.

Development within the recharge area can affect the quality as well as the quantity of groundwater. As human activities within such areas intensify, the potential for infiltration into aquifers of contaminants from waste facilities, leaky sewage pipes, chemical spills, or street runoff increases. A growing realization of the importance of protecting groundwater resources has prompted many state governments in recent years to enact laws regulating the types of development and activities permitted within the critical recharge area of aquifers. In some areas land acquisition plans, funded by either state or local governments, have been instrumental in preserving sensitive recharge areas from potentially harmful development and local citizens' groups have been extremely effective in generating the public support necessary for developing and implementing such programs.

Water Management: Increasing Supply versus Reducing Demand

In the past, as population increase and industrial development boosted urban water demand, cities typically sought to quench their growing thirst by searching for new sources to augment dwindling local supplies. Frequently their reach extended far beyond municipal borders to exploit previously untapped resources in the rural hinterlands. Doing so seemed an obvious solution for a number of reasons: the potential supply appeared limitless and, therefore, relatively cheap; such water generally was of high quality and required little expenditure for treatment; and legal rights to the watershed lands could usually be obtained easily, especially since rural

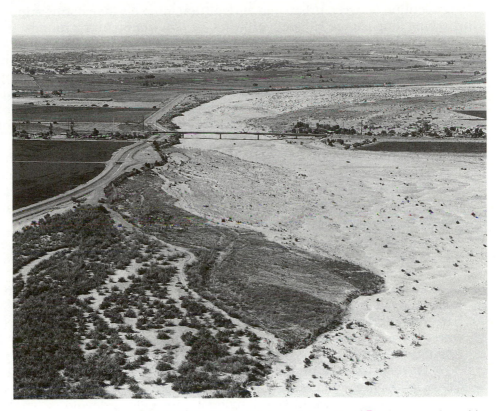

By the time the Colorado River reaches the Southern International Border, there is nothing but dry riverbed. The last of the river's water was diverted 20 miles upstream at the Morelos Dam during the 1950s. [U.S. Department of the Interior, Bureau of Reclamation]

residents seldom had the political savvy necessary to outmaneuver the urban interests which frequently dominated state legislatures. Thus today in places like southern California, where local sources supply only a third of the demand generated by a burgeoning population, the water that maintains lawns, fills swimming pools, and makes life pleasant in the Golden State is imported from the Colorado River, 170 miles to the east, and from sources in northern California as far as 400 miles distant. Similarly, when New Yorkers turn on the tap in Manhattan, the liquid that flows out could have originated from one of a thousand streams in the Catskills, Hudson, or Delaware River valleys. Hetch Hetchy Valley in Yosemite National Park provides much of the water supply for San Francisco; Denver taps the headwaters of the Colorado on the opposite side of the Rocky Mountains; and Oklahoma City pipes its supplies from reservoirs in the northeastern Oklahoma hill country more than 100 miles away (Ashworth, 1982).

Since the 1970s, however, city planners have tempered their once-automatic response of pursuing supply-side solutions. Such modern realities as the scarcity of new untapped sources; the sharply escalating costs of building dams and reduced federal funding for the same;

competition between urban and agricultural interests for existing supplies; growing opposition to such projects on environmental grounds; plus organized legal resistance by groups in areas targeted for water development have basically brought to a close the era in which city planners attempted to solve water problems through a supply augmentation approach. Today, in metropolitan areas as diverse as Los Angeles and Boston, the emphasis for ensuring adequate water resources has shifted decisively from increasing *supply* to managing *demand* (Dziegielewski and Baumann, 1992).

Demand management, more commonly referred to by environmentalists as **water conservation**, can include several components: reducing overall use of water, reducing wastage of water, and recycling used water so it can be made available for other purposes (Dziegielewski and Baumann, 1992).

Water Consumption

To understand how demand management strategies can help meet increased water needs, it is necessary to examine current water use patterns. Worldwide, irrigated agriculture accounts for the lion's share of water consumption—almost 69% of the total. (In Asia, farmers account for fully 82% of all water use; in the United States, 41%; and in Europe, just 30%.) Industries constitute the second largest consumers of water at 23% (more in heavily industrialized areas, less in others), while household use averages about 8% worldwide (obviously, in regions devoid of irrigated agriculture, the percentage of water use attributed to household and industrial use are considerably greater than world averages indicate). Focusing on these three major categories of water consumers, what opportunities do water managers have for reducing demand?

Agriculture.   As the largest user—and the largest waster—of water, agriculture also offers the greatest potential for substantial reductions in water demand, in most cases without reducing crop yields. Because irrigation water is almost everywhere priced far below its true value, farmers are given the impression that the supply is plentiful and thus have little incentive to invest in more efficient irrigation technologies. As a result, in most parts of the world irrigators continue to channel or flood water across their fields in a manner that would have looked entirely familiar to their ancestors thousands of years ago. Such practices waste, on average, more than 60% of the water applied, as evaporation or seepage from unlined channels robs thirsty plant roots of the moisture intended for them. More widespread use of advanced techniques such as the automated ''drip irrigation'' method developed by Israeli scientists can cut water loss to 5% and reduce energy expenses in the bargain. Since the 1980s, farmers in West Texas have achieved dramatic savings by adopting techniques of ''surge irrigation'' or by installing low-energy precision application (LEPA) sprinklers that can achieve water use efficiencies as high as 95%. Experts estimate that if the world's farmers could reduce water losses due to

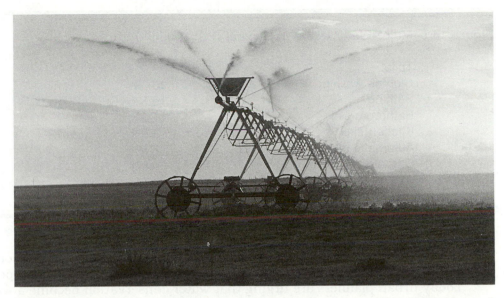

Agricultural irrigation is the largest user—and waster—of water. [U.S. Department of Agriculture]

inefficient irrigation practices by as little as 10%, the amount saved would be enough to double current domestic use (Postel, 1992).

Industry. The huge amount of water needed by factories and power plants for processing, cooling, or generating steam accounts for a sizeable portion of total water use in Europe (54%), North America (42%), and other highly developed areas of the world (World Resources Institute, 1992). Since water used by industry is not "consumed" in the traditional sense (i.e. it may become heated or polluted but isn't used up), industrial water use can be substantially reduced by recycling. Within the past decade or so, increasingly stringent federal mandates requiring treatment of industrial wastewater prior to discharge, coupled with the escalating costs of waste treatment and disposal, have given industry a strong incentive to embark on waste minimization strategies that entail recycling and reuse of process waters. Such efforts have resulted in sharp declines in water withdrawals in many industries. In spite of steadily rising industrial output, water use by industry in the United States and Japan has dropped by 36% and 24%, respectively, during the past several decades (Postel, 1992). Further savings are likely in the years ahead as more and more industries recognize the advantages of climbing aboard the pollution prevention bandwagon.

Households. Although domestic water consumption averages far less than that used for agricultural and industrial purposes, societal norms and public health considerations require that such water be of very high quality, necessitating expensive treatment and distribution systems. In past years, municipal efforts in some areas to restrict residential water

Figure 14-5 Major Water Users in Typical U.S. Home

Toilet	33.0%
Clothes washing	26.0%
Bathing	19.6%
Bathroom sink	11.3%
Kitchen sink	5.8%
Automatic dishwasher	2.5%
Garbage grinding	1.8%

Source: Water Pollution Control Federation, 1986

consumption were launched as a temporary reaction to drought conditions, largely abandoned when the rains returned or new supplies were tapped. Today urban planners are urging that water conservation become a way of life, even in areas of adequate rainfall, as a means of enhancing water availability and containing rising water costs. Contrary to popular belief, a call for water conservation is not a demand for citizens to change their life-style radically, nor does it necessarily imply deprivation. Rather, water conservation means making more efficient use of the resource available.

A number of years ago when a lengthy drought in the Northeast had dangerously lowered the levels of reservoirs supplying water to New York City, officials of the Big Apple sponsored a contest for the best water conservation slogan. One of the catchiest advocated "Save water: take a bath with a friend!" Those who value their privacy can take heart from the fact that today's options for stretching scarce water supplies are far more sophisticated and entail considerably less personal sacrifice than the old Saturday night frontier practice of everyone bathing in the same progressively dirtier tub!

Water Conservation

Some of the major elements in an effective water conservation program include the following.

Rational Water Pricing. Pricing water to reflect its true cost is fundamental to the success of all other water conservation efforts. Ironically, in many cities current price structures reward profligate users through a system of declining block rates, whereby the cost of additional water units above a certain point is lower than the cost of the initial units. An opposite approach, now used in 15% of the major U.S. metropolitan areas, imposes *higher* unit costs on water use above a specified level, thereby encouraging conservation. Peak demand pricing (e.g. summer: winter price ratio of 3:1) can also help curtail profligate use of water for nonessential purposes. Studies conducted in the United States and elsewhere have shown that when water prices increase by 10%, household water consumption drops 3 to 7% (Bhatra and Falkenmark, 1992). Of course household water use can't be priced appropriately if it isn't metered. The failure of cities in many parts of the world to meter home water use actively discourages water conservation efforts, since consumers see no connection between the amount of water they use and the price they pay. Cities such as New York, Buffalo, Denver, and Sacramento witnessed declines in water use ranging from 10%–30% after they installed residential water meters.

Leak Detection/Correction Programs.   Both at the household and municipal level, leaky plumbing can waste enormous volumes of water. In homes, leakage accounts for 5-10% of all residential water consumption. A faucet that loses 1 drop per second due to a worn out washer is wasting 7 gallons of water each day; that figure rises to 20 gallons per day with a steady drip. A leaky toilet tank can waste fully 200 gallons per day without making a sound. (To check for toilet tank leakage, simply pour a small amount of food coloring into the tank; if color appears in the toilet bowl before it is flushed, leakage is occurring, probably caused by a worn-out or defective flush ball.) Correcting these leaks is the easiest and cheapest way to reduce home water consumption.

Cities as well as households may be plagued by leaky plumbing. In many older communities the pipes that carry water from a central treatment plant to thousands of homes, institutions, and businesses were installed during the 1800s or early 1900s and have for decades been in serious need of replacement. The current fiscal plight of many urban areas has resulted in short-sighted postponement of these urgently needed renovations. In those cities that have made the necessary investment, however, results have been striking. Prior to a major leak repair program, Boston was losing an estimated 20% of the water entering its distribution system each day; following recent completion of that program, officials credit leak repair with saving the city 35 million gallons daily.

Installation of Water-Saving Plumbing Devices.   Technology already exists for reducing household water use by a minimum of 50% with no loss of comfort or convenience. Prime targets for water-saving household fixtures include low-flow showerheads, faucets, and toilets. Using 5–7 gallons per flush (gpf), the conventional toilet is the single largest "water hog" in American homes. In recent years low-flush (3.5 gpf) and ultra-low flush (1.6 gpf) toilets have come onto the market and offer significant water savings. Since Jan. 1, 1994, by mandate of the 1992 federal Energy Policy Act, all toilets, urinals, showerheads, and faucets produced in the United States have been required to comply with uniform water efficiency standards. It is estimated that by the year 2026 these newer water-conserving fixtures will have replaced the older pre-1994 stock currently in use, at which time household water use will be less than half of current levels (55 gallons per day for the average 2–3 person household versus 121 gallons per day at present) (Vickers, 1993). Some communities experiencing drought-induced water shortages have attempted to accelerate this

---

Figure 14-6 States Mandating 1.6 gpf Toilets for New or Replacement Plumbing

California	New York
Connecticut	North Carolina
Delaware	Oregon
Georgia	Rhode Island
Maryland	Texas
Massachusetts	Utah
Nevada	Washington
New Jersey	

---

phaseout by offering citizens financial inducements to replace older models now. A case in point is Santa Monica, California, which several years ago imposed a $2 monthly "conservation incentive" fee for all single-family homes that hadn't installed low-volume toilets and showerheads.

Altered Landscape Practices.   Americans' deeply-held conviction that a broad, verdant expanse of weed-free, neatly manicured grass is an essential component of any respectable residence constitutes a major obstacle to meeting urban water conservation goals. Across the United States, approximately 25 million acres are covered with cultivated lawns that annually consume prodigious amounts of fertilizers, pesticides, and high-quality treated water. In some communities in the western United States, fully 40–50% of household water use is devoted to maintaining lawns and gardens.

In an effort to discourage water wastage associated with landscaping practices, a number of communities have initiated some innovative programs aimed at changing American attitudes toward yard maintenance and design. In southern California, where a six-year drought (1987–1992) prompted major changes in water supply planning, the Metropolitan Water District has implemented landscape water conservation regulations for commercial, industrial, institutional, and multifamily properties; MWD is also encouraging similar practices for single-family residences and urging homeowners to select plantings that can thrive with minimal watering. Elsewhere, some communities have enacted legislation restricting the amount of yard space property owners can devote to grass. On Long Island, the town of Southampton, concerned about groundwater pollution by lawn chemicals, mandates that no more than 15% of a residential lot be devoted to fertilizer-requiring lawns or vegetables, while a minimum of 80% must be retained in its natural wooded condition; in Tucson, Arizona, an

BOX 14-4
Water Conservation in Your Own Back Yard

Since lawn and garden maintenance typically account for as much as half of all household water use during the warmer months of the year, it is not surprising that the first action taken by many drought-stricken communities is to impose limitations—or an outright ban—on the use of sprinkler systems or hoses for landscape irrigation. Such mandates certainly are effective in terms of water savings but they can exert a heavy economic and aesthetic burden on areas targeted by the restrictions. Expensive horticultural plantings may shrivel up and die, while whole neighborhoods assume a parched yellow-brown appearance. Landscaping firms, nurseries, and lawn-care companies see their profits evaporate as potential customers postpone purchase of water-thirsty sod or shrubs. Are community efforts to ensure their water security through effective water conservation programs incompatible with the desire of property owners to surround themselves with natural beauty? Not for those familiar with the principles of **Xeriscape landscaping**, a concept that has been spreading rapidly in recent years.

The term Xeriscape™ (derived from the Greek *xeros*, meaning "dry"), was coined and trademarked in 1981 by a group in Colorado searching for a creative new approach to landscaping that would be compatible with and, indeed, enhance water conservation strategies. Convinced that the effects of future droughts could be lessened by water-saving landscaping practices without any sacrifice in landscape beauty, the task force developed and publicized guidelines for Xeriscape landscaping that, if widely adopted, could significantly reduce urban water demand, save home gardeners long hours wielding a hose, and ensure that the periodic dry spells which virtually every region experiences at one time or another (or the long-term climate change many fear is coming) can be weathered with minimal effect on natural surroundings.

Contrary to popular misconceptions, Xeriscape landscaping does not mean a yard composed of pebbles sprayed with green paint nor does it limit one's choice of plants to cactus and yucca. Xeriscaping means designing an outdoor environment that minimizes the need for water input and selecting those plant varieties that can thrive on the amount of natural precipitation characteristic of the region in question. This amount can vary from 8 inches per year in parts of the Southwest, to 30–50 inches in the New England states, to nearly 100 inches per year in the Pacific Northwest. It should be kept in mind that while certain regions of the country may appear to be abundantly well-watered in terms of annual rainfall statistics, many experience prolonged periods of the year during which there is little or no precipitation. Thus in places like proverbially damp Seattle, xeriscaping can be a boon to gardeners during the summer when, in an average year, only 6–10 inches of rain fall from May until October. In such places, Xeriscape landscaping is being actively promoted as "drought insurance."

Just as a xeriscaping approach to landscape design is appropriate in every region of the country, it is also adaptable to virtually any style of landscaping, from the most formal to the most natural. Similarly, there are varying degrees of stringency for executing a xeriscape approach; practitioners may find that they need to water on occasion, but by following certain guidelines they can still achieve considerable reduction in water use (depending on the specific situation, xeriscaping can result in residential water savings of 20–80%). Best of all, when properly carried out, xeriscaping can greatly enhance the visual appeal of one's surroundings. By using a variety of plants appropriate to and reflective of the natural environment of the local area, one can create surroundings far more pleasing aesthetically than the sterile monoscapes of generic grass and shrubs so often the standard choice of homeowners across the country. As proponents of the concept insist, "If it isn't beautiful, then it isn't a Xeriscape landscape."

While "xeriscaping" is not yet a household word, the concept has been gaining adherents rapidly through the combined efforts of gardeners and water managers, both of whom share a common goal: conserving water resources and enhancing the beauty of urban landscapes. In 1986 the Xeriscape trademark was transferred to the National Xeriscape Council, Inc. (NXCI), a nonprofit group that serves as a clearinghouse for information about xeriscaping and supports demonstration gardens throughout the United States to promote Xeriscape landscaping. People interested in "how to" information and plant lists suitable for their own locality may contact NXCI at P.O. Box 767936, Roswell, GA 30076.

Reference

Ellefson, Connie Lockhart, Thomas L. Stephens, and Doug Welsh. 1992. *Xeriscape™ Gardening*. MacMillan.

ordinance passed in 1991 prohibits planting grass on any more than 10% of the landscaped area in new developments (Dziegielewski and Baumann, 1992).

Methods of managing water demand such as those just described, accompanied by intensive public information and conservation education programs, will play a major role in meeting future water needs. Encouraging results are already evident from recently launched programs in such disparate regions as southern California and metropolitan Boston, providing convincing evidence that water conservation not only will provide our largest single source of additional water within the next 20 years but will become an accepted way of life. Provided with appropriate technologies and a cost incentive, citizens, farmers, and industrialists alike will validate the assertion of water managers that the cheapest, quickest, most environmentally benign way to meet future water needs is to use existing supplies more efficiently.

References

Ashworth, William. 1982. *Nor Any Drop to Drink*. Summit Books.

Bhatra, Ramesh, and Malin Falkenmark. 1992. "Water Resource Policies and the Urban Poor: Innovative Approaches and Policy Imperatives." *International Conference on Water and the Environment: Development Issues for the 21st Century*. Dublin, Ireland (January 26–31).

Briscoe, John. 1993. "When the Cup is Half Full: Improving Water and Sanitation Services in the Developing World." *Environment* 35, no. 4 (May).

Council of Environmental Quality. 1981. *Contamination of Groundwater by Toxic Organic Chemicals* (Jan.).

Dziegielewski, Benedykt, and Duane D. Baumann. 1992. "The Benefits of Managing Urban Water Demands." *Environment* 34, no. 9 (Nov.).

Ehrlich, Paul, Anne Ehrlich, and John Holdren. 1977. *Ecoscience*, W. H. Freeman and Co.

Falkenmark, Malin, and Carl Widstrand. 1992. "Population and Water Resources: A Delicate Balance." *Population Bulletin* 47, no. 3 (Nov.).

Linden, Eugene. 1990. "The Last Drops." *Time* (Aug. 20).

Maurits la Riviere, J. W. 1989. "Threats to the World's Water." *Scientific American* (Sept.).

McCaffrey, Stephen C. 1992. "A Human Right to Water: Domestic and International Implications." *Georgetown International Environmental Law Review* 5, Issue 1 (Fall).

Miller, G. Tyler, Jr. 1991. *Environmental Science: Sustaining the Earth.* Wadsworth.

Postel, Sandra. 1992. *Last Oasis: Facing Water Scarcity.* W. W. Norton & Co.

Pringle, Lawrence. 1982. *Water: The Next Great Resource Battle.* MacMillan.

Rail, Chester D. 1989. *Groundwater Contamination: Sources, Control, and Preventive Measures.* Technomic Publishing Co.

Sanford, Cynthia, and Joe Oosterhout. 1991. "Protecting Groundwater: The Unseen Resource." *The National Voter* 40, no. 5 (June/July).

U.S. Water Resources Council. 1978. *The Nation's Water Resources, 1975–2000* 1, Summary. U.S. Government Printing Office.

Vickers, Amy. 1993. "The Energy Policy Act: Assessing Its Impact on Utilities." *Journal of the American Waterworks Association* (August).

World Bank. *The World Development Report 1992: Development and Environment.* Washington, D.C.

World Resources Institute. 1992. *World Resources 1992–93.* Oxford University Press.

CHAPTER 15

Water Pollution

If there is magic on this planet, it is contained in water.

—Loren Eiseley

Back in the "good old days" when human settlements were relatively small and far apart, the issue of water contamination seldom occupied much attention on the part of the general public. Prevailing sentiment insisted that "the solution to pollution is dilution," and popular wisdom held that "a stream purifies itself every ten miles." While such statements have a certain amount of validity, they lost their relevance as villages mushroomed into crowded cities and as the expanse of countryside between towns steadily contracted under the impact of urban sprawl. The rapid growth of human population and of industrial output has resulted in a corresponding decline in water quality, as both municipalities and industry regarded the nation's waterways as free, convenient dumping grounds for the waste products of civilized society. During the present century our careless waste management practices have turned most rivers into open sewers and many once-healthy lakes into algae-covered cesspools. It is estimated that most of the world's water drainage basins are polluted with such contaminants as toxic chemicals, human and animal excrement, heavy metals, pesticides, silt, and fertilizers. These contaminants are carried downstream where they are discharged into coastal waters that have become increasingly degraded over the past two decades. The problems posed by such pollutants involve far more than unpleasant sights and odors. Waterborne disease outbreaks, massive fish kills, long-lasting changes in aquatic ecosystems, and severe economic loss to sports and recreation-based industries are all directly related to degradation of water quality by human activities.

Controlling Water Pollution: The Clean Water Act

Although water pollution had been recognized as a major environmental problem in the United States for many decades, it was not until 1972 that a tough, comprehensive federal program to deal with this issue was enacted by Congress. Known originally as the Federal Water Pollution Control Act Amendments (Public Law 92–500), this landmark piece of legislation underwent some "mid-course corrections" in 1977, at which time its name was changed to the Clean Water Act. Prior to passage of this law, our nation's water pollution control strategy, such as it was, focused on attempts to clean up waterways to the point that they could be used for whatever purpose state governments had determined their function should be (e.g. drinking water, swimming, fishing, navigation, etc.). Thus each stream or portion of a stream might have a different water quality standard, and if that standard was not being met, it was up to the state water pollution control agency to determine which discharger was responsible for the violation and to seek enforcement action. This system was totally ineffective for a number of reasons: designations of desired stream use were frequently modified to retain or attract industrial development; insufficient information was available on how pollutant discharges were affecting water quality; blame for violation was difficult, if not impossible to assess when more than one source was discharging into a waterway; little attention was paid to the effects of pollution on the aquatic environment as a whole; and only contaminants entering a waterway through pipe discharges were given much attention. Undoubtedly the most serious drawback of the pre-1972 water pollution control strategy was the lack of enforcement power. State agencies had to negotiate with all the polluters along a given waterway, trying to persuade each individual source to reduce its discharges to the point at which water quality standards for the particular river or lake in question could be met. Not uncommonly, when industries disliked what they were being told, they would threaten to close down and move to a less-demanding state. Also, due to the nature of river basins, many states discovered that in order to improve their own water quality, they had to persuade states upstream to pollute less.

Passage of the Clean Water Act radically altered this approach to water pollution control and took a new philosophical stance toward the problem, reflected in the 1972 Senate Committee's statement that "no one has the right to pollute . . . and that pollution continues because of technological limits, not because of any inherent right to use the Nation's waterways for the purpose of disposing of wastes." Stressing the need to "restore and maintain the chemical, physical, and biological integrity of the Nation's waters," Congress declared as national goals the attainment, wherever possible, of water quality "that provides for recreation in and on the water" (popularly referred to as the "fishable-swimmable waters" goal) by July 1, 1983, and the elimination of all pollutant discharges into the nation's waterways by 1985 ("zero discharge" goal). These goals are not the same as legal requirements—they cannot be enforced and certainly were not attained by the dates indicated; nevertheless, they have been useful in providing objectives toward which to strive and against which progress in improving water quality can be measured.

Progress in moving toward the goals set forth by Congress is monitored by the Environmental Protection Agency's National Water Quality Surveillance System, consisting of approximately 1000 fixed stations nationwide, and by the U.S. Geological Survey's National Stream Quality Accounting Network, a system of about 500 stations. At each of these sites a wide range of variables (e.g. fecal coliform bacteria, dissolved oxygen, phosphorus, lead, mercury, cadmium) are measured on a regular basis. An analysis of the data collected by these stations since 1975 indicate that so far as river quality is concerned, there has been little overall change. Some waterways, such as the Potomac River near Washington, D.C., the Mississippi at St. Paul, Minnesota, and the Delaware River at Philadelphia have shown marked improvement in levels of dissolved oxygen and less frequent algal blooms. In the Great Lakes, PCB concentrations in fish have been declining; phosphorus loadings to Lake Erie have dropped by 50%, largely due to improved sewage treatment. On the other hand, the quality of many other waterways has worsened over the past two decades. Nutrient and toxic chemical overloads in Chesapeake Bay threaten the continued productivity of that most valuable estuarine environment; the lower Mississippi remains grossly polluted; the degraded condition of Boston Harbor became a subject of national attention during the 1988 Presidential campaign (and is now undergoing a massive cleanup, thanks to a multimillion dollar project to upgrade sewage treatment, renovate sewers, and eliminate combined sewer overflows into the harbor). In contrast to phosphate concentrations which, on a nationwide basis, appear to be holding steady, nitrate levels have been rising. In some locations arsenic and cadmium levels have increased, while lead and mercury have declined.

While progress in restoring the quality of our nation's waterways shows a mixed bag of results, the fact that overall surface water quality has not deteriorated during a period when both population and the GNP have continued to grow gives evidence that the billions of dollars spent on water cleanup efforts are having a positive impact. Nevertheless, the nation still has a long way to go before the goals of the Clean Water Act are fully met. While many of the conventional sources and types of water pollution are now being dealt with fairly adequately, newer problems such as toxic chemical pollutants and difficult-to-control runoff from farms, construction sites, and city streets have stymied pollution abatement efforts. A sustained and costly public commitment to water cleanup is essential if the lofty aims of the Clean Water Act are to be realized (Sheiman, 1982; Wolman, 1988).

Elsewhere in the world, water quality issues rank high on the list of international environmental concerns. Not surprisingly, progress in controlling water pollution varies widely from one country to another. Most developed nations have imposed controls on industrial dischargers similar to those in the United States and the majority have helped finance the construction of sewage treatment plants. As a result, at least two-thirds of all Europeans and North Americans are served by wastewater treatment facilities (Switzerland, Denmark, Netherlands, Sweden, and western Germany provide such services to nearly all their citizens), while Japan, too, has made considerable progress (about 40% coverage). The picture in the developing nations and in parts of the former Soviet empire is much less promising, however. Rapid industrial growth has given rise to numerous toxic "hotspots" of pollution, as industrial dischargers dump poisonous effluent into nearby waterways, unhindered by nonexistent or seldom-enforced water pollution laws. In the Czech Republic, for example, government reports describe 70% of all surface waters as grossly contaminated, with 30% too polluted for fish to survive. Unfortunately, deteriorating economic conditions throughout central and eastern Europe suggest that water quality improvements in this part of the world will be slow in coming. Untreated sewage, as well as salt- and fertilizer-laden irrigation return flows further contaminate lakes, rivers, and coastal waters. In South Asia, the South and Southeast Pacific, and in Africa modern sewage treatment is virtually nonexistent; in Latin America and the Caribbean, according to the World Health Organization, only 41% of the *urban* population is served by sewer systems, and over 90% of the

BOX 15-1
An Old Killer Returns

The River Rimac which flows through the Peruvian capital of Lima is the source of 70% of the city's drinking water supply; it is also choked with sewage which it flushes untreated into the sea. Compounding the problem, raw wastewater is also carried to coastal discharge points by sewers which pour their fetid contents onto beaches adjacent to densely populated settlements, areas frequented by children who bathe and play in the contaminated water. One of the poorest countries in South America, Peru is 40 years behind more advanced societies in basic sanitation investments. Although Lima, a metropolis of seven million people, has an up-to-date water purification plant and a good water distribution system, 40% of its residents nevertheless lack access to the treated water it provides. Many slum dwellers must rely on the river or on house-to-house delivery by government tank trucks which collect their cargo from polluted surface and groundwater sources.

While the provision of potable water is inadequate, the provision of sewage treatment is virtually nonexistent. These factors proved a fatal combination when, in January of 1991, Lima was hit by the first outbreak of epidemic cholera seen in the Western Hemisphere for more than a century. Within a month after the first cases were confirmed, over 10,000 patients, most of them slum dwellers, were being treated each week. The epidemic spread rapidly from Peru to Ecuador, Colombia, Chile, and Brazil—almost monthly another country reported the appearance of the dread disease. By the end of 1991 the Pan American Health Organization had received reports of 391,000 cases and nearly 4000 deaths—more than had occurred

throughout the entire world during the five years preceding the Peruvian outbreak. The return of cholera, one of the most feared 19th century killers, reminded public health officials in the waning years of the 20th century that neglect of basic aspects of sanitation—sewage treatment, provision of safe drinking water, food hygiene—can have disastrous consequences. In this modern "Chemical Age," microbial hazards still lurk, ready to exact their toll of death and disease among the careless or the unwary.

Typically an ailment associated with poor living conditions, cholera is caused by the bacterium *Vibrio cholerae*, an organism that lodges in the intestines, producing a toxin that causes rapid onset of severe watery diarrhea, vomiting, and cramps. The sudden loss of huge amounts of body fluids and salts results in complete dehydration and collapse of the vascular system, frequently killing its victims in less than a day unless treatment is promptly initiated. Exclusively a human pathogen, the cholera bacterium is transmitted from one person to another via water or food contaminated with human fecal material. In Peru, most cases seemed to be associated with consumption of fish or shellfish harvested from sewage-tainted coastal waters. *Ceviche*, a local dish made of raw fish, marinated in lemon juice and onions, was targeted for special blame (since *V. cholerae*, like most bacteria, is sensitive to heat, well-cooked fish would not have transmitted the infection). The disease continued to spread because as many as three-fourths of those who became infected never showed symptoms or received treatment; nevertheless, they became carriers, perpetuating the epidemic when the bacteria were passed in human feces. Progress of the epidemic could have been slowed by rigid adherence to good sanitary practices such as boiling drinking water and frequent handwashing, but at a time of severe economic hardship, when both fuel and water were priced beyond the means of many of the city's poor, such measures were seldom followed. As an official with the Agency for International Development (AID) remarked, "When you have to buy water to drink, it is very difficult to think of using water to wash your hands."

Although, untreated, cholera may kill 50% of those severely stricken, if sufferers are quickly hospitalized most can be saved by administration of fluids and salts ("rehydration therapy"), either orally or intravenously. Antibiotics may be given to shorten the course of illness but generally aren't essential to recovery.

While the peak of the epidemic has now passed, poor levels of sanitation throughout Latin America suggest that the disease will become endemic throughout the region, permanently established in such environmental reservoirs as plankton, shellfish, water, and the human intestinal tract, posing a public health problem well into the future. In the meantime, a new, more virulent strain of cholera has emerged in Asia, sweeping across India, Bangladesh, into Thailand, and threatening to cause a global epidemic wherever sanitary precautions are deficient (health authorities doubt that cholera will spread in the U.S. because of near-universal sewage treatment). Existing vaccines are ineffective against the new strain, giving added urgency to ongoing efforts to develop an oral prophylactic superior to the current inoculation which provides limited protection and is not recommended by either the U.S. Public Health Service or the World Health Organization.

Resurgence of this fearsome disease has focused renewed attention on the as-yet unmet sanitary needs of Third World countries. These needs are immense; simply providing potable water and sewage treatment to Peru's 23 million citizens would cost that government over $300 million each year for the next decade—an amount more than 10 times the sum currently being invested. Beyond the provision of large engineered facilities, fighting cholera will require intensive efforts to improve hygienic practices among the poor through expanded health education programs and through widespread construction of inexpensive latrines. Unless such projects are successfully undertaken within the near future, cholera is likely to become a permanent fact of life throughout South America and the Caribbean just as it is in Asia and Africa.

References

Altman, Lawrence K. 1993. "Doctors Say a New Cholera Poses a Worldwide Danger." *New York Times*, August 13.

Brooke, James. 1991. "Feeding on 19th Century Conditions, Cholera Spreads in Latin America." *New York Times*, April 21.

Glass, R. I., et al. 1992. "Epidemic Cholera in the Americas," *Science*, 256 (June 12).

wastewater collected by these sewers flows directly into surface waters without receiving any treatment whatsoever. And everywhere in the world, in rich and poor nations alike, polluted runoff is only beginning to attract the attention it deserves (World Resources Institute, 1992).

To understand the worldwide impact of water pollution on the health of both ecosystems and their human inhabitants requires a look at the major sources and types of pollution and the problems posed by each. The remainder of this chapter will examine these issues and will describe the pollution control policies developed by the U.S. Congress and regulatory agencies as they strive to protect public health through improving water quality.

Sources of Water Pollution

Pollutants can enter waterways by a number of different routes. Strategies for preventing water contamination must take into consideration the nature of the pollutant source and must devise appropriate methods of control for each source category. Congress has coined two terms—**point source** and **nonpoint source**—to refer to the two general types of water pollution and pollution control regulations adopted within recent years have by necessity been tailored according to source.

Point Sources

Pollutants that enter waterways at well-defined locations (e.g. through a pipe, ditch, or sewer outfall) are referred to as point source pollutants. Characterized by discharges that are relatively even and continuous, typical point sources of water pollution include factories, sewage treatment plants and storm sewer outfalls. Point sources have been the most conspicuous violators of water quality standards, but because effluent from such sources is relatively easy to collect and treat, considerable progress has been made during the past decade in reducing this type of pollutant discharge. The two major categories of point source pollution are sewage treatment plants and industrial discharges. Each will be discussed in greater detail later in this chapter.

Nonpoint Sources

Until recently nonpoint source (NPS) pollutants—those which run off or seep into waterways from broad areas of land rather than entering the water through a discreet pipe or conduit—were largely overlooked as significant contributors to water contamination. However, when stringent effluent limitations on point sources failed to result in dramatic improvements in water quality, it became increasingly evident that in many waterways the largest pollutant contribution was coming from nonpoint sources. Indeed, in its 1990 *National Water Quality Report* to Congress, the EPA identified nonpoint source pollution as the main reason why many

Approximately half of our water quality violations can be traced to stormwater runoff from broad land areas. Controlling pollution from these diverse sources is proving far more difficult than reducing pollutants from point sources.

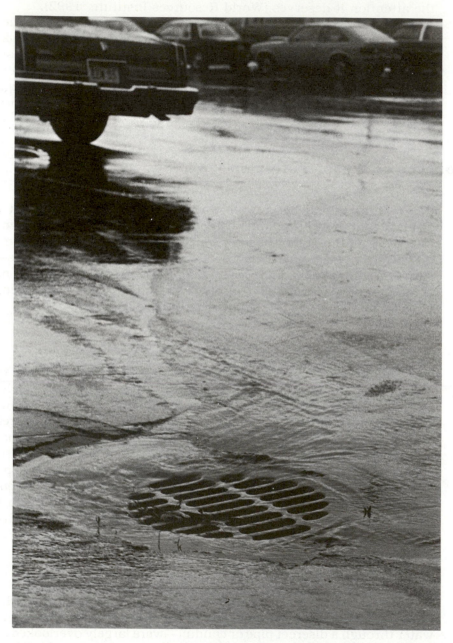

Nonpoint source of water pollution: urban street runoff. [Illinois Environmental Protection Agency]

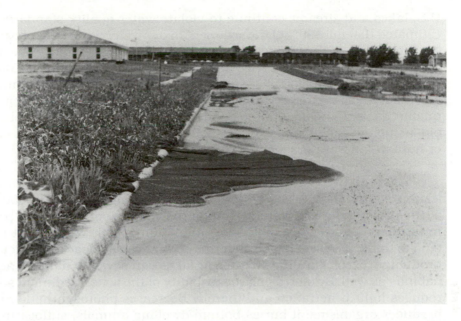

Nonpoint source of water pollution: construction site runoff. [Gary Fak, Soil Conservation Service]

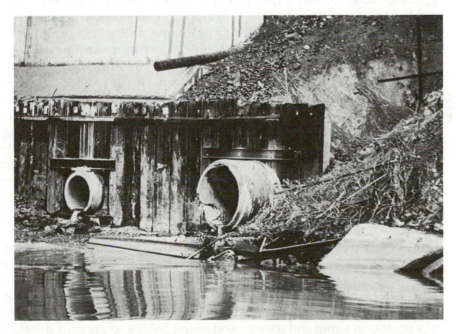

Point source of water pollution: effluents entering a waterway directly from a factory outfall, pipe, ditch, or sewage treatment plant outlet are the most visible source of water pollution. [Illinois Environmental Protection Agency]

U.S. lakes and streams continue to violate water quality standards. It is estimated that fully 99% of the sediment in our waterways, 98% of bacterial contaminants, 84% of phosphorus, 82% of nitrogen, and 73% of biochemical oxygen demand are contributed by nonpoint sources (Gianessi et al., 1986). The majority of states have now identified pollutants from such sources as the main reason they have been unable to attain their water quality goals. Nonpoint source pollution (really just new terminology for old-fashioned runoff and sedimentation) results primarily from a variety of human land-use practices and includes the following.

Agriculture. In the United States as a whole, agriculture is the leading source of water pollution, adversely affecting the quality of 50–70% of the nation's surface waters. Among the various contaminants present in farmland runoff, the single most abundant is soil. While most people tend to think of erosion largely in terms of its adverse impact on agricultural productivity, soil entering streams or lakes can severely damage aquatic habitats as well. By increasing the turbidity of the water, sediment sharply reduces light penetration and thereby decreases photosynthetic rates of producer organisms; it buries bottom-dwelling animals, suffocating fish eggs and aquatic invertebrates. Stormwater runoff from fields and pastures carries more than just sediment into waterways, however. Manures from grazing lands located adjacent to streams or lakes can contribute five or six times as many nutrients to waterways as do point sources. Manure spread on fields can cause similar problems unless it is promptly worked into the soil. In the same way, chemical fertilizers and pesticides, when applied immediately prior to a storm or in amounts exceeding the assimilative capacity of the crop in question, can be carried by runoff water from fields into adjacent lakes or streams. Upon entering a waterway, farm chemicals can poison fish or promote algal growth; if runoff seeps through the soil into shallow aquifers, chemical contamination of drinking water wells can occur. Since these toxic pollutants generally enter waterways attached to soil particles, they can best be controlled by the same strategies used to prevent soil erosion—conservation tillage, terracing, contour plowing, etc.—which aim to keep soil on the land and out of the water. Additional management strategies include: applying pesticides when there is little wind and the potential for heavy rain is low; using nonpersistent, low-toxicity pesticides; disposing of containers properly; applying fertilizers only when they can be incorporated into the soil (i.e. not when the ground is frozen); and using any type of chemical in the proper amount and only when field checks indicate they are needed. Controlling runoff from pasturelands can be managed relatively easily by maintaining a buffer zone of vegetation along waterways and using fences to prevent livestock from walking into streams.

Construction Activities. Acre for acre, runoff from sites where homes, shopping centers, factories, or highways are under construction can contribute more sediment to waterways than any other activity—typically 10–20 times more than the amounts from agricultural lands. More than 500 tons of sediment per acre per year can wash off such sites into streams during the construction period, frequently carrying with them cement wash, asphalt, paint and cleaning solvents, oil and tar, and pesticides. These contaminants from construction sites have impaired an estimated 5% of U.S. surface waters. Fortunately the actual construction time during which land surfaces are unprotected is relatively short and the amount of land exposed is small in comparison with farm acreage. Nevertheless, damage to water quality due to construction site runoff can be severe and long-lasting. Many municipalities are now mandating the use of readily available erosion control techniques on construction sites, the basic approach being to expose the smallest area of land possible for the shortest period of time and scheduling construction activities so that the minimum amount of land is disturbed during the peak runoff period in the spring. Using mulches and fast-growing cover vegetation, retaining as many existing trees and shrubs on the site as possible, roughening the soil surface or constructing berms to slow the velocity of runoff, and building retention basins to detain runoff water long enough to promote settling out of suspended sediment are all well-established management practices for reducing pollutant runoff from construction sites.

Urban Street Runoff.   Although people seldom consider city streets and sidewalks as important sources of water pollution, studies have shown that during storm episodes, particularly storms that terminate a long dry spell, very large amounts of sediment and other pollutants are carried by runoff water into adjacent rivers, streams, or lakes. The Natural Resources Defense Council, a nonprofit environmental organization, recently reported study results demonstrating that in many cities the total pollutant load from urban runoff exceeds that from industrial discharges. Contaminants commonly found in urban runoff include sand, dirt, road salt, oil, grease, and heavy metal particles (lead, zinc, copper, chromium, etc.) from paved surfaces; pesticides and fertilizers from lawns; leaves, seeds, bark, and grass clippings; animal and bird droppings; and other substances too numerous to mention. The Nationwide Urban Runoff Program (NURP), conducted by the EPA, documented discharge of suspended solids from storm sewers in amounts far exceeding those entering waterways from sewage treatment plants. EPA also cited urban runoff as a major contributor of oil to surface waters. Reducing pollution from this source requires broad-based cooperation and effort on the part of both municipal officials and citizens: more frequent street-sweeping to prevent sediment accumulation on streets; proper disposal of pet wastes; careful and limited application of lawn and garden fertilizers and pesticides; litter control on both public and private property; judicious use of road salt and sand; application of organic mulches to reduce erosion on bare ground; incorporating more green space within the urban areas and along waterways to allow runoff to filter into the ground; use of surface ponds, holding tanks, rooftop catchments, subsurface tunnels, or similar structures to hold, retain, and gradually release stormwater.

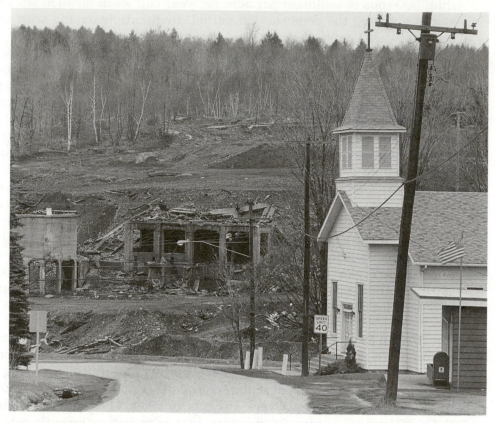

Acidified water flowing out of abandoned mines such as the one in the center of this photo constitutes an important nonpoint source of water pollution. [U.S. Department of Agriculture]

Acid Mine Drainage.   When the iron pyrite found in association with coal deposits is exposed to air and water during mining operations, a series of chemical reactions is initiated, culminating in the formation of a copper-colored precipitate (iron hydroxide) and sulfuric acid. The precipitate frequently covers the bottom of streams in mining regions, smothering bottom life and giving such streams a characteristic rusty appearance. The sulfuric acid lowers the pH of the water, eliminating many aquatic species that cannot survive or reproduce in the acidified water. Both operating and abandoned coal mines of either the underground or surface type are characterized by acid drainage, although only *abandoned* mines are termed nonpoint sources (*active* mines are classified as point source polluters). In West Virginia, the third largest coal-producing state in the United States and home to thousands of inactive mines, acid mine drainage constitutes the leading nonpoint pollution source—a problem shared by many other mining areas as well. Acids, however, are not the only water quality problem posed by abandoned mines. Under the low pH conditions prevailing in such regions, metals such as iron, aluminum, copper, zinc, manganese, magnesium, and calcium are leached from soil and rock, contaminating streams. Large amounts of silt and sediment from slag heaps or refuse piles erode into waterways, clogging streams and burying bottom-dwellers under a thick layer of silt. Legislatively mandated regrading and revegetation of abandoned strip mines have been helpful in reducing runoff of sediment from abandoned mine sites, but have had minimal impact on acid drainage. Sealing openings to abandoned underground mines, thereby cutting off the supply of oxygen and water that permit acid formation, has been the chief means of combatting acid mine drainage. Although this practice significantly reduces acid loadings, it doesn't eliminate them and efforts to find better ways of dealing with the problem continue. In recent years, the use of engineered wetlands to remove toxic chemicals from mine leachate have yielded promising results, as have alkaline recharge zones incorporated into more advanced artificial wetlands designed to neutralize acids. These and other innovative approaches to abating acid mine drainage are undergoing active investigation and offer hope that a solution to this challenge will eventually be found (Bennett, 1991).

Fallout of Airborne Pollutants.   The situation represented by acid rainfall (see chapter 12) is but one example of pollution from the sky causing water quality problems. A great many of the particles released into the atmosphere through human activities eventually return to earth and enter rivers, lakes, or oceans either directly or in runoff. These airborne particles include many hazardous chemicals such as lead, asbestos, PCBs, beryllium, fluorides, and various pesticides. The contribution to water pollution by synthetic chemical fallout is surprisingly large—the major portion of PCBs and other toxic chemicals in the Great Lakes and a substantial amount of the hydrocarbons found in the oceans entered these waters through airborne deposition.

As point source pollutants decline in importance, thanks to improved pollution control technology and enforcement of effluent limitations, nonpoint sources such as those just described present the greatest single challenge to attaining our nation's clean water goals. The "top down" strategy, whereby federal and state governments promulgate regulations with which individual polluters must comply under threat of civil or criminal penalties, has served us well in reducing pollution from point sources but is entirely inappropriate for controlling poison runoff from broad land areas. Recognizing the near-impossibility of requiring discharge permits for every farm field or parking lot, regulators striving to control NPS pollution thus far have focused their efforts on altering harmful land use practices. In 1987 Congress required states to conduct surveys and develop "assessment reports" describing the nature and extent of NPS pollution within their jurisdictions. Subsequently they were to implement management programs to combat the problems identified. Control strategies to deal with NPS pollution fall into one of two possible categories:

- increasing the land's capacity to retain water, thereby reducing runoff (e.g. a wide variety of erosion control measures), or

BOX 15-2

Too Much of a Good Thing

Aquatic plants, like their terrestrial cousins, require certain mineral nutrients for healthy growth and metabolism. An excess of these essential elements, however, can result in a plant population explosion that leads to serious degradation of water quality and radical changes in the species composition of the overfed lake, pond, or stream. The process by which a body of water becomes overenriched with nutrients and as a result produces an overabundance of plant life is known as **eutrophication**, a classic and easily recognized form of water pollution. Although eutrophication can occur in sluggish streams, bays, and estuaries, it is most common in lakes and ponds. This is so because lakes, unlike flowing bodies of water, flush very slowly; thus nutrient-laden wastewaters or runoff introduced into a lake tend to remain there for many years, causing serious pollution problems.

The most characteristic sign that a lake is undergoing eutrophication is the formation of a green scum, consisting of millions of microscopic algal cells, on the surface of the water. This is only the most visible outward indication that something is amiss, however; a closer look reveals that a number of drastic changes in lake ecology are taking place. An analysis of the eutrophication process reveals the following sequence of events:

1. water becomes nutrient enriched with dissolved nitrates and/or phosphates contributed by sewage treatment plant discharges, septic tank seepage, urban street runoff, or runoff from fertilized agricultural lands or animal feedlots.

2. algal "blooms," stimulated by these nutrients, occur near the surface of the water and overpopulate the aquatic environment with enormous numbers of aquatic plants, particularly species of cyanobacteria (previously known as blue-green algae).

3. large numbers of algae die off and then settle to the bottom of the lake or pond.

4. decomposer organisms, primarily bacteria, multiply rapidly in response to the great increase in their food supply (dead algae); as they break down the algal tissues in a low-oxygen environment, they release methane and hydrogen sulfide gas, which accounts for the unpleasant odor frequently associated with algae-choked ponds.

5. levels of dissolved oxygen in the water are depleted due to the very high rate of metabolic activity of the decomposer organisms; the drop in oxygen content is particularly rapid in summer because high temperatures promote more rapid metabolism and because warm water holds less dissolved oxygen than does colder water.

6. fish and insect species requiring high levels of dissolved oxygen die and are replaced by species more tolerant of low oxygen conditions. The kinds of fish and invertebrate species typical of a balanced aquatic ecosystem (e.g. bass, sunfish, trout) cannot live in waters where the dissolved oxygen concentration is below 5 or 6 ppm for any length of time; under low oxygen conditions, these species will give way to less desirable (from a human point of view) organisms such as sludgeworms, which can tolerate oxygen concentrations as low as 0.5 ppm and whose presence inbottom sediments is commonly used as a biological indicator of organic pollution.

7. toxin secreted by cyanobacteria imparts a foul taste to the

water and may poison fish and livestock drinking from the lake if concentrations become sufficiently high.

Although eutrophication is a natural process of aquatic succession, its rate is greatly accelerated by the introduction of human-generated pollutants into aquatic ecosystems. Since people seem to prefer the cleaner water and more varied fish populations characteristic of the early developmental stages of a lake, it is in society's best interest to forestall the described course of events by preventing the nutrients which initiate the eutrophication process from entering the water in the first place.

- minimizing the amount of pollutants available for runoff during storms (e.g. keeping manure piles away from streams, judicious application of farm chemicals, regular street sweeping, capturing potential air pollutants before they become airborne and subject to fallout).

Controlling nonpoint pollution unfortunately demands more than just a technological "fix"; it requires instead the cooperation of farmers, ranchers, municipal officials, developers, homeowners, and others in implementing better land management practices to prevent these diverse pollutants from running off the land and into the water.

Regulatory efforts to deal with NPS pollution have thus far not been very successful. State runoff control programs vary widely and, not surprisingly, focus on different priority activities. Few, however, emphasize the watershed protection approach that is needed for an effective program; most continue to rely on *voluntary* compliance by landowners with recommended water-sensitive practices (a stance which is politically popular but frequently ineffective); few have adequate monitoring data; and, perhaps most important, all lack sufficient funding to hire additional staff needed to carry out meaningful programs. In contrast to the $75 *billion* the U.S. has spent on sewage treatment plant construction alone over the past 20 years, federal dollars allocated for the control of nonpoint pollution—which constitutes a much more serious water quality problem—totaled just $200 million during the four years following initiation of the congressionally-mandated state NPS programs. Major changes in the current governmental approach to NPS pollution control are urgently needed if the biological integrity of our lakes, rivers, and estuaries is not to be further degraded by poison runoff (Adler, Landman, and Cameron, 1993; Griffin, 1991).

Municipal Sewage Treatment

In 1854 the city of London was reeling under a severe epidemic of Asiatic cholera, a disease characterized by the sudden onset of profuse watery diarrhea and vomiting, resulting in rapid dehydration and death of approximately half of those afflicted. Not all parts of the city were equally affected, however. Within a district called St. James Parish, the cholera death rate hit 200 per 10,000 population, while in neighboring Charing Cross and Hanover Square districts fatalities were considerably lower. Dr. John Snow, a member of the commission of inquiry appointed to investigate the outbreak, noted that the vast majority of individuals who had died of cholera obtained their drinking water from a well on Broad Street; in other respects there seemed to be no fundamental difference between conditions in St. James Parish and nearby districts where cholera rates were low. Although the cholera bacillus and its method of transmission had not yet been discovered, Snow recommended that the handle of the Broad Street pump be removed to prevent further consumption of water from the well. Shortly thereafter, the cholera epidemic subsided. Subsequent investigations disclosed that prior to the outbreak, residents of one house on Broad Street had been ill with an unidentified disease. Their fecal wastes had been dumped into an open cesspool near the well, a common method for disposing of human wastewater in those years. Unfortunately, the brick lining of the cesspool had deteriorated to the point that the liquid wastes could readily seep through the ground and contaminate the well water with still viable pathogenic organisms. The connection between poorly managed human wastes and serious human disease was clearly demonstrated (Cholera Inquiry Committee, 1855).

London's use of open cesspools as a method of sewage disposal was a well-established practice in many parts of the world until the late 19th and early 20th centuries. These pits in the ground simply collect wastes which are then stabilized by bacterial action. Seepage of liquids into the soil from such holes was common, and since no disinfection was used, contamination of wells and aquifers with human fecal pathogens frequently occurred. During the 19th century the growing popularity of flush toilets in urban areas resulted in greatly increased volumes of wastewater requiring disposal. This additional influx produced frequent overflowing of public cesspools and caused a further spread of filth and waterborne disease, particularly cholera and typhoid fever. Installation of sewer systems which carried wastes directly from homes into nearby rivers helped to alleviate problems of well contamination but caused severe degradation of surface water quality, resulting in the elimination of many forms of aquatic life and enhancing the risk of waterborne disease in communities downstream which used surface water supplies for drinking.

By the end of the 19th century rapid urban growth convinced city planners that sewage treatment facilities were needed to alleviate the health and aesthetic problems created by dumping raw sewage into waterways. Today in the United States approximately 70% of the population live in areas where domestic wastes pass through a sewage treatment plant before being discharged. The remainder, for the most part, rely on on-site wastewater disposal systems—usually a septic tank and soil absorption field or sand filter. Provision of adequate methods of sewage treatment, along with the chlorination of drinking water, has done far more to reduce the incidence of epidemic disease and to upgrade standards of public health than has the more widely acclaimed introduction of modern medicines and vaccines.

The aim of sewage treatment is to improve the quality of wastewater to the point that it can be discharged into a waterway without seriously disrupting the aquatic environment or causing human health problems in the form of waterborne disease. Achieving these goals requires killing pathogenic organisms present in human wastes (within any human population there will always be some individuals suffering from various gastrointestinal diseases and releasing the causative bacteria, protozoans, etc., in their excreta; it is assumed, therefore, that domestic sewage entering the treatment facility is contaminated with pathogens capable of causing disease outbreaks) and, to the greatest possible extent, removing organic wastes or converting them to inorganic forms so that after discharge they will not deplete the oxygen content of the receiving waters as they decompose. To accomplish these ends, several levels of sewage treatment are necessary.

Primary Treatment

The used water supply of a community, averaging about 100 gallons/person/ day in cities having separate storm and sanitary sewers, flows from homes and institutions into the municipal sewer system which carries the wastes to a treatment plant (in regulatory jargon a "**POTW**"— **publicly owned treatment works**). At this point sewage consists not only of human feces and urine, but also of wastes from laundry, bathing, garbage grinding, and dishwashing, as well as all the miscellaneous articles that find their way into the sewer system—sand, gravel, rubber balls, leaves, sticks, dead rats, etc. Primary sewage treatment consists of several mechanical processes designed to remove the larger suspended solids through screening and sedimentation. Though there may be minor variations in the methods used by different treatment plants, in general the incoming flow first passes through one or more screens to remove large floating objects. Comminutors (grinders) may be used to reduce the solids to a uniform size so they cannot damage or clog equipment. After the waste-laden water has passed the screens, it enters a grit chamber where the reduced velocity of flow permits sand, gravel, and other inorganic material to settle out. Air is sometimes injected into the tank to maintain aerobic conditions and to remove trapped gases. Following several hours in an additional sedimentation tank (a "primary clarifier"), the wastewater enters the secondary treatment system or, in those POTWs having only a primary level of treatment, is chlorinated and discharged into the receiving waters. The solid material (sludge) that settles out in the sedimentation tank is regularly removed, dried, and disposed of by one of several methods.

While primary treatment is unquestionably better than no treatment at all, it does not result in an effluent of sufficiently high quality to prevent degradation of the receiving waters. During primary treatment approximately 50–65% of suspended solids are removed and the BOD (see Box 15-3) is reduced by about 25–40%. Because the pollution potential of

Box 15-3

BOD

The most commonly used measurement of the amount of pollutant organic material in water is a parameter referred to as **biochemical oxygen demand** or **BOD**. When bacteria act upon the organic matter in sewage or certain industrial wastes discharged into waterways, large amounts of dissolved oxygen are rapidly used up; this can result in fish kills and drastic alterations in the aquatic environment. Biochemical oxygen demand basically is an indication of how much putrescible organic material is present in the water or wastewater, with a low BOD indicating good water quality and a high BOD reflecting polluted conditions.

BOD is calculated by taking a sample of water, diluting it with fully-oxygenated water, and determining the amount of oxygen present at that time. The sample is then incubated in the dark at 20°C (68°F) for five days, after which the oxygen content is again measured. The difference between the initial and final readings, expressed in milligrams per liter (mg/l), is the BOD. Some representative BOD values are:

Pollutant	5-day BOD (in mg/l)
raw sewage	150–250
cannery wastes	5000–6000
discharges from pulp mills	10,000–15,000
wastewater from wool scouring	>20,000
treatment plant effluent	
(EPA standard—maximum average for 30 consecutive days)	30

such wastewater is still quite high, the Environmental Protection Agency does not consider primary treatment by itself an adequate level of sewage treatment.

Secondary Treatment

Whereas primary treatment is based upon physical and mechanical methods of removing suspended solids from wastewater, secondary treatment depends on biological processes, similar to naturally occurring decomposition but greatly accelerated, to digest organic wastes. Microorganisms, predominantly aerobic bacteria, are utilized in the presence of an abundant oxygen supply to break down organic materials into inorganic carbon dioxide, water, and minerals. This can be accomplished by means of **trickling filters**—beds of crushed stone whose surfaces are covered with a microbial slime consisting of bacteria, protozoans, nematodes, etc., which absorb the organic material as the wastewater is sprayed over the surface of the rocks—or by the more modern **activated sludge process**. This involves "seeding" a tank of sewage with

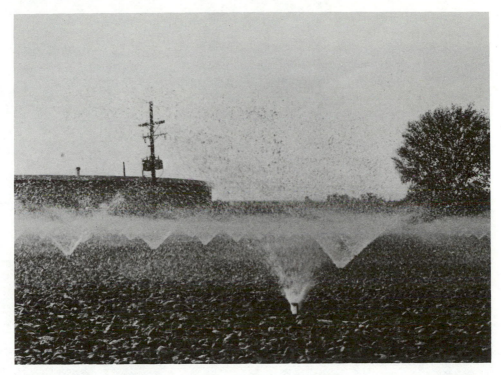

Trickling filter: a method of secondary sewage treatment in which wastewater effluent is distributed over a bed of rocks, the surfaces of which are covered by microorganisms that metabolize the organic nutrients in the wastewater, breaking them down into carbon dioxide and water. [Author's Photo]

bacteria-laden sludge, pumping compressed air into the mixture and agitating it for 4–10 hours. During this time the microbes adsorb most of the colloidal and suspended solids onto the surfaces of the sludge particles and oxidize the organic material. After the process is complete, the sludge is separated from the remaining liquid by settling ("secondary clarification"). Most of this sludge, consisting primarily of masses of bacteria, is removed, but some must be retained and fed back into the incoming sewage to perpetuate the process.

After wastewater has passed through both primary and secondary treatment, the level of suspended solids and of BOD has been reduced by about 90–95% (however, cold weather can reduce the efficiency of pollutant reduction because it slows the metabolic rate of the microorganisms on which secondary treatment depends). Secondary treatment is not effective in removing viruses, heavy metals, dissolved minerals, and certain other chemicals (Koren, 1980). In the United States, a federally-imposed mandate requiring that all POTWs provide at least secondary wastewater treatment took effect in July 1988.

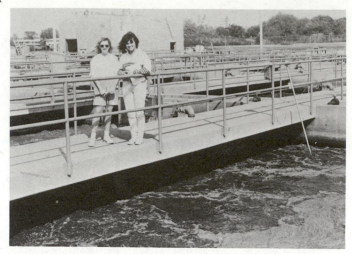

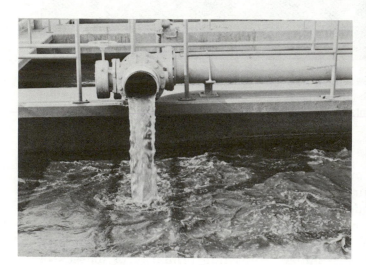

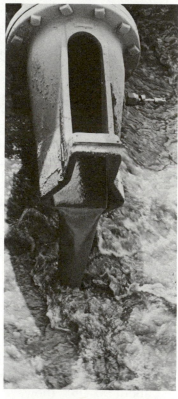

Activated sludge method: (top) a form of secondary sewage treatment in which wastewater effluent from primary treatment is mixed in aerated tanks with large numbers of bacteria ("activated sludge"). These bacteria feed on the organic nutrients, converting them to simpler inorganic substances. This process is energy-intensive, due to power requirements for running the pumps, but can achieve a very high degree of pollutant removal; (bottom left) wastewater entering tank; (bottom right) introduction of activated sludge. [Author's Photos]

Advanced Wastewater Treatment ("Tertiary Treatment")

A third level of sewage treatment may be required in situations where effluent from the secondary treatment process still contains substances that are causing water quality problems; when the sheer volume of effluent is large enough that the remaining 10% of suspended solids and BOD are sufficient to initiate eutrophication; or if the treated wastewater is to be used for purposes of drinking, irrigation, or recreation. Advanced wastewater treatment involves either one or a combination of several biological, chemical, or physical processes designed to remove such pollutants as phosphates, nitrates, ammonia, and organic chemicals. It also further reduces the concentration of remaining suspended solids and BOD to about 1% of that present in raw sewage. Some examples of tertiary treatment processes can be seen in Figure 15-1.

Disinfection

Since the most common waterborne diseases are caused by pathogenic bacteria, viruses, or protozoans present in human excrement, one of the primary purposes of sewage treatment is to kill such organisms before they can infect new victims. Simple exposure to the hostile environment outside the human intestine is sufficient to reduce the number of bacteria appreciably as they pass through the treatment process. However, because a substantial number of live organisms still remain in the wastewater after

Figure 15-1 Tertiary Treatment Processes

Tertiary Treatment Method	Pollutant Removed
Chemical coagulation, followed by filtration or sedimentation	phosphates, tertiary suspended solids, and BOD
Activated carbon adsorption	synthetic organic chemicals, tastes, odors
Nitrifying towers	ammonia
Air stripping	ammonia
Oxidation ponds and aerated lagoons	BOD, phosphates
Reverse osmosis	BOD, nitrates, phosphates, dissolved solids
Electrodialysis	dissolved minerals
Oxidation	organic material
Foam separation	organic chemicals
Land application	phosphates, nitrates, BOD, suspended solids

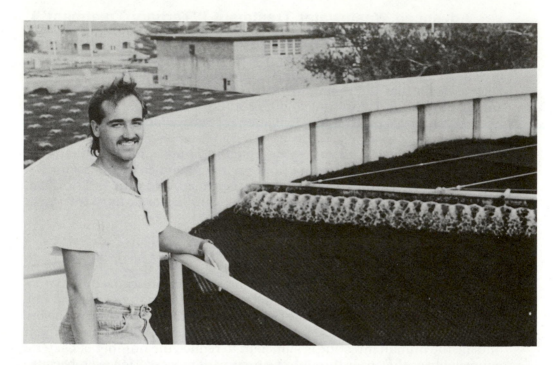

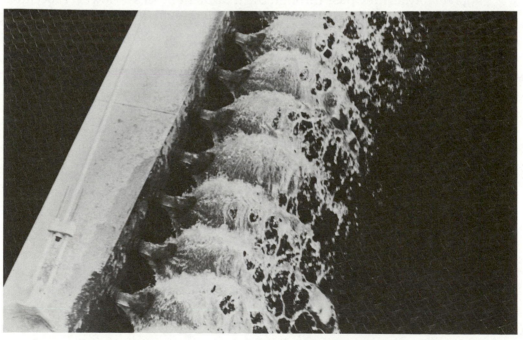

Nitrification tower: a method of advanced wastewater treatment for reducing the ammonia content of wastewater; (top) rotating bars distribute treated wastewater over the upper surface of a 40–50 inch high honeycomb-like plastic grid; as water trickles downward, aerobic nitrifying bacteria on the surfaces of the grid convert ammonia to nitrate; (bottom) closeup of nitrification tower grid surface. [Author's Photos]

primary and secondary treatment are complete, it has been standard procedure for many years to disinfect treated effluent by adding chlorine prior to discharge in order to eliminate any remaining disease-causing organisms. More recently, the policy of chlorinating all sewage treatment plant discharges has met with increasing resistance and today more than half of all states no longer require chlorination of wastewaters. There are several reasons for this change in accepted practice.

1. Chlorine is effective in killing bacteria, but less so in relation to viruses, many of which survive this treatment.

2. Chlorine is very destructive of fish and other forms of aquatic life, many of which are eliminated for a considerable distance downstream from sewage treatment plants due to the presence of this chemical in the water.

3. Chlorine treatment is expensive and poses safety problems at the treatment plant in the eventuality of cylinder leaks or system disruption.

4. Chlorine disinfects only a fraction of the wastes in streams because bacteria-laden runoff from farmland and urban areas enters waterways untreated.

Proponents of chlorinating POTW discharges correctly point out, however, that this practice helps reduce outbreaks of disease that have been associated with swimming in sewage-polluted water or with consuming shellfish taken from contaminated waterways. Although disinfecting such effluent with chlorine does not sterilize the water, in the sense of killing every last microbe, it reduces their numbers significantly and thereby enhances the self-purifying capacity of natural waterways. As the controversy between wastewater chlorination opponents and proponents continues to rage, a compromise solution has been reached in some states where disinfection of discharge waters is required only during the summer bathing season, with the practice being discontinued during the winter when recreational contact with water is unlikely (Shertzer, 1986). In certain other states, requirements for disinfecting POTW effluent have been dropped altogether, except in those situations where a drinking water intake point or a bathing beach is located a short distance downstream.

Sludge Management

Ironically, the high degree of pollutant removal achieved at modern sewage treatment plants has created a new challenge for POTW operators—how to manage the steadily growing volumes of sludge which our increasingly efficient sewage treatment technologies are producing. In the United States, municipal treatment plants cumulatively generate approximately 5.4 million dry metric tons of sludge annually, the equivalent of 47 pounds for every man, woman and child each year. This amount, almost double that produced during the early 1970s, will inevitably increase in the years immediately ahead, thanks to continued population growth, further gains in the efficiency of wastewater treatment, and more widespread compliance with Clean Water Act requirements. Because sewage sludge itself can be a pollutant if improperly managed, its treatment, ultimate disposal, and potential use must be handled in ways that will not endanger public health or the environment.

Routinely removed at each step in the sewage treatment process, the watery sludge (before treatment, sludge consists of 93–99% water) generally is first thickened through the use of coagulant chemicals or dissolved air flotation. It is then stabilized through a two-step anaerobic digestion process in order to reduce problems associated with odors and the presence of pathogenic organisms—a process that takes approximately 60 days to complete. To reduce its volume for ease in handling, the sludge is then dewatered, either by mechanical processes or by drying on sand beds. At this point sludge has the appearance of rich black dirt and is largely odor-free. In fact, because treated sludge is not at all the offensive substance its rather inelegant name suggests, the Water Environment Federation, a nonprofit technical organization working to improve water quality worldwide, is spearheading an effort to change existing nomenclature. In place of ''sludge,'' the Federation is actively promoting use of the term

Figure 15-2 Schematic Municipal Wastewater Treatment Process

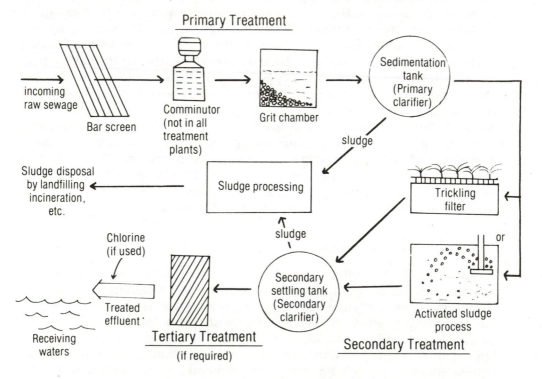

"**biosolids**," asserting that such a designation emphasizes that sewage sludge should not be regarded as an objectionable *waste* but rather as a valuable *resource*.

Indeed, the nitrates, phosphates, and organic matter present in sludge make it useful as a fertilizer and as a soil conditioner. Sludge has a long history of use for improving marginal lands, increasing forest productivity (studies have shown that the rate of tree growth doubles on sludge-enriched soil), boosting home garden yields, and reclaiming lands devastated by strip-mining. Nevertheless, results of the *National Sewage Sludge Survey* conducted in 1988 (though now six years old, this survey constitutes the most recent EPA data available) indicate that many communities fail to take advantage of the resource potential inherent in biosolids. A breakdown of the sludge disposal methods utilized by more than 13,000 POTWs nationwide reveals the following:

- landfilling   33.9%
- land application 33.3%
- incineration   16.1%
- surface disposal 10.3%
- ocean disposal   6.3%

Since this survey was taken, ocean dumping of sludge has been terminated. New York City, the municipality responsible for most of the sludge dumped at sea, is now disposing of its biosolids through land application. Thus reuse strategies currently account for approximately 40% of total U.S. sludge disposal practices rather that the 33.3% indicated in the 1988 data.

Since sewage treatment plants, particularly those in the larger metropolitan areas, generate enormous amounts of sludge during their normal course of operations, finding a place in which to dispose of this material poses major dilemmas for many such facilities. Incineration of sludge can present problems of air pollution and in many communities where landfill space is at a premium, burying sludge is increasingly controversial—and increasingly expensive. In fact, so expensive has sludge management become that, whatever the disposal option chosen, treatment and disposal of sludge now account for over 50% of the operating costs of a typical POTW providing secondary sewage treatment.

Within the past several years, new EPA regulations have encouraged a marked trend toward "**beneficial reuse**" of sewage sludge, particularly forms of land application. The 1987 Clean Water Act amendments established a comprehensive program for reducing potential environmental risks posed by sludge through requirements that EPA 1) identify toxic substances that may be present in sludge at potentially dangerous levels, and 2) promulgate regulations that specify acceptable management practices and numerical limitations for sludge containing those pollutants. These regulations, referred to as the **Part 503** standards, were issued in February of 1993 and are now being implemented nationwide. The main concern that has limited beneficial reuse of biosolids in the past is the fact that sewage sludge often contains toxic chemicals and pathogens as well as desirable nutrients such as phosphates and nitrates. In particular, sludge from POTWs receiving industrial wastewater discharges in addition to residential sewage may contain potentially dangerous concentrations of heavy metals and other toxics—cadmium and lead are of special concern, but copper, zinc, nickel, PCBs, and a number of other contaminants may also be present. EPA addresses this issue by setting maximum loading rates on soils for sludge containing these contaminants, advising POTWs to police industrial discharges in their communities in an effort to eliminate toxic pollutants at the source. While some fears have been expressed regarding the possible presence of pathogens, the number of organisms in *digested* sludge is relatively low and can be further reduced by such management practices as composting or heat drying. Sludge scientists downplay concerns, attesting that there has never been a documented case of human infection due to the use of processed sewage sludge on agricultural lands. As confidence grows that biosolids can be used safely and profitably to increase production on farm fields, forests, and pasturelands, beneficial reuse practices will inevitably grow in popularity among municipal water reclamation districts as the most environmentally acceptable, cost-efficient method for disposing of their sludge.

Although agricultural lands are currently the destination for approximately 70% of the biosolids being land applied, farmers are not the only ones interested in taking advantage of this "black gold." While some municipalities are giving processed sludge away to anyone who will take it, the majority are selling the stuff to home gardeners, nurseries, or landscaping firms at prices ranging from $1.00–$22.00/cubic foot! Milwaukee and Madison, Wisconsin, and Austin, Texas, have employed imaginative marketing skills in promoting their products, selling sludge under such catchy tradenames as *Milorganite, Metrogro,* or *Dillo Dirt* (EPA, 1993; Tenenbaum, 1992).

New Approaches to Wastewater Treatment

Financing the improvements in municipal sewage treatment required by the 1972 Clean Water Act would have been impossible had Congress not included, in that same piece of legislation, the creation of a massive **Construction Grant Program**. This fund provided federal monetary assistance to communities which could not otherwise have afforded the multimillion dollar expenditures necessary to construct new or upgraded POTWs capable of providing the mandatory secondary level of sewage treatment. Under the Construction Grant Program, the second-largest public works project in U.S. history (exceeded only by construction of the interstate highway system), the federal government agreed to provide fully 75% of the cost of such projects, an amount that was subsequently reduced to 55% by the Reagan Administration in 1981. Over nearly two decades Washington contributed $57 *billion* for sewage treatment plant construction (state and local expenditures during the same period exceeded an additional $70 billion); as a result, by the late 1980s, 58% of the U.S. population was served by POTWs providing either secondary or secondary and advanced wastewater treatment. Since POTWs cumulatively serve about 70% of the American population (most of the remainder utilizing on-site wastewater disposal systems), it is obvious that domestic wastewaters in the majority of sewered communities now receive a commendably high level of treatment prior to discharge.

Nevertheless, remaining sewage treatment needs are considerable. In the late 1980s, approximately one out of every ten Americans lived in communities providing less than secondary treatment—and some towns still had no sewage treatment at all, discharging raw wastewaters directly into streams. In 1990, EPA estimated the total cost of bringing all municipal dischargers into compliance with CWA water quality requirements could exceed $110 billion—yet by 1990 the federal well had run dry (Adler et al., 1993). Amendments to the Clean Water Act passed by Congress in 1987 called for a phaseout of the federal Construction Grant Program by 1994, replacing it with a **State Revolving Fund** providing low-interest *loans* (no more free gifts from Uncle Sam!) to municipalities with unmet sewage treatment needs. Unfortunately, the demand for such loans exceeds the supply—but federal deadline dates for compliance with CWA requirements remain unchanged and potential penalties for violation of such standards can be severe. Thus the fiscal and legal realities of the 1990s provide a major incentive to develop new, less costly, yet equally effective methods of treating sewage—alternatives to the highly engineered, energy-consuming, sludge-producing, exorbitantly expensive POTWs which offered a convenient "technological fix" during the era of free-flowing federal dollars but which constitute an unrealistic option for communities of limited means.

Fortunately, the old adage, "Necessity is the mother of invention," is as valid in relation to emerging wastewater management technologies as it is in other spheres of life. In recent years a variety of innovative approaches to solving wastewater problems have attracted considerable interest and a number are now in the pilot-project stage, undergoing extensive field studies; several are in full-scale use, having proven their ability to produce good quality effluent at a fraction of the cost of conventional sewage treatment. The majority of new systems are based on the concept that wastewater effluent, like sludge, should be viewed as a nutrient-laden resource to be utilized rather than as a pollutant to be discarded.

One of the earliest and most widely adopted approaches to alternative treatment was land application of wastewater. This method involves spraying effluent from secondary treatment onto forest, pastures, or crop lands. Land application not only helps to prevent stream pollution by keeping nutrients out of the water, it also utilizes those same nutrients as fertilizer for the plants on which it is applied. A further advantage of this method is that the wastewater is largely purified as it percolates through the soil to recharge the groundwater supply. Early health concerns that dissolved metals or pathogens in the effluent might contaminate soils or vegetation have been dispelled by many years of problem-free experience with land application at Pennsylvania State University; in communities in Texas, Michigan, California, and New York; and in Germany, France, Israel, and Australia.

More recently, emphasis has shifted to the potential for artificial wetlands ("designer swamps"), duckweed systems (*Lemna spp.*), and water-purifying hydroponics-type systems inside greenhouses. In the United States, the Tennessee Valley Authority (TVA) has been at the forefront of research and development efforts focused on wetlands treatment. TVA views such systems as a viable wastewater treatment option for small communities that lack the expertise, as well as the financial resources, to operate highly sophisticated mechanical plants. Since the mid-1980s, TVA has designed and constructed engineered wetlands for a number of small towns in southern Appalachia, enabling such communities to comply with federal water quality standards at a fraction of the cost of conventional facilities. Although the sizeable land requirements for engineered wetlands have deterred many communities from giving such systems serious consideration, some larger cities such as Orlando, Florida, and Columbia, Missouri, have opted to utilize wetlands as one element in their treatment process.

Of the more than 50 municipalities nationwide currently employing wetlands systems to treat sewage, the most renowned is Arcata, California, a community of 20,000 located on the north shore of Humboldt Bay. In the early 1980s, Arcata faced a serious fiscal dilemma: effluent from the town's POTW consistently violated discharge permit limitations and Arcata was being pressured by the state environmental agency to close the plant and join with neighboring municipalities in constructing a large regional facility. Wary of the exorbitant costs such an undertaking would entail, Arcata opted for a radically different solution to its problem. Assisted by faculty at Humboldt State University, the town proceeded to develop a series of ponds and marshes to remove the troublesome pollutants remaining in its effluent following primary treatment at the POTW. Today Arcata's wastewater receives secondary treatment in a 50-acre stabilization pond where suspended solids settle to the bottom, while dissolved organic materials are broken down through a symbiotic association between bacteria and algae. From here the effluent flows into a three-celled, five-acre "treatment marsh" where rooted aquatic plants such as cattails (*Typha latifolia*) and bulrushes (*Scirpus acutis*) flourish. The submerged stems of these plants harbor countless numbers of microorganisms that further metabolize dissolved organic nitrates and phosphates. Passage through the marsh also effectively breaks down pesticides, industrial solvents, and most of the heavy metals in wastewater. After passing through the treatment marsh, the effluent is pumped to a chlorine contact tank for disinfection and is subsequently discharged into an "enhancement marsh" for additional wetlands treatment. This enhancement marsh, open to the public, is interlaced with jogging and hiking trails, picnic areas, and a nature center; it also serves as a wildlife sanctuary, annually attracting more than 130,000 visitors and 160 species of birds and other wildlife— living proof that the imperatives of providing for society's urgent wastewater management needs and restoring valuable ecosystems are mutually compatible.

Figure 15-3 Types of Constructed Wetlands

SURFACE FLOW SYSTEMS

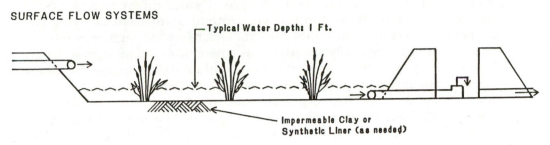

SUBSURFACE FLOW SYSTEMS

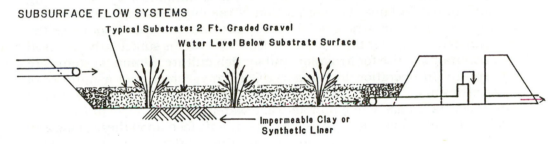

Source: Tennessee Valley Authority

After treatment in the enhancement marsh, the effluent is chlorinated once again and finally discharged into Humboldt Bay (source of 60–70% of California's oyster crop), its levels of suspended solids and BOD by now well below the NPDES limits of 30 mg/L.

Completed in 1986, Arcata's wetland system has been both an environmental and financial success. Once a polluter of Humboldt Bay, Arcata's wastewater treatment process produces an effluent which not only exceeds water quality standards but is even cleaner than the seawater into which it flows—and it has managed to do so at a cost far lower than that of a standard treatment facility. Residents of neighboring Eureka, faced with similar sewage treatment imperatives, opted for the more familiar conventional technology and are now paying wastewater treatment bills more than double those in Arcata.

Why haven't more communities followed Arcata's example? The major limitation to such systems is the amount of land they require—about 20 acres for a town of 10,000 people. Unless a community already owns land on its outskirts, being able to afford, or even find, this much land may present serious difficulties. Perhaps the biggest obstacle to a rapid increase in the number of communities using artificial wetlands is sheer ignorance and inertia. Only recently have adequate design guidelines become available for engineers and regulators; municipal officials frequently are unaware of the advantages such systems offer; conventionally trained engineers are frequently reluctant to embark on new, little-tried technologies and often lack the understanding of environmental conditions needed to factor these into their designs. Cynics might also wonder if engineers' general lack of enthusiasm might stem from the fact that cheaper artificial marshes translate into lower fees for engineering firms, since payment is typically calculated as a percentage of total project cost. Nevertheless, with the evaporation of federal funds for sewage treatment plant construction and upgrading, and with stringent penalties for non-compliance with effluent requirements, it's likely that economically attractive, easy-to-operate "designer swamps" will become a fashion trend in the years ahead ("Small Community," 1993; Dillingham, 1989; Goldstein, 1988).

Elsewhere in the world, a variant on wetlands treatment is the use of fish ponds for treating sewage while simultaneously supporting aquaculture. In Lima, Peru, a portion of the city's sewage is directed to stabilization ponds where solids settle out and bacteria decompose the organic wastes. After three or four weeks the water is sufficiently cleansed of pollutants to use for irrigation and for fish culture. Similar systems are currently in operation in Hungary, Germany, Israel, and a number of countries in South and Southeast Asia. The largest of these can be found in Calcutta, India, where human wastewaters nourish algae in two large lakes. Herbivorous fish such as carp and tilapia feed upon these algae and are subsequently harvested to provide Calcutta markets with approximately 7000 metric tons of fish each year. Obvious concerns about the potential for contamination of fish with human gastrointestinal pathogens can be allayed by retaining sewage in the stabilization lagoons for at least 20 days before allowing it to enter the fish ponds or by transferring the fish to clean waters for a period of time prior to harvesting (World Resources Institute, 1992).

Septic Systems

Approximately 30% of all Americans live in unsewered areas where they must utilize on-site septic systems for the disposal of wastewaters from bathrooms, kitchens, and laundries. Most on-site wastewater disposal systems consist of two basic parts: 1) a septic tank, buried in the ground at some distance from the house, to which it is connected by a pipe, and 2) a soil absorption field or sand filter.

The septic tank itself is a watertight container made of concrete or fiberglass with a minimum capacity of 750 gallons. Sewage entering the septic tank is partially decomposed by bacteria under anaerobic conditions. During this process, sludge settles to the bottom of the tank, while lighter solids and grease, as well as gases from the decomposing sludge, rise to the top to form a floating scum. The partially clarified liquid then passes through an outlet and the effluent is evenly dispersed among several perforated pipes in a carefully designed absorption field, which must be of adequate size and proper soil porosity to ensure that the effluent seeping out of the perforated pipe moves quickly enough to prevent ponding, but not so rapidly as to infiltrate aquifers, wells, or surface water supplies before contaminants in the effluent have been filtered out or oxidized.

Since more than half of the solids in the wastewater settle out during the retention period in the septic tank, the accumulation of sludge at the bottom, as well as the scum layer at the top, must be removed periodically (usually every 3–5 years). If this is not done, the sludge build-up reaches the point that solids are discharged into the absorption field, resulting in clogging and ponding. This accumulation of particulates and scum in the pores of the soil prevents proper drainage of the effluent and eventually results in failure of the system. In addition to improper maintenance of the septic tank, other reasons for septic system failure may be: use of a septic tank that is too small for the householders' needs, excessive household water use (large parties in homes on septic systems can be disastrous; repair men jokingly comment that they routinely notice garbage containers overflowing with beer cans when on a call to deal with sewage backups!), insufficient size of the absorption field, soil too impervious to receive effluent, or tree roots clogging the effluent distribution lines.

Although a well-located, carefully constructed, and properly maintained septic system can be a perfectly adequate method of sanitary waste disposal (and is the only feasible option in most rural areas), malfunctioning septic systems frequently give rise to serious nonpoint source water pollution, as leachates containing pathogenic organisms and nutrients seep from absorption fields into water supplies. The rapid growth of rural subdivisions, many of which rely on septic systems installed on lots too small to provide adequate waste dispersal, ensures that pollution problems related to septic systems will continue to plague public health officials.

Industrial Discharges

Effluent discharges from industry comprise the second major category of point source water pollution and consist of a wide range of pollutants which, for regulatory purposes, have been subdivided into three major groups:

- *Conventional Pollutants*—Include organic wastes high in BOD, suspended solids, acids, oil and grease, etc. Such pollutants originate from food processing plants, pulp and paper mills, steel mills, oil tanker spills and cleaning operations, accidents involving offshore oil drilling, and so forth.
- *Toxic Pollutants*—A list of 129 priority toxic pollutants was developed by EPA in 1976 (3 subsequently have been de-listed); substances listed include heavy metals such as cadmium, mercury, and lead, PCBs, benzene, chloroform, cyanide, arsenic, 2,4-D, and a number of other pesticides. The electroplating and metal-processing industries, plastics manufacturers, and chemical

companies are but a few of the industries discharging toxic effluents.

- *Non-Conventional Pollutants*—All the other pollutants not classified by EPA as either conventional or toxic are grouped into this third category—substances such as nitrogen and phosphorus, iron, tin, aluminum, chloride, and ammonia. As in the preceding categories, the sources of such pollutants can be traced to a wide variety of industrial processes.

The Clean Water Act requires EPA to develop technology-based national treatment standards for each category of industrial discharger (e.g. petroleum refiners, textile mills, iron and steel, leather tanning, etc.), directing that standards be reviewed periodically and made increasingly stringent as pollution control technologies advance. Industries discharging directly into the nation's waterways must obtain an NPDES permit, specifying the allowable amounts and constituents of pollutants in their effluent. Dischargers are required to monitor their effluent on a routine basis and violations of permit limitations can result in serious civil or criminal penalties.

For the most part, industry has a better record of compliance with existing water pollution control regulations than do municipal dischargers (i.e. POTWs); EPA estimates that the use of best available pollution control technologies in 22 targeted industrial categories has reduced releases of certain toxic organic chemicals by 99% and heavy metals by 98% since passage of the Clean Water Act in 1972. Altogether, controls imposed on toxic industrial discharges have, according to EPA estimates, prevented the release of more than a billion pounds of toxics yearly into U.S. surface waters; even larger amounts of conventional pollutants have been controlled. Nevertheless, in spite of significant improvements, toxic releases into rivers, lakes, and coastal estuaries by industrial dischargers remain a serious water quality concern. Due to EPA's tardiness in promulgating the industry-specific effluent guidelines mandated by Congress, many industries continue to discharge toxic pollutants without violating federal standards; such industries technically are in compliance with the law because the categorical standards pertaining to them have not yet been issued. A related problem is the fact that many of the control regulations which *have* been promulgated are now more than 10 years old and in need of revision to incorporate recent improvements in approaches to pollution prevention (Adler et al., 1993). Nevertheless, in spite of such regulatory shortcomings, stream monitoring data and self-reporting by industry both indicate a steady downward trend for industrial discharges in recent years—slow but encouraging progress toward the elusive goal of "zero discharge."

Direct Versus Indirect Discharges

Current water pollution laws distinguish two categories of industrial waste discharges: **direct discharges** which flow directly into a receiving stream or lake and **indirect discharges** which go into the sewer system, where they first pass through the municipal sewage treatment plant before

BOX 15-4

"Deep Tunnel"
Chicago's Response to Combined Sewer Overflows

Deep under the streets of Chicago the 31-mile Mainstream Tunnel System constitutes a visionary—and highly successful—effort to solve a major water pollution problem facing many of our older cities: how to manage combined sewer overflows during periods of heavy rainfall. While most sewer systems installed in recent decades feature separate sanitary and stormwater conduits, the older sections of many urban areas still have combined sewers which carry not only sewage from households, but also stormwater runoff from city streets, rooftops, and lawns—all the water which isn't absorbed into the ground when it rains. Most sewage treatment plants are designed to accommodate the usual domestic wastewater flow (referred to as "dry weather flow"), usually with some built-in excess capacity. During storm episodes, however, water volume in combined sewers may be as much as 100 times greater than usual. Because the excess water would overwhelm the treatment capacity of the sewage plant, it is diverted past the facility and enters the receiving stream untreated. Laden not only with human wastes but also with the wide variety of contaminants characteristic of urban runoff, combined sewer overflows seriously degrade the aquatic environment and are a common cause of water quality violations in older cities.

Beset by approximately 100 storm episodes per year that discharged raw sewage and stormwater into Chicagoland waterways and frequently caused flooding of streets and residential areas as well, the Windy City began looking for a long-term solution to its problem. Efforts to deal with this challenge in other communities suggested several alternative approaches: 1) separation of sewer systems in areas with combined sewers—a massive construction project presenting almost insurmountable difficulties in highly developed urban areas; 2) enlargement of POTW capacity to permit treatment of entire stormwater plus sanitary sewage flow—technically possible but not cost-efficient, since this approach would require enormous capital investments for excess capacity that would sit idle most of the time; 3) construction of retention basins to hold stormwater runoff, gradually releasing it to the treatment plant in volumes which can be accommodated.

Chicago eventually settled upon one of the most ambitious and innovative public works projects ever undertaken. In 1975 the city began construction on its Tunnel and Reservoir Plan (TARP), the key segment of which is the Mainstream Tunnel, completed in 1985 and chosen by the American Society of Civil Engineers as the Outstanding Civil Engineering Achievement for 1986 (technologies developed for TARP have facilitated construction of the recently opened "Chunnel" connecting France and England). The "Deep Tunnel," as it was promptly dubbed by the media, captures sewage-polluted stormwater from a 204-square mile urban area and stores it temporarily in 31 miles of tunnels at depths ranging from 240–300 feet below ground. After a storm has ended, this water is pumped back to the surface and sent at a controlled rate to sewage treatment plants prior to subsequent discharge into a waterway. Since the Mainstream Tunnel came on line, the frequency of combined sewer overflows and flooding throughout most of Chicago and 15 neighboring communities dropped dramatically—down 80% in its first year of operation.

When the tunnel construction phase

of TARP is complete, sometime early in the next century, about 85% of the pollution caused by combined sewer overflows will be captured (of the 131 miles of tunnels planned, slightly over 50 miles have been completed thus far, with another 25 under construction). A second phase of the project, designed to control flooding, is already underway; the first of three huge reservoirs designed to store combined sewer overflows captured by the tunnel system is now under construction. When finished, these reservoirs will increase TARP's water storage capacity by 41 billion gallons. Upon completion, TARP will make it possible for Chicago to capture and contain entire storms, eliminating forever fears of flooding and pollution whenever skies darken over Chicagoland. No longer do engineers from around the world come to the Windy City just to view its skyline—now they come to admire its sewer system as well!

Reference

Metropolitan Water Reclamation District of Greater Chicago.

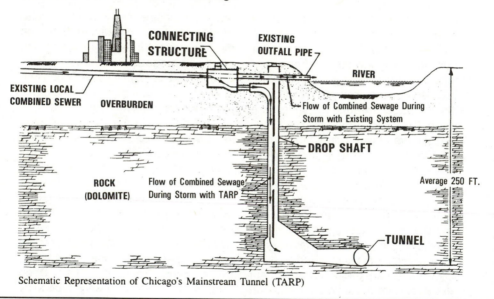

Schematic Representation of Chicago's Mainstream Tunnel (TARP)

entering a waterway along with sanitary wastewater effluent. When citizens think about industrial pollutant discharges, they generally envision the direct type—pipes from a factory leading straight to the water's edge, pouring a poisonous brew onto the back of some hapless fish. In point of fact, however, the majority of industrial dischargers, some 160,000 in the United States, are of the indirect type, discharging at least 448 million pounds of hazardous chemicals into sewer systems every year, according to EPA estimates. Such discharges represent fully 12% of the entire wastewater flow entering the nation's POTWs. In cases where indirect industrial discharges consist primarily of biodegradable organic wastes, sending them to the sewage treatment plant is appropriate, since the same processes that decompose human excreta are effective on other organic materials as well. In situations involving toxic substances, however, indirect discharges via the sewer system can cause a number of very serious problems.

Structural Damage to Sewer System and Treatment Plant. Industrial discharges of strong acids or alkalis can corrode both sewer pipes and equipment at the POTW. Some chemicals react to produce toxic fumes which can present a serious health threat to workers at the treatment plant, and certain volatile substances can generate a build-up of gas in the sewers, occasionally resulting in explosions. An event of this type occurred in Louisville, Kentucky, in February of 1981 when an industrial discharge of hexane exploded in the sewers, injuring four people and causing over $10 million worth of damage (Banks and Dubrowski, 1982). A similar situation took place the same year in Cincinnati when wastewater containing both hydrochloric acid and volatile organic solvents was discharged into city sewers by a large paint factory. The acid corroded the concrete sewer pipe, causing it to collapse and leaving a hole in the street 24 feet in diameter. When workers entered the sewer three days later to try to repair the damage, several were overcome suddenly by nausea, dizziness, vomiting, and eye and nose irritation due to exposure to chemical vapors. All work had to be stopped until the discharges were halted and fumes had dissipated ("Sewer Collapse," 1981).

Interference with Biological Treatment Processes. When toxic chemicals such as the synthetic organic pesticides pass through a sewage treatment plant, they have the same effect on the microbes responsible for the secondary treatment process as they do on the target pests—they kill them, and in so doing render the sewage treatment plant ineffective. In 1977, again at the ill-fated Louisville POTW, pesticide wastes illegally dumped into a city sewer caused a total breakdown in treatment at the huge plant. As a result, for nearly two years until the cleanup was completed, 100 million gallons of untreated sewage were discharged into the Ohio River every day and taxpayers were confronted with a repair bill amounting to millions of dollars.

Sludge Contamination. Certain toxics such as cadmium, mercury, lead, and arsenic may pass through the sewage treatment plant without damaging equipment or interfering with biological treatment. Nevertheless, they pose major problems because they can be assimilated by the bacteria that provide secondary treatment and subsequently accumulate in the sludge, seriously limiting disposal options for biosolids. Sludge containing excessive concentrations of heavy metals cannot be land-applied due to concerns that toxics may be taken up by plants or leach into groundwater. Similarly, there are restrictions on incineration of metals-contaminated sludge (Banks and Dubrowski, 1982).

Violation of POTW Effluent Limitations. Because sewage treatment plants, like industries, must comply with the terms of their NPDES permit, toxic chemicals which pass through the treatment plant and pollute the receiving waters make it necessary for the POTW to install methods of advanced wastewater treatment to prevent such violations from occurring. This, of course, is a costly undertaking, the expense of which will be borne by the taxpaying public.

Need for Pretreatment of Indirect Discharges

Problems such as those just described led Congress to legislate a national **pretreatment program** which would require indirect dischargers of industrial wastes to detoxify their effluent before it entered the sewage system. EPA has been charged with setting categorical pretreatment standards for groups of industries, comparable to the effluent limitations requiring best available technology for controlling pollution from direct dischargers. The work of developing, implementing, and enforcing the program has been assigned to 1500 local POTWs (those treating five million gallons of wastewater or more on a daily basis) which also have authority to set additional discharge requirements above and beyond the federal standards if such action is deemed necessary. Although originally mandated in 1972, the pretreatment program was extremely slow in getting started, in part because EPA did not formulate basic rules for the program until 1980. Implementation of the program by local sanitary districts moved into high gear by the mid-1980s and today most industries discharging wastewaters to municipal sewers have some form of pretreatment program in place. This program is having a significant impact in reducing problems caused by indirect discharges, but it hasn't yet eliminated toxic woes at treatment plants. Problems persist not only because some industrial dischargers are in significant non-compliance with pretreatment program requirements but, more importantly, because many categorical standards have not yet been promulgated by EPA. The agency reports that only about 10% of all industries discharging toxics to POTWs are covered under national pretreatment standards (they may, however, be subject to locally imposed requirements). Certain as-yet unregulated commercial establishments such as car washes and photo-processing plants also contribute a significant percentage of certain toxics to a treatment plant's incoming flow. Finally, not all of the hazardous chemicals flowing into sewage treatment plants are of industrial origin. Of the regulated toxics entering POTWs, about 15% come from residences—all those bleaches, toilet bowl cleaners, paint thinners, outdated medications, etc., that we flush down the drain don't simply disappear but merge with the myriad of other substances moving through the sewers and eventually arrive at a sewage treatment plant. We all contribute to the problem.

Industrial Accidents, Spills, and Stormwater Runoff

In addition to direct and indirect effluent discharges, some industrial pollutants enter waterways due to transportation accidents, leaks in chemical containers, tanker spills or oil rig blow-outs, or chemical runoff from industrial waste sites during storm episodes. In 1987 mounting concerns about the adverse environmental impact of urban stormwater runoff prompted Congress to mandate a far-reaching new program to control stormwater discharges. These regulations, which will be phased in over a period of several years during the mid- to late-1990s, will require that more than 170 cities (those with populations of 100,000 or more), 47 counties, approximately 100,000 industrial facilities, and construction sites identify the sources and types of pollutants which could be present in stormwater runoff from their premises and subsequently implement controls to prevent potential contaminants from washing into storm sewers. For municipalities, required preventive measures will include programs to detect and remove illegal connections, ending the improper dumping of used oil and other wastes into storm sewers, preventing and controlling spills, and adopting street de-icing methods less environmentally damaging than the use of road salt. Affected industries, which include those engaged in activities as diverse as manufacturing, airport operations, recycling, mining, wood treating, landfilling—virtually any facility where stormwater

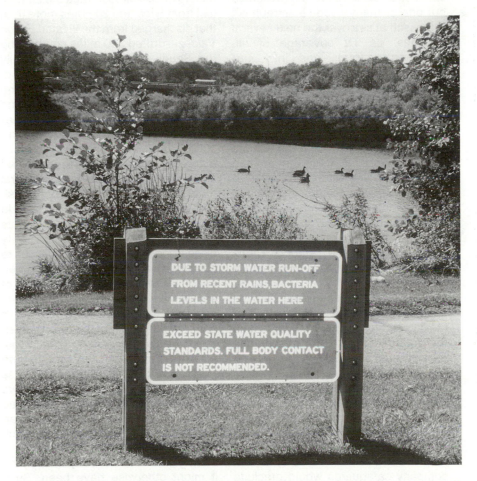

Would-be swimmers are warned of high bacterial levels due to stormwater runoff. [Thomas A. Schneider]

BOX 15-5

Saddam's Toxic Terrorism

For sheer drama, few eco-events compare with a massive oil spill. The spectacular blowout of Union Oil Company's drilling rig off the southern California coast in 1969 was a major media event that galvanized public opposition to thoughtless environmental exploitation and helped to launch a nationwide movement that has continued to grow ever since. Unfortunately, the three million gallons of sticky crude that fouled the scenic beaches at Santa Barbara represented but one of many "eco-catastrophes" witnessed at sea over the next several decades, as TV coverage of oil-drenched seabirds and inky surf became an all-too-familiar sight in coastal areas around the world. The 1976 breakup of a Liberian-registered tanker, the *Argo Merchant*, off Nantucket Island during a winter storm released more than twice the volume of oil discharged at Santa Barbara and represented the worst spill ever to occur in U.S. waters up to that time. The grounding of the *Amoco Cadiz* off the French coast in 1978 still ranks as the world's largest tanker spill. Dwarfing even the *Amoco Cadiz* release, the blowout at Mexico's *Ixtoc I* offshore oil platform in 1979 discharged over 600,000 tons of petroleum into the once-sparkling waters of the Gulf of Mexico and for the next 12 years held the world record as the largest marine oil spill ever. In 1989 Alaskans witnessed the worst spill to date in American waters when the *Exxon Valdez* hit a reef in Prince William Sound, fouling the once-pristine waters with more than 10 million gallons of North Slope oil and enraging residents who had been assured that oil company safeguards would preclude any such accident.

All these events, however, horrific as they appeared at the time, pale by comparison with the environmental travesty deliberately perpetrated by Iraqi troops during the 1991 Persian Gulf War. On January 19th, three days following the outbreak of hostilities between United Nations' forces and the army of Saddam Hussein, Iraqi soldiers began pumping crude oil from Kuwait's Sea Island Terminal into the Persian Gulf. The world watched in fascinated horror as an estimated 950,000 cubic meters of oil—almost twice the amount lost from *Ixtoc* and 20 times more than that discharged from the ill-fated *Exxon Valdez*—drifted 350 miles south along the Saudi Arabian coast, eventually washing ashore near the peninsula of Abu Ali. The oil caused extensive damage along the Saudi coast, inundating the region's numerous saltwater marshes and tidal flats, killing 20,000–30,000 seabirds, as well as all mangrove trees within the affected areas. Algae, sea grass beds, and coral reefs were hard-hit and countless fish died in the aftermath of the spill. In other situations where large amounts of oil have been accidentally discharged into the sea, quick action to contain the spill has often been effective in limiting the extent of ecological damage. In this case, however, cleanup efforts were hampered by the fact that the affected region was at the center of a war zone, making any remedial action too hazardous to attempt, and because Saudi Arabia and Kuwait, the two countries most directly affected, had neither the technology nor the expertise to cope with a disaster of such magnitude. As a result, environmental damage was substantially worse than it might otherwise have been. Such cleanup efforts as were initiated met with limited success. The water intake pipes leading to Saudi desalination plants and to the oil refineries were protected by the rapid deployment of skimmers, booms, and nets, but similar protection was never extended to coastal wetlands which subsequently suffered severe degradation. As petrochemical residues gradually move up the food chain, marine life in the Gulf may be adversely affected for years to come.

However, if experience from earlier events is any indication, the long-term ecological impact of the spill may be less serious than many fear. Studies of past marine spills show that while petroleum is toxic to many organisms, there is no strong evidence that oil spills have done any permanent damage to the world's ocean resources. Such spills, in fact, comprise a relatively small portion of the oil entering the seas each year—routine tanker operations (e.g. tank cleaning, ballasting, etc.) contribute almost twice as many petro-pollutants to the ocean on an annual basis as do spills, even though they attract much less attention. While tanker accidents or offshore rig blowouts can have a catastrophic short-term impact on biotic communities, recovery begins within a matter of months and many such communities have returned to their pre-spill appearance within a year or two. The extent of destruction caused by a particular release depends on such variables as:

Time of Release—If a spill occurs during the spring spawning season or when birds or marine mammals are migrating, the impact will be much more severe than if it occurs at a less ulnerable time of year; the fact that the *Exxon Valdez* accident occurred in late March may explain, at least in part, why a spill which doesn't even rank among the top 10 for volume of oil released nevertheless killed more wildlife than any other.

Type of Petroleum—Since the toxicity and physical characteristics of various crude and refined oil products differs widely, the impact of any particular spill will vary accordingly.

Proximity of Spill to Shoreline— Since biotic communities are much more diverse and complex in coastal ecosystems than in the species-poor open ocean, spills along the coast will have much more serious environmental consequences than similar accidents far offshore.

Shoreline Topography—The persistence of oil released during a spill will be much greater along a sandy, protected coastline than on an exposed, rocky shore.

Weather Conditions—Temperature, wind direction and velocity, and amount of wave action all influence how far the oil will spread and how quickly it will break up and disperse.

At present, the long-term outlook for environmental restoration of polluted Gulf waters is cloudy. Natural cleansing is likely to be a very slow process, not only because of the vast amounts of oil involved but also because of the waterway's configuration; relatively shallow, the Gulf is almost entirely enclosed and requires a long period for self-flushing, its current taking about three years to circulate completely. Thus far, researchers have been unable even to measure the full environmental and health consequences of the 1991 spill with any degree of accuracy. Although hostilities ended several years ago, cleanup activities have been stymied by the reluctance of Saudi officials to experiment with techniques of bioremediation (utilizing oil-munching bacteria to clean up petroleum-contaminated areas) and by the difficulty of obtaining financing for cleanup efforts. It is highly unlikely that Saddam Hussein will respond to a U.N. Security Council resolution demanding that Iraq pay reparations for the damage it caused. Despite worldwide condemnation of the Iraqi regime for flagrant violation of international environmental law, the U.N. lacks effecive means for dealing with acts of eco-terrorism such as that inflicted on the Gulf. The world can only hope that a growing realization among peoples everywhere that "fouling our own nest" will bring tragic consequences to all will help to forestall future acts of environmental warfare.

References

National Research Council. 1985. "Oil in the Sea: Inputs, Fates, and Effects." *National Academy Press*.

World Conservation Monitoring Centre. 1991. "Gulf War Environmental Information Service Environmental Briefing." Cambridge, UK, June 7.

World Resources Institute. 1990. *World Resources 1990–91*. Oxford University Press.

could come into contact with raw materials or wastes—must devise improved methods for handling and storing materials and for preventing spills. All potential contributors to stormwater contamination, municipalities and industries alike, are required to obtain discharge permits stipulating exactly how they intend to minimize polluted runoff by developing and implementing comprehensive management programs. Due to the protracted schedule for filing permit applications and extended timetables for achieving compliance, it will likely be years before all sources of urban stormwater are regulated. Nevertheless, after a decade of hand-wringing over urban water quality problems caused by stormwater runoff, meaningful steps to tackle this problem are finally underway (Goldberg, 1993; Gray, 1991; Adler et al., 1993).

Water Pollution and Health

If a pollster were to conduct sidewalk interviews on what major concerns the average man or woman might have regarding water pollution, it's a safe bet that eutrophication of Chesapeake Bay, fish kills in the Mississippi, or New York City's sludge disposal headaches would rank far down on the list. Among the vast majority of respondents, the number one water quality priority undoubtedly would be assurance that the water flowing from their kitchen or bathroom faucet was safe to drink. Such public concerns stem from the recognition that human health is directly threatened by impure drinking water. There exists today a growing realization that the quality of drinking water is inextricably linked to the quality of our environment as a whole, inasmuch as air pollutants, agricultural chemicals, leachates from landfills, sewage, and industrial effluents all can invade public water supplies. While the nature of drinking water contamination problems differs somewhat in the developing nations versus more industrialized societies, the extent to which polluted water adversely affects health and well-being is a worldwide source of concern. Many health authorities now speculate that unless and until water quality is substantially upgraded, there will be little further improvement in public health and life expectancy such as that witnessed during the past 75 years.

These experts estimate that perhaps 80% of all illness in the world today could be prevented if everyone had access to safe water supplies and argue that it makes little sense to invest large amounts of money in building hospitals and training physicians if the people they intend to serve face renewed risk of disease every time they take a drink of water (Quigg, 1976).

Microbial Waterborne Disease

Prior to the late 19th century, outbreaks of epidemic waterborne disease in every part of the world claimed a heavy toll in human lives and suffering. As late as the 1880s, typhoid killed 75–100 people per 100,000 population in the United States each year. A major outbreak of the disease in Chicago in 1885 claimed 90,000 victims and persuaded city officials to divert the flow of Chicago's sewage from Lake Michigan, also the source of municipal drinking water supplies, into the Sanitary and Ship Canal (completed in 1900) and ultimately to the Illinois River and the Mississippi—a policy decision which had the unintended side effect of seriously degrading the quality and attractiveness of the Illinois River. Cholera also was a feared disease in 19th century America; a major outbreak in the Mississippi Valley during the 1870s claimed many lives and large numbers of westward-bound settlers died of cholera along the wagon trails.

In the Third World, contamination of waterways with a wide range of microbial pathogens found in human body wastes constitutes the most pressing environmental health problem confronting developing nations. It is estimated that worldwide approximately 250 million cases of waterborne disease are reported annually, 75% of them in tropical countries. Each year three million young children die of waterborne diarrheal diseases, a problem directly stemming from lack of adequate sewage disposal facilities. The gastrointestinal infections which occur when such pathogens are ingested are the leading cause of illness and death in most developing countries. Reducing the incidence of such disease requires not only the installation of water purification technologies, but also provision of sanitary wastewater disposal and public education regarding personal and household hygiene. During the 1980s, designated by the U.N. as the "International Drinking Water Supply and Sanitation Decade," significant gains were made in expanding access to safe water supplies, particularly in rural areas where the number of people served increased by 240% worldwide (150% increase among city dwellers). Access to sanitation facilities improved as well, but these gains were largely offset by the continued rapid rate of population growth and urbanization in nations throughout the developing world. After a decade of heroic effort, there remain 1.2 billion people in the world lacking safe drinking water and 1.7 billion without adequate sanitary facilities—largely a reflection of the inability of public works projects to keep pace with burgeoning human numbers (Nash, 1993).

In industrialized countries, disease caused by fecal pollution of waterways is much less common now than it was several generations ago.

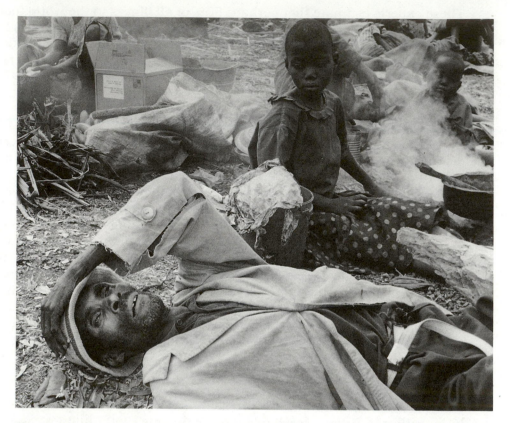

Thousands of Rwandans were struck down by cholera in the squalid, teeming refugee camps to which they fled when civil war broke out in Rwanda in 1994. [A/P Wide World Photos]

Nevertheless, outbreaks of gastroenteritis traced to microbial contamination of drinking water do occur from time to time, occasionally in headline-provoking magnitude. In the United States, despite the impression that waterborne disease is a thing of the past, the Centers for Disease Control and Prevention has documented 554 waterborne disease outbreaks between 1972–1990. Although most such occurrences in recent years have been associated with small water systems where financial resources preclude the sophisticated equipment and highly trained personnel generally found in larger communities, a 1993 outbreak in Milwaukee, Wisconsin, sickened almost 400,000 people. These numbers, of course, represent only those illnesses which are reported to public health authorities. EPA estimates that for every case of waterborne disease identified, 25 more never appear in the statistics because of haphazard reporting.

Diarrheal illness may be caused by any of a large number of microbial species associated with sewage-tainted drinking water and fall roughly into one of the following groups.

Bacteria.   Typhoid fever and cholera are the most notorious of the bacterial enteric diseases and over the centuries have been responsibile

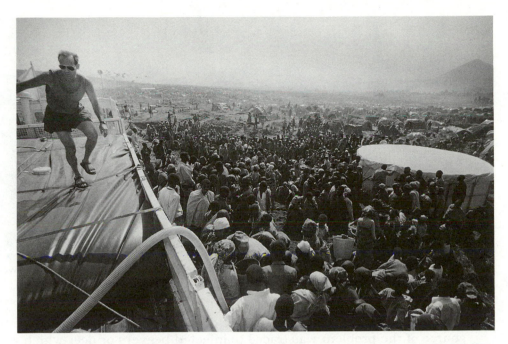

Relief workers pump purified water into a storage tank at the refugee camp near Goma, Zaire. By late July 1994 the fatality rate from cholera at the camp had been dramatically lowered due to improved water supplies. [A/P Wide World Photos]

for millions of human deaths and illnesses worldwide. Other bacterial waterborne ailments include dysentery (*Shigella*), paratyphoid, salmonellosis, *Campylobacter*, and some forms of *E. coli*—ailments which, like typhoid and cholera, can also be contracted by eating food harboring pathogens of fecal origin. Whereas typhoid and paratyphoid are characterized by headache, muscle pains, high fever, and constipation alternating with diarrhea (all symptoms being less severe in paratyphoid), cholera, dysentery, and salmonellosis are all typified by severe diarrhea (bloody in the case of dysentery) and vomiting.

Viruses.   Hepatitis A, poliomyelitis, and Rotavirus diarrhea are all examples of waterborne pathogenic viruses. Several major outbreaks of hepatitis A have occurred in various parts of the world in recent years, one of the largest, in China, severe enough to prompt warnings to tourists planning visits to that country. Outbreaks of infectious hepatitis can occasionally occur even after drinking water has been disinfected because the virus is much more resistant to chlorine than are bacteria.

Protozoans.   While more than 30 species of parasites may infect the human gut, only a few present a serious disease threat. Of these, the most common is giardiasis, caused by the flagellated protozoan *Giardia lamblia*, an inhabitant of the intestines of a wide variety of vertebrate animals. Over the past 25 years *Giardia* has been blamed for close to 100 reported

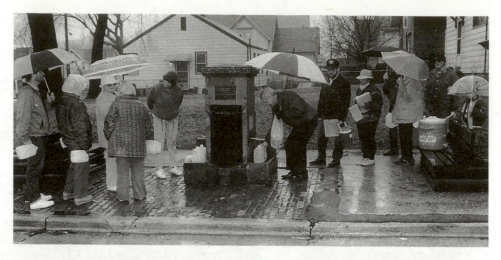

Milwaukee residents stand in line to obtain fresh water after protozoa in the public water supply caused a massive disease outbreak in 1993. [Milwaukee Sentinel Photo]

outbreaks in the United States, some of them in remote areas where the source of the problem was traced to infected beavers or deer which were polluting the water with feces containing protozoan cysts. Since *Giardia* is largely resistant to chlorination, filtration of drinking water supplies is important in forestalling outbreaks of giardiasis. Another chlorine-resistant protozoan parasite causing serious concern is *Cryptosporidium*, the culprit responsible for the massive disease outbreak in Milwaukee in April 1993, as well as for two other major outbreaks a few years earlier in Georgia and Oregon. Finally amoebiasis (amoebic dysentery) is another widespread parasitic infection afflicting an estimated half billion people worldwide. Amoebic dysentery constitutes a major health problem in Mexico, eastern South America, western and southern Africa, China, and throughout Southeast Asia (Nash, 1993).

Water Purification

Toward the end of the last century, a growing awareness of the link between waterborne pathogens and disease outbreaks prompted municipal officials in North America and Europe to institute various methods of drinking water treatment—primarily filtration and chlorination—which largely succeeded in eliminating the serious water-related epidemic diseases of the past. Nevertheless, the organisms which cause typhoid, cholera, dysentery, and other gastrointestinal ailments are still in our midst, ready to make their presence known whenever a breakdown in water treatment processes affords opportunity for such pathogens to penetrate our technological lines of defense.

Unlike sewage treatment, which is intended to reduce levels of wastewater contamination to the point where the effluent can be returned to a stream without provoking serious health or ecological damage,

Box 15-6

Water Woes

Milwaukee pharmacists were the first to notice that something was very much amiss in the city that beer made famous. Already for several days in early April 1993, there had been a run on anti-diarrheal medicine all over town and the drugstore shelves were bare. Hospital emergency rooms were also doing a brisk business; from across the city, Milwaukeeans suffering from watery diarrhea, abdominal cramping, fever, and nausea flocked in seeking relief. On April 6th officials from the Public Health and Water Departments met to compare notes and confer as to the nature of the widening outbreak. They soon decided the problem wasn't foodborne and suspected "something in the water" but were baffled as to what it could be. Results of bacteriological testing were negative, but one hospital reported that several patients had tested positive for *Cryptosporidium*, a protozoan parasite which, until 1976, was not even recognized as a human pathogen. On April 7th a citywide "boil order" was announced and the following day the Howard Avenue water treatment plant, serving the area of Milwaukee where the largest number of illnesses had been reported, was closed, leaving one other plant in operation to meet the city's needs. On April 10th the presence of *Cryptosporidium* in water from both plants was confirmed, although there was still no solid evidence on the origin of the problem. Several days later, by April 14th, tests for the parasite registered negative for the second consecutive day and the boil order was lifted, leaving Milwaukee officials with the daunting task of assessing the damage and figuring out how things had gone so wrong.

The toll was staggering—contaminated water had sickened almost 400,000 people and had hastened the deaths of several AIDS patients whose immuno-compromised status made them especially vulnerable to the ravages of cryptosporidiosis. Milwaukeeans took a crash course on parasitology, learning that the protozoan responsible for their misery is a pathogen which infects many different species (the first reported incident of *Cryptosporidium* as a disease agent came in 1955 when the parasite was blamed for an outbreak of fatal enteritis in turkeys) and is now the cause of serious gastrointestinal disease worldwide. Characterized by a fecal-oral route of transmission, *Cryptosporidium* can readily infect humans when drinking water supplies are polluted with sewage or animal manures. The protozoa multiply inside the host organism and resistant oocysts are then passed in the feces, ready to infect a new host. Virtually all communities which obtain their water from surface supplies are at risk of having their drinking water contaminated with *Cryptosporidium* (as well as with *Giardia*, for that matter). While watershed protection—prohibiting the sort of activities likely to generate polluted runoff—offers the best safeguard for minimizing outbreaks of waterborne pathogens, good filtration practices can remove the protozoan cysts responsible for most outbreaks. For those cities not practicing filtration, chlorination constitutes the sole line of defense against infectious organisms, but chlorine is of questionable value in combatting *Cryptosporidium*. While chlorine quickly kills bacteria and most viruses, it is not as effective at destroying protozoan cysts. *Giardia* frequently survives disinfection with chlorine; *Cryptosporidium* is even tougher, requiring doses of chlorine 100 times stronger than those needed to kill *Giardia*. If the water is clouded with tiny soil particles, as is often the case in waters contaminated with runoff, chlorination frequently is ineffective. By combining filtration with disinfection, a much higher level of water safety can be achieved. In general, those communities which rely solely on disinfection experience waterborne disease outbreaks eight times more often as do communities employing both disinfection and filtration. Even these measures are not foolproof, however. Milwaukee, ironically, *did* filter its water, as did three other cities subsequently experiencing outbreaks, yet *Cryptosporidium* still managed to wreak havoc. Although the cause of Milwaukee's outbreak has never been conclusively established, officials suspect that runoff due to heavy spring rains throughout the watershed area washed large quantities of animal manures into reservoirs, increasing turbidity levels (oocysts can survive in moist soil for 2–6 months, enhancing the danger posed by erosion into waterways). The appropriateness of certain procedures at the city's filtration plant have also been questioned. Since the outbreak, Milwaukee has taken several steps to ensure against any repetition of the 1993 debacle, setting stringent new effluent goals for turbidity; discharging, rather than recycling, filter backwash waters; and testing raw water for the presence of *Cryptosporidium* on a bimonthly basis. Other communities are less well-prepared and officials at the Centers for Disease Control and Prevention worry that what happened in Milwaukee could be repeated elsewhere. As a CDC epidemiologist remarked, "There's nothing in the present system as I see it that would prevent future outbreaks."

Reference

King, Jonathan. 1993. "Something in the Water." *Amicus Journal* 15, no. 3 (Fall).

drinking water treatment theoretically should entirely remove all contaminants in the water, or at least reduce them to acceptable levels. All drinking water, regardless of its source, should be treated prior to consumption, since it can never be safely assumed that such water is totally free from contamination.

Although the precise details of drinking water treatment vary from plant to plant, depending largely on the quality of the local raw water supply (i.e. water from polluted surface sources will require more extensive treatment than does well water drawn from a high quality uncontaminated aquifer), the basic steps in the process can be described as follows:

1. *Sedimentation*—Incoming raw water is detained in a quiet pond or tank for at least 24 hours to allow heavy suspended material to settle out.
2. *Coagulation*—Alum (hydrated aluminum sulfate) is added to the water to cause smaller suspended solids to form flocs which then precipitate to the bottom of the tank.
3. *Filtration*—Filtration through beds of sand, crushed anthracite coal, or diatomaceous earth further reduces the concentration of

remaining suspended solids, including many bacterial cells and protozoans.

4. *Disinfection*—Most commonly accomplished with chlorine (ozone, bromine, iodine, or ultraviolet light can also be used for disinfection), disinfection is the most important method utilized for killing pathogens in water. However, disinfection in the absence of the preceding steps is not highly effective because organic materials and suspended solids in the water interfere with the germicidal action of the chlorine. In addition, occasional outbreaks of hepatitis, giardiasis, and cryptosporidiosis in cities where water has been disinfected indicate that chlorine is not as effective in killing viruses as it is against other disease organisms.

In many water treatment plants, particularly those utilizing well water, preliminary treatment also includes aerating the water to remove iron and dissolved gases such as hydrogen sulfide which impart objectionable tastes and odor to the water. In parts of the country where water contains excess amounts of dissolved calcium or magnesium (i.e. where the water is "hard"), lime and soda ash are added to precipitate these minerals out of solution, thereby "softening" the water. Ion exchange is an alternative method which can be used for this purpose. Finally, many treatment plants today add fluoride to the finished water to reduce the incidence of tooth decay (Koren, 1980).

To ensure that the water treatment process is working efficiently, laboratory tests of finished water samples are carried out on a regular basis. Historically, the presence of appreciable numbers of coliform bacteria in a water sample has been used as an indication that the water is unsafe to drink. In fact, coliforms themselves rarely cause disease; however, because they are common inhabitants of the intestines of warm-blooded animals, present in greater numbers than the pathogenic bacteria, and because they can survive for longer periods of time in water than do the latter, coliforms serve as indicators that the water is contaminated with fecal material and hence potentially hazardous. In other words, the presence of fecal coliform bacteria in a water sample warns health officials that less abundant, but more harmful organisms such as the dysentery bacillus or hepatitis virus might also be present, since all of these organisms live in the intestinal tract and are expelled with fecal material. Recently, however, the validity of the coliform test in establishing the safety of a water supply has been called into question with the finding that pathogenic viruses may still be present in samples which the standard coliform test indicated were bacteriologically uncontaminated.

Chemical Contaminants in Drinking Water

Standard water treatment processes, designed primarily to remove bacteria, hardness, and odors from water supplies, have been outstandingly successful in reducing the incidence of acute waterborne disease throughout the industrialized world. However, in spite of the considerable improvement in drinking water quality from a bacteriological perspective, the public today is justifiably alarmed about the safety of water supplies due to recent revelations of toxic chemicals in drinking water. With purification processes aimed at preventing the microbial diseases of the past, few water treatment plants are equipped to remove—or even to detect—the 100,000 or more synthetic organic chemicals now in use, many of which are known to be present in drinking water supplies across the country. Although these substances may be present in concentrations measured in parts per million (ppm) or even parts per billion (ppb), the fact that many of them are known to be mutagenic or carcinogenic raises unanswered questions concerning the long-term health effects of ingesting small amounts of poison on a daily basis. Indeed, the fact that some organic chemicals can be harmful to human health and to aquatic organisms at levels well below those currently detectable by standard analytical methods makes the issue of chemical contamination of water supplies particularly worrisome. A direct cause-and-effect relationship between toxic chemicals in drinking water and human health damage has not yet been conclusively demonstrated, but circumstantial evidence and the testimony of people who, unknowingly, consumed high levels of poisonous chemicals with their water for a number of years, indicate no reason to be complacent about the situation.

Synthetic Organic Pollutants.   The kinds of synthetic organic chemicals (SOCs, as they are now called) contaminating surface waters and aquifers worldwide consist of a vast array of pesticides, industrial solvents and cleaning fluids, polychlorinated biphenyls, and disinfection by-products. They originate from a wide range of activities such as chemical manufacturing, petroleum refining, iron and steel production, coal mining, wood pulp processing, textile manufacturing, and agriculture. They enter surface waters through direct and indirect discharges, by surface runoff, or by volatilization and subsequent fallout during precipitation episodes. Wellwaters can concentrate high levels of SOCs as a result of poor waste disposal practices or downward percolation of farm chemicals after heavy rains. The presence of SOCs in drinking water supplies has been a steadily growing source of public concern since the mid-1970s when several epidemiologic studies suggestively, though not conclusively, linked the presence of these chemicals with an elevated incidence of various types of cancer among exposed populations. While a number of the more than 100,000 SOCs currently in use (e.g. chloroform, benzene) are known or suspected carcinogens, establishing a direct causal relationship between polluted drinking water and cancer has been problematic. At present, the human health impact of exposure to organic chemicals in water supplies is thought to be relatively minor. However, because sampling for the presence of such chemicals has been quite limited, both geographically and in numbers of chemical contaminants surveyed, it is possible that their impact may be underestimated. The fact that so many different SOCs are being discharged into waterways and that many of them are highly toxic and may have additive or synergistic effects suggests that in the years ahead SOCs in drinking water may emerge as a serious global public health issue.

Box 15-7

Blue Baby Disease

Fecal pathogens and organic chemicals are not the only drinking water contaminants capable of causing illness. A number of inorganic substances—arsenic, heavy metals, and road salts, to cite a few—are known to have caused illness among unknowing consumers. In 1945, a young pediatrician in Iowa City published a landmark article in the Journal of the American Medical Association in which he attributed the cause of a mysterious ailment called "blue baby disease" to contamination of drinking water supplies with nitrates. In the years following this discovery, numerous cases of blue baby disease were reported, primarily from rural areas of the Midwest. In 1950, Minnesota alone listed 144 cases with 14 deaths during one 30-month period. Worldwide, about 3000 cases of blue baby disease have been documented since 1945 (almost half of them in Hungary during the six-year period from 1976–1982).

Blue baby disease, more correctly termed methemoglobinemia, is induced when an infant is given powdered formula or other infant foods mixed with nitrate-contaminated water, generally water from shallow wells polluted by fertilizer or feedlot runoff or by seepage from septic systems. Nursing mothers who drink water with high nitrate levels could possibly pass this on to their babies in breast milk, but such an occurrence is very rare; in fact, where surveys have shown private wells to be polluted with nitrates, doctors urge new mothers to breast-feed their infants. It should also be noted that, unlike situations involving bacteria or other pathogens in drinking water, boiling nitrate-polluted water to rid it of contamination is not advised, inasmuch as this simply results in concentrating any nitrates present.

Where wells are polluted, all residents of a household consume the contaminated water, yet only infants under the age of six months are at risk of acquiring blue baby disease. This is because during the first few months of life babies typically possess low levels of the enzyme which reduces methemoglobin. Concentrations of the enzyme increase with age and reach adult levels about six months after birth.

Better understanding of the disease and regular monitoring of public drinking water supplies for nitrate content since 1945 have reduced the incidence of methemoglobinemia in recent years. Nevertheless, random surveys in the Plains states have revealed a high proportion of private farm wells containing nitrate levels in excess of the 10 ppm EPA standard. Methemoglobinemia thus remains a potentially dangerous problem for babies in rural America—a fact tragically underlined in June of 1986 when a seven-week-old baby girl in South Dakota died of the disease, making her the first such victim in the U.S. in over two decades. When her family's well water was subsequently tested, laboratory results showed 150 ppm nitrate.

Given this history, evidence from many countries that freshwater concentrations of nitrates have been rising steadily over the past 30 years is quite worrisome. Most of this increase can be traced to heavier farm use of nitrogen fertilizers and manures, though industrial discharges and urban stormwater runoff are contributors also.

Because groundwater is more likely to accumulate high concentrations of nitrates than is surface water, the U.S. Geological Survey has estabished a sampling network to monitor nitrate levels in wells. Survey reports published in 1991 revealed that in 5% of the counties investigated, over one-fourth of the wells had nitrate levels exceeding the federal drinking water standard (in some wells, nitrate concentrations were more than 100 mg/L—ten times the legal limit).

Lead. That ingestion or inhalation of lead can cause human poisoning resulting in a wide range of health problems has been known for many years (see chapter 7). Government initiatives to lower the lead content of housepaint and to phase out the use of leaded gasoline were prompted specifically by the desire to reduce human exposure to this toxic metal. However, recent scientific findings have identified a hitherto-unrecognized source of environmental lead—water from our own kitchen or bathroom sinks. Indeed, in many areas of the country, household drinking water is the major route of lead exposure. EPA estimates that more than 40 million Americans are drinking water containing more than the legally permissible level of lead (50 ppb).

This situation does not mean that municipal water treatment plants are doing a poor job, for in almost all cases lead enters drinking water after it leaves the purification plant or private well. The problem arises within the home plumbing system as a result of corrosion when water passes through lead pipes or through pipes soldered with lead, when brass fixtures are used, or in situations where the water itself is corrosive (i.e. low pH). This type of reaction is particularly likely with "soft" water; corrosion is also increased by the common practice of using water pipes for the grounding of electrical equipment, since electrical current traveling through the ground wire hastens the corrosion of lead in the pipes.

The age of a home's plumbing system is a major determinant of whether or not a lead problem exists. In older structures—those built prior to the 1930s—lead was commonly used for interior piping as well as for the service connections that joined the house to a public water supply. Obviously if a home has lead plumbing, a potential problem exists. After 1930, copper piping largely replaced lead for residential plumbing, but such pipes were typically joined with lead solder; it is this solder that many authorities consider the main contributor to drinking water contamination with lead. Over time, the amount of lead leaching into water from plumbing decreases because mineral deposits gradually form a deposit on the inside of the pipes, preventing water from coming into direct contact with the solder. For this reason, homes with the greatest likelihood of having high lead levels are those less than five years old (unless the plumbing is made of plastic, in which case there's no problem).

Although telltale signs of corrosion (rust-colored water, stained dishwasher or laundry, frequent leaks) or recognition that the house falls into one of the high-risk age categories mentioned above can alert residents to a potential problem, the only way to make a definite determination of excess lead levels is to have the water tested at a certified laboratory (unfortunately, this is not a cheap procedure).

If lab analysis confirms high lead levels, abatement options short of total replacement of the plumbing system are somewhat limited. Reverse osmosis devices and distillation units can be installed at the faucet but are quite expensive and of variable effectiveness (faucet filters containing carbon or sand, as well as cartridge filters, are totally useless for removing lead). Lead exposure can be minimized by two simple actions that should be taken by anyone who has, or suspects, a lead problem:

1. Don't drink water that has been in contact with pipes for more than six hours. The longer water has been standing, the greater the amount of lead likely to be present. Before using such water for drinking or cooking, flush out the pipes by allowing water to run for several minutes or until it is as cold as it will get (this water can be used for washing, watering plants, etc.).

2. Don't consume or cook with hot tap water, since lead dissolves more readily in hot water than in cold. If you need hot water, draw it cold from the tap and use the stove to heat it.

In response to this newly recognized health hazard, Congress has prohibited the use of solder containing more than 0.2% lead (formerly, solder was 50% lead) and has banned any pipe containing more than 8% lead in new installations or for repair of public water systems. In addition, a number of states have now banned all use of lead materials in drinking water systems (EPA, 1987).

The realization that lead in drinking water presents a health hazard in many homes has prompted regulators to take a look at the school environment as well. In 1988, under the Lead Contamination Control Act, Congress urged both schools and day care centers to test water from electric water coolers (some models of which were believed to have lead-lined tanks or other components made of lead) to ensure that children attending those facilities were not receiving excessive lead exposure. While the recommendations for testing and remediation were purely advisory and thus not legally enforceable, many schools complied with the government's request. Unfortunately, other potential sources of lead-contaminated water such as ice machines, non-cooled water fountains, and classroom and kitchen sinks were not mentioned in the advisory.

Continuing concerns about lead in drinking water have led to further EPA actions to reduce this hazard. In May of 1991 the agency promulgated the Lead and Copper Rule, setting an "action level" (not the same as an enforceable standard) of *15 ppb* lead at the water's point of use. In cases where that level is exceeded, the new rule calls for the water treatment plant to take steps to reduce the corrosivity of the water—an action designed to reduce the leachability of lead within the plumbing system (Gnaedinger, 1993). New alarms were sounded in the spring of 1994 when EPA issued a warning to millions of private well owners, advising them to have their drinking water tested for possible high levels of lead contamination after research carried out by environmental groups at the University of North Carolina-Asheville revealed that the toxic metal was leaching into wellwater from lead-based brass and bronze alloys in submersible pumps, particularly from those recently installed (of the 11.8 million U.S. homes with private wells, approximately half feature submersible pumps, though not all such pumps have brass components). Environmental groups promptly urged pump manufacturers to recall all pumps containing lead components and replace them with safe, readily available lead-free models made of stainless steel.

Safe Drinking Water Act

Until 1974 regulation of drinking water supplies was the prerogative of the individual states, with federal involvement limited to developing advisory standards (which the states, for the most part, ignored) and to ensuring that interstate carriers such as railroads and airlines provided safe water to their passengers. In 1969 a study of community water supplies conducted by the U.S. Public Health Service revealed that 56% of nearly 1000 public waterworks surveyed were not constructed or operating properly, 51% failed to disinfect their water, and 16% exceeded one or more of the federal drinking water standards. Most of the violations, it was pointed out, were found in small communities that lacked the funds to provide the trained employees and modern equipment necessary to improve their operations; as a result 2.5 million people in the areas surveyed were provided with water of inferior quality, while 300,000 of these were drinking water that was potentially dangerous. Concerns raised by these findings were augmented by EPA revelations a few years later that public drinking water supplies in New Orleans, drawn from the heavily polluted Mississippi River, were contaminated with a number of toxic organic chemicals. A follow-up study by the Environmental Defense Fund reported that New Orleans residents drinking treated city water exhibited the second-highest rate of bladder and intestinal cancer in the country. While it cannot be proven that carcinogenic chemicals in drinking water are the direct cause of cancer incidence in Louisiana, the EDF report helped spur passage of the 1974 Safe Drinking Water Act—the only federal law which focuses on drinking water in a comprehensive manner.

Under the Act, EPA must establish **maximum contaminant levels (MCLs)** for specified pollutants found in the drinking water of any community water system (defined as one having at least 15 service connections used by year-round residents or regularly serving 25 or more people). The Safe Drinking Water Act sets uniform guidelines for drinking water treatment and requires that public water systems follow a prescribed schedule for monitoring and testing the quality of their treated water and report the results of such testing to the appropriate state agency.

The law as enacted in 1974 allowed EPA to decide which contaminants in drinking water required a primary standard. When the Safe Drinking Water Act came up for reauthorization in 1986, Congress

BOX 15-8
"To Chlorinate or Not to Chlorinate . . ."

If Hamlet could suddenly be reincarnated as the director of a modern water treatment plant, the subject of his soliloquy might well be the same issue which water experts and a concerned public have been debating for almost two decades—do the health benefits of using chlorine to disinfect drinking water outweigh the risks?

Ever since 1908 when it made its U.S. debut in Chicago (five years earlier, Belgium was the first country to begin using chlorine as a water disinfectant), chlorine's ranking as the top disinfectant for ensuring the safety of public water supplies has been unchallenged. Swiftly adopted by larger communities nationwide, chlorination of drinking water, along with municipal sewage treatment, can take the lion's share of credit for the precipitous decline in deaths due to infectious gastrointestinal diseases since the beginning of the 20th century. Chlorine, which is currently the disinfection method of choice for 75% of the U.S. water supply, attained its position of preeminence for several reasons: it is relatively inexpensive, highly effective at killing bacteria (though less effective against viruses and some protozoans), and, most important, it leaves a residual in the water that continues to provide germ-killing potential as the water travels through the distribution system to its point of use (the distinctive odor of chlorine in some public water supplies gives evidence of this chlorine residual; while consumers may find the odor objectionable, it does offer reassurance that, in the event of cross-contamination due to faulty plumbing or a break in water lines, some disinfectant is still present to kill intruding pathogens).

Unfortunately, for all its attributes, chlorine has a downside as well. In the mid-1970s it was discovered that adding chlorine to water containing naturally occurring humic substances found in virtually all surface waters can result in unintended chemical reactions, culminating in the formation of **disinfection by-products (DBPs)**, the most common of which are **trihalomethanes (THMs)**. Including such substances as chloroform and bromoform, THMs, unlike other synthetic organic chemicals, are formed at the water treatment plant itself when chlorine is added to the water. Any drinking water supply that has been chlorinated, particularly if the raw water was from a surface source containing substantial amounts of organic material, is likely to contain THMs. In fact, the presence of chloroform has been detected in almost every water system tested for this chemical—and chloroform, at least in high doses, is known to cause liver and kidney disorders, central nervous system problems, birth defects, and cancer.

However, since THMs usually are present only in very small amounts, many water experts argue that they pose a minimal health risk. Others contend that while the dangers inherent in exposure to each individual chemical may be low, over the long term cumulative exposure to the variety of DBPs in drinking water may indeed be a problem. Such individuals point to unexplained "cancer clusters" and reproductive abnormalities in areas where concentrations of organic chemicals in drinking water are higher than usual, suggesting a possible cause-and-effect relationship. In 1992, supporting evidence for the "perhaps we ought to be worried" faction was provided in the form of a statistical survey, based on a number of earlier studies, which revealed a link between drinking chlorinated water and a small increase in the rates of rectal and bladder cancer—approximately 6,500 additional cases of rectal cancer and 4,200 additional bladder cancers each year during the study period. While the studies in question had been conducted during the 1970s when the levels of chlorine added to water were substantially higher than they are today (meaning that the cancer/chlorinated water connection is weaker now than survey results suggest), these results have given added impetus to the search for methods of reducing THM levels in chlorinated water as well as for alternative methods of disinfection which avoid the formation of hazardous by-products.

Research results demonstrate that THM concentrations in finished water can be reduced substantially simply by adjusting the chlorine dose, improving filtration practices to remove as much of the organic material in the raw water as possible, or by adding chlorine after filtration rather than before, in order to reduce contact time between the chlorine and any organic compounds in the water, thereby preventing THM formation. In most areas measures such as these will be sufficient to keep THM levels within the maximum contaminant levels prescribed by the Safe Drinking Water Act. For a few cities with very severe THM problems, however, it may be necessary to adopt more advanced technologies such as **granular activated carbon (GAC)** treatment, recognized as a feasible method for removal of many synthetic organic chemicals. Unfortunately, while effective, GAC treatment is quite expensive, a factor which has delayed its widespread adoption.

Other disinfection alternatives are rather limited. **Chloramination**, the second-most commonly used method, involves a reaction between chlorine gas and ammonia, the latter substance being added to water supplies in order to generate chloramines. A precise proportional relationship must be maintained between the amounts of the two chemicals; if the dose varies, results will be poor. Use of chloramines as a disinfectant tends to result in the generation of fewer DBPs than chlorination does, but their value is limited by the fact that they are 50 to 100 times less effective at killing microbes than is chlorine gas.

Another option to replace chlorine is **ozone**. Ozone is quite effective at killing waterborne pathogens, but since it dissipates within minutes after being introduced into the water, it affords no residual protection. Recent studies have shown that, like chlorination, ozonation produces small amounts of disinfection by-products, in this case organic peroxides that may be more hazardous than trihalomethanes. It also increases the concentration of certain bacterial nutrients through the conversion of nonbiodegradable materials. Ozone destroys materials in water that cause unpleasant tastes and odors (thus its commonplace use as a disinfectant for high-priced bottled waters), but it also costs five to ten times as much as chlorination.

Yet a third disinfectant alternative to chlorine gas is **chlorine dioxide (ClO_2)**, but here, too, residuals are a problem: 50–70% of the chlorine dioxide applied remains in the form of chlorite ions.

Anticipating the likelihood of stringent new federal controls on disinfectant/disinfection by-products, researchers at a number of institutions are hard at work devising ways to surmount the identified limitations of the various disinfection methods. As one EPA regulator remarked, ''. . . we're trying to minimize one type of contaminant while simultaneously trying not to increase the risk for another. . . .'' Striking a balance between the known health risks of microbial waterborne disease and the less well-defined threats posed by trihalomethanes and other DBPs won't be easy. Should society jettison a proven bulwark (i.e. chlorination) against the bacterial killers of the past to rely on possibly less effective, more expensive defenses to ward off a small increased risk of cancer? Hamlet might well ponder the question.

Reference

Morris, R.D., et al. 1992. "Chlorination, Chlorination By-Products, and Cancer: A Meta-analysis." *American Journal of Public Health* 82, no. 7 (July).

expressed profound displeasure that in more than a decade MCLs had been set for only 23 drinking water contaminants—and most of these had been established by the Public Health Service in the 1960s prior to EPA's existence. Recognizing that over 700 organic, inorganic, biological and radiological contaminants had been detected in water supplies around the United States, Congress amended the Act, identifying 83 contaminants for which it required EPA to promulgate standards.

At the same time that Congress was calling for tighter regulation of chemicals in public water supplies, it also demanded that more be done to protect Americans against waterborne microbial pathogens. The SDWA's 1986 amendments require that water suppliers employ filtration to remove pathogens such as *Giardia* and *Cryptosporidium* unless they can prove that they have effective watershed protection programs in place to prevent pathogen-contaminated runoff from entering drinking water reservoirs and that their disinfection controls are stringent enough to remove 99.9% of all viruses and *Giardia* cysts. These are difficult parameters to meet; EPA estimates that only 12% of the 125,000 unfiltered public water systems serving populations over 10,000 will be able to comply with these criteria and thus manage to avoid the enormous expense of installing filtration technologies.

Nowhere is the filtration issue more pressing than in New York City, a metropolis which obtains 80% of its municipal water supply from six reservoirs in the Catskill Mountains. Long known for the excellent taste and quality of its water, New York is nevertheless one of the few large cities in the United States that does not filter its drinking water, relying on the remote location of these reservoirs to protect them from sources of contamination which would necessitate further treatment. However, in the years since its watershed regulations were issued in 1953, population growth and commercial development have altered the once-pristine nature of the region. Today 450,000 people live in the watershed areas serving New York City—as do 70,000 cows and uncounted numbers of wild geese and sea gulls whose droppings have been identified as significant sources of reservoir contamination. More than 100 POTWs, some of which are regularly in violation of their discharge permit standards, also constitute potential sources of watershed contamination. Under such circumstances, can New Yorkers be confident that the minimal level of drinking water treatment which served them adequately in the past will continue to do so in the years ahead? Many water experts think not. In the late 1980s EPA told New York City officials that they would have to construct an $8 billion water filtration plant unless they could prove to agency satisfaction

Figure 15-4 Contaminants Targeted for Regulation Under the Safe Drinking Water Act*

Microbiological Contaminants

Turbidity*	Viruses
Total Coliforms*	Standard Plate Count
Giardia lamblia	*Legionella*

Volatile Organic Chemicals

Trichloroethylene*	Vinyl Chloride*	Trichlorobenzene(s)
Tetrachloroethylene	Methylene Chloride	1,1-Dichloroethylene*
Carbon Tetrachloride*	Benzene*	cis-1, 2-Dichloroethylene
1,1,1-Trichloroethane*	Chlorobenzene	trans-1, 2-Dichloroethylene
1,2-Dichloroethane*	Dichlorobenzene(s)*	

Synthetic Organic Chemicals

Endrin*	Carbofuran	Pentachlorophenol
Lindane*	1,1,2-Trichlorethane	Picloram
Methoxychlor*	Vydate	Dinoseb
Toxaphene*	Simazine	Alachlor
2,4,-D*	PAHs (Polynuclear Aromatic	EDB (Ethylene Dibromide)
2,4,5-TP (Silvex)*	Hydrocarbons)	Epichlorohydrin
Total Trihalomethanes*	PCBs (Polychlorinated	Dibromomethane
Aldicarb	Biphenyls)	Toluene
Chlordane	Atrazine	Xylene
Dalapon	Phthalates	Adipates
Diquat	Acrylamide	Hexachlorocyclopentadiene
Endothall	DBCP (Dibromochloropropane)	2,3,7,8-TCDD (Dioxin)
Glyphosate	1,2-Dichloropropane	

Inorganic Chemicals

Arsenic*	Silver*	Vanadium
Barium*	Fluoride*	Sodium
Cadmium*	Aluminum	Nickel
Chromium*	Antimony	Zinc
Lead*	Molybdenum	Thallium
Mercury*	Asbestos	Beryllium
Nitrate (as N)*	Sulfate	Cyanide
Selenium*	Copper	

Radiological Contaminants

Radium 226 and 228*	Beta Particle and Photon	Natural Uranium
Gross Alpha Particle Activity*	Radioactivity*	Radon

*Substances are currently regulated; all except the VOCs may be revised.

Source: U.S. Environmental Protection Agency

that the city could safeguard its water supply through an upgraded watershed protection program. Officials quickly responded with a draft proposal to protect the quality of Catskill streams and reservoirs by restricting both residential and commercial development and by regulating farming operations—suggestions vociferously opposed by residents of the upstate region. Although in January 1993 EPA gave the city a temporary waiver from the filtration mandate, an advisory panel convened by the agency questioned the effectiveness of New York's efforts at watershed protection and recommended that the city not be allowed to evade filtration requirements. Several months later, then-Mayor David Dinkins announced New York would spend $750 million over the next decade to improve the municipal water system, upgrading local infrastructure and acquiring additional land holdings around reservoirs and along stream corridors to prevent degradation of drinking water quality at the source. Some local environmentalists in the Big Apple fear that forcing the city to install filtration will result in municipal neglect of the watershed protection approach—in effect, causing the city to settle on a "technological fix" as a solution to drinking water uses. EPA, by contrast, insists that the filtration versus watershed protection debate shouldn't be viewed as an "either/or" situation—both are essential to ensure the safety of public water supplies (King, 1993; Terry, 1993; Wapner, 1993).

While the 1986 Safe Drinking Water Act amendments represent an important step forward in national efforts to ensure drinking water quality, several problems persist—the most serious of which is limited financial resources. State regulatory agencies, which bear the lion's share of responsibility for implementing and enforcing safe drinking water regulations, simply have not been given the money and personnel to do the job. A recent survey of state agency performance by the federal General Accounting Office found that inadequate funding is preventing almost half the states from conducting the comprehensive surveys of public water treatment facilities which EPA recommends be done at least every three years. Even when such sanitary inspections are performed, GAO found that 45 states neglect one or more key elements of such inspections and two states (Alabama and Washington) have no routine surveys. This situation means that the drinking water in some communities may be coming from systems that haven't been checked for years and that may be experiencing undetected treatment deficiencies. Another target of GAO criticism is the lack of strict state certification requirements for those who operate water purification facilities. While most states require certification of personnel at large plants, at least 11 exempt operators of systems serving less than 500 people (60% of the nation's 60,000 community water systems fall into this category). Employees in these small treatment plants frequently have minimal training and qualifications, a fact which may explain why a disproportionate share of waterborne disease outbreaks are associated with small public water systems. Beyond lapses in employee certification requirements and inspection procedures, the sheer number of contaminants now being regulated has overwhelmed many state regulatory agencies. With most of the 83 new MCL standards now in place, the number of samples that must be taken—and the cost of analyzing such samples—

has escalated sharply within the past few years. Even when these sampling tasks are assigned to local water departments, the state agencies still are responsible for managing the data collected and seeing that any violations of drinking water standards are corrected. Although by law EPA is authorized to reimburse states for 75% of the cost of their drinking water programs, the federal agency consistently underfunds these efforts (Terry, 1993). In 1992 the National Governors' Association complained that states face a $200 million shortfall annually in resources to fund regulatory activities required under the Safe Drinking Water Act and pleaded with Washington for more flexibility in carrying out the intent of the law. Water utilities and communities, too, face serious financial difficulties as they strive to comply with new water treatment regulations. Just as New York City is balking at EPA's filtration demands, many water suppliers argue that they can't afford to comply with the scores of new drinking water standards (King, 1993). As new requirements take effect within the next few years, the burden on regulatory agencies, water suppliers and taxpayers alike will continue to grow. Nevertheless, events such as Milwaukee's bout with cryptosporidiosis may convince a once-complacent public that safety at the tap, so long taken for granted, faces new threats which must be aggressively confronted. Consumers may not cheer at the prospect of higher water fees to support regulatory programs, but in the long run they're a small price to pay for the assurance that a long drink of cool water will bring refreshment rather than disease.

Looking Ahead

As the 20th century draws to a close, enormous water quality challenges confront societies worldwide. In the United States, despite significant improvement over the past 25 years, 40% of our rivers, lakes, and estuaries have yet to attain the "fishable, swimmable" goal set forth in the Clean Water Act. Clinton Administration proposals for revising the nation's water pollution control laws recognize that we must do far more to reduce the poison runoff largely responsible for the continued degradation of American waterways. A consensus is emerging among researchers, policymakers, and the general public that discharges of persistent toxics which bioaccumulate in aquatic organisms must be prohibited altogether; that more federal dollars must be allocated for State Revolving Funds; that enforcement actions be strengthened; that technological innovation and market-based approaches to pollution control should be encouraged; and that our regulatory emphasis must shift from its past focus on "end-of-pipe" controls to a broad-based comprehensive watershed approach, using in-stream biological indicators as a yardstick for measuring progress in cleaning up the nation's surface waters.

In Europe, Japan, Canada, and most other industrialized regions of the world, water quality challenges parallel those in the United States. All have relied heavily in the past on expensive treatment technologies which

BOX 15-9

Pass the Perrier, Please!

Like Europeans who say they drink wine because the local water makes them sick, Americans in droves have been turning to bottled water because they don't like what's coming from their kitchen tap. Although the current 3% annual growth rate for sales is now well below its late-1980s peak of 500%, a bottling industry survey revealed that by the early 1990s Americans were consuming an average of eight gallons of bottled water per person yearly—double the amount they were drinking ten years earlier. With over 700 brands from which to choose, consumers collectively spend nearly $3 billion each year for a beverage whose labels evoke such back-to-the-wild imagery as "natural alpine spring water," "glacier water," or "nature's perfect beverage." Demand is greatest in the Southwest, with trendy California buying three times the national average—one out of every six residents in the Golden State now drinks bottled water.

Why the rush to the supermarket for a product much more cheaply available from public water supplies? Primarily because many consumers perceive bottled water as safer and tastier than tapwater—and because skillful marketing, particularly of certain imported brands, has made consumption of bottled water fashionable. That health and aesthetic factors are important determinants of bottled water's appeal is obvious from the fact that demand is highest in those areas where taste and odor problems are prevalent or where reports of groundwater contamination have prompted health concerns among consumers. But can health-conscious buyers be sure that the bottled water they're purchasing is any safer than the tap water they spurn?

Many public water commissioners vigorously argue that promotional claims of bottled water being more "wholesome" than tapwater are misleading, citing the fact that public water supplies are strictly regulated and monitored, hence are every bit as "healthy" as the commercial brands—and cost a fraction of the price. They also point out that certain bottled "mineral waters" contain levels of dissolved minerals (e.g. barium) high enough to threaten the health of some consumers. The 1990 scandal involving the recall of 160 million bottles of Perrier mineral water when traces of benzene were discovered in the product demonstrated that sources of bottled water are no less vulnerable to contamination than are public water supplies (Perrier's once-stellar image has yet to recover from its fall in public esteem; more than three years after the benzene fiasco, Perrier's U.S. market share for bottled water sales was just 2%—half of its pre-scare level). Nor are health concerns regarding bottled waters focused solely on chemical pollutants. A 1991 congressional committee investigation found that 31% of bottled waters marketed in the U.S. exceed the maximum allowable levels for microbial contamination.

Even from a taste standpoint, many municipal supplies are as good or better than the highly touted bottled product. The public water supply in cities such as New York and Los Angeles, for example, consistently rank among the best-tasting waters in the nation, commercial brands included. However, it is true that bottled waters are free of the taint of chlorine detectable in some municipally-supplied waters. This is because the vast majority of bottling facilities disinfect their product with ozone, a chemical that leaves no residual which might impart an unpleasant taste or odor to the water.

Bottled waters, like community water supplies, are heavily regulated by the federal government, in this case by the Food and Drug Administration, which classifies the product as a "food." FDA regulations require that water be bottled in facilities which follow food plant regulations, that they be processed under federally approved manufacturing processes, and that they be delivered to customers in sanitized containers. While bottling companies are required to take water from protected sources, until 1993 they were not required to reveal on the label what the source of that water was. When the congressional investigating committee learned that fully 25% of water brands were simply drawn from municipal supplies and put into fancy bottles (at fancy prices!) and that another 25% couldn't document where their water was obtained, the FDA tightened its regulations. Under the new rules, if bottled water is derived from a municipal source, this information must be clearly stated on the label. The revised regulations also establish standard definitions for all bottled water products (e.g. "artesian water," "spring water," "purified water," "distilled water," etc.) and set

new maximum contaminant levels for approximately 50 contaminants that may occur in bottled water. (Note: FDA regulations apply only to firms operating in more than one state). In addition to FDA-imposed requirements, domestic bottled water must meet EPA's drinking water standards and must comply with any state-imposed regulations. Like any food processing facility, all bottled water plants in the U.S. are visited by government inspectors at least once a year (imported brands, however, are not subject to Safe Drinking Water Act standards nor to FDA plant inspections).

While it is probably true that in most communities the public water supply is of high enough quality to make bottled water a nonessential status symbol, the industry fills an important role as a provider of an alternative source of safe drinking water when emergency situations render a public supply unsafe, when special health or dietary needs require low sodium or low nitrate water, or when consumers' demands that their water taste good and look clean are not met by their municipal source of supply.

References

Lambert, Victor. 1993. "Bottled Water." *FDA Consumer* (June).
McCarroll, Thomas. 1993. "Testing the Waters." *Time*, April 26.

deal with pollution problems after the fact and all need to refocus efforts on pollution prevention strategies and regional watershed management.

In the developing world the problems are far more daunting. Water quality is steadily deteriorating under the combined assault of human population increase, rapid urbanization, and growing volumes of toxic pollutant discharges. Simply quantifying water quality problems in Third World countries is difficult, since monitoring is virtually nonexistent and little data has been collected even on such basic concerns as sewage contamination and the frequency of microbial waterborne disease. Virtually nothing is known about the extent of toxic chemical pollution beyond anecdotal accounts of sickness and death wherever Third World residents are forced to utilize waters tainted with industrial effluents. For the immediate future, data collection and interpretation will be high on the priority list for those concerned with water quality in the developing world. At the same time, however, existing knowledge must be used to protect as-yet undegraded waters since widescale construction of expensive treatment facilities to deal with pollution problems after damage has occurred is beyond the means of most Third World nations (Nash, 1993).

Around the globe, in developed and developing countries alike, unrelenting human pressures on the environment have created unprecedented water quality challenges. Confronting these challenges will be expensive and will require some fundamental changes in our traditional approach to environmental protection. Nevertheless, the importance of clean water to human well-being—indeed, to our very survival—is so great that we have no choice but to make the effort. A quarter-century ago the U.S. Senate's leading environmentalist, Senator Ed Muskie of Maine, urged his legislative colleagues to override then-President Nixon's veto of the Clean Water Act. His stirring appeal rings as prophetic today as it did in the autumn of 1972:

> Our planet is beset with a cancer which threatens our very existence and which will not respond to the kind of treatment that has been prescribed for it in the past. The cancer of water pollution was engendered by our abuse of our lakes, streams, rivers, and oceans; it has thrived on our half-hearted attempts to control it; and like any other disease, it can kill us ■

References

Adler, Robert W., Jessica C. Landman, and Diane M. Cameron. 1993. *The Clean Water Act: 20 Years Later*. Natural Resources Defense Council. Island Press.

Banks, James T., and Frances Dubrowski. 1982. "Pretreat or Retreat?" *The Amicus Journal* (Spring). Natural Resources Defense Council.

Bennett, Lyle. 1991. "Abandoned Mines: Report from West Virginia." *EPA Journal* 17, no. 5 (Nov./Dec.).

Cholera Inquiry Committee. 1855. *Report on the Cholera Outbreak in the Parish of St. James, Westminster, During the Autumn of 1854*. J. Churchill, London.

Dillingham, Susan. 1989. "Letting Nature Do the Dirty Work." *Insight* (Jan. 16).

Environmental Protection Agency. 1993. "Standards for the Use or Disposal of Sewage Sludge; Final Rules." *Federal Register, 40 CFR Part 257 et al.* (Feb. 19).

Environmental Protection Agency. 1987. *Lead and Your Drinking Water*, OPA-87-006 (April).

Gianessi, L.P., et al. 1986. "Non-Point Source Pollution: Are Crop Land Controls the Answer?" *Resources for the Future*. Washington, D.C.

Gnaedinger, Richard H. 1993. "Lead in School Drinking Water." *Journal of Environmental Health* 55, no. 6 (April).

Goldberg, Rob. 1993. "EPA Expands Stormwater Control Permitting." *Water Environment & Technology* 5, no. 7 (July).

Goldstein, Bruce E. 1988. "Sewage Treatment, Naturally." *WorldWatch* 1, no. 4 (July/August).

Gray, Robert. 1991. "Washington News." *Water/Engineering & Management* (Feb.).

Griffin, Robert, Jr. 1991. "Introducing NPS Water Pollution." *EPA Journal* 17, no. 5 (Nov./Dec.).

King, Jonathan. 1993. "Something in the Water." *Amicus Journal* (Fall). Natural Resources Defense Council.

Koren, Herman. 1980. *Handbook of Environmental Health and Safety: Principles and Practices*. Pergamon Press.

Nash, Linda. 1993. "Water Quality and Health." In *Water in Crisis: A Guide to the World's Fresh Water Resources*, edited by Peter H. Gleick. Oxford University Press.

Quigg, Philip W. 1976. *Water: The Essential Resource*. National Audubon Society.

"Sewer Collapse and Toxic Illness in Sewer Repairmen—Ohio." 1981. *Morbidity and Mortality Weekly Report*, 30, no. 8 (March 6). U. S. Department of Health and Human Services/Public Health Service.

Sheiman, Deborah A. 1982. *Blueprint for Clean Water*. League of Women Voters Educational Fund, Pub. 639.

Shertzer, Richard H. 1986. "Wastewater Disinfection—Time for a Change?" *Journal of the Water Pollution Control Federation* 58, no. 3 (March).

"Small Community Benefits from Constructed Wetlands." 1993. *Water Environment & Technology* 5, no. 8 (August).

Tenenbaum, David. 1992. "Sludge." *Garbage* 4, no. 5 (Oct./Nov.).

Terry, Sara. 1993. "Drinking Water Comes to a Boil." *New York Times Magazine* (Sept. 26).

Wapner, Kenneth. 1993. "A Tale of Calves, Catskills, and E. coli." *Amicus Journal* (Fall).

Wolman, M. Gordon. 1988. "Changing Water Quality Priorities." *Journal of the Water Pollution Control Federation* 60, no. 10 (Oct.).

World Resources Institute. 1992. *World Resources 1992–93*. Oxford University Press.

CHAPTER 16

Solid and Hazardous Wastes

Nowhere in the world is there such a waste of material as in this country. In our eagerness to get the most results from our resources, and to get them quickly, we destroy perhaps as much as we use. Americans have not learned to save; and their wastefulness imperils their future. Our resources are fast giving out, and the next problem will be to make them last.

—Austin Bierbower, "American Wastefulness,"
Overland Monthly 49, April 1907

The above quotation from a popular magazine in the early years of this century gives evidence that the "waste not, want not" attitude so highly valued in our nation's younger days has long since been replaced by the ethic of a "Throwaway Society." The inevitable result of Americans' proclivity to "use once and throw away" has been an ever-increasing volume of waste material which, for both sanitary and aesthetic reasons, must be regularly collected and disposed of in a manner which will not degrade the environment or threaten public health.

Waste Disposal—A Brief History

Human generation of wastes is, of course, as old as humanity itself. Anthropologists and archaeologists have gleaned illuminating information about the everyday lives of our primitive ancestors by excavating the rubbish heaps outside early cave dwellings and other ancient settlements. Among rural or nomadic peoples, however, discarded wastes seldom accumulated to an extent great enough to threaten human well-being. The advent of the first cities after the Agricultural Revolution of approximately 10,000 years ago presented humankind with its first serious problems of refuse disposal. The poor sanitary conditions and frequent epidemics which characterized city life from ancient times until the late 19th century derived primarily from the perpetuation of country habits in a crowded urban environment. Human body wastes, garbage, and discarded material items alike were typically left on the floors of homes or thrown into the streets. A rudimentary awareness of the link between refuse and disease led to the establishment in Athens, Greece, of what was perhaps the first "city dump" in the Western world around 500 B.C.; this innovation was accompanied by what is believed to be the world's first ban against throwing garbage into the streets, as well as by a regulation requiring scavengers to dump wastes no closer than a mile from the city walls. The Athenian example regarding waste management was not widely emulated, however. Throughout the Roman period and the Middle Ages in Europe open dumping of wastes in streets or ditches remained the prevailing method of urban waste disposal. Attempts by municipal authorities to cope with their citizens' slovenly habits were limited and sporadic. In 1388 the English Parliament prohibited dumping of wastes in public waterways; after the 13th century, Parisians were no longer permitted to throw garbage out their windows (they obviously pitched it elsewhere, however, for by A.D. 1400 the mounds of garbage outside the city gates of Paris were so high that they obstructed efforts by the military to defend the city). As medieval towns gradually developed into modern cities, and particularly after the onset of the Industrial Revolution in Europe at the end of the 18th century, the solid waste problem became even more acute. Urban areas became grossly overcrowded, polluted, noisy, and dirtier than ever. Rising levels of affluence among some segments of society, as well as sheer growth in population size, resulted in the generation of increasing amounts of waste. It gradually became apparent to civic leaders that the accumulation of filth and refuse in urban centers was directly related to disease outbreaks. Thus by the late 19th century, city-sponsored efforts at improving urban sanitation were launched both in Europe and North America. Refuse, previously regarded simply as a nuisance, was finally perceived as a major pollution problem which posed a serious human health threat—a problem so massive that it could be effectively tackled only by municipal governments, not simply by private individuals acting on their own initiative (Melosi, 1981).

Throughout the 20th century the "garbage problem" has continued to mount, in spite of steadily rising expenditures to manage such wastes in an acceptable manner. Unfortunately, victory in our war against waste is nowhere in sight. The rate of solid waste generation continues to increase several times more rapidly than the rate of population growth, suggesting that the major forces determining waste output today are an affluent life-style and changes in marketing techniques (e.g. multiple packaging) which result in more waste materials to be discarded. While tossing garbage into the streets is no longer considered socially acceptable, modern methods of waste disposal, for the most part, are not a great deal more advanced than they were a century ago. Today steadily increasing volumes of refuse, coupled with the realization that many of these wastes are of a toxic or hazardous nature, have lent renewed urgency to the need for finding safer, more effective methods of collecting, storing, transporting, and disposing of the unwanted by-products of modern society.

Municipal Solid Wastes (MSW)

All over the nation it's as plain as the eye can see or the nose can smell that we have to change our ways.

—Robert P. Casey
Governor of Pennsylvania, 1988

The tragi-comic voyage of the Islip, New York, "garbage barge" during the spring and summer of 1987 did more than any other single event to focus national attention on America's rapidly mounting problems of urban waste disposal. Loaded with over 3000 tons of commercial trash banned from a local landfill reserved for residential refuse, the "Mobro" cruised the Atlantic and Gulf coasts for five months, searching for a disposal facility which would accept the odorous cargo. Its odyssey well-chronicled by a bemused national media, the barge's load was angrily rejected in North Carolina, Florida, Alabama, Mississippi, Louisiana, Texas, Mexico, Belize, and the Bahamas. This modern-day version of the "Flying Dutchman"

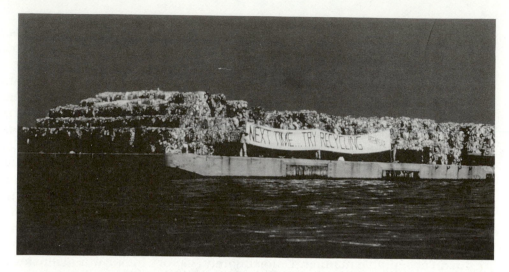

The infamous "garbage barge" from Islip, New York, cruised the Atlantic and Gulf coasts for five months in 1987 searching for a disposal facility for its overripe cargo. It ultimately returned to New York, by which time it sported a Greenpeace banner urging recycling. [© Dennis Capolongo, Greenpeace 1987]

finally returned to New York (festooned with an enormous Greenpeace banner advising, "Next Time Try Recycling!") where its overripe cargo was ultimately burned in a Brooklyn incinerator. The public interest generated by this spectacle raised hopes among beleaguered municipal administrators that perhaps at last citizens would begin to heed their warnings about an impending garbage crisis in our nation's cities.

Every sector of the national economy—farms, mines, and factories as well as businesses, institutions, and households—contributes to the mounting mass of unwanted materials requiring disposal. Nevertheless, municipal wastes, although proportionally far smaller in amount than agricultural and mining wastes, arguably represent our greatest waste management challenge (with the possible exception of industrial hazardous wastes). This is because urban wastes are generated where people live and must be quickly removed and properly disposed of in order to prevent serious environmental health problems. Municipal wastes are also much more heterogeneous than are the wastes produced by agriculture, mining, or specific industries. Paper and paper products constitute the single largest portion of household rejects, but an examination of a typical garbage container would also reveal glass, metal, and plastic containers; rubber, leather, and cloth items; food wastes; grass clippings, tree trimmings, discarded appliances, and numerous other items.

The quantity of these discards has been steadily increasing over the past several decades. By the early 1990s, municipalities were generating over 300 million tons of nonhazardous solid wastes each year (Steuteville, 1994a). Wastes from households and businesses alone accounted for nearly 200 million tons—equivalent to 4.3 pounds of refuse tossed away daily by every man, woman, and child in the United States (EPA, 1990). Since the

Figure 16-1 What's in Our Trash?

41%	Paper
18%	Yard Trimmings
8%	Glass
9%	Metals
7%	Plastics
8%	Food Waste
9%	Other

(As of 1988)

Source: EPA.

late 19th century, Americans have regarded the collection and disposal of urban wastes as a primary responsibility of municipal governments. Unfortunately, the ever-growing volume of such wastes is beginning to surpass the ability of some cities to cope with the problem, while at the same time more stringent state and federal requirements for sounder methods of waste management have increased the costs of disposal and have presented city officials with new challenges to improve their waste management practices. Many a beleaguered city manager, confronted with the question of what his or her most pressing environmental concern might be, would probably reply, "Where to put all that garbage!"

Municipal Waste Collection and Disposal

The piles of refuse and unsightly, unsanitary conditions that quickly accumulate during the garbage workers' strikes which occasionally plague some cities provide a dramatic illustration of the importance to public health of regular, frequent urban refuse collection. Any breakdown in this essential service, particularly during the warmer months of the year, can result in odor and litter problems or in the rapid growth of fly and rat populations. To prevent such problems, the Public Health Service recommends that refuse be collected twice weekly in residential areas and daily from restaurants, hotels, and large apartment complexes. This is particularly important during the peak of the summer fly-breeding season when eggs may hatch in less than a day and larval stages can be completed in three to four days. Historically, because the public has been far more concerned that refuse be regularly removed than with what happens to it once the garbage truck rounds the nearest corner (the "out of sight, out of mind" philosophy), municipal solid waste budgets have traditionally allocated about 80% of their resources to refuse collection, and only 20% to disposal.

From a public health and environmental quality standpoint, proper disposal of urban refuse is just as important as regular collection. Until the 1970s this aspect of solid waste management was given scant attention, resulting in cities utilizing the cheapest method available, with little or no consideration given to the often severe pollution problems thereby created. A new ecological awareness on the part of both the public and policymakers has brought many of these long-established practices into disfavor and some are now legally prohibited or are gradually being phased out. Some of the once-common municipal waste disposal methods now regarded as environmentally unacceptable include the following:

Hog Feeding. From ancient times until the 19th century, freely roaming pigs, goats, cows, and poultry scavenged garbage from city streets; however, since they left behind their droppings while removing food wastes, it might be argued that public thoroughfares were scarcely any cleaner for their efforts. Eventually regulations prohibiting livestock within city limits were enacted, but municipal governments frequently found it expedient to sell, or even donate, food wastes to nearby farmers for use as hog fodder. This practice was most prevalent in parts of New England (at the turn of the century, 61 towns in Massachusetts disposed of at least a portion of their garbage in this manner), but was employed profitably in several Midwestern and Western cities as well (Melosi, 1981). As late as 1941, a survey of American cities whose populations exceeded 25,000 revealed that more than 25% of the garbage collected was used for feeding hogs (Stolting, 1941). The popularity of this method was diminished, however, by the recognition that garbage-fed hogs were frequently unfit for human consumption because they harbored the parasite which produces the disease trichinosis in people eating the pork. In addition, the practice often resulted in outbreaks of diseases such as hog cholera and vesicular exanthema among herds of swine fed on raw garbage. By the late 1950s the U.S. Public Health Service and some state health departments passed regulations prohibiting the feeding of uncooked garbage to hogs. Since cooking the wastes made the practice uneconomical, this method of urban refuse disposal has by now virtually disappeared.

Ironically, since the late 1980s the practice has enjoyed a minor resurgence, thanks to the desperate shortage of landfill space in some areas. In southern New Jersey about 50 farmers have been licensed to feed their hogs food wastes collected from the tourist resorts and gambling casinos of Atlantic City and Cape May. The scraps are first ground and steam-cooked, then mixed with grain before feeding to livestock. So far the arrangement appears to be a win-win situation: restaurant owners get rid of their wastes, farmers obtain free feed (and are sometimes paid to carry it away), and the state saves desperately needed landfill space. And the pigs? A USDA extension agent, commenting on the gourmet scraps being channeled to the hog farms, remarked that, "These hogs eat better than most of the people in Third World countries" ("Impact of Hogs," 1988).

Water Dumping. Another widely condemned and now largely abandoned practice was the dumping of municipal wastes into the nearest body of water. Until 1933 New York City relied on ocean dumping as a primary method of garbage disposal, a practice bitterly resented by New Jersey shoreline residents whose beaches were regularly littered with Manhattan's cast-off mattresses, old shoes, banana peels, and sewage sludge. In the late 1800s, Chicago dumped much of its waste into Lake Michigan about three miles from the mouth of the Chicago River; New Orleans utilized the Mississippi River in a similar manner. Gradual recognition that such dumping was damaging to the aquatic environment and was generating serious shoreline nuisances caused the method to fall into disfavor in most communities or led to legal prohibitions against its continuance. A court suit filed against New York by several New Jersey coastal cities in 1933 resulted in the U.S. Supreme Court's 1934 ban on municipal waste dumping at sea (certain industrial and commercial wastes were exempted from this ruling, however). By the end of the 1960s, 50 million tons of wastes annually were still being dumped into the ocean off U.S. shores, most consisting of dredging wastes from harbor-deepening activities and sewage sludge. The Marine Protection, Research, and Sanctuaries Act, passed in 1972 and subsequently strengthened by a series of amendments, gradually imposed increasingly strict limitations and now prohibits ocean dumping of industrial waste, sewage sludge, radioactive wastes, and all radiological, chemical, and biological warfare agents. It does permit ocean disposal of dredged spoil, authorizing the Army Corps of Engineers to issue permits for the transport of such material to EPA-designated ocean dump sites.

Open Dumping. By far the most common method of urban refuse disposal until quite recently, open dumping epitomizes the problems that can arise when solid wastes are mismanaged. Employed primarily because they are cheap and convenient, open dumps support large populations of rats, flies, and cockroaches that frequently invade nearby dwellings. They contaminate adjacent surface or groundwater supplies when **leachates** (liquids resulting from the interaction of water with wastes) containing dissolved pollutants run off or seep downward through the soil from the dumpsite. If burned over to prevent litter from blowing about or to reduce the volume of wastes, open dumps can pose air quality problems. They are odorous, unsightly, and have a negative impact on property values of adjacent lands. Open dumping as a method for disposing of municipal refuse was outlawed by the federal government in 1976 (earlier by some state governments), and there has been a concerted effort, largely successful, to phase out all open dumping in the United States. In many less-developed areas of the world, however, open dumping remains the most prevalent form of urban waste disposal.

Current Waste Disposal Alternatives

Sanitary Landfilling

In recent decades, most municipalities seeking an economically feasible yet environmentally acceptable alternative to open dumping have opted for sanitary landfills as their refuse disposal method of choice. A sanitary landfill differs from an open dump in that collected refuse is spread in thin layers and compacted by bulldozers. When the compacted layers are 8–10 feet deep, they are covered with about 6 inches of dirt, which is again compacted. At the end of each working day another thin layer of soil is placed over the fill to prevent litter from blowing about, to keep away

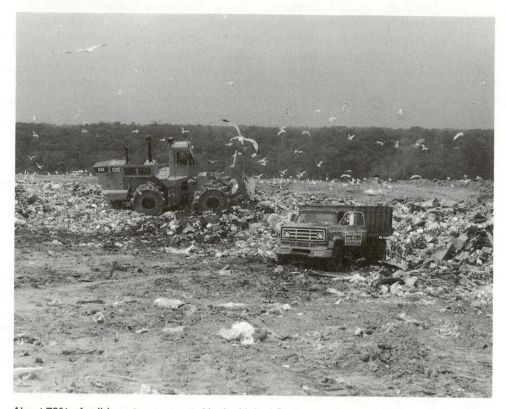

About 70% of solid wastes generated in the United States are disposed of in sanitary landfills. Rapidly dwindling capacity at existing facilities, the difficulty in siting new landfills, and increasing public disfavor have caused many municipalities to explore alternative disposal methods. [Author's Photo]

insect and rodent pests, and to minimize odor problems. When the landfill has reached its ultimate capacity, a final earth cover two feet deep is placed over the entire area and the land can then be used for a park, golf course, or other kinds of recreational facilities.

When properly sited, well designed, and efficiently operated, a sanitary landfill can be a perfectly adequate means of urban refuse disposal, free from offensive odors, vermin, or pollution problems. Unfortunately, in the past most so-called "sanitary" landfills were *not* well sited, properly designed, or well run. As a result, many landfills caused environmental contamination problems little different from those of open dumps and made sanitary landfills unwelcome neighbors wherever they were located. In the mid-1970s it was reported that of 17,000 land disposal sites surveyed, 94% failed to meet the minimum requirements of a sanitary landfill—requirements which in the 1970s were far less stringent than those prevailing today.

Nevertheless, landfills became the overwhelming waste disposal method of choice nationwide, largely because they were (and still are in

Figure 16-2 Where Does Our Trash Go?

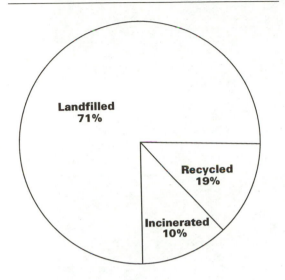

Total weight: 200 million tons, or the equivalent of 4.3 pounds per person per day.

most places) the most economical of the legal options. In 1993 the average cost for burying a ton of MSW at a U.S. sanitary landfill (i.e. the "**tipping fee**") was $28, considerably cheaper than the cost of other management methods (in states such as New York, New Jersey, and Massachusetts, landfill tipping fees are in the $65/ton range, making other alternatives economically attractive). Landfills also appealed to municipal officials because they were capable of receiving any type of waste and could, after completion, be used for facilities popular with the public such as parks, ski slopes, or golf courses. Landfills, of course, are not trouble-free: uneven settling of the land may occur, making them unsuitable as sites for constructing buildings after operations have ceased; anaerobic decomposition of landfilled materials may result in the accumulation of dangerous amounts of methane which can cause explosions or fires if the gas migrates into nearby structures; perhaps the most serious environmental impact associated with landfills is their potential for polluting nearby surface streams or underlying aquifers with leachates. This problem can be minimized by careful site selection, choosing locations underlain by impervious clay formations and far removed from any bodies of surface water. In the past such considerations were frequently neglected, with siting decisions typically based on the price of the land. Unfortunately, in many communities wetland areas, once considered "worthless" because of the cost of developing them for residential or commercial purposes, have been utilized as cheap landfill sites. Aside from the fact that wetlands have intrinsic value for their biologic productivity and flood control attributes, the fact that they are usually in hydrologic contact with groundwater makes wetland areas the least appropriate siting choice for a sanitary landfill.

Although landfills have been regarded with increasing public disfavor in recent years, largely due to the long-term environmental liability they represent (17% of federal "Superfund" sites slated for multimillion dollar cleanup efforts are former municipal landfills), sanitary landfilling remains the most prevalent method of MSW disposal in the United States. According to the most recent estimates published by *BioCycle* magazine, based on surveys of state waste management programs, 71% of the solid waste

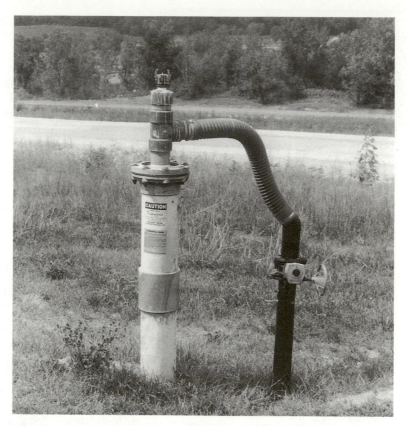

A methane recovery well at a sanitary landfill prevents the gas (a by-product of anaerobic decomposition) from accumulating in dangerous amounts. [Author's Photo]

generated in this country is landfilled (EPA puts this figure a bit lower at 67%, but does not include construction and demolition wastes which comprise a substantial amount of the refuse being landfilled each day) (Steuteville, 1994a). In the mid-1980s, anxious talk about a so-called national "garbage crisis" dominated discussion of MSW issues in the United States. Pointing to still-rising rates of waste generation, a rapidly dwindling number of landfills, and sharply escalating tipping fees at those still operating, many commentators warned that by the early 1990s over half of all American cities would have no place to send their garbage. Compounding the problem—indeed, the essence of the dilemma in a country where open spaces still abound—is the political reality of intense public opposition to landfill siting, a situation which time and again has stymied efforts by local government officials or private waste management firms to develop needed replacement facilities.

The new public focus on MSW concerns sparked intensive efforts by local and state officials to develop new, more sustainable waste management strategies for the decades ahead—and to insist that new and existing landfills be better designed and operated than the earlier facilities responsible for so many environmental horror stories. A major step toward the latter objective was EPA's promulgation of its new **RCRA Subtitle D** landfill requirements, now in effect nationwide. Mandating that all landfills install groundwater monitoring wells and methane detection systems, Subtitle D will sharply increase the cost of landfill operations but will also ensure that leachates or potentially explosive gases migrating from the fill don't go unnoticed and neglected. Requirements that new cells within a landfill be constructed with double liners and a leachate collection system to remove standing water means that in the future MSW landfills will be virtually indistinguishable in design from land disposal facilities licensed to accept hazardous wastes. Compliance with such requirements, of course, is expensive and owners of many smaller landfills opted to go out of business rather than invest the sums necessary to continue operations under the new regulations. As a result, after the federal rules went into effect in October 1993, the number of operating U.S. landfills dropped from 5,386 to 4,482 (compared to approximately 8000 in 1988). The sharp decline is much less of a problem than the statistics might suggest, however, for while the *number* of landfills has fallen, remaining landfill *capacity* has not taken a similar nosedive. In fact, of 26 states providing data on remaining landfill space, only Vermont reported an imminent space crunch, while the others indicated adequate capacity for periods ranging from 9 to 20 years. Current trends indicate that for the foreseeable future, MSW will be transported longer distances to fewer, large regional facilities designed and operated in a manner that provides a considerably higher level of environmental protection than the leaky landfills of the past (Steuteville, 1994a).

In the meantime, waste planners are broadening their perspective, searching for more environmentally friendly MSW management approaches and striving to bring about a paradigm shift in societal attitudes toward the materials we use and throw away. Rather than focusing on one "technological fix" or single disposal alternative to solve every community's problems, most waste management experts view the solution as a combination of approaches, tailored to the specific needs and realities of individual municipalities. While recognizing that there will always be a need for some amount of landfilling to accommodate specific wastes which can't be handled in any other manner, current philosophy regards landfilling as the method of last resort, to be replaced to the greatest extent possible by a mix of the following alternatives.

Source Reduction

The best—and cheapest—way of managing wastes is not to produce them in the first place. Accordingly, policies of reducing wastes at their source are top-ranked in every priority listing of waste management options. First raised as a possible approach for dealing with U.S. solid waste problems at a 1975 EPA-sponsored Conference on Waste Reduction, the goal of conserving materials and energy through waste prevention or by reducing the volume or toxicity of wastes generated was given little more than lip service until recently. The present sense of urgency to relieve pressures on existing disposal facilities has prompted a more serious look at the potential for source reduction strategies, which most advocates estimate could cut present urban waste streams by about 5%. Approaches to source reduction variously target consumers, manufacturers, or government and can include either voluntary or mandatory components.

Appealing to consumers to use their considerable purchasing power in a more environmentally aware manner has been a key component of source reduction efforts for years. By shopping selectively—buying only the amount of a product that will be used, choosing items without excessive amounts of packaging, buying products that have fewer toxic ingredients than comparable items used for the same purpose, avoiding single-serve disposable packages, or participating in waste exchanges (yard- or garage-sales might be regarded as an effective source reduction strategy!) are all ways of reducing the garbage we throw away. Another approach involves substituting reusable consumer items for single-use throwaway products—cloth napkins and terry towels instead of paper ones; china or plastic dishes instead of paper plates; handkerchiefs instead of Kleenex; cloth diapers in lieu of Pampers; refillable pens in place of disposable Bics.

Opportunities for source reduction of wastes in the business or institutional setting are similarly plentiful. Simply by asking employees to use their own coffee mugs rather than the ubiquitous styrofoam cup, daily waste volume can be noticeably reduced. Copy-machines designed to print on both sides of a sheet of paper can save thousands of dollars in business expenditures on paper supplies—as well as on reduced waste disposal fees. Using e-mail rather than paper for interoffice memos, or simply circulating one document rather than making multiple copies, are practices being adopted by thousands of waste-conscious firms.

Manufacturers must play a pivotal role in any national source reduction effort, since their decisions regarding product composition, design, packaging, and durability have such far-reaching implications. Already industry's efforts to reduce packaging and transportation costs through "lightweighting" have had a positive impact on waste reduction trends. When General Mills reduced the thickness of the plastic liners in its cereal boxes, it simultaneously cut the amount of plastic used—and thrown away—each year by half a million pounds. Similarly, lightweighting has increased the number of beverage cans which can be manufactured from a pound of aluminum from 23 in 1976 to 29 today. Many observers feel that manufacturers could do much more, however, by substituting less hazardous components for toxic ones (e.g. Apple Computer several years ago began using brown cardboard packaging containers to replace chlorine-bleached white boxes) and by designing products for easier repair and increased durability, thereby moving away from a corporate policy of "planned obsolescence."

Finally, there are a number of options government could pursue, should it choose to do so, to advance source reduction goals. Aside from efforts at public education—providing citizens with the information they need to make wise purchasing decisions—governments could employ a mix of economic incentives and disincentives, fees, taxes, subsidies, or outright bans to influence consumer choice or manufacturers' behavior. For example, more than 200 communities have adopted unit-based pricing (variously referred to as "bag & tag," "pay-as-you-throw," etc.) rather than the traditional flat fee for residential garbage pickup. Essentially a user fee based on the amount of waste discarded, this approach to funding waste management services provides a financial incentive to householders to reduce waste generation and simultaneously encourages more environmentally desirable behavior such as recycling and composting (in Perkasie, Pennsylvania, wastes headed for the landfill plummeted by 41% after a per-container fee was imposed; in Ilion, New York, a drop of 37% was recorded, according to a 1990 EPA survey). Although most unit-based pricing schemes are volume-based (i.e. per-container fees), a few communities have recently begun to experiment with weight-based systems. While a number of municipalities have hesitated to opt for unit-based pricing for fear it would encourage illicit dumping, experience in the communities which have chosen this approach indicates minimal or short-lived problems in this regard. Taxes at the time of purchase on certain hard-to-dispose-of items may not deter their purchase, but can at least provide funds to help offset recycling or disposal costs. At least 18 states now impose such a tax on tires; motor oil, automobiles, lead-acid batteries, anti-freeze, and major appliances are additional products upon which certain states levy taxes which reflect their environmental impact. Outright bans on the use or disposal of certain troublesome items have been more difficult to impose due to possible conflict of such mandates with laws governing regional or interstate commerce. Nevertheless, several have been success-fully adopted, perhaps the least controversial of which was the nationwide prohibition on flip-top openers for beverage cans. At the local level there have been bans on the use polystyrene food packaging in Berkeley, California, Portland, Oregon, and Newark, New Jersey.

The ultimate success of fledgling national source reduction efforts hinges upon a fundamental shift in society's basic approach to waste management—a refocusing of attention toward ways to *prevent* wastes from being generated in the first place rather than trying to deal with our discards after-the-fact. Source reduction, if wholeheartedly pursued, would also necessitate a different national life-style, though not necessarily a less satisfying one. While the concept has yet to capture the hearts and minds of most Americans and has encountered resistance from certain industries which would be directly affected by such policies, the benefits of source reduction programs in reducing waste management costs, saving natural resources, and easing humanity's impact on the environment guarantee a growing commitment in the years ahead to the *practice*, not just the *promise*, of source reduction (League of Women Voters, 1993).

Recycling

More broadly referred to as **resource recovery**—any productive use of what would otherwise be a waste material requiring disposal—recycling ranks second on everyone's list of preferred waste management alternatives. Perceived by many environmentally aware citizens as "the right thing to do" and by local officials as a way of extending the remaining lifespan of existing land disposal facilities (thereby postponing politically prickly decisions regarding the siting of new landfills or incinerators: the NIMTOO—Not In My Term of Office—response), recycling of MSW has made impressive gains within the last few years. In its 1994 report on "The State of Garbage in America," *BioCycle* magazine reported that recycling rates, including composting, more than doubled between 1989 and 1993—from 9% to the current 19% nationwide. EPA projections indicate another doubling of resource recovery rates by the end of the decade.

Recycling, of course, is not a new phenomenon. The highest rates of resource recovery witnessed in this nation occurred during World War II, when saving valuable resources to aid in the war effort was widely regarded as a patriotic duty. However, interest in resource conservation waned during the prosperous 1950s and 1960s and only revived with the emergence of the ecology movement and the energy "crisis" of the 1970s. At that time increased emphasis on recycling was promoted primarily for its very real ecological benefits:

1. *Resource conservation*—recycling reduces pressure on forest resources and extends the nation's supply of nonrenewable mineral ores.
2. *Energy conservation*—recycling consumes 50–90% less energy than manufacturing the same item from virgin materials.
3. *Pollution abatement*—manufacturing products from secondary rather than virgin materials significantly reduces levels of pollutant emissions. For example, recycling scrap metal, as opposed to processing iron ore in a coke oven, reduces particulate emissions by 11 kg/metric ton and eliminates the mining wastes generated in extracting iron ore and coal. Recycling aluminum has an even greater environmental impact—both air pollution and energy use are thereby cut by 95%.

In recent years, while acknowledging the environmental advantages of resource recovery, advocates point to a more direct impact municipal recycling efforts could have in their own communities. Not only do such programs have the potential to reduce dependence on landfills and incinerators by diverting a portion of the waste flow—they also promote individual responsibility for waste-generating behavior and may eventually help to forge a new public ethic regarding consumerism and sustainable life-styles.

To encourage more aggressive development and implementation of municipal recycling programs, most states, as well as a few cities, have set recycling goals, with deadline dates for achievement (so-called "**rates and dates**"). Many have also enacted legislation requiring that local units of government develop long-range comprehensive waste management plans, detailing how they intend to comply with state-mandated recycling goals. These planning requirements have forced local officials and citizen

Figure 16-3 State Recycling Goals

State	% Recycling Goal	Target Date
Alabama	25	1995
Arkansas	40	2000
California	50	2000
Connecticut	25	1991
District of Columbia	45	1996
Florida	30	1994
Georgia	25	1996
Hawaii	50	2000
Illinois	25	2000
Indiana	50	2001
Iowa	50	2000
Kentucky	25	1997
Louisiana	25	1992
Maine	50	1994
Maryland	20	1994
Massachusetts	50	2000
Michigan	40–60	2005
Minnesota	30	1996
Mississippi	25	1996
Missouri	40	1998
Montana	25	1996
Nebraska	50	2002
Nevada	25	1994
New Hampshire	40	2000
New Jersey	60	1995
New Mexico	50	2000
New York	50	1997
North Carolina	40	2001
North Dakota	40	2000
Ohio	25	1994
Oregon	50	2000
Pennsylvania	25	1997
Rhode Island	70	-
South Carolina	30	1997
South Dakota	50	2001
Tennessee	25	1995
Texas	40	1994
Vermont	40	2000
Virginia	25	1995
Washington	50	1995
West Virginia	50	2010

advisory groups to look much more closely at waste management problems and solutions in their own communities, leading to a number of innovative approaches for reducing the amount of refuse destined for landfill burial or incineration.

To attain these admittedly ambitious goals, waste managers must devise innovative strategies for eliciting greater participation in recycling efforts by householders, businesses, and institutions. One of the most successful approaches to increasing rates of residential recycling in recent years has been the introduction of curbside collection programs which make household recycling as easy as setting out the weekly garbage. From just 1000 programs nationwide in 1988, curbside collection was provided by nearly 6700 U.S. municipalities in 1993, serving over 100 million people. Pennsylvania currently is the curbside champion, with 755 programs (Minnesota in second place with 651), but fully 19 states can boast 100 or more such programs, while only Alaska lacks any. Because many cities (e.g. New York, Houston, Philadelphia, Los Angeles) are expanding existing programs to cover additional neighborhoods, growth in curbside service is even greater than the number of new cities participating would suggest. If current trends persist, as expected, it is likely that over half the U.S. population will have access to curbside pickup of recyclables within the next few years.

Once materials are collected through **source separation** programs (which can include curbside collection, neighborhood recycling centers, community drop-boxes, or periodic recycling drives), they must be sorted and baled prior to being shipped to buyers for reprocessing. Forty-five states now have one or more **materials recovery facilities (MRFs**—referred to in recycling jargon as "murfs") where mixed recyclables are prepared for marketing.

In some regions of the country, municipal leaders have opted for an alternative approach to source separation as a means of complying with state-mandated recycling goals. Since even curbside programs, convenient though they are, almost never achieve 100% public participation, some cities don't even make an attempt to involve citizens in recycling efforts. Instead, they simply collect the mixed residential wastes jumbled together in the garbage can—food scraps, old newspapers, dirty diapers, junk mail, empty milk cartons, and so on—and truck them off to a mixed waste recycling facility (not-so-affectionately known in recycling circles as a "**dirty MRF**"). There the recyclable components are pulled out of the waste stream and diverted for processing, while the remainder is either landfilled or made into pellets for burning in an incinerator. Proponents of "dirty MRFs" admit that the facilities are expensive to construct and operate, but point out that, in comparison with source separation programs (i.e. separation by the person who generates the waste, as in curbside collection or neighborhood drop-boxes), mixed waste recovery facilities are theoretically capable of diverting a much higher percentage of recyclables from the waste stream. This is because *all* of a community's refuse is delivered to them, not just that portion removed voluntarily by household waste generators under the source separation scenario. Some local officials favor such facilities because they don't require any public education efforts to persuade

BOX 16-1
In Germany, the Polluter Pays!

Among Europeans, Germans lead the pack in waste generation. Now, thanks to a 1991 law which some describe as "the world's most ambitious solid waste policy," they also have become the world's champion recyclers. Confronted with a population density of more than 600 per square mile (compared to just 74 in the U.S.), the German government realized that space for land disposal of refuse was in short supply. With resource constraints in mind and with the active support of an already environmentally aware citizenry, German lawmakers enacted the "Ordinance on the Avoidance of Packaging Waste," mandating that manufacturers, distributors, and retailers collect and recycle all 7–8 million tons of packaging wastes they generate annually. Since packaging materials comprise fully half the volume of all residential waste in Germany (one-third by weight), requiring those who create the waste to be responsible for its ultimate recovery has had a revolutionary impact on waste management practices in that country—an impact that is being closely monitored by Germany's European neighbors and followed with interest by recycling advocates in the United States.

The German law has a 3-pronged focus:

1. *Transport packaging*— shipping containers, pallets, corrugated cardboard or any other containers used to deliver products to stores must be taken back by the manufacturer of those products; alternatively, the manufacturer or distributor can arrange for a third party to pick up the material or pay the retailer to have it recycled. Faced with this imperative, some manufacturers have developed new forms of reusable packaging; one recently patented shipping container designed for a leading German supermarket chain promises to save a million metric tons of waste annually and could become the standard container of its type across Europe.

2. *Secondary packaging*—the extra cardboard, plastic wrap, blister-packs, and so on, which help the product "sell itself" or prevent pilfering becomes the responsibility of the *retailer*, who must either remove these materials prior to sale or provide specially marked bins near the check-out counter so that customers may discard such packaging themselves if they so choose (and, avid recyclers that they are, many German shoppers do just that, leaving piles of cellophane and other wrapping materials as a not-so-subtle hint to store managers that they would prefer less useless packaging with their purchases!). A number of retailers have responded with such sensible waste-minimization tactics as stocking supermarket shelves with toothpaste tubes minus their boxes. Though a small decrease in the sales of isolated products and a slight increase in thefts have been reported, retailers are solving such problems by changing the location of such items within their stores. Estimates for the amount of secondary packaging reduction achieved under this program range from 40 to 80%. While the overall impact of this decline on Germany's total solid waste stream is relatively minor (even before diversion, secondary packaging constituted less than 0.5% of MSW in Germany), it is symbolic of consumers' commitment to the ideal of a more environmentally sustainable economy.

3. *Primary packaging*—the myriad cans, bottles, boxes, tubes, and other types of containers which constitute two-thirds of all packaging wastes pose by far the largest collection and recycling challenges. The most controversial aspect of

Germany's 1991 ordinance was its requirement that retail stores take back primary packaging wastes unless German industry can meet stringent recycling targets, phased in over a several-year period. Under the law, product *manufacturers* are to cover all costs of collecting and recycling used packaging material.

The prospect of having to cope with mountains of paper, plastic, and foil spurred nearly 600 German companies to form a new not-for-profit consortium, **Duales System Deutschland (DSD)**, and to implement Germany's acclaimed "**Green Dot**" system. Under this arrangement, officially initiated on January 1, 1993, DSD has provided specially designed yellow collection bins in neighborhoods throughout the country where any used packaging material bearing the Green Dot logo can be deposited for collection and recycling (thereby relieving individual retailers of this responsibility). In order for their packages to carry the Green Dot symbol, manufacturers must pay a variable licensing fee, dependent on the type and recycling costs of the packaging material in question (highest fees are for plastic, the lowest for glass). Signing on with DSD guarantees manufacturers a recycling market for their packaging; as a result, less than a year after the ordinance was enacted, 5000 licenses had been purchased and today at least 90% of the packages on German store shelves are emblazoned with a Green Dot. Licensing costs paid by manufacturers are, predictably, passed on to consumers in the form of higher product prices.

Unfortunately for DSD, the original fee schedule considerably underestimated the costs of implementing the program and repeatedly during 1993 financial arrangements had to be renegotiated to stave off bankruptcy; even with its new lease on life, however, the program is expensive (it is estimated that in 1995 DSD expen-

ditures will amount to approximately $30 for every resident of the country). Shaky finances were not the only problems to develop during the program's first year in operation. DSD had seriously underestimated the German penchant for recycling. Since prevailing fees for residential waste collection services are quite high in Germany, householders enthusiastically utilized the "free" services provided by DSD bins and deposited a much greater volume of materials than the company had anticipated—including items they never intended to pick up! Consistently plastics have posed the most vexing problems. Whereas DSD had expected to collect 100,000 of the 928,000 tons of plastic packaging sold during 1993, the company was deluged with nearly 400,000 tons—an amount far exceeding Germany's plastic recycling capacity. To the chagrin of Germany's neighbors, much of this excess was dumped on world markets (some was found illegally stockpiled in French quarries!), depressing secondary materials prices as far away as East Asia. While domestic recycling capacity thus far has been adequate for absorbing the volumes of glass, paper, and steel packaging DSD has collected, it remains seriously lacking for plastic, aluminum, and aseptic (composite) containers. Recycling quota schedules established by the 1991 legislation, calling for the amount of plastic recycled to rise from a mandated 9% in 1993 to 64% in July 1995, caused such dismay within German business circles that in 1994 the timetable was revised, reducing the targeted plastics recycling rate to 60% and extending the date for compliance to 1998. Requests by the plastics industry that the government recognize incineration with energy recovery as a form of "recycling" for plastics have been rejected, but officials have agreed to permit half the quota to be met through "hydration"—heating plastic waste to produce oil—a process which can be carried out at existing oil refineries at a considerably lower cost than conventional plastics recycling.

Despite complaints that the program was implemented too quickly, before needed infrastructure was in place, it remains popular with the German public and has served as a model for similar new laws in France and the Netherlands. By "internalizing" the environmental costs of packaging in the price of the product, Germany has provided manufacturers with a marketplace incentive to incorporate pollution prevention concepts into the design of their products. Though ostensibly intended to boost recycling rates and thus ease pressure on landfills and incinerators, Germany's innovative ordinance may be most significant in its impact on waste reduction. Already four out of five German manufacturers are reportedly shifting to lighter packages, making drastic cuts in hard-to-recycle packaging materials such as polyvinyl chloride, blister packs, and polystyrene, and in some cases—as with large appliances—avoiding the use of packages altogether. As a result, the total amount of packaging in Germany dropped by 4% during 1993, with plastic steadily being replaced by paperboard and glass. If nothing else, Germany's ongoing experiment with the Green Dot system has shown that when financial incentives or disincentives are built into the cost of a product, consumers and manufacturers alike respond in ways that noticeably impact the composition of the municipal waste stream.

References

Fishbein, Bette. 1994. *Germany, Garbage, and Green Dot: Challenging the Throwaway Society*. Inform, Inc.

LWVEF. 1993. *The Garbage Primer*. Lyons & Burford.

or coerce residents into altering long-established waste-generating behavior. Conversely, opponents contend that, aside from their high cost, "dirty MRFs" are environmentally unsound because the *quality* of potentially recyclable materials pulled from the mixed waste stream is so poor as to have little or no value to a secondary materials industry which demands as clean and homogeneous a waste stream as possible (i.e. who would want to buy paper for recycling once it's smeared with tomato sauce from discarded pizza? How could glass be recovered for shipment to a processor when scattered in small fragments among banana peels, dirty facial tissue, and used tea bags?). Despite such objections, there are currently 74 "dirty MRFs" operating throughout the United States, as compared with 776 materials recovery facilities that process recyclables only (Steuteville 1994a).

Although public response to the concept of resource recovery has generally been enthusiastic, several obstacles have prevented Americans from realizing the full potential of "turning garbage into gold." While increasing the percentage of households actually participating in recycling programs is one challenge, an even greater one is developing strong, reliable markets for secondary materials. Unfortunately, collection is not synonymous with recycling—"it's not recycled until it's reused!" If the tons of paper, glass, and metal brought to a drop-off center or set out for curbside pickup have no market, or if the prevailing price for such items is less than the cost of transporting materials to the buyer, resource recovery efforts are doomed to fail. In recent years the oversupply of recyclable materials—a surfeit of riches brought about largely due to the proliferation of curbside collection programs—has caused a precipitous decline in market prices for scrap over the past several years, imperiling the economic viability of recycling efforts. In many communities the cost of collecting and processing recyclables far exceeds their resale value. Even taking the avoided costs of disposal into consideration, most municipal recycling programs operate at a substantial loss. Reversing this situation requires stimulation of market demand, or "closing the loop" in a cyclic process in which products are used, collected, fabricated into new products, purchased, and used again. Weakness in the demand side of the equation is the greatest obstacle to increasing U.S. recycling rates and exists due to a number of factors:

1. Virgin materials are generally cost-competitive with, or cheaper than, secondary materials and are usually perceived by manufacturers as superior in quality.

2. The composition of virgin materials is usually more homogeneous than that of secondary materials.

3. Technology to utilize virgin materials is well established, while that to process waste materials is not perfected to the same extent.

4. Synthetics are often combined with natural materials, making it difficult or impossible to recycle the latter.

5. Artificial economic barriers (e.g. tax depletion allowances, differential freight rates, government subsidies to producers of virgin materials) discriminate against secondary materials.

In an effort to promote recycling, governments at the federal, state, and local levels are pursuing a number of options to boost the supply of high-quality recyclables or to stimulate market demand. Among the legislative approaches to increase the amounts of material diverted through source separation efforts are the setting of "rates and dates" as previously described, as well as the passage of "**Bottle Bills**," laws currently in effect in nine states (Oregon, Vermont, Maine, Michigan, Iowa, Connecticut, Massachusetts, Delaware, and New York) which require consumers to pay a refundable deposit on beer and soft drink containers. First adopted by Oregon in 1972, bottle bills were originally intended to combat littering, a task at which they were resoundingly successful. Surveys performed a few years after bottle bills took effect documented a 75–86% drop in the number of beverage containers discarded along roadsides in comparison with predeposit days (although some slovenly individuals persist in tossing cans and bottles away even in bottle bill states, there is now financial motivation for others to retrieve them). Bottle bills have subsequently proven themselves equally effective at boosting recycling rates for aluminum, glass, and PET plastic. Data from bottle bill states indicate that over 80% of the beverage containers sold in these states are ultimately recycled—a considerably higher proportion than prevails in states without bottle bills. California has adopted a modified bottle bill which avoids payment of a deposit at time of purchase but allows consumers to collect 2½–5 cents (depending on container size) for each bottle or can they return to a designated redemption center. Florida recently pioneered a slightly different concept in fee legislation targeted at container packaging. In 1993 the state implemented its **advance disposal fee (ADF)** which assesses one cent (collected at the wholesale, rather than the retail, level) on bottles, cans, jars, and beverage containers ranging from five ounces to one gallon in size—*if* that form of packaging is not being recycled at a minimum rate of 50% (since aluminum and steel containers already feature recovery rates in excess of 50%, they are not affected by Florida's mandate).

Another popular legislative trend in recent years has been the prohibition of landfill disposal of such materials as yard wastes, lead-acid batteries, whole tires, and used motor oil. While the main purpose of these bans has been to conserve landfill space or to prevent the formation of toxic leachates, their enactment has greatly enhanced the amount of these materials diverted to recycling centers or composting facilities since there's now nowhere else for them to go!

Minimum recycled content mandates have become an increasingly popular method of creating market demand for old newspaper, glass, and plastic—even telephone directories! Such laws require that targeted products contain a certain percentage of recycled material. For example, 13 states mandate that newspapers contain a specified minimum percentage of recycled fiber, while an additional 15 have negotiated voluntary agreements with newspaper publishers on recycled content of newsprint (Steuteville, 1994b). While unpopular within the newspaper industry, these mandates were adopted in an attempt to ease the glut of old newsprint, caused by an oversupply and too little demand. Florida has opted for a somewhat different solution to the same problem by imposing a 50-cent per ton tax on newsprint containing less than 50% recycled fiber. The success of these initiatives is evident in forecasts that U.S. newspaper publishers will increase their purchases of recycled content newsprint from the current 15% level to 40–50% by the end of the decade (Alexander, 1994).

Government procurement policies which require government agencies, state universities, and public schools to purchase supplies that are recyclable or contain recycled material have long been advocated as a means to promote market demand for recyclables. Since the purchases of goods and services by federal, state, and local governments in the United States cumulatively amount to 20% of the GNP, use of government purchasing power in favor of secondary materials could provide an important boost to the recycling industry. Accordingly, by the early 1990s, 16 states were allocating a portion of their procurement budget to buy recycled products, while 27 permitted government offices to pay somewhat more for recycled products than for comparable items made of virgin material (League of Women Voters, 1993). In a move widely praised by recycling advocates, President Clinton in 1993 signed an executive order requiring that all agencies of the federal government purchase paper containing a minimum 20% recycled content by 1995, a figure slated to rise to 25% by the year 2000. Since the federal government currently uses

BOX 16-2

At ISU, Campus Recycling Is for the Cows!

At Illinois State University, students who grew up with admonishments to "Clean your plate!" ringing in their ears no longer need feel guilty if their "eyes are bigger than their stomachs" when passing through the cafeteria line. Wasteful pitching of half-eaten sandwiches, overcooked "mystery meat," or picked-over salads into garbage dumpsters is now a thing of the past, thanks to an innovative campus recycling experiment attracting attention nationwide. Today, students in ISU's four largest residence hall complexes can discard unwanted food, content in the knowledge that their rejects are not destined for landfill disposal. Instead, their bread crusts, orange peels, dirty napkins, paper cups, and virtually all the rest of the approximately 1½ tons of food and paper waste generated daily at campus dining centers are used to supplement the diets of cattle at the ISU farm.

The unusual project, the first of its kind in the United States, is intended to demonstrate the potential for beneficial reuse of cafeteria wastes, thereby easing pressure on landfill space and cutting university expenditures for waste disposal. Directed by Professor of Agriculture Dr. Paul Walker, in cooperation with ISU's Office of Residential Life, the five-year demonstration project was initiated during the 1993–94 academic year.

The process of resource recovery commences in the residence hall kitchens where uneaten or discarded foods, along with paper wastes, are run through large Hobart pulpers, producing a homogenous slurry which Dr. Walker describes as having "the consistency of strained vegetable soup." Virtually all the biodegradable cafeteria wastes are pulped in this manner, with the exception of grease, which is sent off-campus for rendering, and bones, which are diverted for composting. The pulped material is then transported to the ISU farm where it is mixed in a 50:50 ratio with corn silage (some corn is added also); the resultant mixture is then fed to cattle. Preliminary data indicate that this novel approach to food waste management is highly successful. Cattle accept the pulped food waste without hesitation and, in terms of weight gain and general performance, do equally well on either pulped food wastes or conventional rations. Thus the potential for using pulped food wastes as a feed supplement for animals on a maintenance diet appears quite good. If results at the conclusion of the project are as promising as early data suggest, many other institutions, as well as large hotel/restaurant complexes, may decide that the food waste management approach pioneered by Illinois State could cut their food waste disposal costs as well.

In the meantime, Dr. Walker has several other "irons in the fire" in an effort to reap agricultural benefits from recycling programs. Research is underway to assess the feasibility of combining pulped food wastes with ground newspapers—another waste material in over-abundant supply—then spreading the materials in windrows (long rows piled outdoors) to produce compost. Investigations are also proceeding on the feasibility of combining pulped food wastes with raw corn and putting the mixture through an extruder in a process which heats and then dries the material, resulting in a more digestible, pelletized product amenable to shipping. Yet another project focuses on ensiling food wastes with ground newspapers to produce cattle feed (an earlier project had demonstrated that up to 25% of a cow's diet can consist of newsprint when mixed with grass clippings and ensiled for several weeks prior to feeding).

While the final results of these investigations won't be known for several years, the residence hall food recycling efforts are already saving the university substantial sums in landfill costs and lower feed bills at the university farm. More significantly, ISU is blazing a trail which many other institutions may emulate in the years ahead as "reduce-reuse-recycle" becomes more than just a catchy slogan.

Reference

Dr. Paul Walker, Professor, Dept. of Agriculture, Illinois State University, personal communication, 1994.

300,000 tons of paper annually (about 2% of all the printing and writing paper produced in the U.S. each year), this requirement will generate significant new market demand for recycled fiber—a demand that will be further enhanced if states opt to follow the federal lead.

Whether such active government support for "demand-side" recycling efforts is economically justified remains a matter of intense controversy. Recycling advocates contend that the environmental and resource conservation benefits of recycling, along with avoided costs of disposal (i.e. the money saved by avoiding landfill or incinerator tipping fees), make recycling a better deal than a comparison of costs and revenue would suggest at first glance. Critics respond that recycling can benefit society in many ways, but only when programs are carried out in an economically efficient manner. They argue that government policymakers should not try to skew marketplace decisions through such demand-side measures as minimum recycled content legislation, but rather should pursue whichever waste management method is most efficient and cost-effective, even if this means reverting to landfill disposal or incineration of those materials for which the cost of collection and processing far outstrips their market value (Boerner and Chilton, 1994). As Congress begins reauthorization hearings on federal waste management legislation, these differences in viewpoint will undoubtedly be topics of hot debate.

Composting

Since the late 1980s, proliferation of state mandates prohibiting the landfilling of yard wastes has led to an explosive increase in municipal composting facilities in the United States. By the end of 1993, 23 states had enacted such bans, and over 3000 city-sponsored programs are now in effect nationwide (bans on the landfilling of yard wastes have also contributed to booming sales of mulching mowers; results from a four-year demonstration project conducted by the Rodale Institute concluded that use of mulching mowers produces healthier lawns with fewer weeds and no thatch buildup). While a number of European countries have long recognized that composting of organic household waste can reduce the amount of refuse requiring disposal, consideration of composting as a viable waste management alternative in the United States is a much more recent phenomenon. Even though readily decomposable food and yard wastes make up about 30% of the U.S. urban waste stream (considerably more during the warmer months of the year, less during the winter), perceived lack of demand for the finished product, plus the ease and low cost of landfilling, led city officials to dismiss composting as an impractical venture. That attitude has now been transformed by the realization that it makes little sense to devote valuable landfill space to grass clippings and autumn leaves when such materials could be converted into a useful and environmentally beneficial product. Nor are yard wastes the only potentially compostable materials in MSW. Several dozen communities have proceeded to build composting plants to process the entire organic portion of residential and commercial wastes—food scraps, soiled paper, etc.—removing only noncompostable (but still recyclable) glass, metal, and plastics, as well as any hazardous materials. Though questions have been raised about the quality of mixed waste compost and thus its acceptability to end-users, efforts to educate citizens on the importance of source separation have helped to prevent contamination of the final product and to avoid the loss of potentially compostable materials.

A form of resource recovery, composting utilizes natural biochemical decay processes to convert organic wastes into a humus-like material, suitable for use as a soil conditioner. Although its nutrient content is too low to consider it a fertilizer, compost greatly improves soil structure and porosity, aids in water infiltration and retention, increases soil aeration, and slows erosion. Co-composting of yard wastes with municipal sewage sludge (another increasingly difficult-to-dispose-of waste product), now being practiced in a number of communities, enhances the nitrogen content of the finished product and makes it more valuable for agricultural uses.

A variety of methods for converting wastes to compost are currently in use, ranging from the low-tech, relatively inexpensive **windrow** technique, where long rows of wastes are piled outdoors and mechanically turned periodically to aerate the mass, to highly sophisticated, expensive **in-vessel** operations or processes in which pumps mechanically aerate windrows ("**aerated static pile**"), hastening decay and eliminating the need for frequent turning. Choice of the most appropriate composting method depends on the needs and resources of the community in question: if land is abundant and funding scarce, the windrow method may be the best option—though it often requires two or three years for complete breakdown of wastes to occur if the piles are turned only once or twice annually. If available space is at a premium and rapid turnover of wastes desirable, a community might be wise to choose a more high-tech method, provided it can afford the considerably higher price tag associated with such facilities. Whatever the technology, the composting process consists of four basic steps:

1. *Preparation*—incoming wastes are shredded to a relatively uniform size; in most composting operations, nonbiodegradable materials such as glass, metal, plastics, tires, and so on are separated from the compostable wastes. In some composting

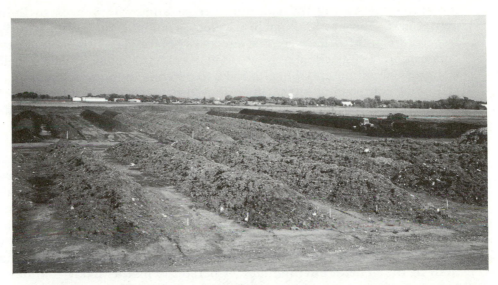

Windrow technique: long rows of composting wastes are piled outdoors and periodically aerated. [Illinois Department of Energy and Natural Resources]

operations, sewage sludge or animal manures are added to the refuse at this point.

2. *Digestion*—microbes naturally present in the waste materials or special bacterial inoculants sprayed on the refuse are utilized to break down organic waste materials. While digestion may be either aerobic or anaerobic, aerobic systems are generally preferred due to shorter time periods required and fewer odor problems. In aerobic decomposition, heat given off by microbial respiration raises the temperature in the windrows well above the 140°F necessary to kill fly eggs, weed seeds, or pathogenic organisms.

3. *Curing*—after digestion of simpler carbonaceous materials is complete, additional curing time is allowed to permit microbes to break down cellulose and lignin in the waste.

4. *Finishing*—to produce an acceptable finished product, compost may be put through screens and grinders to remove non-digested materials and create a uniform appearance. Some composting facilities bag or package the finished product to facilitate marketing or distribution.

While the public rightly regards composting as an environmentally desirable method of organic waste management, composting facilities do not always make good neighbors. Some have been forced to close due to problems with objectionable odors—problems which are gradually being solved as operators compare notes and learn techniques for managing trouble-free facilities. Another recently raised public health issue related to composting operations is their potential to emit **bioaerosols**, tiny airborne particles of microorganisms whose inhalation has been blamed for ailments ranging from a runny nose and watery eyes to flu-like symptoms. Bioaerosols, such as spores of the ubiquitous fungus *Aspergillus fumigatus*, were first cited as a potential environmental health concern in 1992 when a New Jersey epidemiologist testified before Congress about potential health risks to persons living within a two-mile radius of composting sites. Since that time bioaerosols have attracted intensive scrutiny and have prompted organized community opposition to siting of compost facilities in several localities. Representatives of the composting industry argue that any fears are vastly exaggerated, stating that public exposure to *Aspergillus* emissions from composting are negligible when the process is performed correctly. A recently issued report, jointly sponsored by the EPA, USDA, NIOSH, and the Composting Council, tends to support industry's contention. Conceding that exposure to bioaerosols could be life-threatening if inhaled by individuals with suppressed immune systems, the report nevertheless points out that the level of such particles is no higher in the vicinity of composting operations than in the general environment. A person is just as likely to inhale *A. fumigatus* spores while mowing the lawn, raking leaves, or cleaning the attic as by living near a composting facility. Experts report that *Aspergillus* at composting sites originates primarily from the storage of bulking agents such as wood chips, with airborne spores being released at the time of initial mixing (the steam rising off the top of windrows does *not* appear to be a major source). Operational considerations such as moisture and dust control and minimization of handling can significantly mitigate bioaerosol emissions. While authorities agree that more research is needed, the general consensus at present is that bioaerosols *do not* present concerns serious enough to warrant a reconsideration of municipal composting operations (Greczyn, 1994).

In the past, the difficulty of finding outlets for municipal compost was a major stumbling block in convincing local officials to consider composting as a waste management strategy. In recent years, however, cities' marketing efforts and increased public awareness of compost's desirability as a soil conditioner have created sufficient demand among landscaping firms, nurseries, parks departments, and home gardeners to provide a ready outlet. This growing willingness to use compost, coupled with improvements in composting technology and a national need to curtail the flood of urban refuse destined for increasingly valuable landfill space, suggests that municipal composting will constitute an increasingly significant waste management alternative in the years ahead.

Waste-to-Energy Incineration

Prior to passage of the 1970 Clean Air Act, burning of urban refuse at large municipal incinerators was the waste disposal method of choice in a number of communities where the high cost of land, unavailability of suitable sites, or neighborhood opposition to siting made landfilling unfeasible. By the 1960s, almost 300 municipal incinerators were operating in the United States. As the decade of the 1970s ushered in an era of strict air quality control regulations, however, most of these incinerators closed down, unable to comply with the new emission standards. Studies indicated that in some large cities, close to 20% of all particulate pollutants were coming from municipal incinerators (Melosi, 1981).

Today only about 10% of U.S. municipal solid waste is incinerated. However, since the early 1980s as the nation's garbage woes continued to mount, interest in burning as an attractive waste disposal option has been revived by the advent of a new generation of incinerators: **waste-to-energy (WTE)** plants. These facilities not only burn refuse, thereby reducing its volume by 80–90%, but also capture the heat of combustion in the form of salable electricity or process steam. Hundreds of municipalities have already committed themselves to this new technology as the most feasible alternative to disappearing landfill space; at present there are approximately 150 waste-to-energy incinerators operating in 34 states, with 40 more planned for the near future. Ranking third in the established waste management hierarchy, WTE-incineration is expected play an important role in any comprehensive approach to managing municipal solid wastes.

Most WTE plants are "**mass burn**" facilities, accepting unsegregated wastes loaded onto a moving grate which feeds into the furnace; some mass burn plants combine recycling activities with incineration, separating out glass and metals prior to burning. Units come in various sizes; large facilities built on site have capacities ranging up to 3300 tons/day, while modular types can be supplied to be economically feasible for communities producing as little as 100 tons of refuse per day. By contrast, **refuse-derived fuel (RDF)** plants, comprising just 20% of WTE facilities in the United States, first remove noncombustibles, then process the remaining wastes by shredding them with hammermills to produce a pelletized fuel which can be mixed with coal and burned in ordinary boilers.

The euphoria which just a decade ago welcomed WTE incinerators as the ideal solution to our disposal dilemmas is now giving way to a more cautious appraisal, as concerns are raised about possible toxic air emissions, especially dioxins, furans, and heavy metals (e.g. lead, cadmium, and mercury). Proponents of the technology insist such problems can be minimized through good emission controls and proper plant operation; in 1991 tighter emissions limitations required by Clean Air Act Amendments for municipal incinerators were approved by EPA, requiring that facilities install state-of-the-art equipment to control acid gases, metal particulates, and organic products of incomplete combustion, such as dioxin. Smokestacks are now being fitted with acid gas scrubbers, baghouse filters for trapping metal particulates, and activated carbon injection systems for capturing mercury vapors. By utilizing advanced combustion controls, plant operators can maintain furnace temperatures high enough to prevent dioxin formation and to ensure a more complete burn. Disposal of the considerable volumes of incinerator ash generated by large WTE facilities has been another contentious issue. Incineration is not a complete waste management method; in general, for every three tons of refuse burned, a ton of ash remains, requiring disposal. Until recently the most prevalent method for managing incinerator ash was to bury it in ordinary sanitary landfills or in "monofills"—facilities which accepted only incinerator ash for disposal. However, concerns that this material frequently contains dangerous levels of heavy metals (particularly the fly ash captured by pollution control equipment), have led to demands that incinerator ash be classified as "hazardous waste," thereby necessitating its disposal at a hazardous waste landfill—at an anticipated 10-fold rise in tipping fees. In May 1994, the U.S. Supreme Court settled the dispute by ruling that ash from municipal incinerators must be tested, using specified laboratory procedures, and if results indicate that the waste is indeed toxic, it must be managed as hazardous waste. This ruling, while greeted initially with dismay by municipalities currently relying on incinerators as a major component of their waste management program, should give a major impetus to resource recovery programs aimed at removing toxics-containing components of the MSW stream—items such as batteries, paint cans, and electrical equipment. Also, by halting the standard practice of combining the often-toxic fly ash with the far more voluminous but much less dangerous bottom ash, incinerator operators can greatly reduce the amount of ash requiring disposal as "hazardous." Pointing out that the Court decision may have provided the stimulus needed to force incinerator operators to do what they should have been doing already, an attorney for the Environmental Defense Fund remarked, "This is not brain surgery. This decision gives municipalities pollution-prevention incentives that are realistically available" (Greenhouse, 1994).

Nevertheless, opponents remain wary, fearing that cities jumping on the WTE bandwagon are going to find they've simply traded one set of environmental problems for another. Perhaps the major question mark regarding the future of WTE incineration, however, is financing their construction and operation. To remain economically viable, incinerators need a steady supply of trash and a dependable market for the energy they produce—but recent developments make both difficult to guarantee. Competing demands from recycling programs for high-BTU trash and recent court invalidation of local "**flow-control**" ordinances which communities have imposed to ensure incinerators a predictable daily volume of waste have resulted in a number of municipal incinerators operating considerably below their design capacity—a money-losing proposition. WTE incinerators are exorbitantly expensive to construct and operate (as a rough rule-of-thumb, WTE projects average $100,000–$125,000 per ton of daily waste capacity; a city contemplating construction of a typical 1000 ton-per-day facility can thus count on investing well over $100 million). Costs are recovered (hopefully!) through tipping fees (which a *BioCycle* survey of 20 states found averaged $54/ton in 1994) paid by haulers bringing wastes to the facility and through sales of electricity or process steam produced by the plant. Since prevailing regional rates for electricity determine what this amount will be, low power demand reflected in falling prices has caused some communities to cancel plans for incinerator construction, since anticipated revenues from energy sales turned out to be less than originally projected.

The future role of WTE incineration in a comprehensive waste management strategy thus depends not only on how successful source reduction and recycling/composting operations are in minimizing the

BOX 16-3

The Tire Dilemma

The blaze that ignited on Halloween night, 1983, in Winchester, Virginia, was no bonfire for toasting marsh-mallows; the unintended fuel was a stockpile of seven million tires which continued to burn and spew noxious pollutants over the surrounding area until the following June. This incident provided dramatic evidence of the problems posed by one of modern society's most difficult waste disposal challenges—what to do with the more than 240 million car and truck tires which Americans discard every year. When landfilled, tires inevitably work their way up through the soil and pop out at the surface; when piled in waste tire dumps they constitute a fire hazard and mosquito breeding habitat; thoughtlessly scattered about the countryside on rural back roads or along streambanks they constitute a visual blight.

In former years when tires were made almost entirely of natural rubber, worn out tires were generally repro-cessed and used to make new tires. However, with the advent of synthetic rubber and steelbelted radial tires, reprocessing declined and stockpiles of old tires increased dramatically in volume. It is estimated that the United States is currently littered with more than two billion old tires, but relief may be on the horizon with the development of several innovative new approaches to tire recycling.

Although less than a third of the tires discarded each year are now being salvaged, this amount is a considerable improvement over the figures of just a few years ago; while only 24 million tires were diverted from landfills or tire dumps in 1990, by 1992 the number had climbed to 68 million. Over the years a number of imaginative uses have been devised for whole scrap tires: highway crash barriers, play-ground equipment, artificial reefs, even as quick-start planters for tomatoes or squash vines. Other tires have been cut or punched to fashion shoe soles, dock bumpers, or floor mats. Such uses, however, consumed but a minuscule portion of the nation's stockpile of tire discards. In recent years, several new approaches to tire recycling offer much greater hope for beneficial reuse of what today constitutes a troublesome component of MSW.

Of all the various uses for old tires today, **energy recovery** constitutes by far the most important. With a BTU content of 15,000 per pound (one-fourth higher than that of coal), tires release a great amount of energy when burned. Because their sulfur content is lower than that of most coal deposits, substituting tires for coal can reduce pollutant SO_2 emissions. A whole-tire incinerator located in Modesto, California, adjacent to the world's largest tire pile, has been in operation since 1988, burning tires at the rate of 700 per hour to generate power for Pacific Gas & Electric. Other facilities not equipped to incinerate whole tires stoke their boilers with *TDF (tire-derived-fuel)*, produced by shredding tires into small chips 2 inches square or less. In 1994, Illinois Power Company, encouraged by the Illinois Department of Energy and Natural Resources, began burning 7.5 million tires per year at a power plant near St. Louis to test the feasibility of TDF for electrical power generation. In recent years cement kilns have emerged as major potential consumers of both whole tires and TDF. By late 1993, 22 cement plants in 18 states were using tires as supplemental fuel—up from just 2 in 1990; many other cement kiln operators indicate they, too, may opt to burn tires in the near future. Since nearly one-third of the approximately 200 cement plants operating in the U.S. are preheater units, capable of using tires as fuel, the cement industry could emerge as a very significant market for scrap tires. According to some analysts, such a development would represent a win-win situation for both the cement industry, which would get a high-quality fuel at lower cost than it is now paying for coal, and for the environment. Thanks to the high temperature and long fuel residence time in cement kilns, tire combustion is near-total, preventing formation of objectionable by-products such as the inky smoke and offensive odor that plague some tire-burning operations. Another advantage to the industry of burning tires is that the steel content of steel-belted radial tires can substitute in part for the iron oxide required for cement production, constituting an additional saving on material costs. Because nearly all the components in a tire are thus either destroyed, incorporated into the final product, or captured in air pollution control equipment, there is no generation of ash requiring disposal. The Scrap Tire Management Council suggests that if growth trends in tire utilization rates persist, cement kilns could be burning 100 million scrap tires annually by the late 1990s—more than 40% of those generated each year.

A further dent in the nation's heap of discarded tires could result from federal legislation passed in 1991. Section 1038 of the Intermodal Surface Transportation Efficiency Act (ISTEA— dubbed ''Ice Tea'') mandates that, beginning in 1994, states receiving federal funds for highway construction must use rubberized asphalt (made by combining crumb rubber from ground-up tires with asphalt) for at least 5% of the total tonnage applied to roads—a percentage which is to rise by an additional 5% annually until 1997 when it tops out at 20%. The rationale behind this requirement is two-fold: assist in easing the scrap tire glut and build better highways. Proponents of rubberized asphalt insist that the

material is quieter and more durable than conventional asphalt and enhances traction. On the other hand, it is also nearly twice as expensive. However, recent experimentation by the California Department of Transportation suggests that rubberized asphalt can be laid at half the thickness of conventional highway material; if this proves to be the case, any cost differential evaporates. Opponents of mandated rubberized asphalt use charge that not enough is known about potential health danger to highway construction workers exposed to fumes nor about the recyclability of rubberized asphalt—i.e. can such pavement itself be reclaimed and reused again in a new asphalt mixture when the time comes for inevitable highway repairs? Tests conducted in Michigan, New Jersey, and Florida indicate no problems on either count. Indeed, Florida officials were so impressed with test results that in 1994 that state's transportation department began using crumb rubber on a regular basis as a modifier in its asphalt mixtures. In addition to improving pavement quality, Florida's shift toward utilization of rubberized asphalt should help the state to dispose of two million scrap tires each year. New Jersey is similarly excited by the material's potential. In an action going far beyond any federal mandate, the governor has signed an executive order requiring the incorporation of recycled rubber into at least *40% of the asphalt pavement laid by the state starting in 2001*, if the price of the material is competitive with that of conventional asphalt.

Aside from energy recovery and rubberized asphalt, a variety of other end-uses are being explored to deplete the backlog of old tires. A number of state governments have provided grants, loans, or tax credits to businesses or individuals, hoping to spur market development for used tires. Illinois has funded experimentation with scrap tire chips for use as a ground cover beneath playground equipment; Maryland is evaluating tire chips as a replacement for drainage gravel in landfills and as a bulking agent in compost piles, looking at recycled rubber sheets as landfill liners, and experimenting with crumb rubber as a soil amendment; Minnesota is funding studies on the use of crumb rubber mixed with a binder as spray roofing material. The proliferation of state incentive programs, coupled with government procurement mandates and technological advances in

methods of tire recovery all offer promise of an ultimate solution to the tire dilemma.

References

Blumenthal, Michael. 1993. ''The Growing Use of Scrap Tires in Cement Kilns.'' *Resource Recycling* 12, no. 12 (Dec).

Gorman, Jim. 1993. ''Where the Rubber *Is* the Road.'' *Audubon*, (Nov./Dec).

Sikora, Mary. 1994. ''Market Development Is Key to Tire Recovery.'' *Resource Recycling* 13, no. 4 (April).

amount of refuse destined for disposal, but also on such unpredictable factors as the extent of economic recovery (good economy equals good WTE prospects); demand for energy (high demand equals brighter future for WTE); congressional initiatives (will Congress impose a legislative moratorium on incinerator construction?); EPA decisions (will the agency mandate that communities achieve specified recycling goals before building new incinerators?); and trends in landfill tipping fees (sharp increases could make incineration more cost-competitive, and vice-versa!)(Arrandale, 1993). While WTE incineration is the preeminent MSW management method in Japan and a number of European countries, its future on this side of the ocean remains difficult to predict.

Hazardous Wastes

Late in the summer of 1978 the name of a small residential subdivision in the city of Niagara Falls, New York, entered the American vocabulary and became a household word almost overnight, symbolizing the dangers of our chemical age. The tragic sequence of events which unfolded at Love Canal epitomizes the dangers facing millions of citizens in thousands of communities across the nation as a result of our indiscriminate use and careless disposal of hazardous chemicals.

The Love Canal Story

The origin of the chemical dumpsite which became the focus of worldwide attention in the late 1970s can be traced to the mid-1890s when William T. Love began construction of a canal intended to serve as a navigable power channel, connecting the Upper Niagara to the Niagara Escarpment about seven miles downstream, thereby bypassing the Falls.

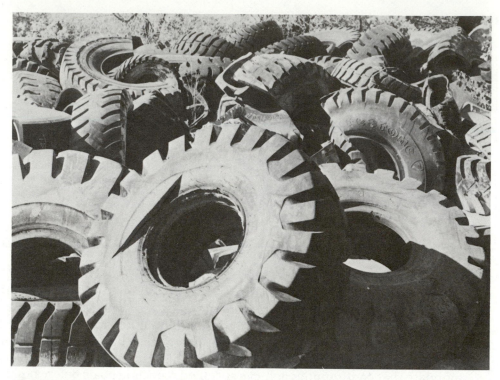

Discarded tires litter the American landscape and pose one of our more difficult solid waste disposal problems. [Author's Photo]

At the point where Mr. Love's canal was intended to reenter the river, the intention was to construct a model industrial city which would be provided with cheap, abundant hydroelectric power. Unfortunately for Mr. Love, his development company went bankrupt shortly after construction of the canal had begun; the project was abandoned, leaving a waterway approximately 3000 feet long, 10 feet deep, and 60 feet wide. For many years, residents of this area on the outskirts of town used the canal for recreational fishing and swimming; in 1927 the land was annexed by the city. In 1942 Hooker Chemical Company (now a subsidiary of Occidental Petroleum), one of several major chemical industries located in Niagara Falls, received permission to dump chemical wastes into the canal, which it proceeded to do from that time until 1952 (in 1947 Hooker purchased the canal, along with two 70-feet-wide strips of land adjacent to the canal on each side). During this time more than 21,000 tons of chemical wastes—acids, alkalis, solvents, chlorinated hydrocarbons, etc.—were disposed of at this site. Only a few homes were present in the area at that time, but old-time residents recall the offensive odors, noxious vapors, and frequent fires which accompanied the dumping.

By 1953 the canal was full and so was topped with soil and eventually acquired a covering of grass and weeds. Hooker then offered to sell the land to the Niagara Falls School Board for the token fee of $1. At the same time company officials pointedly advised school and city administrators that although the site was suitable for a school, parking lot, or playground, any construction activities involving excavation of the area should be avoided to prevent rupturing the dumpsite's clay lining, thereby allowing escape of the impounded chemicals. In 1955 an elementary school and playground were constructed on the site; in 1957 the city began laying storm sewers, roads, and utility lines through the area, disregarding the warnings received a few years earlier. In the years that followed, several hundred modest homes were built in the neighborhood parallel to the banks of the now-invisible canal. Most of the newer residents had no knowledge of the site's past history and, in spite of occasional chemical odors (not considered unusual in a city where chemical manufacturing was a leading industry), few outward signs of trouble were apparent. Unusually heavy precipitation in the mid-1970s, however, was accompanied by some alarming phenomena. Strange-looking, viscous chemicals began oozing through basement walls, floors, and sump holes. Vegetation in yards withered and appeared scorched. Large puddles became permanent backyard features. Holes began to open up in the field which had once been a dumpsite and the tops of corroded 55-gallon drums leaking chemicals could be seen in places protruding from the soil surface. Complaints and fears expressed by citizens were generally downplayed by local authorities who assured them there was nothing about which to be concerned.

By early 1978 pressure from a local congressman and regular critical coverage of events in the Niagara Gazette prompted the U.S. Environmental Protection Agency to undertake a program of air sampling in the basements of Love Canal homes. New York State authorities also began conducting soil analyses and taking samples of residues in sump pumps and storm sewers. The results of these studies indicated that the area was extremely contaminated with more than 200 different chemicals, including 12 known or suspected carcinogens. Benzene, known to be a potent human cancer-causing agent, was readily detected in the air inside many of the houses sampled. Dioxin was subsequently found in high concentrations in some of the soil samples analyzed. State officials in New York estimate that as many as 10% of the chemicals buried at Love Canal may be mutagens, teratogens, or carcinogens. On August 2, 1978, the Health Commissioner of New York publicly proclaimed "the existence of a great and imminent peril to the health of the general public" at Love Canal and advised all pregnant women and families with children under the age of two to leave the area if they could do so. Five days later, President Carter officially declared Love Canal a national emergency.

The months that followed witnessed mass relocation at public expense of residents living closest to the dumpsite, as well as openly expressed fears by those left behind on adjacent streets that their health was similarly endangered. A number of health studies, whose methodology and con-clusions remain highly controversial, suggest that Love Canal residents have experienced statistically significant elevated rates of miscarriage, birth defects, and chromosomal abnormalities. Ultimately 1,004 families were evacuated from Love Canal, their homes purchased by the state. Over 300 of the residences closest to the canal were demolished and the area covered with a protective layer of clay and a synthetic liner to exclude rainwater. Most of the remaining homes were boarded up, awaiting a pending EPA assessment of whether they could ever again be inhabited. Trenches have been dug around the old canal site to capture contaminated groundwater which is then pumped to a treatment center for detoxification. Nearby creeks where high levels of dioxin seepage were detected have been fenced off to protect children and animals. Combined federal and state expenditures for relocating residents, investigating environmental damage, and halting chemical seepage from the site total $150 million, and an additional $32 million has been spent to clean up contaminated creeks and sewers and to determine the future habitability of the neighborhood. The Congressional Office of Technology Assessment estimates that if Hooker had employed current disposal standards and practices, its wastes could have been safely managed for about $2 million in 1979 dollars (Levine, 1982).

Occidental Chemical, which acquired Hooker in a 1968 buy-out, has paid $20 million in out-of-court settlements to affected residents; a federal district court ruling in 1988 held Occidental liable for the cost of previous, ongoing, and future cleanup of the Love Canal site—a figure approximating $250 million. Two years later, the State of New York sued Occidental for an additional $250 million in punitive damages, claiming that its subsidiary Hooker had "displayed reckless disregard for the safety of others." In the spring of 1994, a federal judge ruled against the plaintiff, saying the evidence in the state's case was insufficient; this decision, however, did not alter Occidental's liability for cleanup costs. In the fall of 1988, after reviewing a five-year habitability study of the affected area, New York State Health Commissioner David Axelrod declared that most of the Love Canal neighborhood could be safely resettled by former residents. While the decision was controversial, with some environmentalists warning that "Love Canal is a ticking time bomb," by the summer of 1990 over 200 people had expressed interest in renovated homes selling for 20% less than the prevailing market price. Reassured by government claims that the area no longer presents any threat, new residents have reoccupied several dozen homes in the Love Canal neighborhood, now renamed "Black Creek Village" (Newton and Dillingham, 1994).

The events which transpired at Love Canal cannot be shrugged off as a unique tragedy which unfortunately victimized a few thousand people in western New York State but left the rest of the nation unscathed. Health authorities and environmental agency officials regard Love Canal as but the "tip of the iceberg" in alerting society to the widespread nature of the hazardous waste problem. EPA is currently aware of more than 16,000 hazardous waste dumps scattered across the United States and fear that many of these may be exposing citizens to dangers as serious as those which surfaced at Love Canal. Little wonder that public opinion polls show citizens ranking hazardous waste management issues among their top environmental quality concerns.

What Is "Hazardous" Waste?

In the 1976 Resource Conservation and Recovery Act (RCRA), Congress legally defined hazardous waste as "any discarded material that may pose a substantial threat or potential danger to human health or the environment when improperly handled." EPA has established a two-tier system for determining whether a specific waste is subject to regulation under current hazardous waste management laws:

1. If the substance in question is among the approximately 400 wastes or waste streams itemized in Parts 261.31–33 of the Code of Federal Regulations, it will automatically be subject to regulation as a hazardous waste. Wastes may be placed on the list because of their ability to induce cancer, mutations, or birth defects; because of their toxicity to plants; or because even low doses are fatal to humans. However, the Administrator of EPA can exercise a wide measure of discretion in deciding whether or not to list a particular waste, so a number of potential carcinogens, mutagens, and teratogens are not yet listed as officially "hazardous."

2. In addition to the wastes listed in the federal code, any waste which exhibits one or more of the following characteristics is defined as hazardous and subject to regulation:

    Toxic—wastes such as arsenic, heavy metals, or certain synthetic pesticides are capable of causing either acute or chronic health problems.

    Ignitable—organic solvents, oils, plasticizers, and paint wastes are examples of wastes which are hazardous because they have a flashpoint less than 60°C (140°F) or because they tend to undergo spontaneous combustion. The resultant fires are dangerous not only because of heat and smoke, but also because they can disseminate toxic particles over a wide area.

    Corrosive—substances with a pH of 2 or less or 12.5 and above can eat away at standard container materials or living tissues through chemical action and are termed corrosive. Such wastes, which include acids, alkaline cleaning agents, and battery manufacturing residues, present a special threat to waste haulers who come into bodily contact with leaking containers.

    Reactive—obsolete munitions, wastes from the manufacturing of dynamite or firecrackers, and certain chemical wastes such as picric acid are hazardous because of their tendency to react vigorously with air or water or to explode and generate toxic fumes.

Two other categories of wastes which might logically be considered hazardous—radioactive wastes and potentially infectious medical wastes from hospitals and clinics—are not presently regulated under the same laws as the groups listed above. Radioactive wastes are managed according to regulations adopted by the Nuclear Regulatory Commission under the Atomic Energy Act, while biomedical waste disposal laws vary from state to state. Flagrant incidents of illegal ocean dumping of such wastes during the summer of 1988 attracted widespread media attention, as beaches from Cape Cod to the Carolinas were littered with such unsavory debris as used syringes and blood vials, some of which tested positive for AIDS virus antibodies and hepatitis B antigens. Public outrage generated by this situation resulted in passage of the 1988 Medical Waste Tracking Act, which set up a two-year pilot project to attempt regulation of biomedical wastes through a procedure similar in nature to the manifest system currently required for off-site shipments of hazardous wastes. With the expiration of that program, individual states have, for the most part, adopted medical waste management programs of their own involving the manifesting of such wastes shipped off-site and, in several states, requiring that infectious wastes be "rendered innocuous" in specially licensed high-temperature incinerators—a form of disposal considerably more expensive than sanitary landfilling. Many authorities deplore what they regard as exaggerated public fears about the threats posed by medical wastes. Pointing out that wastes generated by hospitals are no more dangerous than many of the items tossed into the trash by householders (e.g. used syringes from home insulin injections, bloody bandages, outdated medications, etc.) and that not a single case of human illness has been traced to contact with infectious medical waste, they question the public health benefit of strict new regulations which significantly increase national costs for health care.

Generation of Hazardous Wastes

EPA estimates that the United States currently generates approximately 300 million metric tons of industrial hazardous wastes annually, a figure which does not take into account those wastes which are managed illegally. Production of these wastes is not evenly distributed among industries, however. More than 85% of all hazardous wastes are produced by just three major categories of generators: chemicals and allied products, metal-related industries, and petroleum and coal products. Geographic location of these industries, as well as population density, are major determinants of which states are the leading hazardous waste generators.

At the time when new federal waste management regulations went into effect in November 1980, EPA estimated that fully 90% of all hazardous wastes were being disposed of by methods which would not meet government standards. Thanks to what is widely regarded as the most stringent hazardous waste management program in the world, that situation has now markedly improved.

Threats Posed by Careless Disposal

Mismanagement of hazardous wastes can adversely affect human health and environmental quality in a number of ways.

Direct Contact. Direct contact with wastes can result in skin irritation, the initiation of serious chronic illness, or acute poisoning—as in the case of two 9-year-old Tampa boys who were killed in June 1992,

BOX 16-4
Environmental Racism: Dumping on the Poor

In 1982 when civil rights demonstrators in predominantly African-American Warren County, North Carolina, rallied to protest the proposed siting of a PCB landfill in their midst, they may not have realized they were leading the vanguard of a new social movement in the United States. They *did* know they were angry that, once again, a small, poor, politically powerless community of color was being targeted for another **LULU ("locally unwanted land use")**—one which developers would never have dreamed of proposing for a more affluent, white locale. On this occasion, however, the voices of Warren County carried all the way to Congress where Delegate Walter Fauntroy (D.C.) asked the General Accounting Office (GAO) to look into allegations of racial discrimination in the siting of waste facilities. Thus was launched the quest for **environmental equity**—an effort to ensure that environmental risks, where they exist, are fairly distributed across population groups rather than falling disproportionately on those who are already disadvantaged through minority status, low income, or geographic location.

A major contribution to the struggle against environmental racism was the publication in 1987 of a seminal study by the United Church of Christ Commission for Racial Justice, *Toxic Waste and Race in the United States*, detailing for the first time interrelating issues of race, class, and environment across the nation. This work demonstrated that pollution is anything but an "equal opportunity" affliction, blighting and shortening the lives of African-Americans, Latinos, and Native Americans to a far greater extent than white Americans. Some of the more disturbing facts brought to light by this study and by subsequent reports on the same topic by other authors include:

• Although affluent communities tend to generate more waste than poor communities, few waste disposal facilities are proposed and even fewer are actually built in white middle-class areas; in Houston, for example, until the late 1970s all five of the publicly owned landfills and six out of eight municipal incinerators were in predominantly African-American neighborhoods (the 7th was in a Latino section of the city), even though only 28% of Houston's residents are African-American.

• Three-fourths of all U.S. hazardous waste landfills are located in predominantly African-American or Latino communities; a case in point is WMX Technologies' facility in Emelle, Alabama, the largest commercial hazwaste landfill in the United States. Emelle is a small, rural community with a population that is 90% African-American.

• Three out of five African-Americans live in communities with one or more abandoned toxic waste sites; densely populated Southeast Chicago represents a classic example of a highly segregated neighborhood (70% African-American, 11% Latino) which is pockmarked by over 100 abandoned toxic waste dumps and one active commercial hazardous waste landfill.

• Communities where incinerators are proposed have minority populations 60% above the national average; of three WTE incinerators recently proposed for construction in southern California, (two subsequently cancelled), all were targeted for heavily Latino areas.

Federal agencies themselves have been accused of perpetuating environmental injustices. Staff writers at the

National Law Journal charged that EPA was guilty of environmental racism in its implementation of Superfund cleanups, citing evidence of faster action, more thorough remediation, and stricter enforcement of hazwaste regulations in white communities than in areas where large minority populations resided. These inequities prevailed, they asserted, regardless of community income levels—race, and race alone, was the determining factor.

Such findings provided the impetus for a "Conference on Race and the Incidence of Environmental Hazards" held at the University of Michigan in 1990. Following that event, a group of participants wrote to then-EPA Administrator William Reilly, requesting that the agency take action to deal with environmental risks in minority and low-income communities. Reilly responded by forming an Environmental Equity Workgroup, and the agency recently has begun actively investigating environmental discrimination charges under the 1964 Civil Rights Act.

Proponents of environmental justice gained a most important ally in President Bill Clinton who, on February 11, 1994, signed an executive order prohibiting discriminatory practices in any programs receiving federal financial assistance. For the first time, federal agencies must now consider the racial and socioeconomic characteristics of a community prior to launching a new project or issuing new environmental rules. While some business leaders and state regulatory officials worry that the extra layer of review called for by this order will further slow down the facility siting process, environmentalists and civil rights activists praise the President's move as a first step toward preventing the imposition of hazardous waste facilities on the poor and powerless.

Reference

Bullard, Robert D. 1994. "Overcoming Racism in Environmental Decision-making." *Environment*, 36, no. 4 (May).

---

while playing inside a municipal waste bin. Subsequent investigations revealed that the bin, located behind an industrial firm, contained toluene- and acetone-contaminated waste, leading officials to conclude the boys had died due to inhalation of toxic chemical fumes.

Fire and/or Explosions. In April 1980, a spectacular blaze destroyed a riverside warehouse complex in Elizabeth, New Jersey, where 50,000 chemical-containing drums had been sitting for almost 10 years. Such accidents are a constant threat when hazardous wastes are in transit, carelessly stored, or roughly handled. Explosions are a particular threat to workers at landfills accepting hazardous wastes. In Edison, New Jersey, a bulldozer operator who inadvertently crushed a container of flammable phosphorus was burned so quickly that his corpse was discovered with his hand still on the gearshift.

Poison via the Foodchain.   Biomagnification of toxic wastes discharged into the environment can result in the poisoning of animals or humans who consume the toxin indirectly. The tragic outbreak of methyl mercury poisoning at Minamata, Japan, typifies this sort of situation.

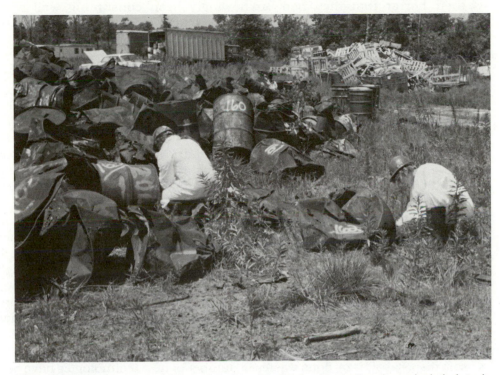

Abandoned hazardous waste dump site where hundreds of corroding drums leak their toxic contents onto the ground, endangering drinking water aquifers below the surface. [Illinois Environmental Protection Agency]

Air Pollution. When toxic wastes are burned at temperatures insufficiently high to completely destroy them, serious air pollution problems can result. Only specialized types of equipment are licensed for the incineration of hazardous wastes, and even these must be carefully monitored while operating to ensure a complete burn.

Surface Water Contamination. Accidental spills or deliberate dumping of hazardous wastes can easily pollute waterways, causing extensive damage to aquatic ecosystems and endangering drinking water supplies. Near Byron, Illinois, a farm stream was seriously polluted with cyanide, heavy metals, and phenols leaching from an abandoned dumpsite where at least 1500 drums of hazardous wastes had been buried. Wildlife, fish, and vegetation along the stream were killed as a result.

Groundwater Contamination. The most common problem associated with poor hazardous waste management is the pollution of aquifers with toxic leachates percolating downward through the soil from landfills or surface impoundments. This type of pollution is particularly insidious because it is seldom discovered until it is too late to do anything about it. Citizens in numerous communities around the nation have discovered to their horror that they had unknowingly been consuming well water contaminated with a variety of toxic chemicals which entered the groundwater supply via seepage from disposal sites.

Methods of Hazardous Waste Disposal

Historically, the largest percentage of hazardous wastes have been disposed of on land, primarily because land disposal, particularly prior to government regulation of hazardous waste management, was by far the cheapest disposal option. During the mid-1970s, for example, almost half of all hazardous wastes, the majority of which were in the form of liquids or sludges, were simply dumped into unlined surface impoundments, technically referred to as "pits, ponds, or lagoons," located on the generators' property (even today, approximately 96% of all hazardous wastes generated in this country are treated or disposed of at the site where they are generated; only 4% of all hazardous wastes are sent off-site for management). These wastes eventually evaporated or percolated into the soil, often resulting in groundwater contamination. Other wastes, about 30% of the total, were buried in sanitary landfills, easily subject to leaching, and another 10% were burned in an uncontrolled manner. None of these methods would be in compliance with current regulations.

Although many citizens are convinced that no methods exist for the safe disposal of hazardous wastes, a number of new technologies have been developed which avoid most of the shortcomings inherent in past hazardous waste management practices. All such methods, not surprisingly, are considerably more expensive than simply dumping wastes in a pit or a municipal landfill, and thus were not widely utilized until strict regulatory action was taken by Congress. A listing of legal hazardous waste disposal options would include the following.

Secure Chemical Landfill. Generally, the cheapest method of hazardous waste disposal is the so-called "secure" chemical landfill, a specially designed earthen excavation constructed in such a way as to contain dangerous chemicals and to prevent them from escaping into the environment through leaching or vaporization. In the past, secure landfills frequently differed from sanitary landfills only in that they were topped with a layer of clay to keep water out of the trenches in which chemical drums had been placed. This of course did not prevent chemical seepage from contaminating water supplies. Under current RCRA standards, a secure chemical landfill must be located above the 100-year floodplain and away from fault zones; it must contain double liners of clay or synthetic materials to keep leaching to a minimum; a network of pipes must be laid to collect and control polluted rainwater and leachate accumulating in the landfill; and monitoring wells must be installed to check the quality of any groundwater deposits in the area (surface water supplies must also be monitored by the landfill operator). In spite of these precautions, most experts agree that there is no way to guarantee that sometime in the future contaminants will not migrate from the landfill site. Liners eventually

Figure 16-4 A Secure Landfill

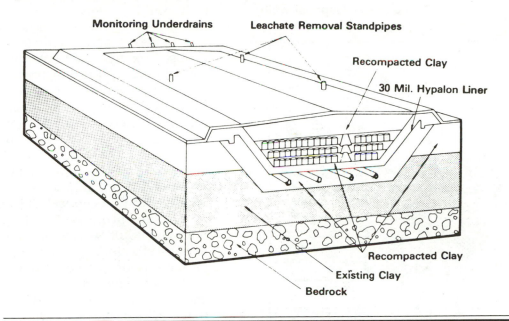

crack; soil can shift or settle. Since many chemical wastes remain hazardous more or less indefinitely, serious pollution problems can occur many years after a secure chemical landfill has been closed and forgotten. Many authorities feel that although chemical landfills are legal, they are the least acceptable method of managing hazardous wastes.

Since 1984 when more stringent requirements for groundwater monitoring, minimum technology standards, and financial guarantees for post-closure activities took effect, the number of operating facilities has dropped substantially. Today there are just 18 commercial hazardous waste landfills operating in the United States and 3 in Canada, compared to more than 1000 during the 1970s Within the past few years, the list of wastes for which disposal in landfills is prohibited has been steadily growing; federal legislation enacted in 1984 and fully implemented by 1990 imposed a ban on the landfilling of virtually all hazardous wastes, unless such materials undergo prior treatment to minimize their toxicity and ability to migrate. The explicit intent of such legislation is to reduce reliance on land disposal and to encourage the use of alternative technologies to the greatest extent possible.

Deep Well Injection.   The use of deep wells for waste disposal dates back to the late 19th century when the petroleum industry employed this method to get rid of salt brine, but its use for liquid hazardous waste disposal began only during the 1940s. A number of industries, most notably

Figure 16-5 Deep Well Injection (subsurface disposal well)

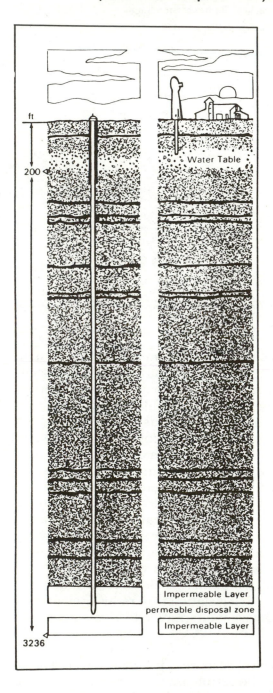

ft

200

Water Table

Impermeable Layer

permeable disposal zone

Impermeable Layer

3236

petroleum refineries and petrochemical plants, now utilize this disposal method. Commercial deep well injection currently is practiced only in the Midwest and in Texas and neighboring states, although many other injection wells operated by private firms solely for the disposal of their own wastes are widely scattered across the United States. Of the total amount of hazardous waste managed each year, the largest portion—about 25% of all such wastes—is disposed of by deep well injection. The process involves pumping liquid wastes through lined wells into porous rock formations deep underground, well below any drinking water aquifers. Some critics point out that cracks in the well casing or undetected faults in the earth which intersect the disposal zone could result in outward migration of wastes. EPA contends that deep wells are safe, provided that they are constructed, operated and maintained in accordance with agency regulations.

Various Chemical, Physical, or Biological Treatment Processes. Processes that render wastes nonhazardous or significantly reduce their volume or toxicity have assumed major importance in recent years, particularly as more and more "**land bans**" have been implemented, prohibiting the landfilling of untreated wastes. With economic motivation spurring invention, a number of promising new technologies are now in the pilot project phase or fully operational, promising safer, more effective ways of cleaning up past mistakes and ensuring that wastes currently being generated are properly managed.

Physical methods include **evaporation** to concentrate corrosive brines, **sedimentation** to separate solids from liquid wastes, **carbon adsorption** to remove certain soluble organic wastes, and **air-stripping** to remove volatile organic compounds from groundwater.

Chemical techniques involve processes such as **neutralization** to render wastes harmless, sulfide **precipitation** to extract certain toxic metals, **oxidation-reduction** processes to convert some metals from a hazardous to a nonhazardous state, and **stabilization/solidification**, in which the waste material is detoxified and then combined with a cement-like material, encapsulated in plastic, blended with organic polymers, or combined with silica to form a solid, inert substance which can be disposed of safely in a landfill or incorporated into road beds. One particularly exciting new technology currently being employed to remediate a federal Superfund site in Michigan is **in-situ vitrification (ISV)**, a process which relies on large amounts of electricity (about 750 kilowatt-hours per ton of soil) delivered by giant electrodes fixed at several locations in the soil surrounding the area undergoing cleanup. Suitable for detoxifying soils contaminated with toxic organics (e.g. chlorinated pesticides), heavy metals, or radioactive wastes, ISV actually melts the soil as the electricity flows through it, fusing the toxics into a solid block of glassified material, similar to natural obsidian. The solidified material can simply be left in place, no longer posing any environmental threat (but perhaps causing immense puzzlement among archaeologists five thousand years hence, trying to figure out what kind of cultural artifact that huge chunk of glass could possibly be!).

Biological treatment, based on the ability of microbes to decompose toxic organic compounds, is increasingly being used for cleanup of oil spills, as well as for remediation of contaminated soil and groundwater (see Box 16–5).

Controlled Incineration.   Because burning at very high temperatures actually destroys hazardous wastes (as opposed to storing them out of sight underground as is essentially the case with various land disposal methods), most hazardous waste management experts regard controlled incineration as the best and, in some cases, the only environmentally acceptable means of disposal. However, due to its relatively high cost compared to other waste management options, incineration until recently accounted for only 1% of all hazardous wastes managed. It is expected that this situation could change dramatically in the years ahead, as land disposal laws become increasingly restrictive and as generators, fearful of legal liability if their wastes migrate from a land disposal site, opt for a management method that ensures waste destruction. A controlled incinerator burns at temperatures ranging from 750–3000 °F, with wastes, air, and fuel being thoroughly mixed to ensure complete combustion. Afterburners, which are part of the incineration system, destroy any gaseous hydrocarbons which may have survived the initial incineration process, while scrubbers and electrostatic precipitators remove pollutant

BOX 16-5

Pollution-Gobbling Microbes: Bioremediation

The concept of utilizing naturally occurring bacteria or fungi to degrade hazardous wastes has intrigued scientists and environmental engineers for at least two decades. Nevertheless, only within the last several years has progress in applying microbiological techniques to the remediation of contaminated soil and groundwater raised hopes that humble "bugs" may offer a valuable new approach to cleaning up chemical pollution.

As far back as 1973, it was suggested that beaches fouled by tanker spills might be effectively cleansed simply by adding inorganic nitrates and phosphates to polluted shorelines, such fertilizers acting as stimulants for resident microbes to gobble up the hydrocarbon wastes. A few years later, researchers observed that when oxygen was pumped into chemically contaminated groundwater deposits, pollutant levels quickly dropped. Subsequent field tests in those years yielded variable results, but demonstrated that **biostimulation**, a process of adding either oxygen or nutrients (or both) to contaminated material, can promote more rapid growth of indigenous microbes, resulting in faster, more efficient metabolism of wastes than would have occurred without human intervention. Techniques have been perfected by years of trial-and-error and today biostimulation of naturally occurring microorganisms has become by far the most widely used method of bioremediation. The process achieved well-deserved acclaim in 1989 when it was successfully used in cleanup operations at Prince William Sound, Alaska, following the *Exxon Valdez* spill. Within two weeks after the application of a fertilizer to the oil-coated cobblestone and sand-and-gravel beaches, obvious reductions in the amount of oil were readily apparent—a clear demonstration of biostimulation's potential for remediation of oil spills in field situations.

A second approach to using microbes for environmental cleanup is **bioaugmentation**, appropriate in situations where resident organisms are too few in number, even with biostimulation, to degrade wastes effectively or when the microbes naturally present are genetically incapable of breaking down a particular waste. In such situations, nonindigenous species may be added to "lend a hand," working in concert with the natural microbes to accomplish pollutant removal more rapidly and completely. In a quest to create new bacterial strains better able to degrade chemicals under specific environmental conditions, scientists have been using the tools of genetic engineering in an effort still in the research and developmental phase. **Genetically-engineered microbes (GEMs)** offer great potential for destroying pollutants which have proven resistant to breakdown by naturally occurring microbes. In order to avoid any possible risk to human health or the environment, the use of GEMs is regulated under the Toxic Substances Control Act which requires that they undergo a rigorous safety review prior to approval for field use. To date, no GEMs have been used for site cleanups in the United States.

Bioremediation projects can be carried out either *in-situ*, treating contaminated soils or groundwater in place, or aboveground in lined treatment beds or in enclosed vessels (bioreactors or biofilters). In-situ treatment can involve the installation of sprinkler systems to deliver liquid fertilizer to the contaminated region or the use of injection wells to pump oxygenated water into a contaminated aquifer. If contamination is restricted to the upper 12 inches of soil, tilling the area for aeration purposes may be sufficient. At greater depths a process known as "**bioventing**"—installing a series of injection wells to force air into poorly oxygenated soil—may be enough to stimulate natural microbial activity; if not, nutritional supplements can be added to further encourage bacterial growth. Bioventing has proven so successful in reducing certain types of petrochemical contamination that the U.S. Air Force now regards the technique as its #1 choice for treating soils contaminated by jet fuels.

Treatment processes in aboveground reactors vary according to the type of material being treated and the desired treatment results, with contaminated soils or liquids being placed into or fed through these systems. In-reactor treatment methods provide a better means than in situ methods for controlling key variables (temperature, oxygen levels, pH, nutrient concentrations) and provide maximum contact between the hungry microbes and the toxic pollutant. Improved understanding of the parameters affecting the success of bioremediation efforts comes as good news to those charged with cleaning up the nation's hazardous waste mess, since bioremediation offers a number of important advantages over other cleanup methods. Perhaps most significant is the fact that, unlike some processes such as air-stripping, in which toxics are removed from one medium (water) only to be released to another (air), microbes *detoxify* the wastes, converting them to such nonhazardous substances as CO_2, water, and salts. Because bioremediation can usually be carried out on the contaminated site, either aboveground or in situ, there is no need to transport contaminated materials elsewhere for treatment,

thereby eliminating concerns about disseminating pollutants over a wider area. When wastes are treated in situ, bioremediation avoids the environmental disruption caused by the excavation, chemical treatment, or incineration and subsequent landfilling involved in other processes. Finally, the expense of biological treatment is usually considerably less than that of other methods, as little as one-tenth the cost of incineration.

Of course there are limitations to the process as well; experience has demonstrated that bioremediation is not suitable in every environment nor are microbes capable of degrading all types of wastes. Whereas bacteria performed admirably in cleaning up the rocky shores of Prince William Sound, there is considerable question whether they would have been as effective on oil-drenched mudflats or tidal marshes where pores between the sediment particles are extremely small. Successful application of bioremediation to subsoil cleanup is highly dependent on soil permeability, since a tight soil inhibits the movement of forced air or remedial liquids into the contaminated zone. Thus a bioremediation method which performs extremely well in cleaning up an oil-contaminated sand and gravel aquifer may give disappointing results in clay soil. Similarly, while microbes have a healthy appetite for a wide range of petrochemical pollutants, creosote, pentachlorophenol—and a number of other organic contaminants, they can't be used to treat metal-contaminated soil.

Nevertheless, the range of potential applications for bioremediation is considerable: hundreds of thousands of sites contaminated by underground storage tanks leaking fuel oil or gasoline into soil and groundwater supplies; up to 15,000 accidental oil spills each year; thousands of industrial sites where solvents, wood preservatives, and pesticide wastes poison the ground; and over 10,000 pesticide dealerships where chemicals are mixed and sold—and spilled—all represent situations where bioremediation could play an important role in restoring environmental quality.

Thanks to active support by EPA, bioremediation research is proceeding at a number of laboratories throughout the U.S., driven by the priority status accorded to cleaning up hazardous waste sites. Currently bioremediation projects are either in the planning stage or being implemented at more than 150 sites under federal or state regulatory oversight. It is expected that the demand for bioremediation services and products will grow at a 15% average annual rate for the next several years and that industry earnings could easily exceed $300 million by 1997. Microbes are well on the way to becoming one of our most valuable assets in the ongoing efforts to detoxify America.

References

Bioremediation: Innovative Pollution Treatment Technology. 1993. EPA, Office of Research and Development, Nov.

Piotrowski, Michael R. 1993. "Bioremediation Milestones." *Water Environment & Technology*, (Dec.).

Swannell, Richard P.J., and Ian M. Head. 1994. "Bioremediation Comes of Age." *Nature*, 368 (March 31).

emissions from the stack gases. Capable of handling solid, liquid, and gaseous wastes, incineration has several distinct advantages over other disposal methods: 1) it can convert toxic compounds to harmless ones, 2) it greatly reduces waste volume, 3) by destroying wastes rather than isolating them, it eliminates future problems, and 4) it offers the potential of energy recovery during combustion of wastes. Several different types are currently being used, each having its own advantages and disadvantages for combustion of specific waste categories.

Waste Exchanges.   The ideal way to manage hazardous materials would be to recycle them, thus preventing their entry into the waste stream and eliminating the disposal problem. This is the idea which prompted the establishment of waste exchanges, which act as helpful third parties in establishing contact between waste generators and potential waste users. For example, a paint manufacturer, faced with the problem of how to dispose of hazardous sludges from a mixing operation, contacts a waste exchange and is referred to another company which willingly purchases the sludge to use as a filler coat on cement blocks. Thus, the paint manufacturer avoids the high cost of disposal in a secure chemical landfill or controlled incinerator and also makes a modest profit on the sale of the waste. The buyer, too, is pleased with the arrangement because a needed raw material is obtained for a lower price than unused filler would have cost; and society is well served because a potentially hazardous substance has been prevented from entering the environment. The waste exchange concept originated in Europe where the first such program began in the Netherlands in 1972. The Midwest Industrial Waste Exchange, started in 1975 in St. Louis, was the first U.S. program, the forerunner of 42 materials exchange programs now operating in North America (with 30 more in the development stage). The most common type of waste exchange is

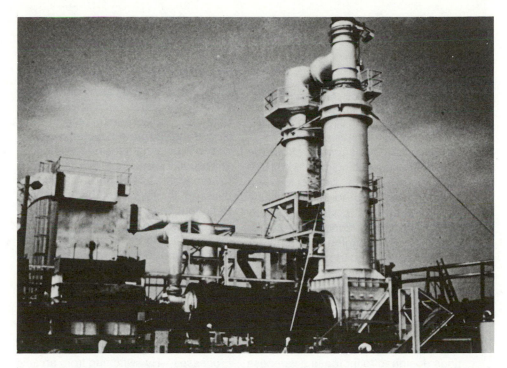

A ''mobile'' incinerator for destroying hazardous wastes. This equipment can be disassembled and moved from site to site on flatbed trucks. Use of such incinerators is becoming more common as a result of SARA requirements to minimize off-site transport of hazardous wastes from Superfund cleanup projects. [Author's Photo]

basically an information clearinghouse which publishes monthly, bimonthly, or quarterly coded listings of waste items available or desired. Interested parties then contact the clearinghouse and negotiations between potential buyers and sellers are initiated. A smaller proportion of waste exchanges act as a direct brokerage service, sometimes actively seeking a buyer or seller for a particular waste material. Although waste exchanges were first developed exclusively for industrial hazardous waste trading, in recent years they have been increasingly involved in marketing nonhazardous solid waste materials as well (though solvents still remain the single most widely swapped item). As waste disposal costs continue to rise and as industries become more familiar with the opportunities for waste recycling, utilization of the services provided by waste exchanges is expected to increase significantly (Gruder, 1993).

Siting Problems: from ''NIMBY'' to ''BANANA''

Everyone wants hazardous wastes to be managed in ways which present the least possible threat to health or the environment, but no one wants to live near the site chosen for such storage, treatment, or disposal. Get rid of such wastes in the next county, a neighboring state, out in the desert, anyplace else—but ''Not In My Back Yard!'' (referred to as the

BOX 16-6

Pollution Prevention

Just as municipal waste management strategies emphasize the value of waste prevention as opposed to clean-up, so does national policy for hazardous waste management stress the importance of reducing the amount and toxicity of waste generated—an approach referred to among waste managers as **P2 ("pollution prevention")**. P2 is a concept that has gradually been winning adherents for more than a decade. In its 1984 Hazardous and Solid Waste Amendments to RCRA, Congress decreed that "the generation of hazardous waste is to be reduced or eliminated as expeditiously as possible." EPA was told to issue waste minimization regulations designed to increase awareness among industrial managers of waste reduction possibilities and to encourage voluntary initiatives aimed at lowering the amounts of waste generated. While the initial response to such urgings was tentative within a corporate world still focused on traditional, end-of-pipe controls, in the past few years P2 has become a buzzword among savvy managerial types who recognize that implementing effective pollution prevention programs is a key to economic competitiveness. Not simply a public-relations ploy to appease the "green faction," corporate policies to reduce waste at the source—to prevent pollution before it's created—constitutes an economically sound business decision, since in today's highly regulated world it is far cheaper and more efficient to avoid the generation of waste rather than try to clean it up after the fact. Not only can effective P2 strategies save money on pollution abatement costs (which, in the U.S. at least, have been rising faster than the growth rate of industrial production), but by using raw materials

more efficiently they also contribute to lower production costs. Fears of potential liability under the federal Superfund program have also been a strong motivating force for the adoption of pollution prevention programs—the fewer wastes shipped off-site for disposal, the less a company needs to fret about being cited as a "potentially responsible party" when a land disposal facility springs a leak!

The opportunities for significantly reducing the industrial waste stream are numerous—and often require little or no capital investment. Methods which can be employed with significant results include:

1. *Changing manufacturing processes*—By switching from an acid spray to a mechanical scrubber using pumice and rotating brushes to clean copper sheeting at its electronics plant in Columbia, Missouri, the 3M Corporation reduced its generation of liquid hazardous wastes by 40,000 lbs. annually. Similarly, American Cyanamid modified a process it had long used for manufacturing yellow dye, thereby totally eliminating the need for a nitrobenzene solvent and its associated wastestream.

2. *Reformulating the product*— In a plastics factory in New Jersey, Monsanto changed the formula for an industrial adhesive it was producing; in doing so, it eliminated the need for filtering the product and thus no longer had any hazardous filtrate or filters requiring disposal.

3. *Substituting a nonhazardous chemical for a hazardous one in the manufacturing process*—In Memphis, Cleo Wrap, the world's largest producer of holiday gift-wrapping paper, switched from using solvent-based printing inks to water-based materials. In so doing, the company

virtually eliminated its generation of hazardous wastes.

4. *Changing equipment*—Simply by adding a condenser to an existing piece of equipment, a USS Chemicals plant in Ohio was able to capture escaping emissions of cumene, returning them to the phenol process unit. By so doing, the company solved an air quality problem and recaptured a major raw material. To recover product being lost during the drying stage for its salicylaldehyde process, Rhône-Poulenc installed in-line condensers which increased product yield by 10 pounds per batch.

5. *Altering the way hazardous wastes are handled in-plant*—Basically housekeeping changes, efforts at minimizing spills and using chemicals more conservatively can make a considerable difference in the amount of hazardous wastes generated. Segregating wastes to reduce contamination can also have a major impact. In Fremont, California, the Borden Chemical Company has reduced the phenol content of its wastewater by 93% simply by separately collecting and reusing rinsewaters used to clean resin-contaminated filters. Formerly the company had allowed this rinsewater to flow into floor drains where it contaminated all the wastewater which flowed from the factory to a sewage treatment plant.

Not only do the approaches just described reduce the amounts of hazardous waste requiring disposal, they also save the companies which utilize them a great deal of money. The catch-phrase "Pollution Prevention Pays," coined by the 3M Corporation, rings true in case after case. In one year after changing its process for cleaning copper sheeting, 3M saved $15,000 in raw materials and in waste disposal and labor costs; the $100,000 which American Cyanamid invested in equipment modification to allow in-process recycling of another solvent substituted for nitrobenzene resulted in $200,000 in annual savings, thanks to reduced costs for energy and waste disposal; by switching to water-based inks, Cleo Wrap recouped $35,000 annually in waste disposal costs; by recovering 400,000 pounds of cumene after installation of a $5000 condenser, USS Chemicals saved $100,000 in raw materials; Rhône-Poulenc's capital costs for its in-line condensers amounted to $10,000—repaid threefold by first-year savings of $30,000.

Until recently, many companies failed to take a comprehensive view of their waste streams—pinpointing precisely where wastes were generated and the exact management cost of each waste. By lumping all waste treatment, disposal, and oversight expenses together, corporate accountants denied themselves the opportunity of identifying specific process control points where considerable savings could be achieved. More recently, assisted and encouraged by state and federal programs as well as by enlightened self-interest, a growing number of firms are conducting intensive waste audits, instituting cost-accounting procedures, and involving employees at all levels to identify opportunities for pollution prevention. While wholehearted endorsement of P2 principles within conservative corporate boardrooms is by no means universal yet, the transition is now well underway.

References

Dorfman, Mark H., et al. 1992. "Environmental Dividends: Cutting More Chemical Wastes." *Inform*.

"State of the Environment: A View Toward the Nineties." 1987. Conservation Foundation.

World Resources Institute. 1994. *World Resources 1994–95*. Oxford University Press.

"NIMBY" problem in agency argot). This, in essence, is the siting dilemma which represents one of the most difficult obstacles faced by those trying to deal with municipal or hazardous wastes (not to mention *radioactive* refuse!) in a safe and responsible manner. Certainly waste disposal horror stories from Love Canal and countless other places across the nation have made citizens understandably nervous at the prospect of seeing hazardous waste management facilities locate in their communities. Nevertheless, if society desires to continue using products whose manufacture entails the production of hazardous wastes, improved waste handling facilities are urgently needed. Inevitably, the best location for some of those facilities will be in someone's "back yard." Responsible decision-making demands that citizens carefully evaluate the pros and cons of a site under consideration before automatically rejecting it. Laws governing the siting of hazardous waste facilities provide for public information and public participation programs during the siting process, though the scope for public input into the decision-making process varies widely from state to state. Before opposing or supporting a proposed facility, citizens should gather information on the following points:

- characteristics of the wastes involved
- nature of the proposed waste management process
- the design and manner of operation of the proposed facility
- the topographical, hydrogeological, and climatic characteristics of the site
- transportation routes to the site
- safeguards to be employed at the facility
- potential for human or ecological exposure to hazardous chemicals released into the air, water, or soil
- location of the site in reference to population centers, farmland, or valuable natural areas (e.g. wetlands, endangered species' habitat, etc.)
- possible uses of site after closure

Public opposition has brought acquisition of new hazardous waste management sites to a virtual standstill in recent years, with objectors mobilizing from far beyond the locality directly affected. Indeed, the sentiment prevailing among many activist groups at present has moved well beyond the familiar NIMBY protests to encompass the ultimate in negative responses: BANANA (Build Absolutely Nothing Anywhere Near Anything!). Unless society is willing to adopt a life-style in which no wastes whatsoever are generated (assuming this is even possible), a more reasonable, middle-ground approach to waste management decisions must be adopted. Protection of public health requires a new willingness on the part of citizens to sanction the siting of new facilities when a thorough review of site and operational considerations indicate that such facilities will not present serious environmental health problems.

Hazardous Waste Management Legislation: RCRA

An evaluation of the types of hazardous waste incidents that have occurred indicate that we are basically dealing with two different categories of hazardous waste problems: how to manage the new volumes of chemical wastes being generated daily by American industry and what to do about wastes improperly disposed of years ago which are only now beginning to make their presence known.

In order to tackle the first of these issues, the problem of newly created wastes, Congress in 1976 enacted the **Resource Conservation and Recovery Act (RCRA**—pronounced "rickra" in bureaucratese) which mandates that EPA:

- define which wastes are hazardous
- institute a "**manifest system**" to track the movement of hazardous wastes from the place they were generated to any off-site storage, treatment, or disposal facility
- set performance standards to be met by owners and operators of hazardous waste facilities
- issue permits for operation of such facilities only after technical standards have been met (operating licenses specify which types of wastes may be managed at that facility; thus most hazardous waste disposal sites are authorized to accept only certain classes of wastes)
- help states to develop hazardous waste management programs of their own which may be more stringent than the federal program, but which cannot be less so.

RCRA took effect in 1980 when EPA finally issued its generator and transporter regulations (i.e. manifest requirements) and marked an important step forward in responsible hazardous waste management. However, it soon became apparent that the 1976 law featured some glaring loopholes which needed to be plugged. There was also mounting sentiment in Congress and elsewhere that land disposal of hazardous wastes is the least desirable method of managing these substances and that legislation should encourage reliance on alternatives. Accordingly, when RCRA came before Congress for reauthorization in 1984, the original legislation was substantially strengthened with the enactment of the Hazardous and Solid Waste Amendments (HSWA). Among the key provisions of this law are mandates which 1) significantly reduce the types of hazardous wastes which can be buried in landfills; 2) strengthen requirements for landfill design and operation; 3) bring into the regulatory framework hundreds of thousands of previously exempt "small quantity generators"—those who produce 100 kg (220 lbs.) per month or more of hazardous wastes (under the original law, only those generators producing 1000 kg or more per month were subject to regulation); and 4) create a whole new program for detecting and controlling leakage of hazardous liquids (mainly petroleum products) from underground storage tanks. Implementation of these new requirements, while making hazardous waste management considerably

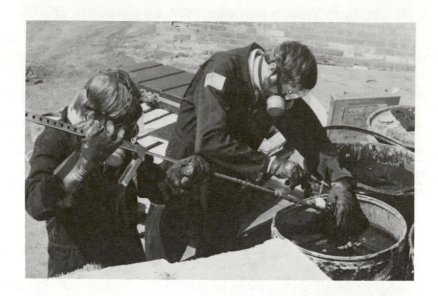

Cleanup of hazardous waste dump sites begins with careful sampling and identification of the abandoned material so that an appropriate disposal method can be chosen. Personnel carrying out the investigation wear protective ''moon suits'' and respirators to guard against personal injury. [Illinois Environmental Protection Agency]

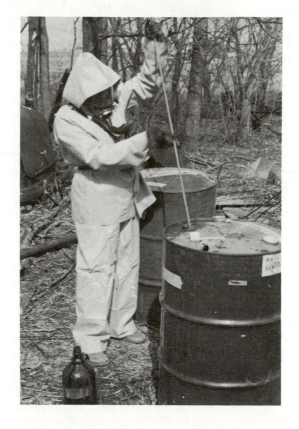

more expensive than it had been previously, gave new impetus to safer, more environmentally responsible waste management strategies.

While confronting the issue of newly generated wastes with an array of regulatory approaches, RCRA does nothing to deal with the serious problem posed by leaking abandoned dumpsites. Even in the relatively few cases where the owners can be found, they often lack the financial resources to clean up the site, making litigation a futile exercise. Since EPA estimates there may be anywhere between 30,000–50,000 abandoned hazardous waste dumps in the United States—more than 2000 of which are thought to present public health risks, the potential for future problems is obviously very great.

"Superfund"

Spurred by public demands that something be done to alleviate problems caused by old, leaking dumpsites, Congress in December of 1980 enacted the Comprehensive Environmental Response, Compensation, and Liability Act (CERCLA, dubbed the "Superfund"), authorizing the expenditure of $1.6 billion over a five-year period for emergency cleanup activities and for the more long-term containment of hazardous waste dump sites (the legislation, however did not include funds to compensate victims for health damage incurred by exposure to such sites—an issue which was the focus of considerable debate). EPA, in cooperation with the states, was charged with compiling a **National Priority List (NPL)** of sites considered to be sufficiently threatening to public health or environmental quality to make them eligible for Superfund cleanup dollars. These funds can be used either to remove hazardous substances from the site (a process which may also include temporary relocation of people in the area and provision of alternative water supplies) or for remedial measures such as storage and confinement of wastes, incineration, dredging, or permanent relocation of residents (such as occurred at Times Beach, Missouri).

The original Superfund bill expired in September 1985, and in spite of public demands for speedy reauthorization so that cleanup work could proceed without interruption, the law was not renewed until late the following year. Extreme congressional dissatisfaction with the excruciatingly slow rate of progress during Superfund's first years led to several significant changes in the 1986 Superfund Amendments and Reauthorization Act (SARA). Realizing that 1980 funding levels were inadequate, Congress in 1986 increased Superfund allocations to $8.5 billion to be spent over the next five years (in 1990 Congress once again reauthorized Superfund until September 1994, allocating an additional $5.1 billion for the program). EPA was given mandatory deadlines for initiating site-specific cleanup plans and remediation activities. Concerned that previous cleanup actions represented little more than moving contaminated wastes from one site to another site, which would itself then become eligible for Superfund status, Congress specified a preference for cleanup actions which "permanently and significantly" reduce the volume, toxicity, or mobility of hazardous substances. This mandate has given a

Figure 16-6 Who Is Responsible for Hazardous Wastes?

At the national level there are a variety of agencies responsible for the control of hazardous wastes. Which agency is responsible and under what legislation is dependent upon whether the wastes are being transported, stored, disposed of, the type of wastes, and where they were found in the ecosystem. The following is a brief summary of federal waste responsibilities:

AREA	AGENCY	LEGISLATION	PROVISIONS
TRANSPORTATION	Department of Transportation	Hazardous Materials Transportation Act P.L. 93-633	Regulates interstate commerce of hazardous materials
	U.S. Environmental Protection Agency	Resource Conservation and Recovery Act of 1976 P.L. 94-580	Sets standards for manifests (shipping tickets and transporters)
	U.S. Coast Guard	Ports and Waterways Safety Act of 1972	The question of bulk shipment of oil and other hazardous materials on the lakes
WASTE DISPOSAL	U.S. Environmental Protection Agency	Resource Conservation and Recovery Act of 1976 P.L. 94-580	Sets standards and issues, permits for producers, transporters, and disposal sites
AIR QUALITY	U.S. Environmental Protection Agency	Clean Air Act of 1970 P.L. 91-604 Amended 95-95	Sets emission standards for 5 hazardous air pollutants
WATER QUALITY	U.S. Environmental Protection Agency	Clean Water Act of 1977 P.L. 95-217	Sets standards for toxic discharges through NPDES permits to achieve fishable and swimmable water
SPILLS	U.S. Environmental Protection Agency	Clean Water Act of 1977 P.L. 95-217	Prepares national contingency plan for spills, coordinates spill response. levies penalties and recovers costs

Category	Agency	Act	Description
NUCLEAR WASTES	Nuclear Regulatory Agency	Atomic Energy Act P.L. 83-703	Sets standards and licenses nuclear waste disposal sites
DRINKING WATER	U.S. Environmental Protection Agency	Safe Drinking Act of 1974 P.L. 93-523	Sets national standards for safe drinking water. Regulates the underground injection of wastes which could contaminate drinking water
FOOD	Food and Drug Administration	Food, Drug, and Cosmetic Act P.L. 75-717	Sets, enforces tolerances for contaminants in food for interstate commerce, bans unsafe foods
OTHER CONSUMER PRODUCTS	Consumer Product Safety Commission	P.L. 92-573 Consumer Product Safety Act Hazardous Substances Act	Sets and enforces tolerances for household products, requires labelling, bans unsafe products
FISH AND WILDLIFE	Department of the Interior Fish and Wildlife Service	Fish and Wildlife Coordination Act of 1965	Research, technical assistance spill response, monitoring for contaminants and effects on fish and wildlife
OCCUPATIONAL SAFETY	Occupational Safety and Health Administration	Occupational and Safety Health Act P.L. 91-596	Sets and enforces standards for worker exposure
CHEMICALS	U.S. Environmental Protection Agency	Toxic Substances Control Act P.L. 94-469	Obtains industry data on product use and health effects of chemicals. Regulation of manufacturer, use, distribution, and disposal of chemical substances
PESTICIDES	U.S. Environmental Protection Agency	Federal Insecticide, Fungicide and Rodenticide Act as amended in 1975 P.L. 94-140	Registration and classification of all pesticides

BOX 16-7

Midnight Dumping

In August of 1978, residents along 210 miles of rural highways in North Carolina discovered an unwelcome gift—31,000 gallons of waste oil containing high levels of PCBs had been deliberately discharged by a tank truck whose driver had simply opened its back spigot while driving along country roads. The pervasive odor caused nausea and headaches among nearby residents and killed vegetation along the roadside. Farmers were advised not to eat or sell vegetables or beef grown within 100 yards of contaminated areas and the Governor offered a $2500 reward for information leading to the arrest of the "midnight dumpers." Within a few weeks three Pennsylvania men, a father and two sons, were arrested and confessed to having accepted $75,000 from a transformer company in Raleigh, the state capital, to haul away the PCB-laden wastes. Since the nearest PCB disposal site happened to be in Alabama, the men decided to maximize their profits by illegally draining the waste along the road where they hoped it wouldn't be noticed.

Although this case was unusual in the volume of waste discarded—and in the fact that the perpetrators were apprehended—midnight dumping (illegal, clandestine disposal of wastes in gullies, fields, streams, abandoned buildings, etc.) had become an all-too-common phenomenon in the months before the RCRA regulations took effect. Many midnight dumpers were involved with organized crime networks; few were arrested, and those who were seldom received a punishment that came even close to matching the public expense of repairing the damage they had caused.

Midnight dumping flourished in the late 1970s, and remains a problem even today, because of the scarcity of approved disposal sites, the high cost of legal disposal, and because, until implementation of RCRA, generators of wastes were not required to document the final disposition of their waste materials (for example, at a time when Illinois had 22 licensed disposal sites, 2 million tons of chemical wastes were legally disposed of annually, but 12 million additional tons could not be accounted for). The manifest system required by RCRA was designed primarily to amend this situation. Under manifest requirements, off-site shipments of hazardous wastes are tracked from "cradle to grave." Waste generators are required to complete an official form describing the amount and composition of the waste material, where it originated, where it is to be taken, and the transportation route to be followed. They must package the material in approved containers with proper labelling and hire a registered hauling company to transport the waste. The vehicle carrying the wastes must be properly placarded and a description of the wastes provided to the transporter. After the waste material reaches the intended waste facility, the completed manifest is returned to the waste generator and must be kept on file for three years. If for any reason the manifest is not returned by the waste management facility, the generator is required to notify state environmental authorities who then launch an investigation into the matter. This system, of course, is not foolproof. Unscrupulous generators or waste haulers may still try to subvert the intent of the law by neglecting to fill out a manifest in the first place, thus leaving no "paper trail" for regulators to follow. Nevertheless, the requirement constitutes a valuable legal tool for prosecutors who may ultimately win a conviction by proving that a generator or hauler broke the law by not manifesting a shipment—regardless of the final disposition of the waste. And in the 1990s, unlike the 1970s, criminal penalties for knowing violation of hazardous waste laws can be stiff indeed—fines up to $50,000 or two years in prison, or both.

In a new twist on an old crime, midnight dumping of *nonhazardous* city garbage has emerged as a vexing problem in recent years, particularly in heavily urbanized sections of the Northeast where escalating landfill tipping fees have provided financial motivation for illegal disposal. New Jerseyites have felt particularly victimized, being left "holding the bag"—literally—when so-called "gypsy" haulers from New York City come calling. The standard *modus operandi* involves an illicit driver with a tractor stealing a box trailer from a freight company yard and filling it with wastes from a generator happy to pay the "gypsy" $250 to haul away a load for which legal disposal might cost as much as $2000. Such loads typically don't travel far—many of them end up, trailer and all, abandoned on the streets of Jersey City, though some have been found in state parks near the New Jersey Turnpike while a few have made it all the way to the southern tip of the state. Since municipal wastes are not required to be manifested prior to shipment and because there is no way to tell whether any given trailer is hauling garbage, apprehending the perpetrators of this type of crime isn't easy. After discovering an abandoned 45-foot long trailer containing 21 tons of trash parked at the edge of Liberty State Park, two frustrated New Jersey park rangers reported that "We had patrolled that area about 6 P.M. and nothing was there. When we came back at 9:30 P.M., there it was!"

References

Brown, Michael. 1980. *Laying Waste: The Poisoning of America by Toxic Chemicals*. Pantheon Books.
Sullivan, Joseph F. 1992. "Dumping Trash, Trucks and All, In New Jersey." *New York Times*, July 30.

major impetus to development of treatment or disposal technologies (e.g. mobile incinerators which can be moved from one Superfund site to another) which permit hazardous wastes to be destroyed or detoxified on site, thereby avoiding the risks of transporting such wastes to another facility where they might cause future problems.

While Americans (72 million of whom live within four miles of a Superfund site) generally support the concept of cleaning up our hazardous waste mistakes of the past, there has been a steadily mounting crescendo of criticism of the accomplishments and expense of the program to date. By mid-1994, the number of officially listed or proposed NPL sites had grown from an original 400 to 1286—yet after more than a decade of on-site work and the expenditure of more than $20 billion by government and industry, construction was complete (i.e. all cleanup equipment was in place) at just 235 and only 58 sites had been delisted, indicating that they no longer presented a threat to human health or the environment. Admittedly, the pace of remedial work has improved during the past several

---

Figure 16-7 "Top 20" Most Prominent Toxic Substances Found at NPL Sites

Lead	Trichloroethylene
Arsenic	DDT
Mercury (metallic)	Arochlor 1254
Benzene	Hexachlorobutadiene
Vinyl chloride	Arochlor 1260
Cadmium	DDE
PCBs	Arochlor 1242
Benzo(*a*)pyrene	Dibenzo(*a,h*)anthracene
Chloroform	Hexavalent chromium
Benzo(*b*)fluoranthene	Dieldrin

Ranking based on: 1) frequency at NPL sites, 2) toxicity, 3) exposure hazard to humans.

Source: Agency for Toxic Substances and Disease Registry.

---

years as regulatory officials and private contractors alike acquired knowledge and expertise in what was, in the early 1980s, a completely new and highly complex undertaking.

Passionate disputes also rage over the extent of remediation necessary—"How clean is clean enough?" Critics complain that it makes no sense to spend millions of dollars to remove every last trace of contamination on a site destined to be paved over for a parking lot; it is quite likely that future amendments to the law will permit cleanup decisions to be based, at least in part, on the probable future use of the site. As EPA Administrator Carol Browner recently predicted, ". . . there will be different levels of clean." Undoubtedly, the most controversial feature of the Superfund program has been its liability provisions, based on the philosophically sound "the polluter pays" principle, but which has resulted in fully one-quarter of all Superfund dollars spent thus far going to pay legal fees. While business interests are demanding fundamental changes in what they regard as inherently unfair provisions, environmental advocates strongly support the status quo, insisting that concerns about "Superfund liability" alone have caused generators to be much more conscientious about managing their wastes properly and have given major impetus to serious efforts toward pollution prevention. As evidence, they point to the fact that between 1987 and 1991, the chemical industry alone has reduced its output of toxic wastes by 35%, largely in response to future liability considerations.

Finally, there is the question of cost. In 1994, fully 22% of EPA's entire budget was allocated to Superfund. The Agency estimates it will cost at least $28 billion to clean up the sites currently on the NPL—and sees an additional 4800 sites as likely candidates for listing in the years ahead.

Figure 16-8 States with the Most NPL Sites (1994)

New Jersey	107	Florida	54	Ohio	34
Pennsylvania	100	Washington	54	Indiana	32
California	91	Minnesota	40	Massachusetts	30
New York	83	Wisconsin	40	Texas	29
Michigan	76	Illinois	37	South Carolina	23

Although Superfund legislation mandates that 10% of site cleanup costs be paid by the state in which the site is located and requires that an attempt be made to find the "**potentially responsible party**" (**PRP**) who caused or contributed to the problem in order to recover cleanup expenses through litigation, the federal government will continue to bear much of the financial burden for site remediation efforts. The ultimate future of the Superfund program obviously will depend on the continued willingness of taxpayers to support the detoxification of America's hazardous waste dumpsites (Schmidt, 1994).

Household Hazardous Wastes

Comforting references to "Home Sweet Home" are slightly less reassuring today than in years past. The invisible hazards posed by radon and other indoor air pollutants make us wonder if we'd be safer inhaling deeply at a busy intersection than in our panelled family room. More recently, the righteous indignation directed at corporate polluters who disregard public well-being by careless disposal of their toxic by-products is being tempered somewhat by the realization that all of us—whatever our occupations—contribute to the nation's hazardous waste woes through our use, misuse, and thoughtless disposal of hundreds of potentially dangerous household chemicals.

It is estimated that the average American generates about 20 pounds of household hazardous waste each year. Typical examples of such discarded materials include pesticides, paints and varnishes, brush cleaners, ammonia, toilet bowl cleaners, bleaches and disinfectants, oven cleaners, furniture polish, swimming pool chemicals, batteries, motor oil, outdated medicines, and many others. Although these substances may be every bit as toxic, corrosive, flammable, or explosive as the industrial wastes regulated under RCRA, federal and state hazardous waste laws do not apply to the comparatively minor household sources. Nevertheless, the cumulative environmental impact of even small amounts of these materials being carelessly discarded by millions of individuals can be significant.

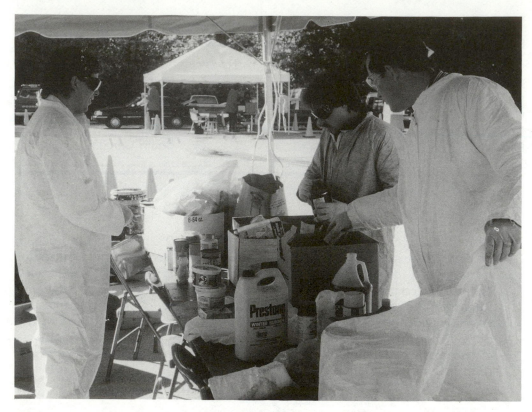

Hazardous household waste collection day: after residents have deposited their old paint cans, motor oil containers, discarded cleaning products, outdated medicine, and the like, workers from the Illinois EPA separate the wastes and prepare them for shipment to a licensed facility for disposal, treatment, or recycling. [Illinois Environmental Protection Agency]

A worker in protective gear examines potentially toxic containers at a hazardous household waste disposal center in Seattle.
[© Steve Schneider/ Greenpeace 1994]

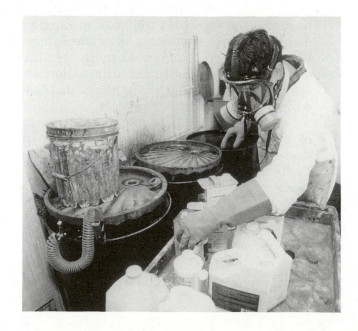

Household hazardous waste disposal practices present a variety of concerns:

1. Stored inside the home, hazardous chemicals pose poisoning risks, particularly for children; some, such as paints and solvents, pose problems of indoor air pollution; others, ammonia and chlorine bleach, for example, can result in highly toxic emissions when inadvertently mixed; still others pose serious fire hazards.

2. The welfare of public employees can be threatened by hazardous household products. Home fires involving hazardous chemicals can result in explosions or the generation of toxic fumes which can kill or seriously injure firefighters. Refuse collectors frequently suffer injury when they throw garbage bags into compactor trucks, unaware that they contain corrosive or flammable materials.

3. The environment itself can be seriously degraded when householders pour hazardous liquids into drains and flush them down toilets or into septic systems. People who pour waste motor oil into storm sewers or dump paint cans in the woods can cause long-lasting damage to ground and surface water supplies. Throwing such materials in the trash may ultimately result in the threat of contaminated incinerator ash and air pollution or in the formation of toxic leachates at municipal landfills.

In an effort to raise public awareness about these problems and to provide concerned citizens with a safe and responsible way of getting rid of hazardous household wastes, an increasing number of communities and public interest groups have been sponsoring household hazardous waste collection programs in recent years. These events have attracted large numbers of householders who are happy to take advantage of the opportunity to clean out the basement or garage and safely get rid of those old bottles of pesticides, paints—even ammunition—that may have been sitting on a shelf gathering dust for 20 years or more. Once wastes are brought to a collection center, they must be separated by type, packaged and manifested as RCRA hazardous wastes by trained personnel (usually licensed hazardous waste transporters), and taken to a licensed facility for treatment, disposal, or recycling. The cost of such programs, as well as concerns about legal liability, have limited their more widespread adoption. Nevertheless, these widely publicized efforts have had an impact far beyond the city limits of their sponsoring communities, enhancing public awareness of the fact that each one of us is a part of America's solid waste problem and pointing the way toward safer, more responsible ways of managing the hazardous by-products of our national life-style ■

References

Alexander, Michael. 1994. "Developing Markets for Old Newspapers." *Resource Recycling* XIII, no. 7 (July).

Arrandale, Tom. 1993. "Waste-To-Energy: Promises and Problems." *Governing* (Feb.).

Boerner, Christopher, and Kenneth Chilton. 1994. "False Economy: The Folly of Demand-Side Recycling." *Environment* 36, no. 1 (Jan/Feb).

Environmental Protection Agency. 1990. *Characterization of Municipal Solid Wastes in the United States: 1990 Update.* Office of EPA, Solid Waste and Emergency Response, June.

Greczyn, Mary. 1994. "Researchers and Community Reps Call for More Bioaerosol Research." *Environmental Health Letter* 33, no. 7 (March).

Greenhouse, Linda. 1994. "Justices Decide Incinerator Ash Is Toxic Waste." *New York Times*, May 3.

Gruder, Sherrie. 1993. "Matchmakers: Materials Exchange Programs." *Resource Recycling* 12, no. 12 (Dec.).

"Impact of Hogs on an Ecological Crisis." 1988. *BioCycle* 29, no. 5 (May/June).

League of Women Voters Education Fund. 1993. *The Garbage Primer.* Lyons & Burford, Publishers.

Levine, Adeline G. 1982. *Love Canal: Science, Politics, and People.* Lexington Books, D. C. Heath & Company.

Melosi, Martin V. 1981. *Garbage in the Cities: Refuse, Reform, and the Environment, 1880–1980.* Texas A&M University Press.

Newton, Lisa H., and Catherine K. Dillingham. 1994. "Toxin's Halloween." In *Watersheds: Classic Cases in Environmental Ethics.* Wadsworth Publishing Company.

Schmidt, Karen. 1994. "Can Superfund Get On Track?" *National Wildlife* 32, no. 3 (April/May).

Steuteville, Robert. 1994a. "The State of Garbage in America: Part I." *BioCycle* 35, no. 4 (April).

———. 1994b. "The State of Garbage in America: Part II." *BioCycle* 35, no. 5 (May).

Stolting, W. H. 1941. *Food Waste Material, A Survey of Urban Garbage Production, Collection, and Utilization.* U.S. Department of Agriculture.

Appendix A

Environmental Agencies of the Federal Government

National policy-making regarding environmental health issues has been delegated among several different federal agencies and cabinet-level departments. Among the more important groups dealing with issues discussed in this book are:

Environmental Protection Agency (EPA)
401 M Street, N.W., Washington, D.C. 20460

Created by President Nixon in December 1970, the EPA is an independent agency formed to coordinate the administration of a wide range of environmental programs which, prior to that time, had been scattered among a number of governmental agencies and departments, several of which frequently worked at cross-purposes. EPA has been charged with setting and enforcing standards pertaining to air and water pollution, solid and hazardous waste management, noise, public water supplies, pesticides, and radiation (excluding that associated with nuclear power plants). The agency also administers the municipal sewage treatment plant construction grant program authorized by Congress in the 1972 Clean Water Act. All EPA actions are published in the *Federal Register* as "proposed regulations," with time being allowed for public comment prior to their adoption as legally enforceable "final regulations."

The Administrator of the EPA is appointed by the President of the United States, as are five assistant administrators who head the five major divisions within the agency: the Office of Planning and Management, the Office of Enforcement, the Office of Air and Waste Management, the Office of Water and Hazardous Substances, and the Office of Research and

Development. All six presidential appointments must be confirmed by the U.S. Senate. Although EPA headquarters are in the nation's capital, the agency has ten regional offices, each with its own regional administrator, responsible for the states within its region.

The Council on Environmental Quality (CEQ)
722 Jackson Place, Washington, D.C. 20006

Established by the National Environmental Policy Act signed by President Nixon on January 1, 1970, the CEQ operates within the Executive Office of the president. Consisting of three members appointed by the president, one of whom functions as chairperson, the CEQ employs a professional staff of scientists and attorneys. Prior to the Reagan Administration, this professional staff consisted of about 30 people; all were dismissed by Reagan (the first time any staff member had been discharged by an incoming administration) and replaced by approximately six new staff people. The CEQ coordinates the environmental impact statements required by the National Environmental Policy Act and assists the president in preparing environmental legislation. It also had conducted extensive studies on the environmental effects of governmental policies and is charged with preparing annual reports for the president on the current state of the nation's environmental quality. Unfortunately, the drastic budget cuts imposed on the CEQ and the dismissal of all experienced staff members under the Reagan Administration seriously limited the council's previously valuable activities.

Nuclear Regulatory Commission (NRC)
1717 H Street, N.W., Washington, D.C. 20555

A five-member civilian board, this agency was created in 1974 by the National Energy Reorganization Act which broke up the old Atomic Energy Commission (AEC) into the research-oriented Energy Research and Development Administration (ERDA—subsequently absorbed by the Department of Energy) and the NRC. The Nuclear Regulatory Commission has jurisdiction over the licensing and regulation of nuclear reactors and also over the processing, transportation, and security of nuclear materials.

Office of Science and Technology Policy
Executive Office Building, Washington, D.C. 20500

Established within the Executive Office of the president, this agency advises the president on scientific and technological considerations involved in a wide range of national concerns, including health and the environment.

Office of Technology Assessment (OTA)
600 Pennsylvania Ave., S.E., Washington, D.C. 20510

An agency within the legislative branch of the government, OTA provides independent, objective information on the impacts of technological applications and identifies policy alternatives for technology-related issues. The main function of the OTA is to provide congressional committees with studies that define a broad range of both social and physical consequences of various policy choices affecting the uses of technologies.

Consumer Product Safety Commission
1111 Eighteenth Street, N.W., Washington, D.C. 20207

This independent regulatory agency seeks to reduce unreasonable risks of injury associated with consumer products by encouraging the development of voluntary standards related to consumer product safety, requiring the reporting of hazardous consumer products and, if justified, recall for corrective action of hazardous products already on the market. The commission conducts research on consumer product hazards, can establish mandatory standards, and, if necessary, has the authority to ban hazardous consumer products.

Public Health Service
200 Independence Ave., S.W., Washington, D.C. 20201

An office within the Department of Health and Human Services, the U.S. Public Health Service assists states and communities in developing local health resources, conducts and supports medical research, and overseas other public health functions. Among the various subdivisions within the Public Health Service which are of particular environmental health interest are:

Centers for Disease Control and Prevention (CDC)
1600 Clifton Road, N.E., Atlanta, GA 30333

This agency is charged with protecting public health by providing leadership and direction in the prevention and control of disease. It administers programs related to communicable and vectorborne diseases, urban rat control, control of childhood lead-based paint poisoning, and a range of other environmental health problems. CDC also participates in a national program of research, information, and education regarding smoking and health. The nine major offices of the CDC are those dealing with epidemiology, international health, laboratory improvement, prevention services, environmental health, occupational safety and health, health promotion and education, professional development and training, and infectious diseases.

Food and Drug Administration (FDA)
5600 Fishers Lane, Rockville, MD 20857

The FDA's activities are aimed at protecting public health against impure and unsafe foods, drugs, cosmetics, and other possible hazards such as radiation. In carrying out its responsibilities, the FDA conducts research and develops standards for food, drugs, medical devices, veterinary medicines, and biologic products. Through its National Center for Toxicological Research, the FDA studies the biologic effects of potentially toxic chemicals in the environment.

Occupational Safety and Health Administration (OSHA)

Operating within the Department of Labor, OSHA develops and promulgates safety and health standards and regulations for the American workforce. It conducts investigations and inspections of workplaces to ensure compliance with those regulations and can issue citations and propose penalties for employers who violate such standards.

Fish and Wildlife Service

A bureau within the Department of the Interior, the Fish and Wildlife Service has jurisdiction over matters regarding endangered species, certain marine mammals, wild birds, inland sports fisheries, and wildlife research. The bureau carries out biological monitoring for effects of pesticides, heavy metals, and thermal pollution; it maintains wildlife refuges, enforces game laws, and carries out programs to control livestock predators and pest species. The bureau maintains a number of fish hatcheries, conducts environmental education and public information programs, and provides both national and international leadership regarding endangered fish and wildlife species.

Office of Surface Mining Reclamation and Enforcement

Another agency within the Interior Department, this office is charged with assisting states in developing a nationwide program to protect society and the environment from the harmful effects of coal mining, while simultaneously ensuring an adequate coal supply to meet the nation's energy needs.

Bureau of Land Management (BLM)

The BLM is responsible for managing the nation's 341 million acres of public lands, most of which are located in the Far West. In doing so, the bureau manages the timber, minerals, rangeland vegetation, wild and scenic rivers, wilderness areas, endangered species, and energy resources of these lands. BLM also is involved in watershed protection, development of recreational opportunities, and programs to protect and manage wild horses and burros. The bureau provides for the protection, orderly development, and use of public lands and resources under principles of multiple use and sustained yield. Criticism in recent years has focused on the bureau's overemphasis on permitting exploitation of public resources for private gain and insufficient protection and conservation of these resources.

Soil Conservation Service (SCS)

An agency of the Department of Agriculture, the SCS develops and carries out soil and water conservation programs in cooperation with landowners and operators, land developers, and community planning agencies. SCS also is active in programs aimed at controlling agricultural pollution and in effecting environmental improvement.

Appendix B

Environmental Organizations

Individuals wishing to influence environmental policy have been greatly helped by public participation provisions in almost all recent federal and state environmental legislation. Prior to adoption of proposed regulations, advertised public hearings offer an opportunity for ordinary citizens to make their views known. However, although a dedicated and informed person can have a surprising amount of influence, one's personal impact can be significantly enhanced by joining forces with one of many environmental organizations operating at the local, state, or national level to inform their members on environmental issues and, in the case of many such groups, to lobby their elected representatives to support the causes they espouse. Quite commonly the national organizations publish informative newsletters, bulletins, or magazines to keep their membership up-to-date on current environmental issues and many people affiliate with such groups simply to receive their attractive and interesting publications. The following list includes the names and addresses of many of the most prominent national environmental organizations which the interested student may wish to contact for further information on membership or publications:

American Lung Association
1740 Broadway, New York, NY 10019
(212)315-8700

The Acid Rain Foundation, Inc.
1410 Varsity Drive, Raleigh, NC 27606
(919)828-9443

Citizens for a Better Environment
407 South Dearborn, Suite 1775, Chicago, IL 60605
(312)939-1530

Citizens' Clearinghouse for Hazardous Wastes
P.O. Box 6806, Falls Church, VA 22040
(703)237-2249

Defenders of Wildlife
1244 19th St., NW, Washington, D.C. 20036
(202)659-9510

Ducks Unlimited, Inc.
One Waterfowl Way, Memphis, TN 38120-2351
(901)758-3825
Publications: *Ducks Unlimited Magazine, Puddler Magazine*

Environmental Action, Inc.
6930 Carroll Ave., Suite 600, Takoma Park, MD 20912
(301)891-1100
Publication: *Environmental Action*

Environmental Defense Fund, Inc.
257 Park Ave. South, New York, NY 10010
(212)505-2100
Publication: *EDF Letter*

Freshwater Foundation
Spring Hill Center, 725 County Road 6, Wayzata, MN 55391
(612)449-0092

Friends of the Earth
218 D St., SE, Washington, D.C. 20003
(202)544-2600
Publications: *Friends of the Earth Newsmagazine, Atmosphere Ozone Newsletter*

Greenpeace USA, Inc.
1432 U St., NW, Washington, D.C. 20009
(202)462-1177

League of Conservation Voters
1707 L St., NW, Suite 550, Washington, D.C., 20036
(202)785-8683

League of Women Voters of the United States
1730 M St., NW, Suite 1000, Washington, D.C. 20036
(202)429-1965

National Audubon Society
700 Broadway, New York, NY 10003-9562
(212)979-3000
Publications: *Audubon, American Birds, Audubon Activist*

National Coalition Against Misuse of Pesticides
701 E St., SE, Suite 200, Washington, D.C. 20003
(202)543-5450

National Environmental Health Association
720 S. Colorado Blvd., Suite 970 South Tower, Denver, CO 80222
(303)756-9090
Publication: *Journal of Environmental Health*

National Wildlife Federation
1400 Sixteenth St., NW, Washington, D.C. 20036-2266
(202)797-6800
Publications: *National Wildlife, International Wildlife, Ranger Rick*

The Nature Conservancy
1815 North Lynn St., Arlington, VA 22209
(703)841-5300

Natural Resources Defense Council
40 West 20th St., New York, NY 10011
(212)727-2700
Publications: *Amicus Journal, NRDC Newsline*

Population-Environment Balance, Inc.
1325 G St., NW, Suite 1003, Washington, D.C. 20005
(202)879-3000

The Population Institute
107 Second St., NE, Washington, D.C. 20002
(202)544-3300
Publication: *POPLINE*

Population Reference Bureau, Inc.
1875 Connecticut Ave., NW, Suite 520, Washington, D.C. 20009-5728
(202)438-1100
Publications: *Population Bulletin, Population Today*

Sierra Club
730 Polk St., San Francisco, CA 94109
(415)776-2211
Publication: *Sierra*

The Wilderness Society
900 17th St., NW, Washington, D.C. 20006-2596
(202)833-2300

Worldwatch Institute
1776 Massachusetts Ave., NW, Washington, D.C. 20036-1904
(202)452-1999
Publications: *Worldwatch Papers*, *World Watch Magazine*, *State of the World* (annual report published by W.W. Norton Co., New York)

World Wildlife Fund
1250 24th St., NW, Washington, D.C. 20037
(202)293-4800

Zero Population Growth, Inc.
1400 Sixteenth St., NW, Suite 320, Washington, D.C. 20036
(202)332-2200

Index